INTENSIVE CARE

of the

SURGICAL PATIENT

with 42
contributors

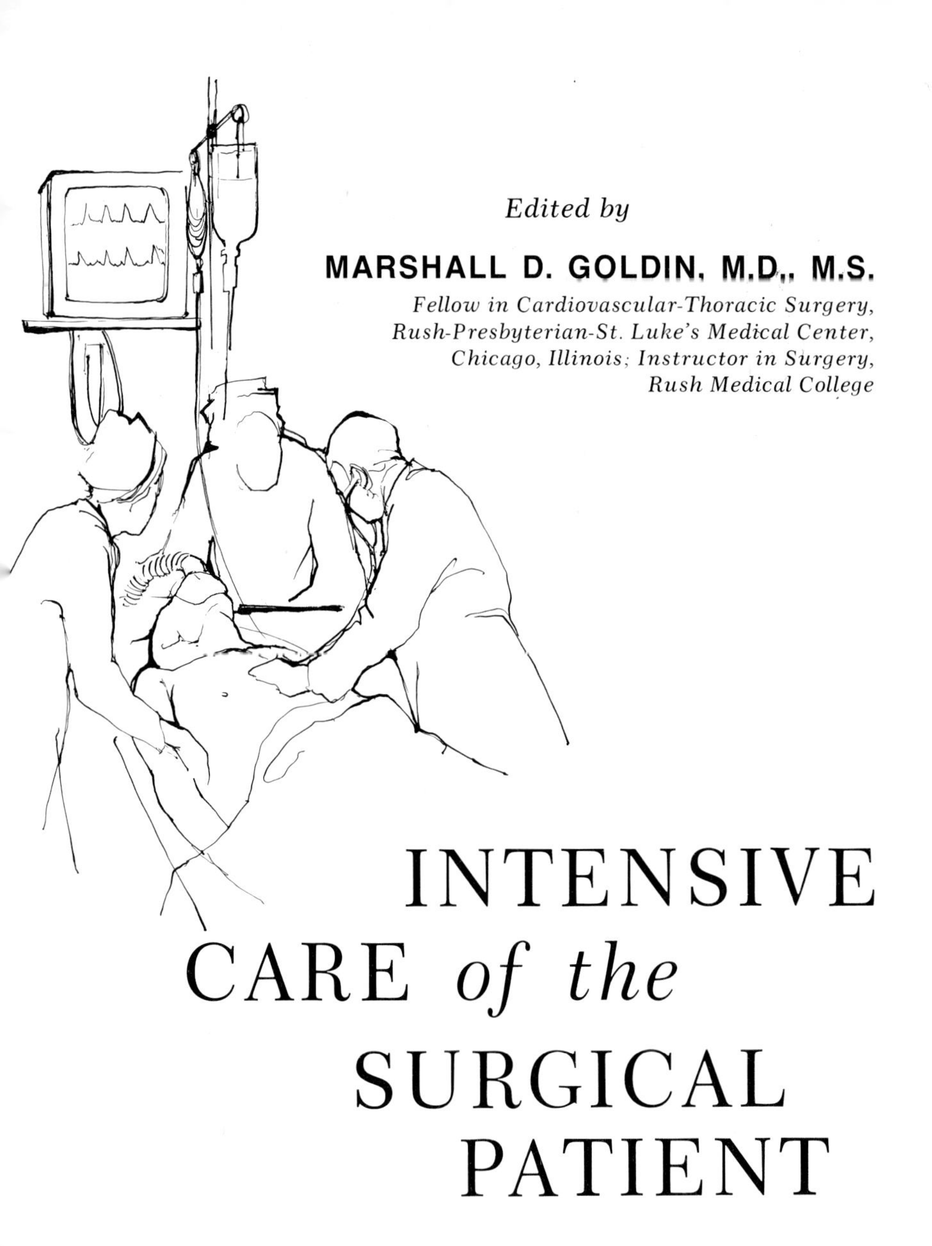

Edited by

MARSHALL D. GOLDIN, M.D., M.S.

Fellow in Cardiovascular-Thoracic Surgery, Rush-Presbyterian-St. Luke's Medical Center, Chicago, Illinois; Instructor in Surgery, Rush Medical College

INTENSIVE CARE *of the* SURGICAL PATIENT

YEAR BOOK MEDICAL PUBLISHERS • INC.

35 EAST WACKER DRIVE • CHICAGO

Reprinted, March 1972

Library of Congress Catalog Card Number: 78-125803

International Standard Book Number: 0-8151-3731-1

Preface

THE OBJECTIVE OF THIS TEXT is to provide a comprehensive source of information to assist those who care for surgical patients in intensive care units. It must be emphasized that the postoperative period is but a portion of the entire sequence of events related to surgical care. Advances in modern surgical technique have evolved to such a degree that an entire new spectrum of problems evolves with each new development.

Intensive care facilities have become more sophisticated over the past decade. Concentration of critically ill patients within a given area allows centralization of facilities, coordination of medical effort, and thereby improved patient care. By the above mechanisms the intricacies of management of such patients become more familiar and permit earlier recognition and therapy of otherwise infrequent episodes.

There is a significant difference between the coronary care unit and the surgical intensive care unit. The former is designed primarily for surveillance of patients and maintenance of nearly basal conditions with minimal stimulation. Surgical units are also designed to detect abnormal alterations; however, by necessity, a major portion of the care requires numerous patient attachments, many personnel, and frequent disturbances. These disturbances include changes in position, dressing changes, coughing, nasotracheal aspiration, etc. While all are essential in postoperative care, they would serve to inordinately increase the stress presented to a cardiac patient who is in proximity to such activity.

For these reasons, it is considered that separation of these patients is necessary. For purposes of efficiency, however, intensive care facilities should be located in adjacent areas. Each will ultimately provide a more efficient service as the personnel become accustomed to the unit.

An intensive care unit requires 24-hour coverage. The personnel staffing the unit should have specialists in all disciplines readily available for consultation. The combined medical and surgical approach to the care of these patients is essential. A combination of attending and resident staff serves to enhance patient care and advance education. Only by cooperative care and freedom of consultation between the various specialties can such comprehensive care be obtained. It is vital that these efforts be coordinated by those with the broadest perspective.

Emphasis is directed toward the clinical aspects of postoperative intensive care. Since the major portion of postoperative care often is the responsibility of the resident and nursing staff, it is largely to this group that this book is addressed. The diversity of the specialties covered should, however, make the book valuable for practitioners at all levels. The editor joins the contributors in hoping that this volume will enable physicians to become familiar with those methods that have been of benefit in the surgical intensive care unit at the Rush-Presbyterian-St. Luke's Medical Center.

The editor extends his deepest gratitude to Dr. Steven G. Economou for his initial impetus and continued encouragement in the planning of this text and to Dr. Ormand C. Julian for his support in this undertaking as well as a profound influence upon my medical career. To the artist – my wife, Jo Ann – I extend appreciation for the illustrations and her understanding, which permitted me to engage in this effort.

The patience of Mrs. Judy Schoolwerth, who did the major portion of the typing, and the efforts of the Rush-Presbyterian-St. Luke's Medical Center Department of Photography are greatly appreciated. Mr. Louis Gdalman, Director of Pharmacies, was most helpful in confirming the doses of the medications.

The contributors have been most cooperative in the preparation of manuscripts from the outlines used in the intensive care lecture series.

To the medical staff, nursing staff, and inhalation therapists, I would like to join the multitude of patients in extending appreciation for their devoted care.

The Year Book editorial staff has been most helpful in providing assistance in every possible capacity.

Support for this work was aided by USPHS Training Grant No. IT 12 HE 05808.

MARSHALL D. GOLDIN

Table of Contents

1

Postanesthetic Management

PETER MURPHY, M.D.

Assistant Attending Anesthesiologist, Rush-Presbyterian-St. Luke's Medical Center; Assistant Professor of Anesthesiology, Rush Medical College

RECOVERY FROM ANESTHESIA is a much longer process than induction. Fat, protein and tissue fluids all absorb anesthetic agents. When administration stops, the blood level falls and the tissues give up their store to the blood according to the concentration gradient. Thus, the time taken for recovery to wakefulness is extended.

Vasomotor and respiratory depression persist for several hours following anesthesia. During this time aspiration or asphyxia may occur. The surgeon and anesthesiologist should be readily available.

Central Nervous System

The return of previously obtunded reflexes is the first indication of recovery from anesthesia. Swallowing or sucking movements indicate the return of pharyngeal and glottic reflexes. A gentle pressure on the eyelashes will provoke a contraction of the orbicularis muscle, but it may be some time before the patient opens his eyes voluntarily. The pupils are usually constricted throughout anesthesia and remain equally small. As the patient wakes up, the pupils enlarge quite suddenly just before the lids open, allowing the eyes to gaze at the surroundings. A pupil that is widely dilated and does not respond to light or accommodation may still be under the influence of belladonna, instilled preoperatively in preparation for eye surgery. If deliberate hypotensive techniques have been used during surgery, the ganglionic blockade will dilate the pupils. Otherwise, dilated unresponsive pupils may indicate cerebral hypoxia resulting from cardiac arrest or severe hypotension.

PROLONGED RECOVERY.—Inhalation anesthesia owes its popularity to the ease with which it can be reversed. Anesthetic gases can be excreted through the lungs quickly and almost completely. If the breathing is not impaired or restricted, recovery should be rapid. Ethers do take somewhat longer to clear from the body than other agents. Premedication which includes a phenothiazine compound or morphine analogue will also prolong recovery.

The treatment of prolonged recovery is primarily supportive. Adequate minute ventilation clears volatile agents from the lungs. Maintaining a good cardiac output will keep the drug moving out of the tissues. Opiate narcosis can be completely reversed by levallorphan, in which event the analgesia is also withdrawn.

BRAIN DAMAGE.—Postoperative edema following craniotomy contributes to prolonged recovery. Careful consideration should be given to the size of the pupils and any variation between them. If an intracerebral hematoma collects, the respiratory rate will slow and eventually cease.

Although not common, strokes may occur during anesthesia. Deep coma persisting more than one hour after the withdrawal of anesthesia may be due to cerebral thrombosis or hemorrhage.

NERVE DAMAGE.—Whenever postoperative weakness is discovered in one arm, a brachial plexus injury must be suspected. The plexus may be injured by the pressure of a shoulder brace or by the stretching that results when the arm is hyperextended, as during thoracotomy. Pressure against the medial epicondyle by the operating table can cause ulnar paresis. A similar injury to the peroneal nerve can occur when the patient is in the lateral position. These paralyzed limbs should be splinted to prevent distortion and further injury. Encouragement and assistance should be given to the patient in exercising the joints and muscles until neuromuscular function returns. Recovery of function is slow but usually complete.

SPINAL AND EPIDURAL ANESTHESIA.—Postural pressor reflexes are absent in anesthetized patients. For this reason and as a prophylaxis against headache, these patients should remain supine for the first 24 hours after surgery. The analgesia lasts only up to the second hour after the injection was given.

CEREBRAL HYPOXIA.—Since the mixture of anesthetic gases is always rich in oxygen, cerebral hypoxia is more often the result of poor blood flow than of low oxygen saturation. Anesthesia in the sitting position is commonly used in neurosurgical, dental and some orthopedic procedures. There is of course a much greater risk of cerebral hypoxia when the patient is erect. If the blood pressure does fall briefly, the patient may be confused and disoriented for 24 hours following arousal. Hypotension lasting for longer than two or three minutes may delay recovery to consciousness for several days, after which some impairment of memory persists. Complete arrest of blood flow to the brain for three minutes will produce coma and convulsions and finally atrophy of the whole cerebral cortex. Until they emerge from coma, these patients need extra care to prevent respiratory insufficiency, skin necrosis and urinary stasis.

FAT EMBOLISM.—Multiple fractures are associated with a high incidence of fat embolism. Typically the onset is delayed 12–24 hours after the injury. The fat may enter nearby veins at the moment of fracture or later during manipulation.

Fat emboli plug pulmonary capillaries, limit alveolar perfusion and can produce cyanosis. The cerebral circulation may be reduced and coma may follow. Petechiae appear over the anterior chest wall and shoulders. The diagnosis can be confirmed by analyzing urine and sputum for fat or by examining the fundus oculi for fat in the blood vessels or hemorrhages.

Because multiple fractures cause more blood loss into the surrounding tissues than is generally realized, patients with multiple fractures must first receive adequate blood by transfusion. Supplementary oxygen inhalation is necessary to minimize tissue hypoxia.

AIR EMBOLISM.—Incisions into the tissues of the head and neck, particularly above the level of the right atrium, may allow air to enter veins which cannot collapse readily because of fascial attachments. The air causes frothing in the outflow tract and blocks ejection of blood from the right ventricle. The physical signs include tachypnea, tachycardia and loud, slapping heart sounds. By turning the patient quickly onto the left side with the head tilted steeply downward, the air block is moved out of the outflow tract, permitting blood to enter the pulmonary circulation.

HYPOGLYCEMIA.—Some brittle diabetics with unstable requirements may be difficult to control for surgery. The best routine is simply to rely on regular insulin given just prior to operation, so that the greatest flexibility in controlling blood sugar levels is achieved. Half the morning dose of insulin is given on the morning of surgery. A dextrose infusion is run throughout the operation to which supplements of dextrose may be added. Rarely does hypoglycemia cause delayed recovery, but the injection of 50 ml. of 50% dextrose is both diagnostic and therapeutic should this possibility be considered.

HYPOADRENALISM.—Following bilateral adrenalectomy the blood pressure does not immediately fall, even though a catecholamine store has been removed. A program of replacement, begun in the preoperative period, is essential. Most commonly, hypoadrenalism is related to previous long-term therapy for other diseases.

There is some evidence that corticosteroids are of value in the treatment of shock. When the more established treatment of fluid and blood replacement has been completed without the anticipated improvement, 100 mg. hydrocortisone should be injected for appraisal.

HYPOTHERMIA.—Some degree of unintentional hypothermia occurs with most major surgery under anesthesia because temperature control is imperfect and shivering does not take place. The skin circulation is inappropriately large for the difference between body and operating room temperature. Ventilation with cool, dry gases carries away the alveolar moisture at body heat, while blood is infused, cool from the refrigerator.

In infants the skin surface is so large in proportion to body weight that the temperature under anesthesia may fall rapidly. Infants tolerate such losses poorly. Postoperatively, the body temperature should be kept above 94 F. by keeping the infant in a temperature-regulated incubator.

In the adult patient, compensation is soon effected postoperatively by a spell of shivering and cutaneous vasoconstriction. Shivering is commonly seen after halothane anesthesia. Cutaneous vasoconstriction and cyanosis persist until the temperature returns to normal.

Cooling severe enough to cause loss of consciousness is uncommon, but it may occur after deliberate hypothermia when the warming phase has not been adequate. The body may then lose more heat, so that the temperature falls below 85 F., at which point consciousness may be lost. Ventricular fibrillation occurs at temperatures below 80 F.

HYPERPYREXIA.—In contrast to excessive cooling occurring in infants during anesthesia, older children may develop an elevation of temperature. Premedication with atropine diminishes sweating. Preoperative apprehension and excitement increase the metabolic rate. Dehydration prevents physiologic cooling by the skin. During the operation, the drapes covering the skin prevent the necessary loss of heat, and the temperature rises.

Tachycardia and excessively dry skin are the first signs of hyperpyrexia. The temperature rises quickly and may reach a peak at 110 F. Initially, the blood pressure is normal, but eventually it falls and the pupils dilate. Convulsions begin soon afterward.

Immediate and thorough cooling is necessary to prevent irreversible brain damage. The simplest technique is to bathe the skin with water from an ice water mixture until the temperature is brought to normal levels. Hypothermia blankets are often the most efficient method of cooling.

Respiration

PATTERNS OF RESPIRATION.—The simplest way to judge adequate ventilation is to feel the breath against the hand held next to the patient's lips. Auscultation will indicate whether the breathing is spread equally over both lungs. If ventilation is inadequate, manual assistance is initiated. In an emergency, mouth-to-mouth ventilation may be needed. Self-inflating respirator bags are available for artificial ventilation via mask or endotracheal tube.

Conscious breathing has a pattern of inspiration-expiration waves separated by short pauses between one expiration and the next inspiration. Surgical anesthesia results in "automatic" respiration in which the waves are "saw-toothed" and there is no pause.

The diaphragm is the most important respiratory muscle and the most powerful. The intercostals are used in deeper breathing. A muscle relaxant drug does not appear to paralyze the diaphragm as thoroughly or as soon as it does striated muscle elsewhere in the body. Deep anesthesia paralyzes the intercostal muscles first. When the diaphragm contracts the chest descends instead of rising, so that "see-saw" or paradoxical respiration appears, with its axis on the xiphisternum.

When obstruction of the airway causes a violent struggle to cough and breathe, the diaphragm makes vigorous pumping efforts to increase the capacity of the chest. Sudden low pressure results, causing the ribs and intercostals to collapse inward. The resulting movement of the chest and abdomen resembles paradoxical respiration.

Hypopnea and hypoventilation.—The most common cause of postoperative hypoventilation is persistent muscle relaxant effect. However, drugs given during anesthesia or as premedication, particularly the opiates, are all offenders.

Reduction in the volume of alveolar ventilation limits oxygen uptake and upsets acid-base balance by retention of CO_2. The limited chest movement and ineffective cough result in mucus plug collection and distal atelectasis.

Muscle relaxant drugs.—This group of drugs produces voluntary muscle weakness by inhibiting neuromuscular conduction. They comprise the depolarizing drugs, such as succinylcholine, which paralyze instantly in the wake of widespread muscular contractions, and the nondepolarizing drugs, such as curare, which produce neuromuscular blockade without prior depolarization.

Succinylcholine has an evanescent action of two to three minutes while curare lasts one-half hour. Succinylcholine paralysis is so profound that faradic stimuli produce only a weak response. A brief tetanic stimulus applied to the motor nerve during curare paralysis will enhance subsequent faradic stimuli. This effect is known as facilitation.

There is no antidote for succinylcholine paralysis. By raising the concentration of acetylcholine at the end-plate, curare blockade is overcome. Neostigmine (Prostigmin), an anticholinesterase, is an antidote. In practice, atropine is combined with neostigmine to inhibit the undesirable bradycardia and salivation that would otherwise result.

Both depolarizing and nondepolarizing types of relaxants are used during anesthesia (Table 1-1). A situation may arise in which the paralysis does not attenuate as the anesthesia draws to an end. Succinylcholine is not destroyed by enzyme action as rapidly as usual in a small percentage (0.3%) of the population, who display an inherited deficiency of serum cholinesterase. Paralysis in this situation may last several hours until succinylcholine is hydrolyzed in due course. Curare paralysis may be extended by the presence of metabolic acidosis. A pos-

TABLE 1-1.—DEPOLARIZING AND NONDEPOLARIZING MUSCLE RELAXANTS

RELAXANTS	DOSE	DURATION	ELIMINATION	ANTIDOTE
Depolarizing				
Succinyl-choline (Anectine)	10–80 mg.	3 min.	Destruction by cholinesterase	None
Nondepolarizing				
Curare (d-tubocurare)	10–20 mg.	30 min.	Excreted in bile and urine	Prostigmin 5 mg. and atropine 2 mg. given simultaneously intravenously
Gallamine	40–100 mg.	30 min.	Excreted in urine	

itive facilitation test will sometimes indicate that the block is nondepolarizing. If a small dose of Tensilon causes no improvement, then the neuromuscular blockade is a depolarizing one. If Tensilon does augment or initiate respiration, then neostigmine may be given subsequently.

OPIATES.—Opiates depress respiration in a characteristic manner. The natural expiratory pause is accentuated. The depth of respiration is increased. Levallorphan or N-allyl-nor-morphine are specific antidotes. The dose is 1 mg. of either antidote per 100 mg. meperidine or per 10 mg. morphine. The analgesic effect of morphine is reversed by the administration of the antidote.

ENDOTRACHEAL TUBE.—At a time when anesthesia is light, the presence of an endotracheal tube in the trachea is enough to cause a reflex arrest of breathing. A slight downward push on this tube will elicit a cough which signifies there is little or no further paralysis and that removal of the tube will be followed by normal breathing.

LUNG COLLAPSE.—Accidental intubation of one or the other bronchus with an endotracheal tube or the insertion of an overlong tracheostomy tube which blocks air exchange to the opposite lung will produce sufficient collapse of the unaerated lung (usually the left) to render that side opaque to x-ray. Patchy atelectasis occurs in an identical manner because smaller air ducts become blocked by mucus. Cilial movement and coughing reflexes, which are normally responsible for the scavenging of this mucus, are arrested by anesthesia.

Treatment is directed to clearing the obstruction. For patchy collapse caused by mucus plug, "springing" the chest removes the block. In this maneuver, the sternum is compressed by pressing firmly on the chest to coincide with the end of expiration. This action decreases the capacity of the chest more completely. The pressure is suddenly released and inspiration allowed to proceed. The routine is repeated some dozen times. This, of course, is not recommended after thoracotomy.

After the obstruction has been removed, the pharynx is suctioned clear of mucus and saliva.

ASPIRATION.—Aspiration of gastric contents into the lungs is not an uncommon postoperative tragedy. The aspiration of blood clot from an operation in the nasopharynx may have similar grave consequences.

Active vomiting requires an active medullary reflex. As the vomiting reflex returns, so does the glottic reflex to protect the lungs from soiling. Aspiration may occur if intestinal reflux or gas accumulation elevate the intragastric pressure prior to return of the protective laryngeal reflexes.

Prophylaxis against vomiting begins before operation. Emergency operations require anesthesia when the stomach may be full. It should be emptied of fluid via a large stomach tube and then neutralized with a sodium bicarbonate wash, using 50 ml. of standard 8% solution.

Elective operations on the biliary tract or those including intestinal resection should include the insertion of a gastric tube. The stomach should be aspirated every five minutes. Fluid should never be allowed to accumulate during the phase when the patient is recovering consciousness, since the very presence of the tube makes regurgitation even more likely because it prevents tight closure of the cricopharyngeal valve.

Aspiration of a small quantity of fluid may result in scattered areas of lung infiltration without a fatal outcome. Massive aspiration causes shock, cyanosis unresponsive to oxygen inhalation and rapid death. In these patients tracheo-bronchial lavage with 1% sodium bicarbonate is beneficial. Oxygen therapy and support to the circulation by infusion of electrolytes or blood as required are needed urgently. Intravenous administration of hydrocortisone will diminish the inflammation of the mucosa and allay bronchospasm.

BRONCHOSPASM.—If the history of the patient's previous health includes attacks of dyspnea in association with allergy or chronic infection, there is an increased likelihood of postoperative bronchospasm and respiratory distress. Noisy breathing is most commonly due to the base of the relaxed tongue occluding the hypopharynx. This situation is corrected with a stiff airway and by pulling the mandible forward. When musical rales are heard widely over the chest wall and the effort of breathing is disproportionate, steps must be taken to relieve the bronchiolar spasm. Aminophylline, 500 mg. intravenously, may excite tachycardia or cardiac irregularity if given rapidly, but it will generally abolish the spasm. Hydrocortisone, 100 mg. intravenously, should be used in refractory cases.

When respiratory therapy is required for these patients, it is vital to give expiration sufficient time to reach completion. If this is not done, air will be trapped in the chest. A negative-pressure machine may sometimes help suck out the expired gases, but weakened bronchioles may collapse under the negative pressure and trap the alveolar air.

Hypotension

There is no substitute for regular blood pressure readings taken postoperatively with a standard pneumatic cuff. However, the degree of filling of the superficial veins, the color of the lips and nail beds and the pulse pressure are indices of peripheral blood flow. If the flow is judged adequate, some slight sacrifice of systolic pressure below the level recorded preoperatively may be allowed.

Persistent tachycardia and hypotension indicate oligemia. Insufficient replacement of blood and fluids remains a common cause of early postoperative hypotension. If the patient survives the first few hours with less than sufficient blood volume, the renal blood flow may be so reduced that renal failure will follow.

ANESTHETIC DRUGS.—Many anesthetic agents have an undesirable hypotensive capacity by central or myocardial depression or by autonomic ganglia blocking. Curare releases histamine which dilates the capillary bed.

Morphine and meperidine both induce hypotension by a central effect, depressing the vasomotor tone. Others which potentiate these drugs, for example the phenothiazine derivatives, will accentuate the hypotension. Levallorphan will reverse the hypotension caused by morphine-like drugs.

HYPOTENSIVE DRUGS.—Knowledge that antihypertensive therapy was used prior to surgery is helpful in the prevention of unexpected hypotension. Although hypotensive drugs are readily countered with a wide variety of vasopressor drugs, the safest course is to prohibit their use during the week before surgery.

Quaternary ammonium compounds (hexamethonium) produce a sympathetic blockade which is readily reversed with adrenergic pressor agents. Reserpine and methyldopa deplete the stores of norepinephrine in peripheral nerves. In this altered state the usual vasopressor response to amphetamine or ephedrine will be much reduced, since they act by stimulating the release of norepinephrine. However, administration of phenylephrine or norepinephrine will produce the desired vasoconstriction of blood vessels.

MONO-AMINE OXIDASE INHIBITORS.—This group of mood elevators (isocarboxazid, nialamide, phenelzine, and tranylcypromine) is derived from iproniazid, which was originally used to treat tuberculosis. Inhibition of normal degradation results in an intracellular increase in catecholamine stores. Thus, the action of central nervous system stimulants is enhanced and their administration may cause convulsions. Phentolamine, 5 mg. intravenously, is the best antidote.

These drugs also inhibit the breakdown of opiates and barbiturates. Ordinary doses of either may produce coma and hypotension. The treatment is administration of 200 mg. hydrocortisone intravenously.

MYOCARDIAL INFARCTION.—Previous history of coronary or cerebrovascular insufficiency requires especially accurate regulation of blood pressure in the normal range. Hypotension can usually be prevented by maintenance of the blood volume and support with a slow intravenous infusion of 0.01% solution of phenylephrine when necessary.

PULMONARY EMBOLISM.—Prolonged bed rest and surgery of the hip and pelvis predispose the patient to pulmonary embolism. Often a change in position or an attempt at defecation immediately precedes the catastrophic event. A severe embolus produces cyanosis which is unrelieved by 100% oxygen.

ADRENAL INSUFFICIENCY.—Previous steroid therapy and chronic stress induce adrenal cortical hypoplasia (Chapter 24). Adrenal insufficiency may be manifest by severe postoperative lethargy and hypotension. The presence of oral pigmentation and loss of pubic and axillary hair indicate the possibility of this condition in the chronic state (Addison's disease). A therapeutic response to the intravenous administration of cortisol is diagnostic in all of these conditions. (See Chapter 24.)

SPINAL AND EPIDURAL BLOCKADE.—Peridural or subarachnoid infiltration with local anesthetics can induce severe hypotension. The hypotension responds when the patient returns to the supine position. Vasomotor tone can be restored rapidly by 0.1 mg. of phenylephrine intravenously. Meanwhile the patient is kept horizontal for two hours after the operation until the anesthetic block wears away.

CARCINOID.—These tumors form from cells in the ileum, appendix, rectum or lung and secrete 5-hydroxytryptamine. The hormone produces widespread smooth muscle contraction. Sudden release by manipulation during intra-abdominal surgery causes flushing of the face and bronchospasm. The vasomotor component of the hormone action acts to produce a transient hypertension, followed shortly by a longer, hypotensive phase. In most cases no treatment is necessary.

Hypertension

The blood pressure will, if fluid has been satisfactorily replaced, stabilize postoperatively at previous resting levels. Postoperative hypertension may be "normal" in some patients and therefore require no treatment.

PAIN.—If blood pressure rises above normal levels and persists after surgery, pain is a probable cause. Restlessness and sweating usually accompany the hypertension. Moderate doses of analgesics help to return the pressure to normal but an excess may reinduce anesthesia.

HYPERCAPNIA AND ANOXIA.—Hypoventilation will soon cause a rise in serum Pa_{CO_2}. The central effect on vasomotor tone overrides the peripheral arteriolar dilation and results in hypertension. Anoxia from the same cause reinforces these effects. Hypercapnia also acts on the adrenal medulla, causing epinephrine release and cardiac irregularities.

Any obstruction to respiration should be removed and respiration supported if necessary.

VASOPRESSORS.—An overdose of vasopressors, with hypertension extending into the postoperative period, is preferably countered with a suitable head-up posturing. If for reasons of renewed bleeding or the risk of stroke or myocardial infarction it is deemed essential to lower the pressure, 10 mg. Thorazine intravenously may be given and repeated several times at 5–10 minute intervals. If this fails, a slow intravenous infusion of 0.1% trimethaphan may be used. However, caution is advised with the latter drug, and the physician must be present during the infusion to take readings of the pressure minute by minute, until the desired level of pressure is attained.

PHEOCHROMOCYTOMA.—This tumor of adrenal tissue or paraganglia produces hypertensive crises. The tumor cells secrete epinephrine and norepinephrine, which may enter the circulation during intra-abdominal manipulation. The hypertension which follows is treated with phentolamine, whereas postoperative hypotension requires supplementary infusion of norephinephrine. (See Chapter 24.)

PRIMARY ALDOSTERONISM.—This tumor of the adrenal medulla secretes aldosterone. The serum potassium level may fall to less than 2 mEq./L., with resulting muscular weakness and tetany. The hypertension which accompanies the electrolyte disturbance is reversed by removal of the tumor.

Analgesic and Anesthetic Medications

UNTOWARD EFFECTS.—*Morphine and meperidine* may induce a shocklike state of pallor and hypotension. Both are powerful respiratory depressants. Chronic pulmonary disease is a contraindication to their use preoperatively, particularly in the elderly, since some patients may be asphyxiated by the usual dosage. Vomiting is not uncommon following the use of both drugs.

Atropine, given to counteract vagal stimulation, stops sweating and increases the metabolic rate. Administration to small children may cause fever which, if increased by heavy blankets or drapes, may reach dangerous levels.

Phenothiazines are used as antiemetics and tranquilizers. When combined with morphine or meperidine, hypotension may follow. The narcosis is also potentiated by the phenothiazines.

Neostigmine is an anticholinesterase used to reverse the action of curare and similar nondepolarizing drugs. Atropine is always given in combination to counteract the bradycardia and intestinal spasm induced by neostigmine. When combined in a single injection atropine and neostigmine produce a decided increase in the secretion of viscid saliva, which is often difficult to expectorate.

INHALATION ANESTHETIC AGENTS.—*Diethyl ether* is an inflammable anesthetic vapor. Administration of ether causes stimulation of the adrenal medulla and release of circulating catecholamines. Respiration is stimulated in the lighter stages of ether anesthesia but becomes depressed as anesthesia deepens. Recovery from the ethers is slow.

Halothane, a fluorinated ethane compound, is a potent drug. Respiration and blood pressure are soon depressed. The blood pressure fall is greatly accentuated by lateral and prone posturing. Venous stasis is so marked that the initial incision may release very dark, desaturated blood, while the bright red color of the tongue and lips indicate that carotid blood is well saturated with oxygen. Shivering and peripheral vasoconstriction with stasis and desaturation occur frequently during recovery, apparently in response to the cooling which occurs during anesthesia.

Cyclopropane is another potent anesthetic drug which exists at room temperature as a gas. Cyclopropane produces hypertension and some carbon dioxide retention, both of which maintain perfusion. Rapid postoperative CO_2 loss may cause hypotension.

LOCAL ANESTHETIC AGENTS.—The toxic effects of *cocaine, lidocaine, mepivacaine*, etc. depend not only on the nature of the drug but on the speed with which it gains access to the blood stream. Spraying a mucous membrane with a local anesthetic results in a higher blood concentration than a subcutaneous injection of a similar amount.

Drug reactions are not rare. All of these drugs excite the medullary area of the brain, stimulating respiration and causing involuntary muscle movement. Hypertension, generalized seizures and respiratory arrest are followed by a phase of medullary depression in which the blood pressure drops and breathing is shallow. The treatment in such a crisis is to paralyze the patient when tremors or twitchings are first seen, using intubation of the trachea, respiratory support and vasopressors as necessary.

UNTOWARD COMBINATIONS OF DRUGS.—The additive effects of a combination of *morphine* and a *phenothiazine* may produce hypotension and respiratory depression.

Previous treatment with *monoamine oxidase inhibitors* may accentuate the hypotensive and narcotic effects of even the smallest dose of *morphine, meperidine* or indeed of any drugs of this group. Care should be taken when countering these effects with stimulant drugs, because the monoamine oxidase inhibitors also enhance the effects of injected catecholamines. The depressant effects of *barbiturates* and monoamine oxidase inhibitors are exaggerated. A state of hypotension and shock may occur when *diuretics* and monamine oxidase inhibitors are given together.

The sensitivity of the myocardium is increased when *halothane* and *epinephrine* are given together. Ventricular fibrillation may occur.

Epinephrine sensitivity of the myocardium is also enhanced when *cyclopropane* is administered. Ventricular fibrillation may occur.

Curare is potentiated by *antibiotic drugs* such as streptomycin, neomycin and polymixin, or by any drug containing quinine. Calcium gluconate (1–2 Gm.) may reverse the block caused by the antibiotics.

Succinylcholine and *neostigmine* are mentioned only to emphasize the fact that succinylcholine has no true antidote. Neostigmine would in fact extend the action of succinylcholine.

DRUGS CONTRAINDICATED BY SPECIFIC DISEASE STATES.—*Morphine* should be avoided when asthma or bronchitis exists. Morphine depresses respiration while histamine release by the morphine causes bronchoconstriction. Barbiturates or phenothiazines may substitute adequately for morphine.

Atropine may precipitate hyperpyrexia. When high fever already exists in a child aged 1 to 5 years, this drug may be replaced by an antihistamine preparation with milder drying effects and some sedative properties.

Barbiturates should be avoided if there is any suspicion of porphyria. These patients exhibit manic episodes which may need sedation, or gastric crises develop which mimic acute abdominal emergencies. A dose of intravenous sodium pentothal may cause an acute postoperative exacerbation of porphyria.

2

Postoperative Monitoring

DAVID L. ROSEMAN, M.D.

Assistant Attending Surgeon, Rush-Presbyterian-St. Luke's Medical Center; Assistant Professor of Surgery, Rush Medical College

THE TYPICAL PATIENT in an intensive care unit will have an acute or chronic debilitating disease on which has been superimposed the physiologic insult of a major surgical procedure. The survival of such a patient often depends on the excellence of postoperative management. One facet of this intensive care is that of surveillance. In some patients, this simply requires that the blood pressure, pulse, respiratory rate and temperature of the patient be measured at regular intervals. In critically ill patients, however, more thorough surveillance is often required. A penalty for increasing the thoroughness of monitoring is that the patient must be subjected to the placement of one or more catheters and must be attached to an increasing number of machines. In this chapter the use of catheters and the electronic machines will be discussed.

Catheters

The sicker the patient the more catheters may be required. In general, the urinary catheter, the central venous catheter and the arterial catheter are placed in that order.

URINARY CATHETER.—*Indications.*—The volume of urine gives information regarding hydration and renal status. This information is of such significant value that urinary catheterization is indicated in almost all critically ill patients. Urinary catheterization is not without complications, such as infection, septicemia and chronic stricture, but the advantages gained usually offset the risks.

Technique.—The placement of a urinary catheter does not require review except that the need for an aseptic technique should be emphasized.

CENTRAL VENOUS CATHETER.—*Indication.*—The central venous pressure can be estimated by observing the patient's neck veins. This estimation will suffice if the patient is thought to be hypovolemic and is responding well to volume replacement. Any patient with persistent hypotension and poor peripheral perfusion who has distended neck veins, or one who does not respond to volume replacement should have a central venous pressure catheter inserted.

Technique.—The best method for placing a central venous catheter is that of percutaneous subclavian puncture, as described in Chapter 22. The tip of the catheter must lie within the thorax. This can be determined at the bedside by noting if the height of the venous pressure column varies with respiration. Occasionally, a high venous pressure that fluctuates with the heart beat will be found; this indicates that the tip of the catheter lies within the right ventricle and that it should be withdrawn into the atrium. A chest x-ray should be obtained to confirm the position of the catheter.

ARTERIAL CATHETER.—*Indication.*—Arterial cannulation is indicated for a patient in whom minute-to-minute knowledge of the blood pressure is required or in whom frequent samples of arterial blood are taken.

Technique.—Arterial catheters are usually introduced via cutdowns. A ready site is the ulnar artery, which is exposed through a short longitudinal incision using the usual cutdown techniques.

Electronic Monitoring

Electronic monitoring devices have had widespread use in the recent past, and since their appropriate use requires some knowledge of their function, this section will attempt to provide the reader with sufficient background to obtain reliable information from these devices. A more comprehensive review of the subject can be found in the literature cited at the end of this chapter. Here, however, an overview is presented, not only of devices in current use, but also of those that will become available in the near future.

The following is a partial list of physiologic variables that may be monitored.

1. Electrocardiogram
2. Electroencephalogram
3. Blood pressure (arterial, venous, various intracardiac)
4. Pulse rate
5. Cardiac output
6. Total peripheral resistance
7. Temperatures
8. Respiratory pressures (airway, esophageal)
9. Respiratory flow rates
10. Respiratory rate
11. Respiratory compliance/resistance
12. Respiratory gases (O_2, CO_2, N_2)
13. Blood gases (Pa_{O_2}, Pa_{CO_2})
14. Blood acid-base values (pH, base excess, etc.)
15. Urine volumes

Because of the ease with which electrical signals can be manipulated and recorded, most monitoring is currently performed with electronic equipment. The goal of electronic monitoring is to convert a physiologic variable into a form that will make it readily available to those caring for a patient. It is convenient to think of these variables as falling into three categories, namely, those which are *electrical* in nature, such as the electrocardiogram; those which may be *converted* to electrical signals, such as blood pressure; and those which may not be measured directly but which must be *calculated*, such as the total peripheral vascular resistance. The variables listed above can be regrouped according to these three categories:

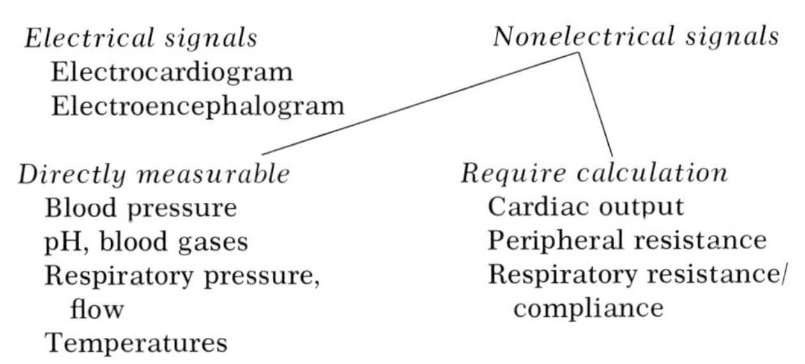

In order for the nonelectrical variables to be handled electronically they must be converted to electrical signals. This is done by various types of *transducers*. For example, blood pressure is, of course, a mechanical variable. It is possible to measure blood pressure in a mechanical way, that is, with a manometer. It is also possible, and often more convenient, to convert the mechanical value into an electrical signal by means of a pressure transducer. The electrical signal generated is proportional or analogous to the mechanical variable, and so it shows as an *analog signal*. The analog signal may be manipulated electronically. The manipulation of the electrical analog values is shown in the accompanying flow diagram.

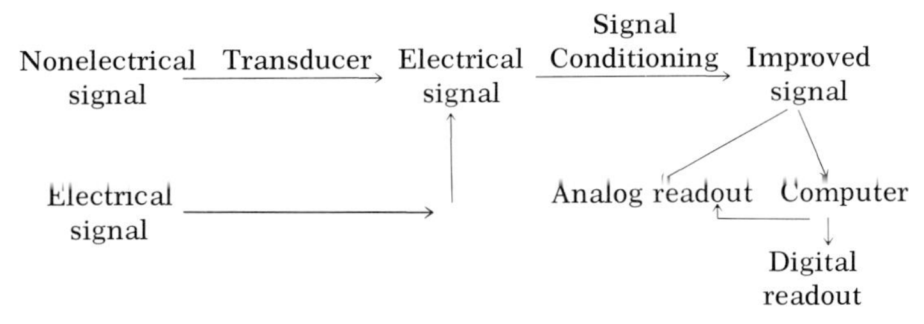

Transduction

A wide variety of transducers are available. The more common types will be described briefly. Detailed discussions are contained in the references listed at the end of the chapter.

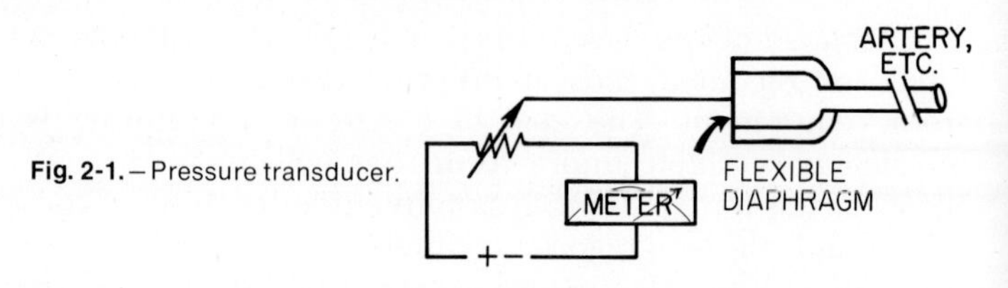

Fig. 2-1. – Pressure transducer.

Pressure transducers. – Pressure transducers consist of an unyielding chamber fitted at one end with a flexible diaphragm. The chamber is filled with the fluid (liquid or gas) whose pressure is to be measured. Connected to the diaphragm is an electrical device which causes a change in the output voltage directly proportional to the pressure within the chamber. This produces an electrical signal analogous to pressure. The general form of this electrical circuit is shown in Figure 2-1.

It is apparent that the transducer does not measure *absolute* pressures. It requires calibration; for example, the electrical signal produced must be checked against manometer measurements before each use and calibration must be performed, as described in the next section. It is not possible to obtain accurate measurements if this step is ignored.

Temperature transducers. – These are currently widely used in monitoring, perhaps because they are so simple and accurate. They operate on the principle that some materials have rather wide variations in electrical resistance with changes in temperature. The devices usually employed are known as *thermistors*. In their simplest form they are connected to a voltage source and a meter, as shown in Figure 2-2. The voltage drop across the thermistor is an analog function of temperature.

Electrochemical transducers. – A detailed description of these transducers is beyond the scope of this book; pertinent references are listed at the end of this chapter. The range of electrochemical measurements is now quite broad and is finding increasing use in monitoring systems. It is possible to measure pH, Pco_2, sodium and chloride quite accurately and to measure potassium and calcium with reasonable accuracy. It soon should be possible to measure such things as blood sugar, urea nitrogen, etc., on a continuous basis with an analog output.

Photocells. – Hemoglobin, percent oxygen saturation, and the

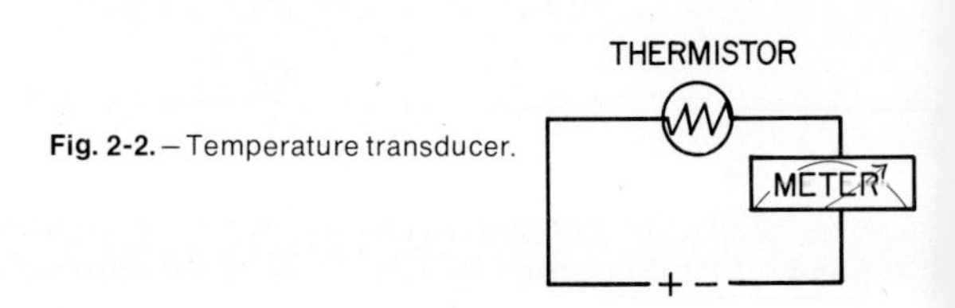

Fig. 2-2. – Temperature transducer.

concentration of various exogenous dyes can be measured by passing a light beam through a blood sample and recording the amount of light striking a photosensitive cell. The voltage output of this cell is a function of the amount of light passing through the sample, and therefore a function of the concentration of the substance in question.

Signal Conditioning

The electrical signals just discussed, whether originating in the patient (for example, the electrocardiogram) or from transducers, are usually of low voltage and current. In order for these signals to be useful they must be conditioned; in most cases this requires *amplification*. A detailed discussion of amplifiers is not feasible. But because intensive care personnel are called upon to use amplifiers, it is necessary that the steps required for calibration of these instruments be understood. There are two controls that are common to most amplifiers. These are the ZERO (sometimes called BALANCE or BIAS) control and the GAIN control. To illustrate their use, a pressure transducer system will be examined. It is recalled that this system consists of a pressure transducer, its amplifier and a voltmeter. The meter, of course, responds to voltages, but the meter face, instead of reading volts, will read mm. Hg. Suppose the face has been marked so that 0 mm. Hg corresponds to 0 volts and 200 mg. Hg corresponds to 5 volts. This relationship is shown by line *B* in Figure 2-3. Suppose that the system is out of calibration so that it corresponds to line *A* instead. In other words, at 0 mm. Hg the meter reads 1 volt instead of 0 volts, and at 200 mg. Hg it reads 4 volts instead of 5 volts. Two types of alterations must be made in the amplifier, namely, changes in both the zero intercept and the slope. In order to alter the zero intercept in the example, 1 volt must be subtracted; this is done by turning the balance (ZERO) control. The transducer is placed at 0 mm. Hg and the amplifier zeroed. The slope is altered by changing the GAIN. A pressure of 200 mm. Hg is applied to the transducer and the GAIN control turned until the meter reads 200 mm. Hg (that is, 5 volts). The device is then calibrated over its en-

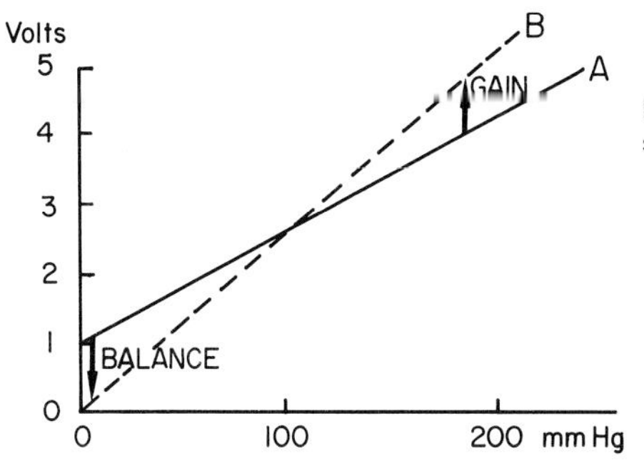

Fig. 2-3.—Amplifier calibration of pressure transducer system.

tire range. The same general procedure is followed for all types of amplifier calibrations.

Analog Readouts

After the signal has been conditioned the next step is that of making it available, in a meaningful way, to those caring for the patient. This, in many cases, e.g., the blood pressure and electrocardiogram, only requires that the electrical signal be converted to some form that can be read visually. For example, the blood pressure may be displayed on a meter, and either the blood pressure or electrocardiogram may be displayed on pen writers or on oscilloscopes. These machines have in common the ability to convert an electrical signal to a visual signal. The simple readouts are feasible if only a few parameters are being monitored in a given patient. If, however, many values are being monitored it becomes very difficult to display these signals in a manner that allows easy discrimination of abnormal values. Also, there are many physiologic variables such as peripheral resistance that cannot be measured directly but must be calculated. In order to facilitate both of these functions it is becoming necessary to employ computers.

Computers

Analog computers.—Analog computers are simply composed of a number of operational amplifiers which do arithmetic manipulations on electrical signals. For example, suppose that it is desired to calculate peripheral resistance, and further suppose that analog signals are available for cardiac output and blood pressure. Since peripheral resistance is equal to blood pressure divided by cardiac output, an analog divider would be employed. The output of this divider would be an electrical (analog) signal proportional to the value of the total peripheral resistance. In order for the signal to be available, one of the simple readout devices mentioned would have to be employed. For example, it would be possible in this situation to have a meter calibrated in peripheral resistance units. This type of computation has obvious advantages over doing the same computations by hand, but it has the disadvantage of adding still another analog readout device.

Digital computers.—The digital computer differs from the analog computer in that, instead of using electrical voltages as inputs, it requires actual numbers or digits, much the same as an adding machine requires actual numbers. In order to use this device to measure peripheral resistance, it is necessary to have a real number value for blood pressure and cardiac output. In return, a real number value for peripheral resistance is obtained. This number cannot be displayed on an ana log recorder, but may be recorded by a *digital readout device*, such as a teletype machine. The digital computer can be *programmed* to provide text in addition to the number readout. For example:

MR. JONES' PERIPHERAL RESISTANCE AT 10:45 A.M. IS 20 PERIPHERAL RESISTANCE UNITS

Since the digital computer is capable of extremely rapid calculations, it can be used to monitor a large number of variables. In addition, it can examine the values for the parameters, decide if they are abnormal and, if so, alert those caring for the patient. Such a device provides the present "ultimate" in patient monitoring and will see increasingly wider use in intensive care.

Most biologic variables are not digital but rather analog in form. Analog signals must be converted to digital values in order to be manipulated by the digital computer. This is done by what is known as *analog-to-digital conversion*. The analog signal is sampled at a rate of up to several thousand times per second, and each sampling is converted to a digital number. This seemingly tedious task is readily performed because of the speed of the digital computer.

Philosophy

The word "monitor" was used interchangeably with the word "surveillance" in the early part of this chapter. Actually, electronic monitoring is only one form of patient surveillance. It is often not as good as, and certainly never replaces, observation and physical examination of a patient. For example, anxiety and restlessness in a patient are sure signs of cerebral hypoxia even if cardiac output, arterial oxygenation, etc., are within normal limits. Cool, sweaty extremities indicate poor peripheral tissue perfusion even if total peripheral resistance happens to be within normal limits, and so on. The main function of monitors is to provide quantitative information about the patient, thus allowing detection of trends. These devices then must be considered as being nothing more than valuable adjuncts in the care of the patient, and the data they provide must always be interpreted in terms of the clinical course.

REFERENCES

1. Butler, J.: Measurement of Cardiac Output Using Soluble Gases, in *Handbook of Physiology: Respiration* (Washington, D.C.: American Physiological Society, 1965), vol. II.
2. Eisenman, G.: Glass Electrodes for Hydrogen and Other Cations, in *Principles and Practice* (New York: Marcel Dekker, Inc., 1967).
3. Malmstadt, H.V.; Enke, C. G., and Toren, E. C., Jr.: *Electronics for Scientists* (New York: W. A. Benjamin, Inc., 1963).
4. Osborn, J. J., *et al.*: Measurement and monitoring of acutely ill patients by digital computer, Surgery 64:1057–1070, 1968.
5. Severinghaus, J.: Blood Gas Concentrations, in *Handbook of Physiology: Respiration* (Washington, D.C.: American Physiological Society, 1965), vol. II.

6. Sheppard, L. C., *et al.*: Automated treatment of critically ill patients following operation, Ann. Surg. vol. 168, no. 4, Jul.-Dec., 1968.
7. Warner, H. R.: Experiences with computer-based patient monitoring, Anesth. & Analg. 47:453–462, 1968.
8. Yanof, H. M.: *Biomedical Electronics* (Philadelphia: F. A. Davis Co., 1965).

3

Central Venous Pressure: Indications and Technique

HAROLD A. PAUL, M.D.

Associate Attending Surgeon, Rush-Presbyterian-St. Luke's Medical Center; Associate Professor of Surgery, Rush Medical College

CENTRAL VENOUS PRESSURE is that pressure recorded in the central venous system within the right atrium or the great veins within the thorax. It is of particular value because it closely reflects the filling pressure and adequacy of the pump. The normal central venous pressure is in the range of 5–12 cm. H_2O. The clinical observer is particularly interested in high venous pressure, reflecting fluid overload or cardiac failure, or in low venous pressure, reflecting a decrease in volume or a disparity between the circulating volume and the circulatory bed.

In the following discussion consideration will be given to anatomic choices available for the introduction of a central venous catheter. Some description of technique and anatomic considerations will be given in each case.

Special attention and illustrations will be given to the technique utilizing the external jugular vein—a convenient and readily available site in most patients.

Indications

The central venous pressure should be monitored in all patients with circulatory failure. It is particularly useful when there is difficulty in stabilizing circulatory hemodynamics or when there is doubt as to the presence or absence of a hemodynamic abnormality. Central venous pressure monitoring should be done in:

1. Shock in which the usual measures have not improved circulation.

2. Conditions in which large volumes of fluid replacement are re-

quired; for example, massive hemorrhage, diabetic acidosis or late small bowel obstruction, especially in the elderly or in those patients with known cardiac disease.

3. Shock in which multiple factors contribute, especially when full information as to the relative importance of cardiac efficiency versus volume adequacy is desirable.

4. Septic shock, especially when therapy includes vasodilatation and infusion into the enlarging "vascular space."

An adequate central venous pressure is important in that it exerts significant influence on the cardiovascular function in the following ways: (*a*) It is one of the factors determining filling of the heart, therefore cardiac output. In any given circulatory state there is a constant relationship between filling pressure and ventricular work. (*b*) Maintaining an adequate venous pressure has an effect on the microcirculation. A low venous pressure will increase the arteriolovenular pressure gradient. This can be expected to increase flow in thoroughfare channels at the expense of lateral pressure. This will result in closure of precapillary sphincters and limited perfusion of the microcirculatory bed.

A natural speculation arises as to whether central venous pressure or the determination of serial blood volumes is the most reliable method of following patients who are critically ill and require volume replacement. The answer is clearly central venous pressure because of the following reasons:

1. There is reason to suspect that blood volume determinations are subject to "mixing errors" when done in shock patients. (This is brought about presumably by "trapping" in the microcirculation.)

2. In replacing blood volume, the rate and amount of loading are clearly dependent on the ability of the vascular system to accommodate that load. This has led to the term "capacity" or "capacitance" vessels, which defines the quality of the highly distensible vessels of the circulatory system – mainly the veins. "Capacitance" is derived from a similar term in electrical terminology meaning an increase in quantity of an electric charge held in a condenser for a given period and for a given increase in electrical potential. The ability of veins to hold progressively larger and larger quantities is particularly important in relation to venous return and therefore venous pressure.

Routes of Introduction of the Catheter

Central venous pressure catheters may be introduced percutaneously or by cutdown through the antecubital vein. Proper positioning is verified by observing appropriate fluctuation with respiration. Further confirmation may be obtained by chest x-ray or fluoroscopy.

The cephalic vein may be used by the cutdown approach, but it is not always desirable since the cephalic vein may be small, it may require more dissection, and it does not always permit easy transit of the catheter to the central point after it is introduced.

The subclavian vein is a useful approach (Chapter 22). Its use requires expertise and should be attempted only after careful study of the method and numerous manipulations in the morgue. There are significant complications of subclavian vein cannulation. The reported complications include pneumothorax, hydropneumothorax, arterial or venous laceration, thrombosis, embolism and thrombophlebitis. The frequency of the foregoing complications diminishes with experience. Proper training and experience can reduce the technique to one of minimal risk. After introduction, a chest x-ray confirms the position.

Technique of External Jugular Vein Cutdown (Fig. 3-1)

A.—Place the patient in the supine position with the head rotated to the opposite side. Place a rolled towel or sheet beneath the shoulders if hyperextension is needed. An oblique lighting angle and digital pressure over the clavicular end of the vein to produce distention assists in locating the external jugular as it traverses the midportion of the sternocleidomastoid muscle. After application of antiseptic, but prior to draping, a small transverse scratch is made to guide the subsequent incision. Infiltrate under the scratch mark with an appropriate local anesthetic. Carry the skin incision through the platysma muscle.

Fig. 3-1.—Technique of external jugular vein cutdown.

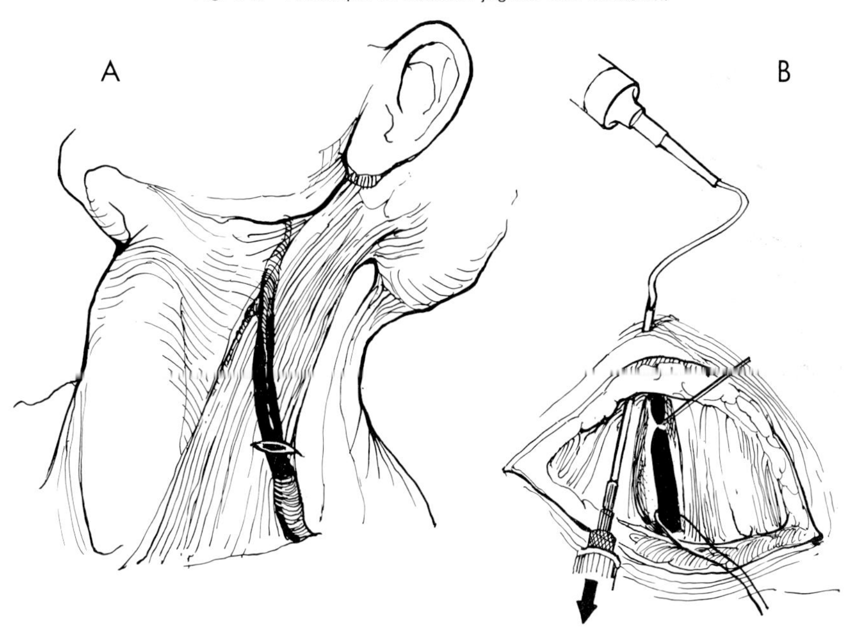

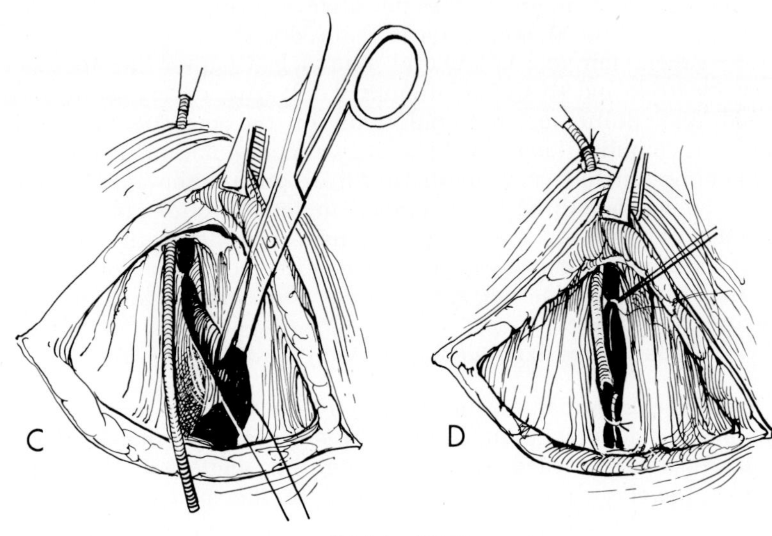

Fig. 3-1.—(*cont.*)

B.—Elevate the vein with two guy sutures of 000 silk. In most adults a 7 in. catheter (available as #1917 Deseret) is of proper length to reach the junction of the superior vena cava and the right atrium.

Attach a syringe containing heparinized saline to the catheter. Be certain to evacuate air from the catheter and syringe before flushing the vessel with saline. Tie the cephalad suture at its highest level. Using the cannula from the Intracath, make a counterpuncture just above the incision. Pass the catheter retrograde through the cannula to achieve transit through the counterpuncture, then withdraw the cannula.

C.—Between the guy sutures make a small opening in the vein with a small dissecting scissors.

D.—Introduce the catheter into the vein. Advance the catheter centrally and secure the lower tie. Aspirate to assure free flow. An extra suture is placed in the skin to secure the catheter. Remove the syringe and attach the catheter to the previously prepared manometer.

4

Tracheostomy and Respiratory Care

STANTON A. FRIEDBERG, M.D.

Chairman, Department of Otolaryngology and Broncho-esophagology, Rush-Presbyterian-St. Luke's Medical Center; Professor of Otolaryngology, Rush Medical College

THE IMPORTANCE of management of the respiratory tract in the intensive care of the surgical patient is taken for granted today. However, the basis of our current concepts became established just over 25 years ago with Galloway's monumental contribution on the use of tracheostomy in the management of the secretional problems of bulbar poliomyelitis patients. It is now universally accepted that proper respiratory tract care may contribute to patient survival in life-threatening medical and surgical situations.

Preoperative counseling, demonstrations and actual practice in deep breathing are important. The conscious patient who has undergone thoracic or upper abdominal surgery usually finds coughing extremely painful and his respiratory excursion will be correspondingly compromised. The patient with chronic bronchitis or emphysema is particularly prone to postoperative respiratory problems. Smoking should be completely eliminated at least one week prior to surgery.

In the following sections, the various methods and techniques of respiratory care and secretional management will be outlined.

Aspiration Techniques

Nasotracheal Aspiration

An ineffective cough, an unexplained fever or a suspicious-appearing chest x-ray in the early postoperative period are indications for nasotracheal aspiration, the first procedure among induced efforts to enhance coughing.

Equipment.—The basic equipment consists of sterile catheters and

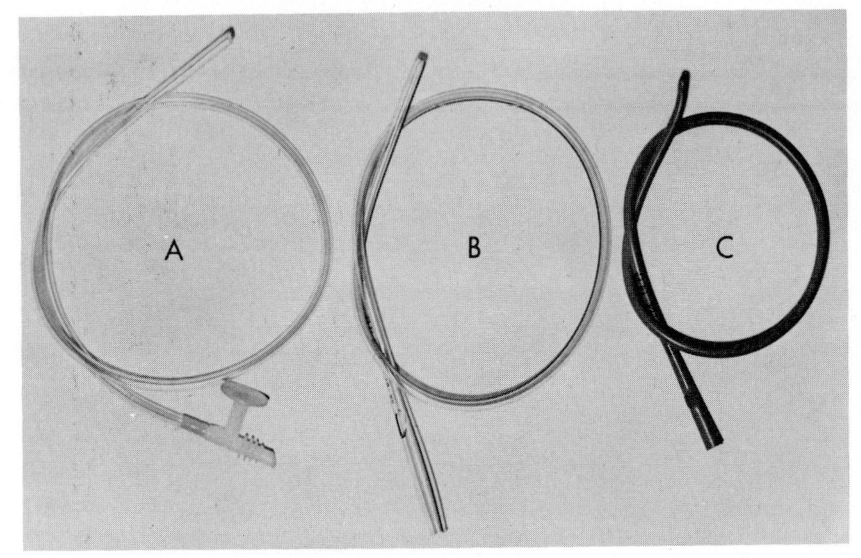

Fig. 4-1.—Types of catheters used for aspiration. **A,** Regu-Vac suction catheter (Bard-Parker), **B,** Tip-Trol suction catheter (Argyle), **C,** Stitt catheter.

an efficient suction apparatus. Some type of valve arrangement is necessary so that the suction can be activated only when needed; otherwise the continuous suction will cause the catheter to adhere to the walls of the trachea and remove air and oxygen from the physiologic dead space. The latter situation may precipitate cardiac arrest.

A popular aspirating technique makes use of a glass or plastic Y tube and a straight catheter with an end hole. Occlusion of the open Y permits intermittent suction. Other comparable catheters include the thumb valve and whistle tip types (Fig. 4-1, *A* and *B*). A Stitt catheter (*C*) with its angulated tip may facilitate insertion through the larynx and direction into the right or left bronchus.

A sterile catheter should be used for each aspiration to prevent contamination of the tracheobronchial tree. Disposable suction catheters are currently being employed with increasing frequency. Masks and sterile gloves are necessary to maintain sterile technique.

Technique.—Passage of a catheter through the nasal passages may be quite painful. This discomfort can be minimized by preliminary nasal application of a cotton-tipped applicator containing 2 ml. of 1% pontocaine or 5% cocaine solution. Figure 4-2 shows insertion of the catheter.

It may become necessary to instill normal saline solution to stimulate the cough reflex or to liquefy dried secretions. The catheter should be high in the trachea. The patient may be tilted laterally to ensure that the solution reaches each main bronchus. Five to 15 ml. of saline can

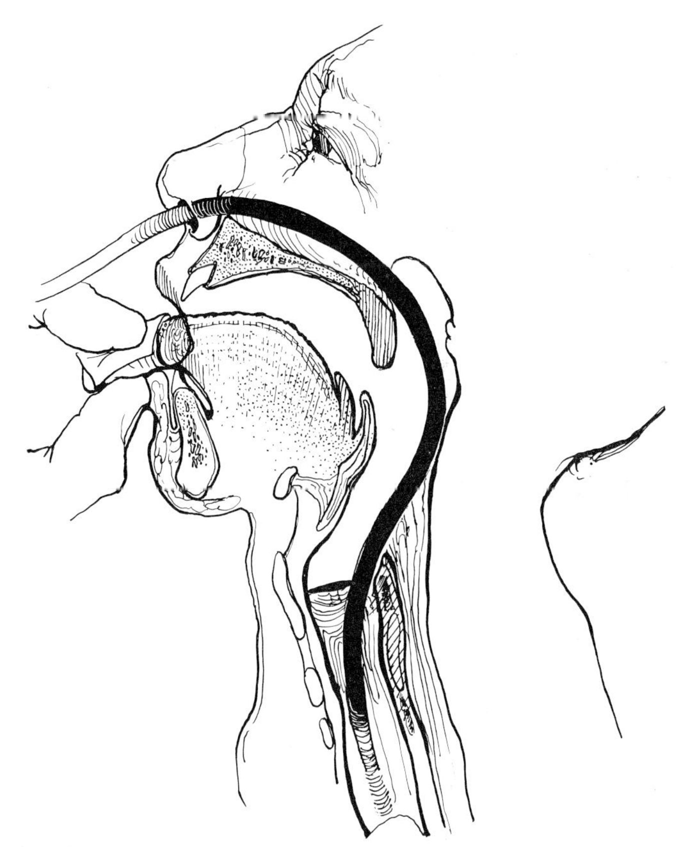

Fig. 4-2.—Nasotracheal aspiration. Extension of the neck and traction on the tongue facilitate entrance into the trachea.

be used safely on each side. The aspiration should not last longer than 15 seconds.

Complications.—One should be very circumspect in performing nasotracheal aspiration in patients with myocardial infarctions or those who have had recent heart valve or aneurysm surgery. Many of these individuals have impaired myocardial blood supply, and nasotracheal aspiration, particularly if prolonged, can precipitate cardiac arrest. It is beneficial to supply oxygen by mask or cannula during the period of aspiration.

Transtracheal Catheterization

This technique is used primarily for those patients who require cough stimulation but who can raise secretions once the cough has been initiated.

Equipment.—Either a large bore needle and polyethylene tube or a standard #14 Intracath may be used. The procedure should be done with sterile technique.

Technique.—A large bore needle (#18) is introduced through the neck into the trachea just below the cricoid cartilage, and a polyethylene tube is threaded downward through the needle. The needle is removed, allowing the tubing to remain in the trachea, and the tubing is then secured to the skin by suture or adhesive tape. A convenient alternative method is to use a standard #14 Intracath (Bard) in the same manner. The needle and catheter must be carefully secured to prevent the needle point from cutting the catheter. The catheter must be capped when not in use to prevent an air leak which would further impair effective coughing.

Since the diameter of the tubing is too small to permit effective aspiration, the usefulness of this method is related to the amount of cough stimulation which results from the introduction of saline or other solutions. Saline instillation is well tolerated and will promote coughing.

If saline alone is ineffective, a combination of Mucomist (1 ml.) and normal saline (2 ml.) will have both an irritating and liquefying action.

Complications.—Caution is required in patients with emphysema because of the increased volume of secretions which may result from the use of mucolytic agents. Other possible complications include subcutaneous emphysema, false passage into the peritracheal area or through the esophagus and occasional bleeding from the thyroid gland or an anomalous vessel.

Bronchoscopy

When nasotracheal aspiration or transtracheal catheterization does not produce the desired clearing of accumulated secretions, bronchoscopy should be performed without further delay. Auscultation, chest x-ray and an otherwise unexplained fever in the postoperative period should establish the diagnosis of early atelectasis. Unfortunately, the tendency is to procrastinate and to repeat x-ray examinations, thus permitting the optimum time for the procedure to pass.

Equipment.—A 7×40 bronchoscope, adequate illumination by fiber optics or standard light carriers, suction tips, suction apparatus, Lukens tubes and topical anesthesia form the basic equipment. Sterile gown and gloves should be used for protection of the patient as well as the physician and his assistant.

Technique.—For the patient who can be moved either in his bed or transferred on a hospital cart, bronchoscopy is ideally performed in an endoscopic suite. Quite often, the patient in the intensive care unit cannot be moved, and the bronchoscopy may then be performed with the operator at the head of the patient's elevated bed. (It is of historic interest that the first bronchoscopies were done with a patient seated on a low chair and the operator standing just behind him.) When the patient must remain supine, the head and shoulders can be moved diagonally off the bed and held by an assistant. The position chosen will often depend upon the patient's physique. The obese individual with a short neck and limited jaw excursion can be bronchoscoped with greater ease and facility in the supine position. Topical anesthesia is used but in less than maximal dosage, taking into account the patient's overall status and the fact that one does not wish to obtund completely the cough reflex.

It is important to collect the aspirated secretion in a sterile container (Lukens tube) for culture (Fig. 4-3). The operator may recognize whether the procedure has indeed been timely by the nature of the aspirate. Mucoid secretion signifies that infection has not yet occurred, while a purulent return indicates that the patient has an infectious bronchitis or pneumonia which will require antibiotic therapy. This should be initiated on the basis of an immediate Gram stain and modified as necessary when the culture report is available.

Valuable guides in assessing whether tracheostomy will be required include the amount of secretion, whether it emanates from one or both lungs, the level of consciousness of the patient and the degree of effective coughing produced by the instrumentation.

Complications.—Care should be taken to avoid dislodging any loose teeth. The lips and gums should be protected from instrument pressure. Gentle manipulation is required to prevent mucosal injury, which offers a portal of entry for infection.

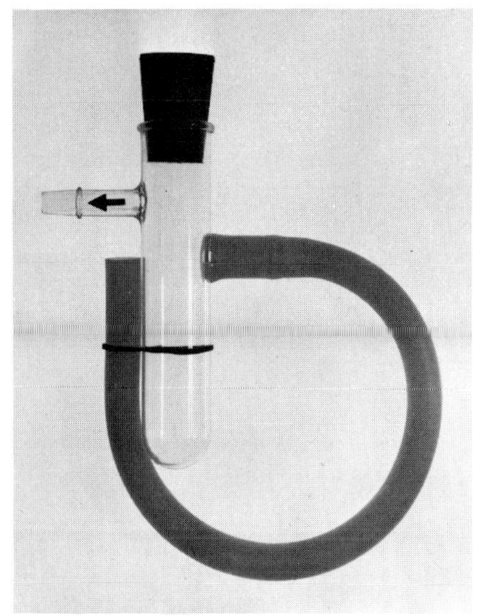

Fig. 4-3.—Lukens tube for collection of aspirated secretions. Secretions first traverse the lower sidearm to permit trapping in the collecting tube.

Aspiration Pneumonia

The extremely irritating effect of gastric juice upon the mucosa of the tracheobronchial tree and the resulting aspiration pneumonia call for preventive measures plus aggressive steps in actual management.

Comatose patients are particularly apt to aspirate and their stomachs should be kept empty by means of nasogastric suction. Patients who have undergone previous esophageal or gastric surgery in the form of resection with pyloroplasty or gastroenterostomy should have the stomach aspirated even before general anesthesia is induced. The same precautions are to be taken in patients with achalasia, esophageal strictures, pyloric or intestinal obstruction when a general anesthetic is contemplated. Additionally, the presence of an endotracheal tube does not guarantee against aspiration and the continued appearance of yellowish secretion via the endotracheal tube either during anesthesia or in the postoperative period should arouse suspicion of aspirated gastric contents.

In diagnosis, testing the pH of the secretion may provide information as to its acid content. A diffuse pulmonary infiltrate seen on x-ray may indicate aspiration pneumonia, whether or not vomiting has been actually witnessed. Bronchoscopy in such a situation will reveal intense hyperemia of the tracheobronchial mucosa, often with serosanguineous exudate having a slight odor.

Bronchoscopy should be performed as soon as possible after a proved episode of aspiration. Thorough irrigation of the entire tracheobronchial tree with 15–30 ml. of normal saline solution may be of value. A combination of aggressive steroid and antibiotic therapy should be instituted, and the progress of the pneumonic infiltrate followed by serial x-ray films.

Tracheostomy

In general, intensive care of surgical patients' respiratory problems involves control of secretions. It is for this reason that elective tracheostomy is being performed with increasing frequency. There are, in fact, situations in which anticipated difficulties in respiratory care are best dealt with by preoperative tracheostomy.

Emergency Airway Obstruction in Postoperative Patient

Emergencies calling for immediate relief of airway obstruction frequently occur in the postanesthesia recovery area and in the intensive care unit. These include:

1. Premature extubation. Stertorous breathing and cyanosis in a patient whose relaxed tongue has displaced the epiglottis to the point where it occludes the larynx can be immediately relieved by drawing

the tongue forward. One should not hesitate to use a towel clip or hemostat if the tongue cannot be held by the finger.

2. Bronchospasm. This may occur and must be dealt with by appropriate bronchodilators (aminophylline, 200–500 mg., given slowly intravenously over three to five minutes).

3. Laryngeal edema. A tracheostomy may be required for laryngeal edema as a result of prolonged intubation, particularly in children. Adrenalin, antihistamines and steroid therapy may be given a therapeutic trial, but unless a beneficial effect is soon apparent, one should proceed with tracheostomy.

4. Vocal cord paralysis. The patient who has undergone thyroidectomy should have direct laryngoscopic visualization upon emergence from anesthesia to rule out the possibility of bilateral abductor vocal cord paralysis, which results from an injury to the recurrent laryngeal nerves. If stridor and intercostal retractions develop in the postoperative period, several skin sutures are removed and a tracheostomy cannula is inserted into the skeletonized trachea. It is a common misconception that some voice alteration must accompany cord paralysis. In bilateral abductor paralysis, however, the voice is excellent and stridorous respiration may be the only sign of the patient's difficulty.

5. Fractured larynx. Although not commonly included in conventional concepts of postoperative care, an airway emergency may occur in a patient with multiple injuries when surgery has been performed for cerebral, abdominal or skeletal trauma. If there is an unrecognized fracture of the larynx or trachea, airway obstruction may develop rapidly when a previously placed endotracheal tube is removed. The clue in this situation is the presence of subcutaneous emphysema. As the tracheostomy is being done, an attempt is made to determine the site and extent of injuries of the larynx and trachea. It may be possible to deal with these directly, but it is important to appraise the degree of damage in planning further therapy.

6. Paradoxical respiration. Patients with chest trauma and paradoxical respiration may also require emergency tracheostomy in order to ensure adequate ventilation.

7. Respiratory burns. The severely burned patient may show signs of laryngeal obstruction and require tracheostomy under such circumstances. Routine early use of tracheostomy in burns, however, is not advocated. It does have a place in the control of secretions which result from bacterial pneumonia developing in two to seven days. In this instance the tracheostomy should be used for a short period only.

Elective Tracheostomy

The major indications for tracheostomy in the postoperative care of the patient are management of secretions and provision for assisted ventilation.

Stagnant secretions in the bronchial tree are obstructive and lead to atelectasis with compromised ventilation of the alveoli. Blood oxygen is reduced and CO_2 accumulates; the latter in turn may result in more secretions, and the systemic effects of hypoxia and acidosis soon complicate the picture.

The decision to perform tracheostomy is usually made: (1) after other aspirating maneuvers have proved ineffective or are too traumatic, or (2) when it becomes apparent that the patient will require assisted ventilation subsequent to removal of the endotracheal tube. In an extreme emergency either a bronchoscope or an endotracheal tube will provide a temporary airway, permitting the operator to perform his task in a tranquil manner. Good light and adequate suction are indispensable for an efficient tracheostomy. Valium given intravenously in 5 mg. increments is useful for agitated patients.

TECHNIQUE (FIG. 4–4)

A.—The type of incision is optional and may again depend somewhat upon the patient's physique. A horizontal skin incision is quite adequate in many instances, but most surgeons prefer a vertical incision. The latter is certainly desirable in the short-necked or emphysematous patient whose cricoid cartilage often seems to lie just above the jugular notch. Chief advantages of the vertical incision are improved exposure of the upper and lower limits of the thyroid isthmus and better delineation of the trachea to permit optimal placement of the cannula.

B.—Separation of the strap muscles is carried out in the midline. The trachea lies beneath the deep cervical fascia. The thyroid isthmus may be evident on its anterior and lateral surface, along with sizable veins which may require interruption. It is helpful to incise the fascia which envelops the thyroid to retract it superiorly or inferiorly. Division of the isthmus between Kocher clamps may occasionally be necessary. Frequent palpation of the trachea is helpful in keeping to the midline.

C and *D.*—An ovoid or rectangular segment of anterior tracheal wall is removed between the second and fourth tracheal rings to permit introduction of the cannula (except in infants and small children where only an incision is made). Thorough aspiration of the tracheobronchial tree is carried out just prior to cannula insertion. Care must be taken to prevent entry of a foreign body (such as the excised cartilage segment) into the trachea during the tracheostomy.

E.—The cannula is stabilized with a secure square knot.

It is advisable to avoid undue skeletonization of the trachea because this opens the deep fascial spaces of the neck and mediastinum. Coughing or mechanical ventilation will then force air into these areas with resulting emphysema. For the same reason, suturing of the deep layers is to be avoided as well as tight skin closure, although one or two sutures may be employed at the outer limits of an unduly long skin incision.

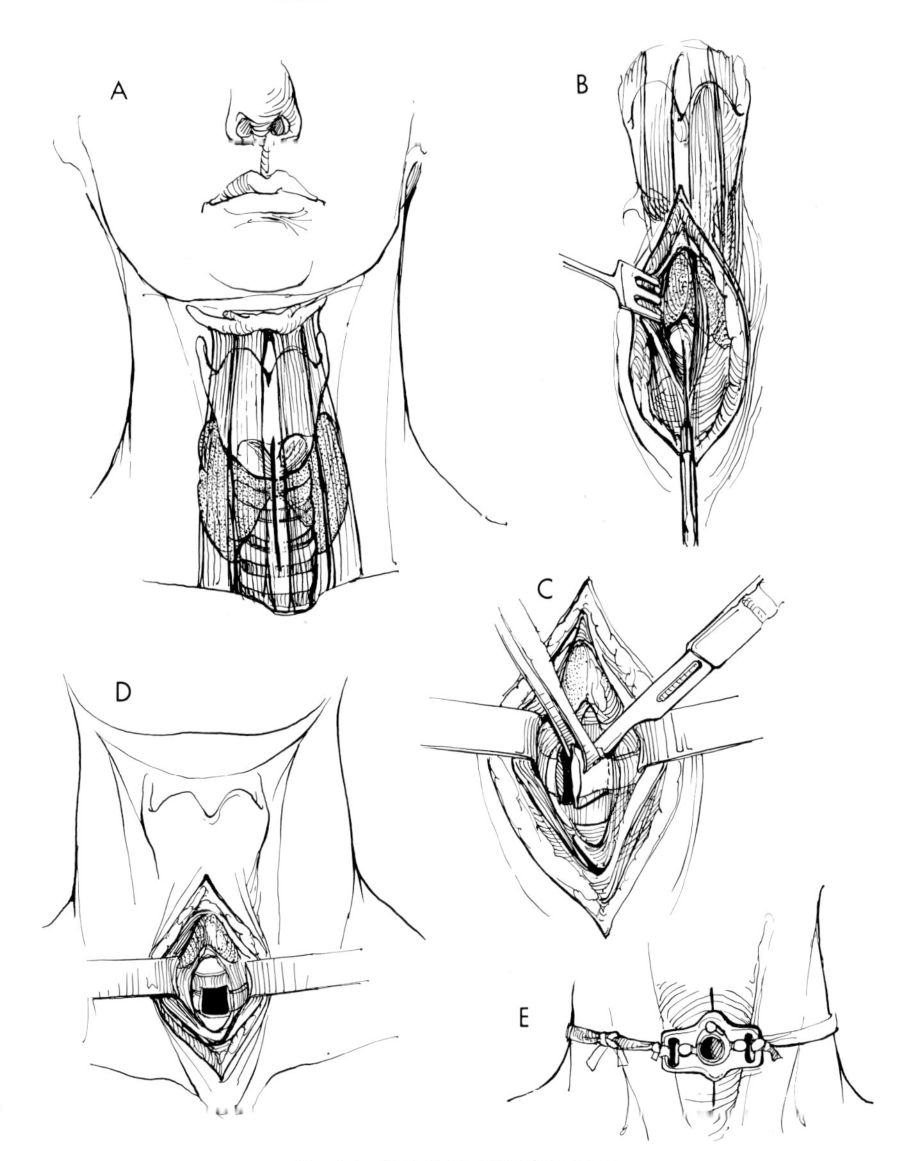

Fig. 4-4. – Technique of tracheostomy.

Certain variations of standard tracheostomy have been advocated, such as suturing the tracheal margins to the skin or turning down an inferiorly based flap of anterior tracheal wall and suturing it to the skin. These may be advisable if adequate postoperative monitoring is not available. In general, these techniques have not found widespread acceptance.

The use of a cuffed tracheal cannula is necessary when intermittent positive pressure ventilation is employed. Further, prophylactic placement of a cuff is indicated in any patient who is even in remote danger of cardiac or respiratory arrest. Therefore, it is wise to attach a cuff to the tracheal cannula and leave it uninflated. This permits use of positive pressure breathing on an instantly available basis.

Postoperative Management

Trained personnel and efficient nursing supervision are mandatory in the care of the patient with a tracheostomy. The patient cannot talk and his cough is unusually inadequate, so some type of signal must be at hand for use by the patient, together with facilities for prompt suctioning. It is readily apparent that no tracheal wound can be kept absolutely sterile, but precautions are required to prevent all avoidable contamination.

A tray at the bedside, adjacent to the suction apparatus, should have several basins, one with normal saline solution and another with a collection of sterile aspirating catheters, individually wrapped. The catheters are depicted in Figure 4-1. Use of gloves and masks during tracheal suction is strongly advocated. Aspiration procedures should be performed as gently as possible, since the tracheobronchial mucosa is easily denuded and this increases the susceptibility to infection.

A portable chest x-ray is taken routinely after tracheostomy and daily to ascertain the position of the tracheal cannula and to rule out the possibility of pneumothorax or mediastinal emphysema, occasional complications of tracheostomy and/or assisted ventilation.

ROUTINE POSTOPERATIVE TRACHEOSTOMY ORDERS

These orders also are applicable to patients with laryngectomy.

1. Place bell, a well-marked signal light, pencil and paper (or Magic Slate) at the patient's bedside. If the patient is unable to signal for help, he *must* be attended at all times.
2. Mark the intercom signal at the nurses' station to indicate that the patient cannot speak.
3. Fasten hospital gown in front of the patient with the top tie unfastened.
4. Aspirate the tracheostomy as often as necessary when secretions collect. This may be determined by bedside observation or auscultation of the chest.
5. Supply continuous humidity by tent or collar.
6. Instill sterile saline (2–5 ml.) into cannula when there is need to soften encrusted secretions.
7. Use a catheter for aspiration of the tracheostomy once only. Use a separate catheter to aspirate the nose or mouth.

8. Remove and clean the inner cannula every 4 to 6 hours, and every 8 hours in patients on assisted ventilation (more adequate humidification). Devices used as temporary adapters for respirators during cleaning of the inner cannula often do not fit well and air loss results unless precautions are taken.
9. Outer cannula and cord tape are to be removed by the physician only. (Tapes are to be tied with square knots, never with bow ties.)
10. Summon a physician if the tracheostomy cannula should become dislodged or if the patient's breathing becomes harsh or noisy. (If the outer cannula becomes displaced, hold the wound open with a hemostat until a physician arrives.)
11. Keep obturator of patient's cannula in a sterile container at bedside.
12. Provide 2 extra complete sets of tracheal cannulas and cuffs of identical size and type at the bedside in sterile jars.
13. Notify a physician immediately if the patient shows signs of restlessness, cyanosis or skin crepitation.
14. Always aspirate the pharynx before deflating the cuff. Deflate cuffed tubes for at least 5 minutes each hour.
15. Report any persistent bloody aspiration.

Additional suggestions for nursing personnel:

1. Place dry sterile gauze dressings around the cannula as required. (These dressings should be plain gauze rather than the cotton-filled type, since the latter may yield particles of foreign material which can be inhaled into the tracheobronchial tree.) It is essential that this dressing be kept dry. A wet dressing will promote infection.
2. Soiled tracheal cannulas with all parts—outer cannula, inner cannula and obturator—should be returned to service area for cleansing and re-sterilizing immediately upon removal from the patient.

Complications

1. Subcutaneous emphysema. In a patient on assisted ventilation, this may be the result of overzealous skin suturing and can be relieved by removal of skin sutures. If subcutaneous emphysema persists, depending upon whether a volume or pressure respirator is being used, the wound opening can be made larger to allow egress of air (volume respirator) or the cuff can be inflated more (pressure respirator).

2. Pneumothorax. This may occur as the result of a pleural wound, from excessive coughing or from the dissection of air from the mediastinum along the hilar structures. Pneumothorax should always be suspected in a patient who does not appear to be doing well after an adequate tracheostomy.

3. Tracheobronchitis. In tracheostomized patients the normal physiologic mechanism for moistening inspired air, namely, the nasal mucosa, is bypassed. Therefore, supplementary humidification is essential to

protect the mucosa from desiccation, tracheobronchitis and atelectasis. Humidity may be supplied via a tent or, better, with a tracheostomy collar. The collar has the advantage of patient accessibility. Saline (5–10 ml.), instilled into the tracheal cannula, is a valuable moistening supplement and cough stimulant. Crusting is often troublesome and calls for vigilant attention to adequate humidification and moistening procedures.

4. Dislodgment. If it becomes necessary to remove a tracheal cannula before a tract is well-established (four to five days) or if a cannula becomes dislodged, no attempt at reintroduction should be made without good light, satisfactory retraction, a tracheal dilator and a tracheal hook. Many tragedies occur as a result of a displaced cannula and the accompanying frantic efforts to replace it by forcing the cannula into the neck or mediastinum.

Once the tract is well-established, a complete change of cannula should be a daily routine or carried out more often, if indicated.

5. Infection. Because there is always some degree of infection, the risk of tracheal perichondritis and subsequent stenosis is ever present. Mediastinitis and pneumonia may also result from wound contamination.

6. Hemorrhage. Any persistent bleeding from an established tracheostomy must be considered potentially serious. Peritracheal inflammation may involve the walls of major vessels, particularly the innominate and carotid arteries, and massive exsanguinating hemorrhage from this type of vessel erosion is by no means rare.

Tension and torsion on the trachea and adjacent structures can be minimized by proper support of respiratory tubing and connections.

7. Tracheoesophageal fistula. This is an infrequent complication of tracheostomy but may occasionally result from infection and ulceration in the presence of an ill-fitting cannula.

Decannulation

Decannulation should be considered: (1) when the physical and x-ray findings indicate improvement, (2) when the need for aspiration diminishes, and (3) when the patient's cough reflex becomes effective. Taping or corking the tube for 24–48 hours will help determine the patient's status. Fenestrated or valved tracheostomy tubes may be used for several days as the patient is being weaned from aspiration and ventilatory assistance. If in doubt, gradual substitution of tubes of progressively smaller diameter is a practical method and also ensures uniform concentric wound healing.

Feeding of Tracheostomy Patients

Some patients may experience swallowing difficulties immediately following tracheostomy. When oral feedings are begun, the patient should be placed in a semiupright position. Custards, jello and other mechanically soft items may be given initially and are often tolerated better than liquids. The latter should be administered in sips only until the patient's confidence and ability to handle more are well established. Precautions must be taken to deflate the cuff before feedings.

Prolonged Intubation

Although it is difficult to establish arbitrary time limits regarding their sojourn, the prolonged use of intratracheal tubes is to be discouraged. Nasotracheal tubes used for ventilatory assistance are uncomfortable and cause trauma to the nasal mucosa, often resulting in troublesome bleeding. In addition, nasotracheal tubes may be of insufficient size for adequate ventilation. For these reasons they should usually not be permitted to remain for longer than 48 hours. Tracheostomy should be performed if assisted respiration is required beyond that time, preferably with the nasotracheal tube in situ so that the airway and mechanical assistance can be maintained during the procedure.

The endotracheal tube, when allowed to remain too long, is capable of causing laryngeal edema as well as contact ulcers or granulomas of the vocal cords. Additionally, the complications associated with the use of cuffed tubes are becoming increasingly apparent and more alarming. The major damage has been shown to occur at the site of the balloon cuff and the degree of damage increases as the period of mechanical ventilation is prolonged. There is a gradual progression from tracheitis to ulceration of mucosa to destruction of cartilage with loss of substance, followed by scarring and tracheal stenosis, which may occur even under optimal management with cuffed endotracheal tubes. These changes begin early and the tendency at present is to limit the use of an endotracheal tube to a maximum of 48 hours. One may elect to substitute tracheostomy before this time has elapsed.

Tracheostomy can be performed safely before the endotracheal tube is removed. It is essential that precise preparations be made with respect to the exact type of connectors needed for attachment to whatever type of ventilatory assistance is to be used. Arrangements should be made for at least five minutes of cuff deflation at one-half to one hour intervals in an attempt to minimize the adverse effects of the cuff inflation. Inflated cuffs, whether used perorally or via tracheostomy, should be employed no longer than absolutely necessary.

Summary

Respiratory tract care is of paramount importance in the management of surgical patients. Carefully performed nasotracheal and bronchoscopic aspiration procedures are valuable adjuncts in dealing with secretional problems. Transtracheal instillations may be helpful for people who require cough stimulation.

Tracheostomy is the procedure of choice when other aspirating measures are inadequate and when patients require prolonged assisted respiration. The care of patients with tracheostomies requires careful attention to many details of postoperative management, particularly when cuffed tubes are used.

Prolonged nasotracheal or endotracheal intubation is to be avoided whenever possible.

REFERENCES

1. Beatrous, W. P.: Tracheostomy: Its expanded indications and its present status, Laryngoscope 78:3–55, 1968.
2. Bendixen, H. H., *et al.*: *Respiratory Care* (St. Louis: C. V. Mosby Company, 1965).
3. Cooper, J. D., and Grillo, H. C.: Evolution of tracheal injury due to ventilatory assistance through cuffed tubes, Ann. Surg. 169:334–348, 1969.
4. Friedberg, S. A.; Griffith, T. E., and Hass, G. M.: Histologic changes in the trachea following tracheostomy, Ann. Otol. Rhin. & Laryng. 74:785–798, 1965.
5. Galloway, T. C.: Tracheostomy in bulbar poliomyelitis, J.A.M.A. 123:1096–1097, 1943.
6. Karlson, K. E.: Respiratory problems in the immediate postoperative period, S. Clin. North America 44:537, 1964.
7. Pearson, F. G.; Goldberg, M., and Da Silva, A. J.: A prospective study of tracheal injury complicating tracheostomy with a cuffed tube, Ann. Otol. Rhin. & Laryng. 77:867–882, 1968.
8. Radigan, L. R., and King, R. D.: A technique for the prevention of postoperative atelectasis, Surgery 47:184, 1960.

5

Postoperative Ventilatory Management

MORTON SHULMAN, M.D.

Anesthesiologist, University Hospital; Associate Professor of Anesthesiology, University of Illinois Abraham Lincoln School of Medicine

VENTILATORY PROBLEMS continue to plague surgeons and anesthesiologists as one of the more common groups of adverse postoperative sequelae. These problems vary in severity from conditions which respond to simple conservative methods of inhalation therapy to the opposite extreme of respiratory failure which requires management with sophisticated techniques and mechanical equipment. It should be recognized that almost all of the conditions that will be discussed can run this spectrum. The astute clinician must constantly be on the alert for these problems, and when they occur, he must be able to assess their severity and to decide whether or not they are progressing in degree. Many of these conditions, although they may progress to respiratory failure, should not necessarily indicate the demise of the patient, provided adequate use is made of the relatively sophisticated techniques and equipment that have been developed for these conditions. The proper use of the intermittent positive pressure respirators in particular has markedly altered the prognosis of severe postoperative pulmonary complications.

ETIOLOGY OF POSTOPERATIVE VENTILATORY PROBLEMS

Most postoperative ventilatory problems are usually due to pulmonary hypoventilation, pulmonary ventilation perfusion disproportions or a combination of these two factors. Indeed, most of the situations to be

TABLE 5-1.—Etiology of Postoperative Ventilatory Problems

I. *Pulmonary hypoventilation*
  A. Secondary to hyperventilation during anesthesia and surgery
  B. Drug effects
    1. Drugs which depress the central nervous system
      a) General anesthetics
      b) Barbiturates
      c) Narcotic analgesics
      d) Overdosage with local anesthetics
    2. Drugs which block the myoneural junction
      a) Muscle relaxants—*d*-tubocurarine, gallamine, succinylcholine
      b) Drugs which interact with muscle relaxants and/or diethyl ether
        (1) Antibiotics—neomycin, kanamycin, streptomycin, polymixin, colistin
        (2) Quinidine
        (3) Pseudocholinesterase inhibitors—hexafluorenium, echothiophate iodide
    3. High spinal anesthesia
  C. Obesity
  D. Mechanical impediments to respiration
    1. Pneumothorax, hemothorax, hydrothorax
    2. Ascites
    3. Abdominal and chest masses
    4. Abdominal and chest packs and binders
  E. Pre-existing diseases
    1. Congenital diseases
      a) Myasthenia gravis
      b) Myotonia congenita
      c) Porphyria
      d) Abnormal serum pseudocholinesterase
    2. Neurologic diseases
      a) Poliomyelitis
      b) Polyneuritis
      c) Idiopathic pulmonary hypoventilation
      d) Multiple sclerosis
      e) Amyotrophic lateral sclerosis
    3. Pulmonary diseases
      a) Bronchial asthma
      b) Chronic lung disease
      c) Chronic cystic fibrosis
    4. Musculoskeletal diseases
      a) Scleroderma
      b) Muscular dystrophy
      c) Scoliosis
      d) Flail chest

II. *Ventilation perfusion disproportions*
  A. Postoperative lung syndrome
  B. Atelectasis
    1. Massive
    2. Patchy
    3. Micro
  C. Others
    1. Bronchial asthma
    2. Chronic lung disease
    3. Acute pneumonias
    4. Respiratory distress syndrome of the newborn

described will have elements of both these conditions. Nevertheless, for practical purposes, we can classify most situations as either one or the other (Table 5-1).

Pulmonary Hypoventilation

Pulmonary hypoventilation is a situation in which alveolar ventilation is inadequate. It is characterized by low tidal volumes and low minute volumes. Arterial blood gas patterns in patients breathing room air will show decreased oxygen tensions and increased carbon dioxide tensions. If the hypoxia is severe enough and of sufficiently long duration, metabolic acidosis characterized by a base deficit will also appear.

One of the commonest causes of postoperative pulmonary hypoventilation is prolonged hyperventilation during anesthesia and surgery. A depletion of total body carbon dioxide stores results, and the patient will hypoventilate during the immediate postoperative phase until the carbon dioxide stores reach normal. Such a patient will show a variance from the blood gas patterns just described. The carbon dioxide tension of arterial blood (Pa_{CO_2}) will be normal; nevertheless, the minute and tidal volumes will be decreased, as will the arterial oxygen tension (Pa_{O_2}), so long as the patient is breathing room air. The enrichment of the inhaled atmosphere with oxygen via one of the many oxygen therapy devices available today usually constitutes adequate therapy for this condition. Oxygen therapy should be continued until the total body carbon dioxide stores, minute volume and alveolar ventilation have reached normal levels.

The drugs used during anesthesia and surgery are another common cause of postoperative pulmonary hypoventilation. Their action may extend to the immediate postsurgical phase and produce hypoventilation. Relative overdosage with long-acting anesthetic agents such as diethyl ether and methoxyflurane can also cause a patient to hypoventilate during the immediate postoperative period. Even halothane, which is usually thought of as a short-acting agent, may have this effect. Narcotics and barbiturates can produce pulmonary hypoventilation, especially when used in conjunction with one of the more potent inhalation anesthetics.

Except for the specific antagonists that are available for the narcotic class of drugs, it is not advisable to treat drug-induced pulmonary hypoventilation by pharmacologic means. The proper use of analeptic drugs is difficult at best. Much more reliable therapy is provided by the use of ventilatory assistance with a positive pressure respirator until the adverse effects of the depressant have waned.

Residual curarization from a muscle-relaxing drug is also a common cause of postoperative pulmonary hypoventilation. Patients are often sent to the recovery room with a partial myoneural blockade still in effect. Proper treatment of this situation will often depend on the type of myoneural blocking agents used during anesthesia. If the relaxant drug that was used was one of the nondepolarizing group of relaxants, such as *d*-tubocurarine or gallamine, then adequate reversal of the myoneural blockade can often be achieved with neostigmine (Prostigmin). On the other hand, if the relaxant was one of the depolarizing groups, such as succinylcholine, quite often neostigmine will not be effective in reversing the block. This is especially true when the patient's ability to metabolize succinylcholine has been impaired, either due to the presence of atypical serum pseudocholinesterase or to prior treatment with drugs which depress plasma pseudocholinesterase, for example, echothiophate iodide. Whenever doubt exists as to whether the effect of a muscle relaxant can be reversed, the safest means of handling the patient is to support ventilation with an intermittent positive pressure respirator until the relaxant effects have worn off.

Neostigmine, when used to reverse muscle relaxation, should never be used alone but should be preceded by atropine to prevent the muscarinic effects of the neostigmine. The usual ratio is 0.4 mg. atropine for every 1 mg. neostigmine. If bradycardia develops during administration of neostigmine, additional atropine should be given. It is probably useless to exceed a dose of 5 mg. neostigmine intravenously. If this dose does not produce adequate reversal of the curarized state, then ventilation should be assisted with an intermittent positive pressure respirator.

In no event should edrophonium be used as a therapeutic drug to antagonize the effects of muscle relaxants. This drug is evanescent in its action and recurarization will inevitably result. Its use should be restricted to that of a diagnostic drug only.

Certain antibiotics have myoneural blocking properties and, when used in conjunction with muscle relaxants during anesthesia and surgery, may produce prolonged myoneural blockade. These drugs are streptomycin, neomycin, kanamycin, polymyxin and colistin. Quinidine, although not an antibiotic, also shares this effect. Prolonged myoneural blockade due to a combination of antibiotics and muscle relaxants is often difficult to treat pharmacologically. Neostigmine seems to work in some cases and not in others. The combination of calcium gluconate and sodium bicarbonate also seems to work in some cases, but is not necessarily effective in all. Here again is an indication for assisted respiration using an intermittent positive pressure respirator until the patient is able to breathe adequately on his own.

A patient arriving in the recovery room shortly after a high spinal anesthetic may be unable to ventilate adequately due to the pharmacologic block of the nerves that lead to the muscles of respiration. The treatment here is quite simple: respirations should be maintained with an intermittent positive pressure respirator until the spinal anesthetic has worn off.

Severe obesity presents ventilatory hazards to patients undergoing surgery. It is not uncommon to see hypoventilation among these patients in the recovery room. The cause is apparently a mechanical impediment due to the obesity. In extreme cases the inability to ventilate adequately may persist for several days or even weeks. The combination of obesity and any of the other factors producing pulmonary hypoventilation often makes management extremely difficult. Proper skill in utilizing intermittent positive pressure respirators may mean the difference between a stormy postoperative course and a relatively smooth one.

Other mechanical impediments to ventilation may occur in postoperative patients. These include pneumothorax, hemothorax, hydrothorax, ascites, the presence of large abdominal masses and tight abdominal or chest binders or packs. The primary treatment consists of removing the causative factors whenever possible. Fluid in the chest and abdomen should be drained. Air in the chest cavity should be aspirated, and restricting packs and binders should be removed when possible. If adequate relief of respiratory distress cannot be achieved in this manner, ventilation should be supported by an intermittent positive pressure respirator.

The surgical patient may have a pre-existing disease which is independent of the condition that necessitates surgery, but which nevertheless can produce postoperative ventilatory problems. Here again the degree of respiratory embarrassment may vary from that needing only conservative supportive care, such as oxygen inhalation, to that requiring prolonged management with an intermittent positive pressure respirator. The conditions may be of several types: primary pulmonary conditions, such as chronic lung disease with decompensation, bronchial asthma with acute exacerbation, or chronic cystic fibrosis; congenital diseases, such as myasthenia gravis, myotonia congenita or porphyria; primary neurologic disease, such as poliomyelitis or polyneuritis; or musculoskeletal diseases, such as scleroderma, severe scoliosis, or flail chest following trauma.

The management of the patient with a flail chest using the intermittent positive pressure respirator represents a marked improvement over previous therapy. The patient may be unable to ventilate the lungs because multiple rib fractures have destroyed the ability of the chest wall to act as a bellows. Former methods of attempting stabilization by the use of sand bags or traction devices were largely unsuccessful, especially in severe cases. An intermittent positive pressure respirator establishes effective ventilation and reduces the rib fractures by internal pressure. Most patients with flail chest must remain on the respirator continuously until sufficient healing has occurred at the fracture sites to stabilize the chest wall. This may require from four to six weeks.

Ventilation-Perfusion Disproportion

In recent years it has been realized that even though tidal and minute volumes of respiration may be normal or greater than normal, alveolar ventilation may still be inadequate. This results when air entering the lung is not properly distributed to all alveoli. Some alveoli may be well ventilated but poorly perfused, resulting in an increase in the physiologic dead space. Other alveoli may be adequately perfused but poorly ventilated, resulting in an increase in the right to left physiologic circulatory shunt.

A relatively common condition which appears to be predominantly a problem of gas distribution within the lung is one I call the "postoperative lung syndrome." This condition usually occurs after major intra-abdominal or intrathoracic surgery in patients with pre-existing pulmonary disease of a chronic nature. It is characterized by a decrease in lung compliance, increased tidal and minute volumes of respiration and either normal or increased respiratory resistance. Arterial blood gas patterns when the patient is breathing room air show low Pco_2, low Po_2 and usually a base deficit secondary to hypoxia. Like the conditions described under hypoventilation, this condition may also vary from one of moderate severity to life-threatening respiratory failure. Loss of normal alveolar surfactant activity may be an etiologic factor. Post-pump lung syndrome following cardiopulmonary bypass is a variant of this condition.

Atelectasis is another situation in which ventilation-perfusion disproportions exist. The pathologic involvement may be scattered in a patchy manner throughout both lungs or may be concentrated, with massive collapse of an entire lobe or even an entire lung. A condition of micro-atelectasis or miliary atelectasis has been postulated, in which the atelectatic areas are so small that they cannot be seen on an x-ray, yet a pathologic effect on blood gas patterns is evident when the arterial blood is examined. Here the blood gas pattern is markedly similar to that in the postoperative lung syndrome. The arterial Pco_2 is relatively normal or even below normal. The arterial Po_2 is quite low.

Other conditions not necessarily related to the surgical procedure but present in the postoperative period may have ventilation-perfusion disproportions as part of their pathology. These include bronchial asthma, chronic lung disease and acute pneumonias. Here again the degree of ventilatory embarrassment can vary from mild to that of acute respiratory failure.

Acute Respiratory Failure

When the patient's ability to maintain an adequate gas exchange is impaired to the extent that life is threatened, the patient has entered the phase of acute respiratory failure. One of the best methods to determine whether acute respiratory failure has developed is to examine the arterial blood gases. An arterial Pco_2 of greater than 55 mm. Hg or an arterial Po_2 of less than 50 mm. Hg while the patient is breathing room air should immediately make one suspect respiratory failure. This is particularly true when repeated arterial blood samples show a progressive rise in arterial Pco_2 or a progressive fall in arterial Po_2.

If the etiology of the respiratory failure is primarily pulmonary hypoventilation, then both an increased arterial Pco_2 and a decreased arterial Po_2 will be seen. If, however, the etiology is primarily a problem of gas distribution within the lungs, the arterial Po_2 will be low, but the arterial Pco_2 can be variable. It may be increased, normal or even decreased. Tidal and minute volumes of ventilation will be decreased in pulmonary hypoventilation, but they are often increased with severe ventilation-perfusion disproportions.

Conservative methods of therapy such as inhalation of oxygen or occasional intermittent positive pressure breathing therapy with aerosols are usually inadequate. In respiratory failure, one must rely upon continuous ventilatory support with an intermittent positive pressure respirator. These machines are capable of providing the increased minute and tidal volumes that are necessary to treat pulmonary hypoventilation and, when used properly, seem capable of more adequately distributing the gas flow into the lungs in conditions with ventilation-perfusion disproportions.

METHODS OF TREATMENT

Oxygen Therapy Equipment

Mild cases of pulmonary hypoventilation and ventilation-perfusion disproportions frequently can be treated adequately by providing the patient with supplementary oxygen. By and large, devices for oxygen therapy can be divided into three major categories: tents, catheters and masks.

The oxygen tent which encloses the entire body is usually a poor method of administering oxygen to a surgical patient. It is difficult to maintain adequate oxygen concentrations inside an oxygen tent and still provide the continuous care which the average postsurgical patient requires, unless very high flows of oxygen into the tent are utilized and flush mechanisms are used each time the tent is opened. The concentration of oxygen inside an oxygen tent is often only slightly above that of the atmosphere.

A more effective method for providing oxygen is that using a nasal catheter or a nasal cannula (Fig. 5-1). Both devices seem to be equally effective for oxygenation of the patient. However, a nasal cannula is better tolerated by the patient because it is more comfortable. Patients can also tolerate higher flows of oxygen with a cannula than with a catheter. With the nasal catheter, oxygen flows should be limited to a maximum of 5 L./minute. When the cannula is used, flows of 10 L./minute are usually well tolerated.

If a device more efficient than the catheter or cannula is desired, a face mask should be used. These masks are available in a wide variety of types, both with and without reservoir bags; those with reservoir bags (Fig. 5-1) provide much more effective oxygenation. Oxygen flows of 10 L./minute delivered into a face mask with a reservoir bag attached constitute an efficient means of oxygen therapy. It is imperative when giving oxygen therapy that measures be taken to assure that the mask or other device being used remains in its proper place. It is often easier to maintain oxygen therapy with a catheter or cannula than with a face mask because the patient is more prone to remove a face mask than he is a catheter or cannula.

ENDOTRACHEAL OXYGEN ADMINISTRATION.—Specialized methods of administering oxygen are necessary if the patient has an indwelling endotracheal tube or a tracheostomy. One of the simplest methods of administering endotracheal oxygen is to place an oxygen catheter into the lumen of the endotracheal or tracheostomy tube. This method provides adequate oxygen supplementation to the patient. However, it has the disadvantage of markedly increasing airway resistance if the catheter diameter approximates the diameter of the lumen of the endotracheal tube.

If the catheter method is used to administer endotracheal oxygen, care must be taken to assure that airway resistance is minimally

Fig. 5-1.—Three common devices for administering oxygen: rebreathing mask, nasal cannula and nasal catheter.

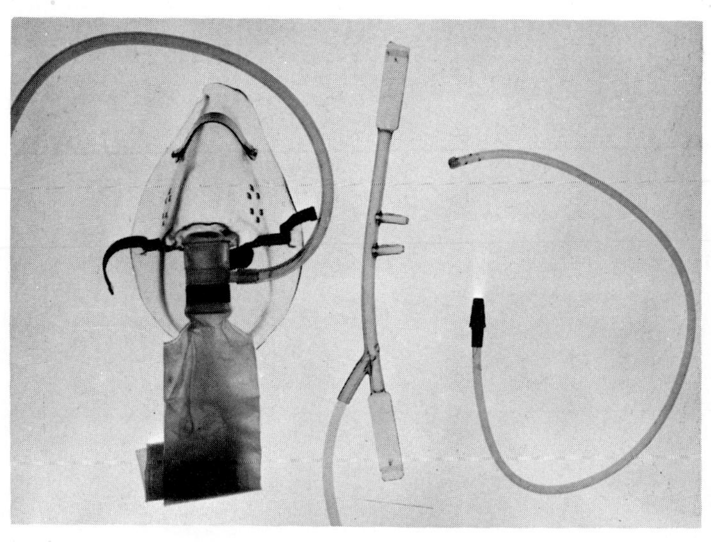

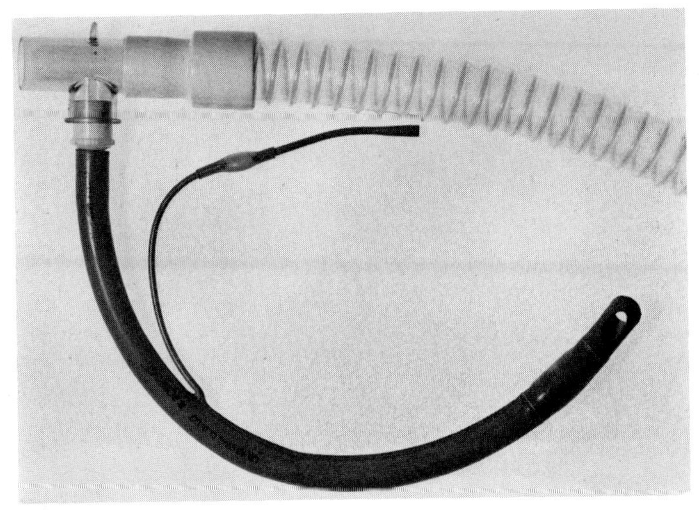

Fig. 5-2.—Plastic T-piece for administering endotracheal oxygen. Wide-bore corrugated tubing from humidifier conducts oxygen to T-piece and attaches to one arm of T. Base of T connects to standard 15 mm. adapter of endotracheal tube.

affected. This can be accomplished with endotracheal tubes of #30 French or larger by using a small catheter to administer the oxygen, for example, a #8 French urethral catheter. The catheter should not be inserted more than 1–2 in. into the lumen of the endotracheal tube. A

Fig. 5-3.—Plastic T-piece connected to metal tracheostomy tube by corrugated rubber tube. A reservoir tube has been added to the arm of the T-piece opposite the oxygen-conducting tube in order to increase the inhaled concentration of oxygen. The humidifier pictured is of the nebulizer type.

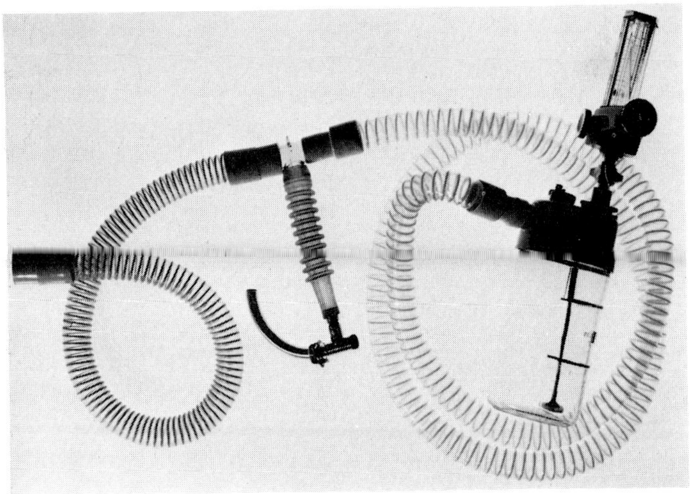

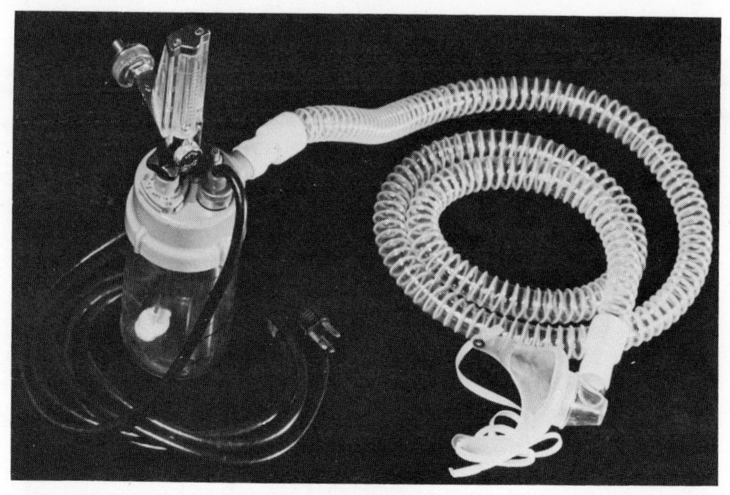

Fig. 5-4.—Plastic collar used to administer oxygen and aerosols to tracheostomy patient.

practical method of giving adequate oxygenation through an endotracheal or tracheostomy tube is to use a small plastic T-piece arrangement (Figs. 5-2 and 5-3). This device, especially when used with a reservoir tube, gives efficient oxygen and aerosol therapy and yet does not increase airway resistance. A plastic tracheostomy collar is also an effective means of administering oxygen and aerosol therapy to patients with tracheostomies (Fig. 5-4).

Whenever oxygen therapy is utilized, the aim should not be to hyperoxygenate the arterial blood, but rather to bring its oxygen content up to a normal range. Because of the particular shape of the oxygen-hemoglobin dissociation curve, the arterial oxygen content does not increase greatly after the arterial Po_2 has reached 70 mm. Hg; it increases very little after the tension reaches 100 mm. Hg. Thus an arterial Po_2 of 100 mm. Hg is a perfectly adequate endpoint to strive for in oxygen therapy. Patients receiving oxygen therapy should have the arterial Po_2 checked periodically to assess the adequacy of therapy.

Humidifiers and Nebulizers

Patients with ventilatory problems are often unable to humidify the inspired respiratory gases adequately. This is due to one or both of the following reasons. First, they may have bronchostasis or inspissated secretions in the tracheobronchial tree because the normal humidification mechanism of the nose does not provide enough moisture to keep secretions liquefied. Second, the normal nasal humidifying mechanism may have been bypassed by the insertion of an endotracheal tube or by the performance of a tracheostomy. In these cases, some means of establishing adequate humidification of inspired respiratory gases must be provided by the physician.

Bubble humidifiers were used for many years in an attempt to add adequate humidity to the essentially dry oxygen used for oxygen therapy. These devices were found inadequate for the job and today have been largely replaced by nebulizers. The nebulizers provide microdroplets of fluid suspended in the airstream which the patient inhales and carries into the airway.

Pneumatic nebulizers utilize the energy of the airstream flowing through them to produce these droplets. The sizes of the available pneumatic nebulizers vary greatly. Some are quite small, with a capacity of only 10–20 ml. These small nebulizers are used predominantly to provide aerosolized medications for inhalation therapy. The patient may inhale the aerosolized medications directly through a face mask or mouthpiece attached to the nebulizer, or the medications may be forced into the lungs by means of an intermittent positive pressure breathing machine attached to the nebulizer. Large nebulizers with a capacity of 500 ml. or greater are often used to provide mist therapy. There may be heaters attached to warm the aerosols emitted. Because a warm aerosol carries more moisture than does a cold one, these nebulizers provide a readily efficient method of enabling the patient to inhale large quantities of moisture.

The recent development of ultrasonic nebulizers has provided a means of adding large amounts of fluid to the tracheobronchial tree by inhalation. These nebulizers have high outputs; most of the brands available are able to nebulize anywhere from 2 to 6 ml. of fluid a minute.

In utilizing nebulizers for inhalation therapy, care should be taken that the liquid nebulized is not plain water. Nebulized water is often irritating to the larynx and tracheobronchial tree and can produce severe spasms of coughing. Half-normal saline is not irritating when inhaled and seems to be the fluid of choice for filling nebulizers.

Inhalation of large quantities of aerosolized saline enables a patient to mobilize and cough up large amounts of secretions from the tracheobronchial tree. Occasionally, however, too much aerosolized fluid may be presented to the patient too rapidly, and the retained secretions will be liquefied at a rate greater than they can be mobilized. When this occurs, an increase in respiratory resistance and respiratory distress may be seen. The rate of administration of aerosols must then be reduced until the patient can adequately handle the liquefied secretions. In some instances, this problem can be solved by attaching the nebulizer to an intermittent positive pressure breathing machine and assisting the patient's respiration.

Usually the administration of aerosols can be readily accomplished by conducting the aerosol to the patient via a wide-bore tube and attaching a face mask or a face tent to the end of this tube. When aerosol therapy is given to infants or small children, it is usually best to place the child in a plastic tent and fill the tent with the aerosol. Because very small infants may absorb significant quantities of moisture through their respiratory tracts, this must be taken into account when calculating fluid requirements. One method of doing this is to weigh the infant every eight hours to see how much fluid has been absorbed.

Intermittent Positive Pressure Breathing Units

Intermittent positive pressure breathing (IPPB) machines have been used extensively for respiratory therapy. Some controversy exists as to whether these units are actually of benefit in the prevention of postsurgical respiratory complications. Nevertheless, many people who are familiar with these units feel that, when used properly, they can be of great value to the surgical patient.

The rationale behind IPPB therapy is twofold. (1) The machines can be valuable adjuncts to the stir-up regimen by actively inflating the lungs and thus opening up alveoli which may have been partially ventilated due to progressing atelectasis. (2) These machines are capable of forcing aerosolized medications deep into the tracheobronchial tree. Since the use of positive pressure distributes gas into those sections of the lung which are normally underventilated, it is an excellent method of delivering aerosolized medications to those areas where they are needed most.

Proper use dictates that patients be properly trained to breathe with these machines, rather than against them. Too often one sees a patient who has not been properly instructed actually fighting the machine with his respiratory muscles. For a beneficial result from IPPB therapy, it is imperative that the patient be properly trained to use these machines. This training is best done preoperatively. It is unreasonable to expect a patient who has had extensive abdominal surgery to use one of these machines adequately for the first time in the immediate postoperative period. On the other hand, if he has learned to use IPPB therapy preoperatively, he will be able to utilize the treatment more effectively.

Once a patient has been adequately instructed in the use of IPPB units, steps must be taken to ensure proper use of the units during each therapy period. This means that each treatment period should not be limited arbitrarily to five or ten minutes, but rather should be sufficiently long to allow complete utilization of the medication prescribed for aerosolization. Also, one should not attempt to set pressure limits arbitrarily in writing orders for IPPB therapy; rather, the therapist should be permitted to determine which pressure the patient seems to tolerate best and to use his judgment in setting the pressures on the machine. Too often orders are written that limit the pressure to such low values that the therapy is virtually worthless. A general rule is to start with pressures that are easily tolerated by the patient (for example, 10–15 cm. of water) and gradually increase the pressure until it reaches the maximum tolerable pressure that the patient can readily accept. The common fear that pressures above 15–20 cm. of water delivered at the airway can cause the rupture of alveoli is unfounded. If these patients are to benefit from IPPB therapy, they must receive adequate pressure during each therapy session. This is especially true in atelectasis, which often responds well to IPPB therapy if adequate pressure (often 30–40 cm. of water, if tolerated) and adequate inspiration time (2–4 seconds) are provided.

Aerosolized Medications

Several classes of drugs have been used for inhalation by aerosolization. The most common are the mucolytics, bronchodilators, decongestants, antibiotics and adrenocorticosteroids.

MUCOLYTICS.—Several types of drugs have been used as mucolytics to lyse inspissated bronchial secretions. Surface-active agents constitute one of these groups. Commonly used among these agents are detergents, propylene glycol, glycerol and ethyl alcohol. Ethyl alcohol has also been used extensively as an antifoaming agent in treatment of pulmonary edema. Commercial preparations of surface-active agents, such as Alevair and Tergemist, have been available for several years. Results from these preparations tend to be somewhat disappointing, however, and in recent years their use has decreased.

The second group of drugs used by inhalation for mucolysis is the proteolytic enzymes. These include trypsin, chymotrypsin and pancreatic dornase. Although these enzymes are often efficient mucolytics, their use is not without significant hazards. Trypsin and chymotrypsin are irritating to the airway and have been known to digest normal tracheal mucosa. For these reasons they have never gained wide popularity in the treatment of retained bronchial secretions. Pancreatic dornase appears to be helpful only when the secretions contain a large quantity of desoxyribonucleic acid, and it has been used predominantly for the treatment of grossly purulent secretions.

Acetylcysteine is an excellent mucolytic and has been used both in aerosolization and by direct instillation into the tracheobronchial tree to produce lysis of thick secretions. However, it is quite irritating and can produce spasmodic coughing and bronchospasm. The degree of irritation produced by acetylcysteine is directly proportional to its concentration. Therefore, a proper balance is attempted between a concentration sufficiently high to produce adequate therapeutic results and sufficiently low to reduce irritative phenomena. A 10% concentration is thought to be a good compromise. Therefore, the commercially available 20% solution of acetylcysteine (Mucomyst) should be diluted. Because the irritancy of acetylcysteine solutions is a result of their high osmolality, dilution should be with distilled water rather than saline.

Bronchodilators and decongestants are often added to an acetylcysteine mixture in an attempt to counteract some of the bronchospasm that it may cause. A commonly used mixture consists of 5 ml. of 20% acetylcysteine, 3 ml. distilled water, 1 ml. of 0.5% isoproterenol and 1 ml. of 1% phenylephrine. This mixture is nebulized in a small nebulizer and inhaled by the patient, often in conjunction with IPPB therapy.

Ascoxal (Ascumist) is another effective mucolytic. This material does not appear to produce as much irritation of the tracheobronchial tree as acetylcysteine. To be effective, it must be freshly mixed from the powdered form each time it is used, and it may be used in concentrations of 9–12%. It is administered by inhalation of nebulized particles or by direct instillation into the tracheobronchial tree. Unfortunately, at the time of this writing, ascoxal is not yet commercially available.

For any mucolytic to be effective, a sufficient quantity must be presented to the secretions upon which the mucolytic must act. In order for this to occur, large quantities must be nebulized or instilled in the tracheobronchial tree. If these agents are used as aerosols, then large output nebulizers should be used and, when possible, they should be given by ultrasonic nebulizers.

Bronchodilators and decongestants.—The bronchodilators and vascular decongestants most commonly used for aerosol therapy are all sympathomimetic amines. Racemic epinephrine is available in concentrations of 2.25% for inhalation use. Epinephrine is itself both a bronchodilator and a decongestant. However, a more commonly used bronchodilator is isoproterenol, which is available for inhalation as a 0.5% solution. Isoproterenol is not a vascular decongestant and is therefore often mixed with phenylephrine, a decongestant. A mixture of 1 ml. of 0.5% isoproterenol, 1 ml. of 1% phenylephrine and 2 ml. normal saline used in a nebulizer with an IPPB unit is an effective treatment for bronchospasm, such as that which occurs during an acute attack of bronchial asthma. If active bronchospasm is not present at the time these agents are being used, concentrations of isoproterenol and phenylephrine may be reduced by at least half. Some controversy exists as to whether the phenylephrine actually has any beneficial effect, and whether bronchial decongestion does occur when it is used. Nevertheless, the incidence of cardiac side effects due to absorption of the isoproterenol is reduced when phenylephrine is added to the mixture.

Isoetharine, a derivative of isoproterenol, is an excellent bronchodilator. It appears to have the advantage of producing fewer cardiac side effects from systemic absorption. Commercially, it is available in combination with phenylephrine and the antihistamine phenyldiamine under the trade name Bronkosol.

Antibiotics.—Antibiotics have not been used extensively in inhalation therapy, although many people feel that in specific instances they would be of value. One such instance is the use of 1% neomycin by nebulization three to four times a day when pseudomonas has been cultured from tracheobronchial secretions. During each treatment 5 ml. of the 1% neomycin solution is nebulized, and the resulting aerosol is either inhaled directly by the patient or is administered by an IPPB machine. Other antibiotics, such as penicillin, streptomycin and bacitracin have also been given by nebulization in the past. The main route of antibiotics for pulmonary infections, however, continues to be systemic rather than topical.

CORTICOSTEROIDS.—Adrenocorticosteroids, such as hydrocortisone, prednisone and prednisolone, have been given by aerosolization, mainly to patients with bronchial asthma. It is felt by many, however, that the topical effect produced by the inhalation of these agents is negligible compared to the effect they exert following systemic absorption from the tracheobronchial tree.

Intermittent Positive Pressure Respirators

There are two main types of respirators: the body-type respirator and the intermittent positive pressure respirator. Body-type respirators such as the chest cuirass and the tank respirator were popular at one time, but this popularity has waned with the development of good intermittent positive pressure respirators. This discussion will be concerned only with intermittent positive pressure respirators.

The term "intermittent positive pressure respirator" should not be confused with the similar term "intermittent positive pressure breathing." The latter refers to a specific type of inhalation therapy, as previously described. The former term refers to a general classification of respirators. The confusion is often compounded because certain devices can perform dual service as an intermittent positive pressure breathing (IPPB) machine or as an intermittent positive pressure respirator.

FUNCTIONAL CHARACTERISTICS

There are many respirators available today. Some are made in the United States, while others are imported, mainly from Europe. The respirators discussed here probably constitute over 90% of the respirators presently used in the United States.

In the past, several classifications have been advanced for positive pressure respirators. Some of these are: flow generators, pressure generators, pressure machines, volume machines and time-cycled machines. These descriptive terms have, however, usually referred only to one functional characteristic of a respirator. In actuality, every respirator has multiple functional characteristics (Table 5-2). In the following discussion, the functional characteristics of 8 commonly used respirators will be presented.

BENNETT PR-1 AND PR-2 RESPIRATORS.—These machines are similar and will be discussed together. The Bennett PR-1 and Bennett PR-2 (Fig. 5-5) use compressed gas as a source of power; thus, they are oper-

TABLE 5-2.—FUNCTIONAL CHARACTERISTICS OF COMMONLY USED RESPIRATORS

Respirator	Power Source	Flow Control Mechanism	Limitation of Inspiratory Phase	Limitation of Expiratory Phase	Patient Circuit	Ability to Assist	Ability to Compensate for Leaks	Automatic Sighing Mechanism	Ability to Compensate for Decreased Compliance or Increased Resistance
Bennett PR-1 and PR-2	Compressed gas	Flow-sensitive valve	Flow, time	Pressure, time	Primary	Yes	Poor	No	Poor
Bird Mark 7,8,10	Compressed gas	Pressure-sensitve valve	Pressure	Pressure, time	Primary	Yes	Good	No	Fair*
Air-Shields	Electric motor	Turbine	Time	Time, pressure	Secondary	Yes	Good	No	Fair†
Mörch	Electric motor	Piston and cylinder	Volume	Time	Primary	No	Good	No	Good
Emerson	Electric motor	Piston and cylinder	Volume, pressure	Time	Primary	Yes	Good	Yes	Good
Engström	Electric motor	Piston and cylinder	Volume, pressure	Time	Secondary	No	Good	No	Good
Bennett MA-1	Electric motor	Pump	Volume, pressure	Time, pressure	Secondary	Yes	Good	Yes	Good‡
Ohio 560	Electric motor	Turbine	Volume, pressure	Time, pressure	Secondary	Yes	Good	Yes	Good

*Compensation must be performed manually. Maximum achievable airway pressure is about 40 cm. H_2O.

†Turbine tends to slip as airway resistance increases or compliance decreases, causing tidal volume to decrease. Maximum achievable airway pressure is about 60 cm. H_2O.

‡Maximum achievable airway pressure is 60 cm. H_2O in the older models and 80 cm. H_2O in the newer models.

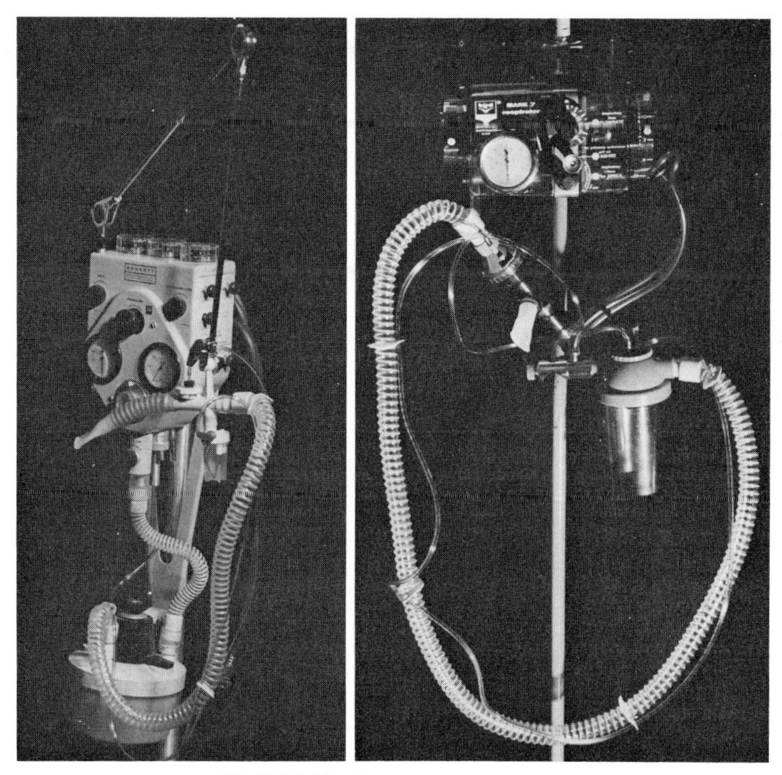

Fig. 5-5 (left). – Bennett PR-2 respirator.
Fig. 5-6 (right). – Bird Mark 7 respirator.

ated either from a tank of oxygen, a tank of compressed air or an oxygen or compressed air line. They are designed to use a compressed gas source with a pressure of about 50 lb./sq. in. Accordingly, when a tank is the source, a reducing valve must be used. Another method of powering these machines is an air compressor driven by an electric motor. Under these conditions, the machines can be operated as electrically driven respirators.

The flow of gas from the machine to the patient is controlled by a flow-sensitive valve. During the early phase of inspiration, this valve allows a relatively high flow of gas to reach the patient; then, as the pressure in the patient circuit downstream from the flow-sensitive valve builds up, this flow decreases. When the flow reaches a critical minimum level, the valve automatically shuts off the flow of gas and thus ends or limits the inspiratory phase of respiration. This critical minimum flow rate is 4 L./minute for the PR-1 and 1.5 L./minute for the PR-2. Hence, the inspiratory phase of respiration of these machines is flow limited. An auxiliary timing mechanism is also present so that the inspiratory phase of respiration can also be time limited.

These machines are capable of sensing a subatmospheric pressure in the patient circuit and responding to this pressure by starting the flow of gases through the valve again. Therefore, the expiratory phase of respiration is pressure limited. Because the generation of the subatmospheric pressure in the patient circuit is usually produced by the patient's attempt to initiate an inspiratory cycle, these machines are capable of assisting the patient's own respirations. An auxiliary timing mechanism is also present to limit the expiratory phase of respiration.

The patient circuit on these machines is a primary circuit; that is, the gas that flows through the flow control mechanism goes directly to the patient's lungs. A Venturi mechanism is present which can be switched in or switched out at the discretion of the operator. When the mechanism is switched out, the gas flowing into the patient circuit comes only from the power source; for example, if the power source is compressed oxygen, the machine will deliver 100% oxygen to the patient. As the Venturi mechanism is switched in, the gas from the power source is diluted with atmospheric air; if oxygen is used as the power source, the resulting gas mixture to the patient circuit usually consists of 40% oxygen. However, the actual concentration of oxygen inspired by the patient may be greater if the nebulizer on the machine is in use, because it is also powered by oxygen. Thus, additional oxygen will be entering the patient circuit downstream from the flow control valve, and the inspired oxygen concentration may be as high as 80%.

The rate of flow of gases through the flow control valve depends upon the amount of resistance in the patient circuit. With high resistances, the flow rate decreases rapidly; as a result, the ability of the machine to compensate for conditions of decreased chest compliance or increased pulmonary resistance is relatively limited. These machines have little ability to handle leaks in the patient circuit; if the leak is greater than the minimum flow rate, the flow control valve will never cycle from the inspiratory to the expiratory phase. Under these conditions, the only mechanical limit to the inspiratory phase of respiration is the timing mechanism. The disadvantage in using the timing mechanism to limit the inspiratory phase is that, although the machine may cycle properly, ventilation may not be adequate because most of the gas can exit through the leak rather than enter the patient's lungs. Matching the amount of leak flow with an additional flow of gas from the nebulizer control system of these machines can occasionally compensate for small leaks. The gas flow from the nebulizer contol bypasses the flow control valve. Thus, if the amount of gas flowing from the nebulizer system matches the amount leaking from the patient circuit, the gases flowing through the flow control valve will reach the minimum critical level. Under these conditions the valve will cycle.

The separate terminal flow control valve of the PR-2, which permits gas to bypass the flow-sensitive valve in an attempt to compensate for leaks, renders the PR-2 somewhat superior to the PR-1 in this respect.

Small leaks can be managed by both machines but neither is able to compensate for large leaks.

Humidification can be provided by attaching a large nebulizer or a heated cascade-type humidifier to the machines. The maximum effective airway pressure that can be obtained is about 45–50 cm. of water.

BIRD RESPIRATOR.—The Bird respirator (Fig. 5-6) is available in several models, of which the Mark 7, Mark 8 and Mark 10, all quite similar, are the most commonly used. The Bird respirator uses compressed gas as a power source. Its flow control mechanism is a pressure-sensitive valve. This valve separates the machine into two main compartments: a high-pressure compartment, and a low-pressure compartment which connects to the patient circuit. During inspiration, gas flows from the high-pressure compartment through the pressure-sensitive valve to the low-pressure compartment. When the pressure in the latter compartment reaches a preset level, the valve closes; thus, the inspiratory phase of respiration is pressure limited. The valve will respond to a subatmospheric pressure in the patient circuit to limit the expiratory phase of respiration, and inspiration will again commence. Therefore, the machine is capable of assisting the patient's own respiratory efforts. An auxiliary timing mechanism is present as a secondary method to limit the expiratory phase of respiration only. The inspiratory phase of respiration cannot be regulated by this means. The patient circuit is a primary circuit.

A separate needle valve controls the rate of gas flow through the pressure-sensitive valve. Gas flow can be adjusted by this needle valve to the individual patient's optimal level. Because of this device, the machine is better able to ventilate lungs having increased pulmonary resistance than is the Bennett. Minor changes in resistance are compensated for automatically by a Venturi mechanism; however, large changes must be managed manually. The variable flow control mechanism also enables this machine to compensate well for leaks in the patient circuit. The maximum effective airway pressure that is achievable is about 45 cm. of water. If pressure greater than this is necessary to ventilate a severely noncompliant chest, the machine is inadequate. Humidification is achieved by attaching a large, gas-driven nebulizer to the patient circuit.

AIR-SHIELDS RESPIRATOR.—The Air-Shields respirator (Fig. 5-7) is powered by an electric motor. This drives an air turbine which provides a flow of air that can be modified by various valves on the machine. This flow of air does not go directly to the patient's lungs but instead is utilized to compress a bellows. Air from the bellows is then conducted to the patient's lungs. This configuration constitutes a secondary patient circuit in contrast to the primary circuits present on the Bennett and Bird respirators.

A valve system modifies the flow of air from the turbine to provide a

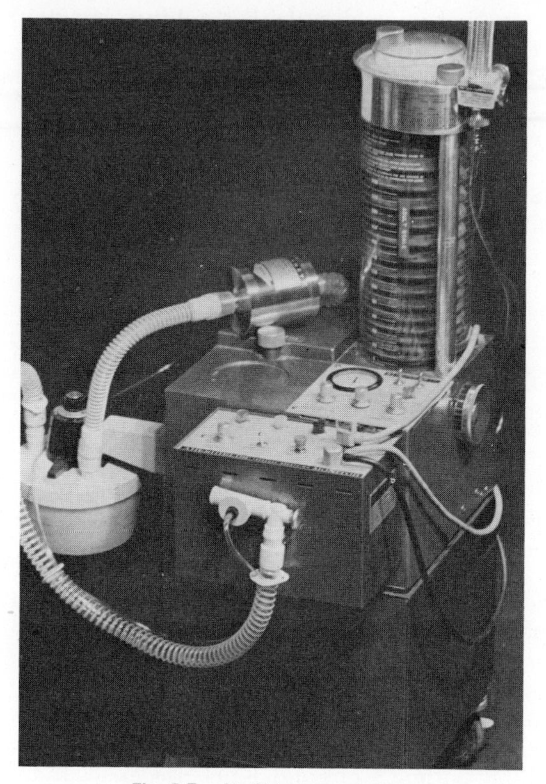

Fig. 5-7.—Air-Shields respirator.

variable flow rate. A timer limits the inspiratory phase of respiration. The limitation of the expiratory phase of respiration is also handled by a timer; however, the machine can limit the expiratory phase should a subatmospheric pressure be generated in the patient circuit. This respirator is therefore capable of assisting the patient's own respirations. It compensates well for leaks in the patient circuit and can be regulated by adjusting the variable flow mechanism to match the flow requirements of each individual.

The Air-Shields respirator adequately ventilates normal lungs as well as those which show a mild-to-moderate decrease in compliance or increase in resistance. Because of a progressive slipping of the turbine when airway impedance increases, this machine falters in response to severe changes in the patient's compliance or resistance. Humidification is provided by a centrifugal nebulizer which is built into the respirator.

MÖRCH PISTON RESPIRATOR.—The Mörch respirator (Fig. 5-8) is powered by an electric motor which is connected to a piston and cylin-

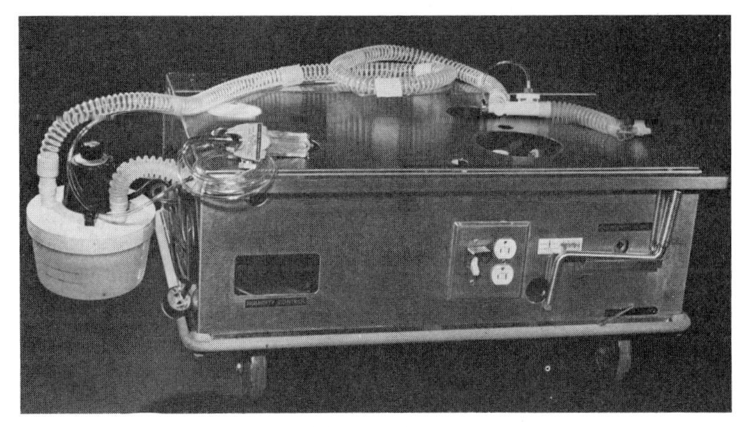

Fig. 5-8.—Mörch piston respirator.

der via a variable gear box. The stroke of the piston in the cylinder generates the air flow. This respirator has only two controls—the volume control on the piston, which varies the length of the stroke of the piston in the cylinder, and the rate control on the variable gear box, which varies the frequency of these strokes. The inspiratory phase of respiration is thus limited by the delivery of a preset tidal volume (the stroke volume of the piston in the cylinder). The expiratory phase is limited by the time necessary for the piston to be withdrawn from the cylinder and to begin the inspiratory stroke again. This time is a function of the rate set on the variable gear box. The flow rate is variable and is a function of both the tidal volume and the respiratory rate. By manipulating the two controls in conjunction with each other, variable flow rates can be produced. Air flow from the piston and cylinder are conducted directly to the patient's lungs via a primary patient circuit.

The pressure developed by the machine varies with the compliance and resistance of the patient's lungs. The necessary pressure is automatically developed for any particular combination of resistance, compliance, tidal volume and flow rate. Leaks in the patient circuit can be easily compensated by increasing the tidal volume. The Mörch respirator cannot assist the patient's own respiration and must be used strictly as a controller. Its ratio of expiration to inspiration is fixed at approximately 1.2:1.0.

This extremely powerful machine can effectively ventilate lungs which are severely noncompliant or have very high pulmonary resistances. The Mörch respirator is also a rugged machine, legendary for its long-term reliability in respiratory management. Early models had a somewhat deficient humidification system that has been corrected in the later models. An accessory humidifier, such as a large pneumatic or ultrasonic nebulizer, is often interposed into the patient circuit.

EMERSON POST-OPERATIVE VENTILATOR.—The Emerson Ventilator (Fig. 5-9) is quite similar to the Mörch. The main difference is that the motor drives the piston via a flywheel and belt arrangement rather than a gear box. Rate variation is controlled by a variable speed motor. A series of microswitches enable this motor to change speed at each end of the piston stroke. Thus, inspiration and expiration times can be varied independently of each other rather than being forced to adhere to a fixed ratio.

This respirator also utilizes a primary patient circuit. Its potential amount of power is similar to that of the Mörch. Limitation of the inspiratory phase of respiration occurs when a preset volume is delivered. A variable pressure relief valve is provided so that this phase also can be pressure limited. The expiratory phase of respiration is time limited. A hot-pot and moisture exchange column are utilized in conjunction to provide an effective humidifier. Early models of this respirator could only control respirations; however, the latest model is able to assist also.

Extensive clinical experience with the Emerson has shown it to be similar to the Mörch in ruggedness and reliability. It is effective for ven-

Fig. 5-9.—Emerson Post-Operative Ventilator.

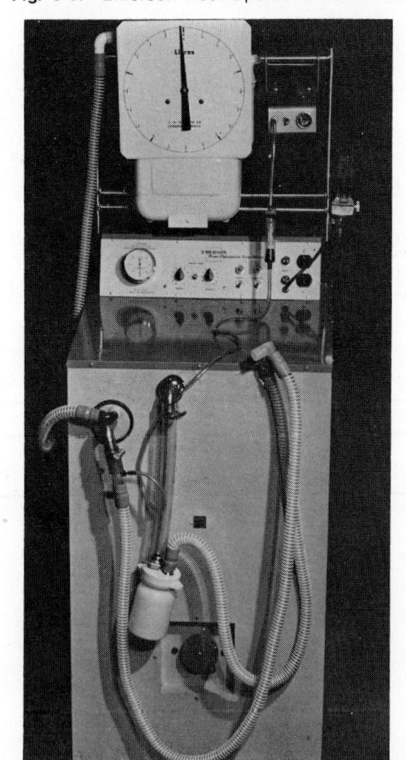

tilating severely noncompliant or highly resistant lungs and automatically compensates for changes in compliance and resistance. It also compensates well for leaks in the patient circuit.

ENGSTRÖM RESPIRATOR.—The Engström respirator (Fig. 5-10) utilizes a piston and cylinder flow-generating mechanism powered by an electric motor. It differs from the Mörch and Emerson respirators in its use of a secondary patient circuit. Gas from the flow generator (piston and cylinder) is led during inspiration into a rigid container, where it compresses a flexible bag. Gas from this bag then flows to the patient's airway. During expiration a preset volume of gas is drawn into the bag; the delivery of this volume limits the inspiratory phase of respiration. A pressure relief system is present which can also act to limit the inspiratory phase. The expiratory phase of respiration is time limited, its duration dependent upon the rate of cycling of the piston in the cylinder. Flow rate varies with changes in respiratory rate and tidal volume. However, the flow pattern differs somewhat from those of the Mörch and Emerson because of the use of the secondary patient circuit.

The Engström respirator also acts strictly as a controller of respiration; it automatically generates the pressure necessary to deliver its preset tidal volume. This machine is able to compensate well for leaks in the patient's circuit and has sufficient power to effectively ventilate severely noncompliant chests. A heated humidifier is built into the machine.

BENNETT MA-1 RESPIRATOR.—The Bennett MA-1 respirator (Fig. 5-11) is a newly developed machine. It is powered by an electric motor

Fig. 5-10.—Engström respirator.

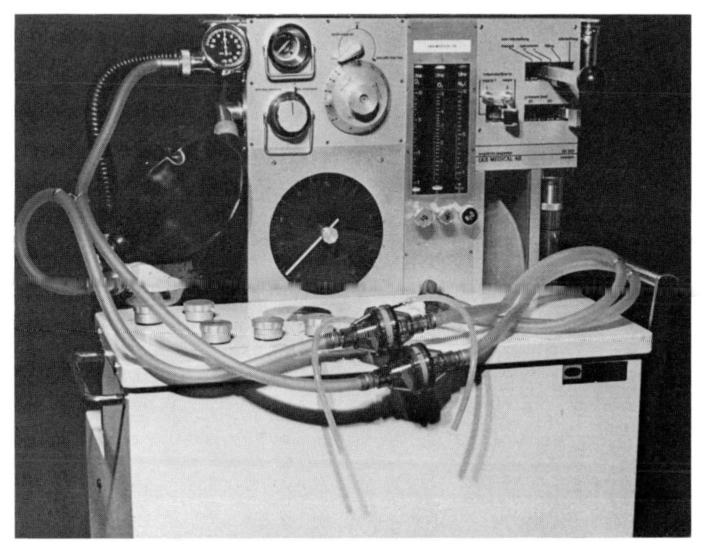

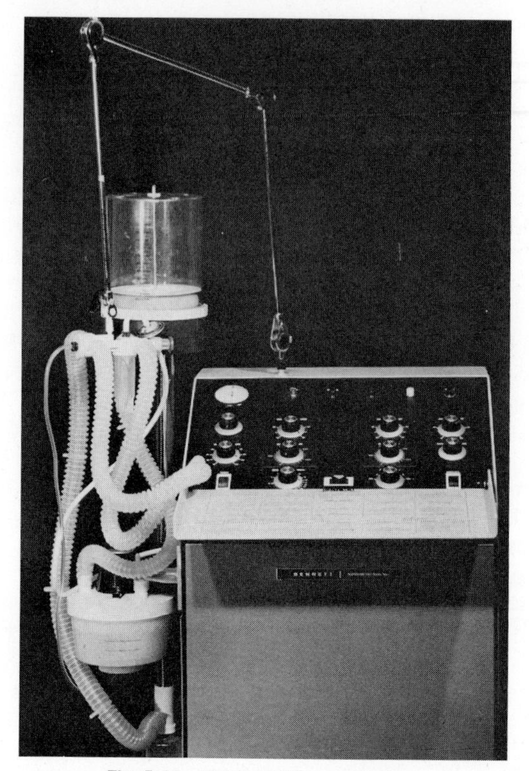

Fig. 5-11. – Bennett MA-1 respirator.

which drives an air pump. The pump compresses a bellows which is part of a secondary patient circuit. During the inspiratory phase of respiration, flow rate, tidal volume and pressure are controlled by a series of adjustable valves. The limitation of the inspiratory phase can be preset by volume or pressure. The limitation of exhalation is time controlled. The machine can also sense a subatmospheric pressure in the patient circuit, and thus will assist the patient's own respirations.

This respirator is able to compensate well for leaks in the patient's circuit and possesses sufficient power to ventilate severely restricted chests effectively. Maximum pressure, generated during inspiration, is limited to 60 cm. of water in the older models and 80 cm. of water in the latest models by a built-in pressure release system. Consequently, in extreme cases of poor thoracic compliance the early model may prove inadequate. A heated cascade humidifier is utilized, and in addition, an auxiliary nebulizer is provided. The machine is also capable of accurately delivering predetermined oxygen concentrations to the patient.

OHIO 560 RESPIRATOR. – The Ohio 560 respirator (Fig. 5-12) is powered by an electric motor. The electric motor is used to drive a turbine

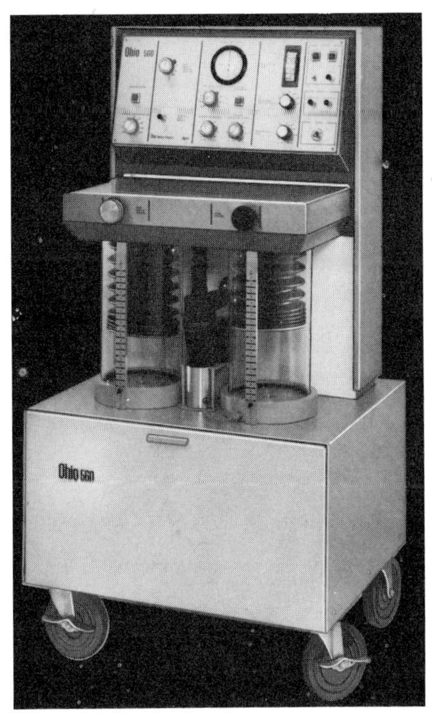

Fig. 5-12.—Ohio 560 respirator.

which provides a source of gas flow. This gas flow then is used to compress a bellows, which is part of a secondary patient circuit. The inspiratory phase of respiration is limited by the delivery of a predetermined volume of air to the patient. An adjustable pressure relief valve is also provided so that pressure limitation of the inspiratory phase can be achieved. The rate of air flow to the patient is controlled by an adjustable valve. The machine is capable of sensing a subatmospheric pressure in the patient circuit. The response to this pressure limits the expiratory phase of respiration. Thus the machine is capable of assisting the patient's own respirations. A time mechanism is also present for limiting the expiratory phase so that the machine can be used as a controller of respiration.

This respirator compensates well for leaks in the patient's circuit and is sufficiently powerful to ventilate severely noncompliant and highly resistant lungs effectively. Accurately controlled oxygen concentrations can be presented to the patient. A variable-output ultrasonic nebulizer, built into the machine, provides an excellent method of responding to the various humidification problems that may arise in individual patients.

Management of Patient on Respirator

The intermittent positive pressure respirators represent the most effective instruments we have today for treating respiratory failure. These machines, however, might be compared to two-edged swords —when they are used improperly, a great deal of harm can result to the patient. It is therefore imperative that the physician using one of these machines be familiar with some of the basic principles of clinical management of a patient on a respirator.

The proper physical attachment of the patient to the intermittent positive pressure respirator is important. This attachment must be accomplished by means of an endotracheal tube; the use of a face mask does not represent an adequate means of attaching a patient to a respirator. The endotracheal tube used may be either an orotracheal tube, a nasotracheal tube or a tracheostomy tube. Orotracheal or nasotracheal tubes are often left in place for several days at a time. In these circumstances, the patient is usually more comfortable with a nasotracheal than with an orotracheal tube.

If prolonged use of a respirator is anticipated, a tracheostomy should be considered. A tracheostomy is usually not necessary if the anticipated time on the respirator does not exceed 2–3 days. However, a tracheostomy is probably indicated if the anticipated time is over 10 days. Clinical judgment should be the deciding factor in regard to tracheostomy when the anticipated respirator time lies between the two extremes.

In attaching the respirator to the endotracheal tube, the use of

Fig. 5-13.—Mörch swivel system for attaching a respirator to a tracheostomy tube. The arrows point to the sites where free swiveling occurs.

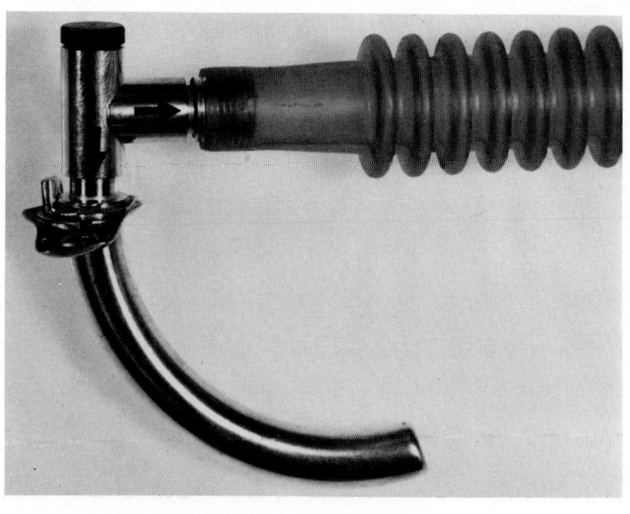

swivel coupling between the respirator and the endotracheal tube (Fig. 5-13) eliminates much of the torque that the respirator can place on the tube in the trachea. This torque is a considerable source of patient discomfort and even damage to the trachea. Torque can be further minimized by interposing a short length of corrugated rubber or plastic tubing between the connector on the respirator and the swivel.

Inflatable cuffs are often used on endotracheal tubes to seal the airway and prevent leaks. These cuffs represent a serious hazard when used improperly. A completely inflated cuff will cause tracheobronchial secretions to collect distal to the cuff, where they may eventually obstruct the tube. When an uncuffed tube is used, the air which is leaking around the tube will sweep these secretions with it into the pharynx. The trachea will thus be automatically cleansed. An overinflated cuff will interfere with the circulation of blood to that area of the tracheal mucosa with which it is in contact. This interference can result in tracheal stricture at the site of the cuff. Attempts to circumvent this problem by placing two cuffs on the tube, alternately inflating and deflating each cuff, can result in two sites of stricture in the trachea rather than none. An uncuffed tube, on the other hand, is devoid of this problem.

If a completely airtight tracheal seal is necessary, as with the Bennett PR-1, then a low-pressure cuff, such as a fluted cuff (Fig. 5-14), should be used. It should be carefully inflated so that just enough air is introduced into the cuff to barely stop the air leak around the endotracheal tube when the respirator is functioning. If the respirator is one which compensates well for a leak in the patient circuit, the best way to manage the airway is to inflate the cuff to the point where the leak that is left is easily compensated for by the respirator. As long as some air leaks around the endotracheal tube with each inspiration, it can be safely assumed that the cuff is not exerting excess pressure upon the tracheal mucosa. Devices are available which automatically inflate the cuff with each inhalation and then allow it to deflate during exhalation.

Adequacy of ventilation must be ascertained whenever a patient is

Fig. 5-14.—The upper endotracheal tube is fitted with a standard high-pressure cuff. The lower one has a fluted low-pressure cuff.

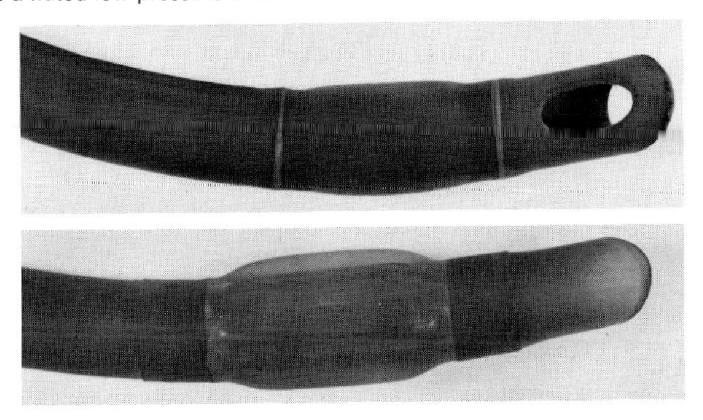

placed on a respirator. One of the best ways of determining adequate tidal volume is simply to observe the motion of the patient's chest during inspiration. This is often a much more reliable guide than the measuring attachment included on many respirators. When spirometers or other meters are used to measure tidal volume, they should be located on the exhalation limb of the patient circuit. Otherwise, they may provide inaccurate measurements of patient tidal volume.

Tidal and minute volumes themselves are not always the best measurement for determining adequacy of ventilation. A patient with a very high physiologic dead space will require much larger tidal and minute volumes than would ordinarily be anticipated. Quite often one of the best ways of determining if the patient is being adequately ventilated is simply to ask if the machine is breathing adequately for him. If the patient is able to communicate, he will often tell you whether the machine is ventilating adequately, underventilating or overventilating.

Arterial blood gas determinations should be made whenever possible to assess ventilation. In any final analysis of ventilatory adequacy, the Pa_{O_2} and Pa_{CO_2} will be two of the most important determinants. Reasonable goals for which to aim are a Pa_{CO_2} of 32–40 mm. Hg and a Pa_{O_2} of 80–150 mm. Hg. If necessary, supplementary oxygen should be added to the respirator to bring the Pa_{O_2} to this level.

When severe ventilation perfusion disproportions are present in the lungs, it may be difficult to achieve an adequate Po_2 in the arterial blood, even though high concentrations of oxygen are being delivered by the respirator. It is often helpful then to prolong the inspiratory phase of respiration. This prolongation serves to distribute gas more adequately within the lungs and can thus increase the arterial Po_2 by more evenly ventilating the alveoli. On occasion, inspiratory durations of 2 and even 3 seconds may be necessary to oxygenate the patient adequately (Table 5-3).

TABLE 5-3.—EFFECT OF CHANGING RESPIRATOR PHASING ON ARTERIAL BLOOD GAS PATTERNS

	A	B
Tidal volume	500 cc.	500 cc.
Respiratory rate	15	15
Minute volume	7,500	7,500
Length of inspiration	1 sec.	2.5 sec.
Length of expiration	3 sec.	1.5 sec.
Inspired O_2 concentration	60%	60%
Arterial pH	7.46	7.45
Arterial Pco_2	35 mm. Hg	36 mm. Hg
Arterial Po_2	43 mm. Hg	225 mm. Hg

White female, aged 63, two days postlaparotomy, with diagnosis of postoperative lung syndrome, was ventilated with the Bennett MA-1 respirator. Column A, inspiration to expiration ratio of 1:3. Column B, 10 minutes after changing ratio to 2.5:1.5. Note marked change in arterial oxygen tension with elevation from hypoxic range to adequate oxygenation. All other settings remained the same and overall pulmonary ventilation remained the same, as evidenced by there being no effective change in arterial Pco_2.

There is good evidence to show that excessively high oxygen tensions over long periods may produce pulmonary damage. Whether this actually occurs is still a controversial subject. However, since a high arterial Po_2 is not necessary, it seems to be safer to utilize only enough oxygen supplementation to keep the arterial Po_2 at about 100 mg. Hg. The actual inspired oxygen concentration necessary to produce this tension can vary greatly from individual to individual. The only way to determine the proper inspired oxygen concentration for any given patient is to rely on arterial oxygen analysis.

The decision to use assisted or controlled respirations will often depend on which respirator is being utilized. Machines such as the Mörch and the Engström can only control. Other machines can do either, and the decision of which type of ventilator to use will rest with the physician. The decision will often be based on the particular set of circumstances present for each patient. In some instances it is easier to maintain a patient with controlled ventilation; in others, it is easier to assist.

At all times, care must be taken to prevent the patient from fighting the respirator. Whenever a patient fights a respirator, inadequate ventilation is almost always the result. Ironically, the usual cause is also inadequate ventilation. In most instances, increasing the minute volume of ventilation is the only corrective measure needed. Routine prophylactic use of sedative drugs to prevent fighting the respirator is not ordinarily needed or indicated. Use of muscle relaxants to paralyze the patient so that he cannot fight the respirator is rarely needed, although on some occasions short-term sedation or even paralyzation of the patient may be necessary until adequate ventilation has been established. Once a mild respiratory alkalosis has been produced, the patient usually relaxes and allows the machine to breathe for him. Adequate ventilation in itself is still the most effective sedative that can be given to a patient who is in respiratory failure.

Generally, a patient, when initially placed on a respirator, will allow the respirator to breathe for him if it is being used in the controlled respiration mode. If adequate tidal and minute volumes are now maintained, the patient will rarely fight the respirator. The patient who does not readily allow the respirator to control his breathing initially will usually stop fighting after a few minutes if the tidal volume is increased to twice the estimated necessary volume and the rate increased to 20–25 breaths/minute. Once the patient has stopped fighting, the rate and tidal volume may be reset to those levels which are deemed proper. If control of the patient cannot be accomplished by these methods, sedation or muscle paralysis should be considered. Sometimes a patient will allow a respirator to assist him when he will not allow it to control. Usually, however, if he fights controlled respirations, he will also fight assisted respirations.

When a patient is on a respirator, the endotracheal tube bypasses the normal humidification mechanisms of the nose. It is for this reason that the supplementary humidifiers previously described have been added to each respirator. It is imperative that these humidifiers be kept constantly filled and in working order. Draw-over type humidifiers should be filled with sterile distilled water. Nebulizer-type humidifiers should be filled with sterile half-normal saline. Sterile precautions should be maintained when filling a humidifier.

Pulmonary infections are an ever present hazard in respirator patients and scrupulous care must be exercised in maintaining cleanliness and sterility whenever possible. Suctioning of the airways should be done frequently and under sterile conditions. Respirators should be cleaned between uses, and all the breathing hoses should be sterilized. Other parts of the patient circuit should be sterilized whenever possible. Those patients who must remain on respirators for more than one day should receive, when possible, fresh sterile breathing hoses daily. Respirator patients should not be placed in proximity to patients with infectious conditions.

Whenever patients are ventilated at a set tidal volume for each breath, there is a tendency toward gradually decreased lung compliance and gradually increased ventilation perfusion disproportion. This results in a gradual decrease of the arterial Po_2. These changes can often be prevented by giving the patient an occasional deep breath—that is, one which has a tidal volume greater than the patient has been receiving. These occasional deep breaths, or sighs, appear to be important in maintaining normal pulmonary function. Prolonging the inspiratory time as described previously may function in a manner similar to intermittent sighs in preventing the progressive development of serious ventilation perfusion disproportions. The Emerson, Bennett MA-1 and Ohio 560 respirators have built-in automatic intermittent sighing mechanisms.

The decision of when and how to remove a patient from a respirator can be difficult. Nevertheless, certain guidelines may be followed. Those patients who have chronic diseases which affect the chest wall bellows mechanism (for example, poliomyelitis) must often be weaned from the respirator. This is accomplished by removing the patient from the respirator for a short period initially, and then gradually increasing the length of time the patient is off the respirator each period. It is in patients with chronic disease of the chest wall that psychologic dependency on the respirator may develop. On the other hand, patients who have normal chest walls but abnormal lungs rarely require weaning. They either need the respirator continuously, or they do not need it at all. Psychologic dependency is uncommon in this group; when suspected, careful study usually shows the problem to be physiologic rather than psychologic. Although these patients are apparently able to ventilate adequately, the gases are not properly distributed within the lungs. Therefore, when they are off a respirator, the arterial Po_2 falls to low levels. It is this resulting hypoxia and their response to it that is sometimes confused with psychologic dependency.

Many times these patients can be adequately treated by giving them supplemental oxygen to inhale. Arterial blood gas studies, especially the arterial Po_2, are extremely valuable in determining when the respirator is no longer needed. If the patient can barely maintain a normal arterial Po_2 while on the respirator and receiving high oxygen concentrations, he can be expected to become hypoxic when off the respirator. If, however, a high arterial Po_2 (200 mm. Hg or greater) is maintained with high oxygen concentrations on the respirator, then a trial period off the respirator is in order. During this trial period, oxygen is given by inhalation, and serial arterial Po_2 determinations are made. If the patient is able to maintain an arterial Po_2 of 70 mm. Hg or greater when off the respirator and receiving oxygen by inhalation, then he may be allowed to remain off. However, periodic checks should be made to ascertain that the tension does not begin to decrease. If in doubt, it is best to leave the patient on the respirator and remove it at a later date.

6

Acid-Base Balance

DAVID L. ROSEMAN, M.D.

Assistant Attending Surgeon, Rush-Presbyterian-St. Luke's Medical Center; Assistant Professor of Surgery, Rush Medical College

DERANGEMENTS IN ACID-BASE balance are frequently present in intensive care patients. The diagnosis of acid-base abnormalities is important for two reasons: (1) Acid-base abnormalities may be detrimental to the patient. (2) Acid-base abnormalities may signal the presence of threatening conditions. Another way of stating these principles is that acid-base abnormalities may be diseases in themselves and that they may be symptoms of other diseases.

In this chapter will be discussed the mechanisms by which the body maintains acid-base balance, the pathogenesis of acid-base imbalances and the diagnosis, implications and treatment of such conditions. A word first about the use of this chapter. Clinical acid-base balance is best understood in the context of general acid-base chemistry, but a discussion of this chemistry and its terminology[16] seems to destroy the continuity of a clinical discussion. This chapter has been written in two major parts. The first part is purely clinical, the second is a review of pertinent acid-base chemistry. Methods of obtaining and storing blood samples are then outlined. For optimal use, the reader is advised to skim both sections first, then to read the chemistry in detail and finally read the clinical part in detail.

CLINICAL ACID-BASE BALANCE

Acid-base balance refers to the relationship between hydrogen ions and the various buffers. A comprehensive understanding of this relationship is essential in the management of acid-base disturbances.

Buffers

The body produces about 28,000 mEq. of hydrogen ion daily, yet maintains the hydrogen ion concentration of its fluids at 0.0001 to 0.00001 mEq./L. This remarkable feat is made possible by the various body buffers, which act by converting strong acids to weak acids. The general reaction is:

$$\underset{\text{strong acid}}{H^+} + \underset{\text{base}}{A^-} \rightleftharpoons \underset{\text{weak acid}}{HA} \qquad (1)$$

By definition, a buffer is composed of a weak acid and its conjugate base. As long as base is available, hydrogen ions are converted to weak acid, thus lowering the hydrogen ion concentration.

Acidosis and Alkalosis

A discussion of acid-base balance centers around the hydrogen ion, for it is the level of this ion which controls the acidity of a fluid. The hydrogen ion concentration, or $[H^+]$, is usually measured as the pH. It is recalled that as the $[H^+]$ increases, that is, as the solution becomes more acid, the pH decreases.

The normal pH of arterial blood is 7.40. A pH of less than 7.35 indicates an increase in the hydrogen ion concentration and thereby an increase in the blood acidity. This condition is known as acidosis. The opposite condition, a pH greater than 7.45, indicates a decrease in the hydrogen ion concentration and is known as alkalosis.

$$\text{Acidosis} = pH < 7.35$$
$$\text{Alkalosis} = pH > 7.45$$

The various mechanisms by which the $[H^+]$ may be affected can best be explained in terms of one of the body's most important buffer systems, the bicarbonate-carbonic acid system. One reaction of this system is:

$$\underset{\text{weak acid}}{H_2CO_3} \rightleftharpoons H^+ + \underset{\text{base}}{HCO_3^-} \qquad (2)$$

This reaction states that carbonic acid, a weak acid, dissociates incompletely to a hydrogen ion and a bicarbonate ion. Carbonic acid can also undergo another reversible reaction:

$$H_2CO_3 \rightleftharpoons H_2O + CO_2 \qquad (3)$$

This reaction is unique in that carbon dioxide is the only gas which is a component of a major buffer system. If reactions (2) and (3) are combined:

$$H_2O + CO_2 \rightleftharpoons H_2CO_3 \rightleftharpoons H^+ + HCO_3^- \qquad (4)$$

The central ion in this system is, of course, the hydrogen ion. Its concentration may be altered in several different ways, each of which has clinicial significance.

Respiratory Acidosis and Alkalosis

Pathogenesis and diagnosis.—First of all, if the amount of CO_2 is increased, reaction (4) would be driven toward the right, thus increasing the $[H^+]$.

$$H_2O + \underset{\uparrow}{CO_2} \rightarrow H_2CO_3 \rightarrow \uparrow H^+ + HCO_3^-$$

Since CO_2 is volatile gas its concentration (Pco_2) is completely under the control of the respiratory system. It is virtually impossible for the body to generate so much CO_2 that the arterial Pco_2 would be increased on a nonrespiratory basis. Since CO_2 is the only major component of any buffer system that is under respiratory control, and since an increased Pco_2 would tend to elevate the $[H^+]$, an increased arterial Pco_2 results in the condition known as respiratory acidosis. The normal arterial Pco_2 ranges from 35 to 45 mm. Hg. Therefore:

Respiratory acidosis = arterial Pco_2 greater than 45 mm. Hg
Respiratory alkalosis = arterial Pco_2 less than 35 mm. Hg

Treatment.—Respiratory alkalosis is generally desirable and seldom requires treatment in the postoperative patient. Respiratory acidosis is the most serious type of acid-base derangement because it indicates respiratory insufficiency and because it causes rapid and potentially profound changes in pH. Hypoventilation is the most common cause. The treatment of respiratory acidosis involves improving the patient's respiration. The steps to be taken are:

1. Exclude pneumothorax. This is done by physical examination and by chest x-ray. If present, pneumothorax is treated by placement of an intrathoracic catheter.

2. Exclude bronchial obstruction. A common perioperative cause of bronchial obstruction is an endotracheal tube which has been passed into the right main stem bronchus. If the patient is ventilating only one bronchus, as determined by physical examination, the endotracheal tube should be withdrawn slightly. The position of the tube can be noted on a chest film.

3. Exclude atelectasis. Diagnosis is made on physical examination in the early postoperative period, because the usual or "patchy" type does not show up on a chest x-ray for a matter of several hours to days after its onset. This diagnosis is made by hearing tubular breath sounds over the bases. Initially, treatment consists of nasotracheal aspiration. If this is unsuccessful or requires repetition, the patient should have bronchoscopy and, finally, if bronchoscopy is only temporarily successful, the patient should have a tracheostomy.

We now have considered four of the six major acid-base disorders, and the tests required for their diagnosis. To repeat: pH distinguishes acidosis or alkalosis; Pco_2 distinguishes respiratory acidosis or respiratory alkalosis. The final two disorders, metabolic acidosis and alkalosis, are less straightforward.

Metabolic Acidosis

All factors which alter the H^+ concentration, other than changes in CO_2, must be nonrespiratory or metabolic in nature. In terms of the bicarbonate system, metabolic acidosis may be produced in one of two ways:

1. The bicarbonate concentration may be decreased with the resulting mass action changes causing an increased H^+.

$$\uparrow H^+ + \underset{\blacktriangledown}{HCO_3^-} \leftarrow H_2CO_3 \leftarrow H_2O + CO_2$$

For example, a biliary fistula with the resultant loss of large amounts of bicarbonate would be one cause of metabolic acidosis.

2. The $[H^+]$ may be directly increased by the endogenous addition of hydrogen ions.

$$\underset{\blacktriangle}{H^+} + HCO_3^- \rightarrow H_2CO_3 \rightarrow H_2O + CO_2$$

This is by far the more common mechanism for the development of metabolic acidosis. These hydrogen ions may come from many different sources, but the most important is the following:

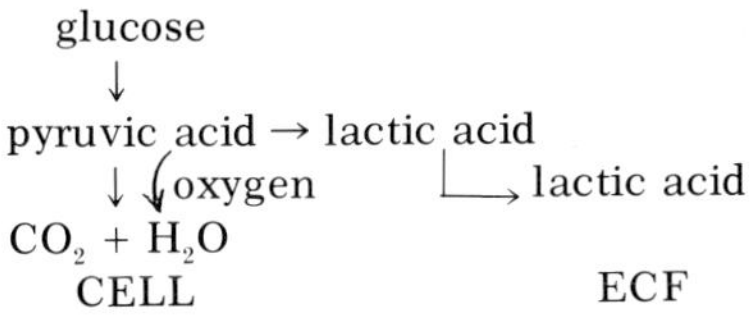

```
glucose
   ↓
pyruvic acid → lactic acid
   ↓ ↓oxygen        └──→ lactic acid
CO2 + H2O
  CELL                      ECF
```

Glucose is metabolized anaerobically to pyruvic acid. Normally (that is, when sufficient oxygen is present) most of the pyruvic acid is converted via the Krebs cycle to CO_2 and H_2O. If the cell is hypoxic, the Krebs cycle is blocked and the pyruvic acid is converted to lactic acid, which then diffuses into the extracellular space and finally into the blood. It is the hydrogen ion of lactic acid which is responsible for the great majority of cases of metabolic acidosis in surgical patients. It is apparent that the villain in the preceding plot is the hypoxia, so every patient with metabolic acidosis is considered to have cellular hypoxia until proved otherwise. This cellular hypoxia may be caused by increased peripheral resistance, arteriovenous shunting, low cardiac output, respiratory insufficiency, etc., all of which are covered in detail in other chapters.

Diagnosis.—The accurate diagnosis of metabolic acidosis is necessary to correct the acidosis and, more importantly, to detect the presence of other physiologic dysfunctions. There is no universal agreement about which test best measures metabolic acid-base derangements. This topic is discussed in detail later in the chapter.

The determination of base excess is widely employed clinically. Base excess quantitates the total amount of fixed base or fixed acid present in the blood in excess of normal. The normal base excess is, obviously, 0. If, for example, 5 mEq. of sodium hydroxide were added to 1 L. of blood, this blood would have a base excess of 5 mEq./L. Similarly, if 5 mEq. of hydrochloric acid were added to 1 L. of blood there would be an acid excess or base deficit of 5 mEq./L. By convention, a base deficit is referred to as a negative base excess, so that in the second example we would say that the blood had a base excess of −5 mEq./L. In vitro, base excess is independent of changes in the P_{CO_2} and is therefore a measure of metabolic acid-base balance. We can tentatively complete our list of diagnostic tests:

Metabolic acidosis = a negative base excess (below −2.6 mEq./L.)
Metabolic alkalosis = a positive base excess (above +2.6 mEq./L.)

The above discussion is workable for clinical purposes although the section on the pertinent acid-base chemistry should be consulted for details. The reader is especially urged to look at Figure 6-8, which shows the effect of rather severe respiratory changes on base excess values.

TREATMENT.—The treatment of metabolic acidosis must be aimed at correcting both the acidosis and its cause. The acidosis is attacked by administering sufficient base to the patient to buffer the excess acid present. The base generally employed is HCO_3^-, given as $NaHCO_3$. Other buffers such as TRIS (tromethamine) have been used but seem to offer more disadvantages than advantages.

The total amount of bicarbonate required to correct the acidosis is determined by:

Body weight (kg.) × 0.3 × (−) base excess[3]

Usually, one half of the solution is administered intravenously immediately, and the remainder is given as an intravenous drip over a half-hour period.

More important than the treatment of the acidosis is the treatment of the cause. It would be impossible to overemphasize the point that every patient with metabolic acidosis has cellular hypoxia until proved otherwise. Administration of bicarbonate to such a patient is no more than a gesture unless the tissue oxygenation is improved.

Also, it must not be assumed that giving a calculated dose of bicarbonate will correct the patient's metabolic acidosis forever. Obviously, patients with persisting tissue hypoxia will continue to generate metabolic acids. For this reason it is imperative that serial base excess determinations be performed, the interval between determinations being adjusted according to the needs of the particular patient.

Metabolic Alkalosis

Metabolic alkalosis in intensive care patients is usually iatrogenic (from bicarbonate replacement) and is usually innocuous and perhaps even desirable. An exception is the state of hypochloremic alkalosis seen in some patients with prolonged loss of gastric contents. The pathogenesis of this state is as follows: The loss of HCl causes alkalosis because of the loss of hydrogen ions; the chloride deficiency temporarily decreases the resorption of sodium from the renal tubules, although this situation is short lived because of the provocation of aldosterone and other sodium-retaining mechanisms. Hydrogen and potassium are then exchanged for sodium in the distal tubules, and it is this inappropriate loss of hydrogen ions which accounts for the paradoxical acid urine in the face of alkalosis.[18]

Other serious causes of metabolic alkalosis include diuretic treatment, diarrhea, Cushing's disease and hyperaldosteronism.[4]

Treatment.—Iatrogenic metabolic alkalosis rarely requires treatment. The treatment of the other forms of metabolic alkalosis is directed to appropriate electrolyte administration. In hypochloremic, hypokalemic alkalosis, chloride, sodium and potassium ions are required and should be given as KCl and NaCl. In so-called hypokalemic alkalosis following diuretic therapy, both potassium and chloride ions are deficient, and KCl should be administered.

Mixed Derangements

Acid-base derangements are often combinations of those detailed. A patient's blood values could be, for example:

pH	7.25
Pa_{CO_2}	30 mm. Hg
Base excess	−15 mEq./L.

This patient is acidotic as a result of metabolic acidosis, and in addition has a respiratory alkalosis. It should be noted that it is not inconsistent to speak of respiratory or metabolic alkalosis in an acidotic patient. This patient's decreased Pa_{CO_2} is helping to maintain the pH, and is sometimes said (in what is often an oversimplification) to be compensatory. This patient obviously requires treatment of his metabolic acidosis, including improvement in perfusion.

A slightly more difficult example of a mixed derangement would be:

pH	7.25
Pa_{CO_2}	50 mm. Hg
Base excess	−10 mEq./L.

This patient has both metabolic and respiratory acidosis. In general, correction of the respiratory status takes precedence over correction of the metabolic acidosis. A patient like this demands immediate improvement in ventilation.

ACID-BASE CHEMISTRY

Buffers

As defined in the introduction, a buffer consists of a weak (incompletely dissociated) acid and its basic salt. The general reaction is:

$$\underset{\text{weak acid}}{HA} \rightleftharpoons H^+ + \underset{\text{base}}{A^-} \tag{1}$$

Since the acidity of a solution is governed by the hydrogen ion concentration, it is useful to examine the manner in which the buffer changes this concentration. It will be recalled that a reaction such as the one shown has an equilibrium constant so that:

$$\frac{[H^+][A^-]}{[HA]} = K \tag{2}$$

The brackets indicate that we are considering the concentrations of the various ions, and K is the dissociation constant. Since we are interested in the H^+, it is useful to solve the equation for this substance:

$$[H^+] = K\frac{[HA]}{[A^-]} \tag{3}$$

Since the hydrogen ion concentration in biologic systems is quite small (in the range of 10^{-7} equivalents/L.), this concentration is often expressed as the negative logarithm of the hydrogen ion concentration, or pH. For example, a hydrogen ion concentration of 10^{-7} equivalents/L. would be a pH of 7, 10^{-8} equivalents/L., a pH of 8, etc. If equation 3 is restated in terms of pH, the following solution obtains:

$$\log [H^+] = \log K + \log \frac{[HA]}{[A^-]} \tag{4}$$

$$-\log [H^+] = -\log K + \log \frac{[A^-]}{[HA]} \tag{5}$$

$$pH = pK + \log \frac{[A^-]}{[HA]} \tag{6}$$

$$pH = pK + \log \frac{[base]}{[acid]} \tag{7}$$

Equation 6 is, of course, the familiar Henderson-Hasselbalch equation, which states simply that the pH of a buffer solution is related to a constant (pK) plus the logarithm of the ratio of the base concentration: weak acid concentration.

Bicarbonate-Carbonic Acid System

CARBON DIOXIDE.—It was pointed out in the section on clinical acid-base balance that carbon dioxide is the only component of a major biologic buffer system which is under respiratory control, and that the level of carbon dioxide in the blood determines the state of the patient's respiratory acid-base balance. This level is generally measured as the partial pressure of carbon dioxide or P_{CO_2}. This is the pressure, usually stated in millimeters of mercury, which would be exerted by the dissolved carbon dioxide if it were in equilibrium at an air-fluid interface. The sum of the partial pressures of all gases dissolved in a fluid is equal to the pressure in the gas portion of this system, this being atmospheric pressure in an open container such as the body. The quantitation of P_{CO_2} is usually done in one of two ways at present.

ASTRUP TECHNIQUE.—The technique of Astrup[1,10] allows determination of all of the pertinent acid-base parameters, although it was originally conceived as a means of determining Pa_{CO_2} in patients requiring artificial ventilation.[6] Astrup rediscovered the fact that the pH of a solution is linearly related to the logarithm of the P_{CO_2}. If this relationship is plotted on semilog paper, the technique of this determination is sim-

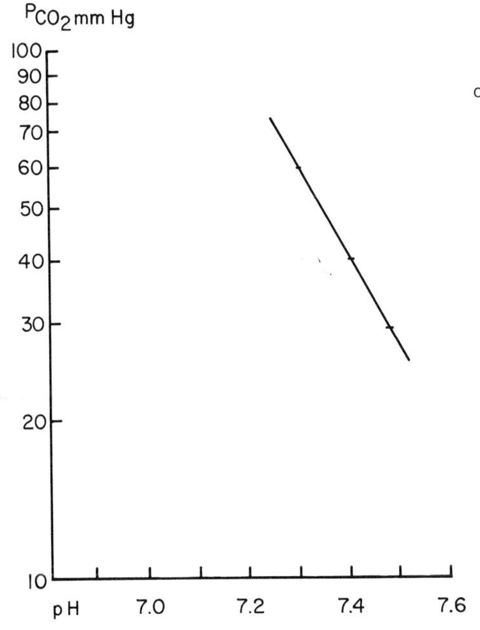

Fig. 6-1.—Linear relation of pH of a solution to logarithm of the P_{CO_2}.

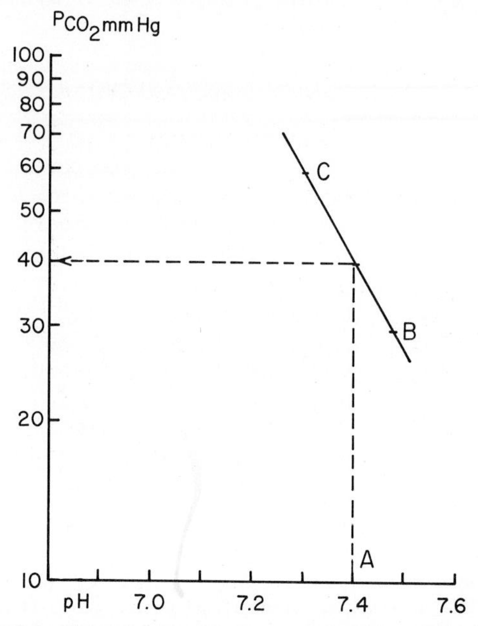

Fig. 6-2.—Determination of Pa_{CO_2} using relationship with pH.

ple (Fig. 6-1). Arterial blood is obtained anaerobically and the pH of the blood is measured (Fig. 6-2, *A*). The blood is then equilibrated with 2 gases of different, known Pco_2, and the pH redetermined on each of the equilibrated samples (Fig. 6-2, *B* and *C*). Two points are thus determined, and the straight line drawn. The patient's actual Pco_2 then is determined by interpolation, using the actual pH value.

SEVERINGHAUS ELECTRODE.—The Severinghaus Pco_2 electrode[9] is employed in a number of commercial acid-base measuring devices. This electrode takes advantage of the relationship between pH and Pco_2 described above. It consists of a pH electrode contained within a rigid chamber, the end of the chamber being enclosed by a membrane which is freely permeable to carbon dioxide. A thin space between the pH electrode and the membrane is filled with a bicarbonate buffer solution. The electrode is placed in a blood sample. The carbon dioxide equilibrates across the membrane, and the resulting pH determined by the glass electrode is a function of the logarithm of the Pco_2 concentration.

CARBONIC ACID.—Carbonic acid values are not readily determined directly. It is recalled, however, that:

$$H_2O + CO_2 \rightleftharpoons H_2CO_3 \quad (8)$$

Since carbonic acid is in equilibrium with carbon dioxide, and since the concentration of carbon dioxide can be measured as described above, it is possible to determine the carbonic acid concentration by knowing the appropriate solubility and dissociation constants for the above reaction. In blood or plasma at 37 C.:

$$Pco_2 \times 0.03 = [H_2CO_3] \text{ (mEq./L.)} \quad (9)$$

BICARBONATE.—Bicarbonate concentrations are also difficult to determine directly. If the Henderson-Hasselbalch equation is stated in terms of the bicarbonate reactions:

$$pH = pK + \log \frac{[HCO_3^-]}{[H_2CO_3] = Pco_2 \times 0.03} \quad (10)$$

it is seen that we have determined two of the three components of this system, namely the pH and the H_2CO_3. Since the pK is a constant (6.1 for blood and plasma at 37 C.), we have an equation with one unknown which can be readily solved for the bicarbonate concentration.

Metabolic Acid-Base Balance

The interpretation of base excess results was described in the clinical section. It will be the purpose of this section to describe some other measures of metabolic acid-base balance and to review the technique for determination of base excess.

We have discussed acid-base balance in terms of the bicarbonate-carbonic acid system. It would appear at first glance that metabolic acid-base derangements could be quantitated by measuring the HCO_3^- concentration. This is inaccurate for two reasons:

1. An increase in the Pa_{CO_2}, that is, respiratory acidosis, causes the reaction (4) to be shifted to the right:

$$H_2O + CO_2 \rightleftharpoons H_2CO_3 \rightleftharpoons H^+ + HCO_3^-$$

so that the hydrogen ion is increased but also the bicarbonate ion concentration is increased. In other words, the bicarbonate ion concentration is not independent of the Pco_2 and so is not a measure strictly of nonrespiratory changes.

2. There are other buffer systems in the body besides the bicarbonate system, so that a determination of bicarbonate excess or deficit is not a measure of the total base excess or deficit.

The following tests are some which have been designed to circumvent one or both of these inaccuracies.

MEASUREMENT OF METABOLIC ACID-BASE BALANCE

CO_2-COMBINING POWER, CO_2 CAPACITY.—These tests differ in technique but not in concept. Basically, the tests are performed on anaerobically separated plasma. This plasma is equilibrated to 40 mm. Hg Pco_2 so that the respiratory component is normalized. The total amount of carbon dioxide—that is, the amount in the form of HCO_3^- as well as in H_2CO_3—is measured and this value expressed in mEq./L. Normally, there is 20 times as much bicarbonate as carbonic acid:

$$pH = pK + \log\frac{[\text{base}]}{[\text{acid}]}$$

$$pH = pK + \log\frac{[HCO_3^-]}{[H_2CO_3]} \quad pK = 6.1 \quad pH = 7.4$$

$$7.4 = 6.1 + \log\frac{[HCO_3^-]}{[H_2CO_3]}$$

$$\log\frac{[HCO_3^-]}{[H_2CO_3]} = 1.3 \qquad 1.3 = \log 20$$

$$\frac{[HCO_3^-]}{[H_2CO_3]} = \frac{20}{1}$$

so it is assumed that the total CO_2 (in mEq./L.) is a measure of the bicarbonate ion concentration. The normal total CO_2 is 25.2 mEq./L.

$$P_{CO_2} \times 0.03 = [H_2CO_3]$$

$$40 \text{ mm. Hg} \times 0.03 = 1.2 \text{ mEq./L.} = [H_2CO_3]$$

$$[HCO_3^-] = 20[H_2CO_3]$$

$$[HCO_3^-] = 24 \text{ mEq./L.}$$

$$\text{Total } CO_2 = 24 + 1.2 = 25.2 \text{ mEq./L.}$$

An elevated CO_2-combining power or capacity indicates metabolic alkalosis; a depression, metabolic acidosis. This test, of course, does not quantitate buffer bases other than bicarbonate.

STANDARD BICARBONATE.—This test, first proposed by Astrup, is similar in concept to those just detailed. If the pH-log P_{CO_2} relationship is determined for a patient's blood, it is apparent that one knows the pH at any given P_{CO_2} for this specimen. If the pH corresponding to P_{CO_2} of 40 mm. Hg is obtained from this analysis, it is then possible to solve the Henderson-Hasselbalch equation for the bicarbonate concentration that would be present if the P_{CO_2} were normal, that is, 40 mm. Hg. The normal value for this determination is 24 mEq./L. Once again, an elevation indicates metabolic alkalosis, a depression, metabolic acidosis (Fig. 6-3).

BUFFER BASE.—The previous tests for metabolic acid-base balance measure only the bicarbonate deficit or excess. Body fluids contain other bases which are available to buffer a hydrogen ion load; these primarily consist of the protein anions. It is recalled that a buffer is defined as a weak acid and its conjugate base; the conjugate base being an anion. Also, proteins are composed of weak acids, namely, amino

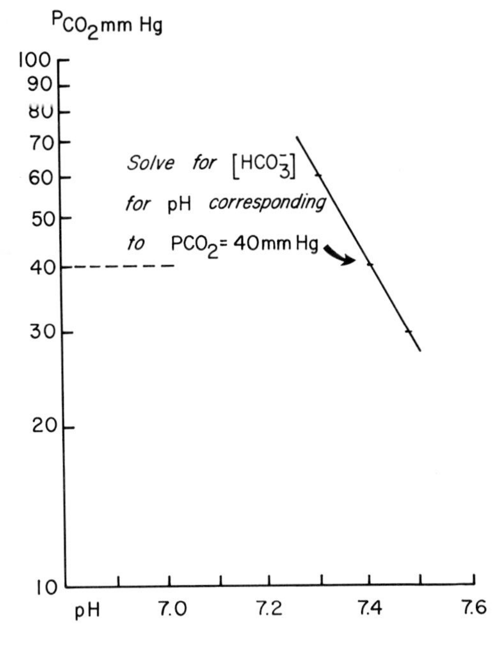

Fig. 6-3. — Standard bicarbonate determination from pH-log P_{CO_2} relationship.

acids. Amino acids may be present in a positively charged, negatively charged or uncharged form.[2]

Weak Acid

$^{+}NH_3 - R - COO^-$

$+H^+$ (to the left) $\quad +OH^-$ (to the right)

$^{+}NH_3 - R - COOH \leftarrow \qquad \rightarrow NH_2 - R - COO^-$

Base

It is obvious that the protein anion may accept hydrogen ion and qualify as a buffer base. A glance at the Gamblegram of the extracellular fluids (Fig. 6-4) indicates that HCO_3^- and protein anions are the only buffer bases. If one measures the buffer base and then varies the P_{CO_2} of the fluid in question, the results in Figure 6-5 are obtained.[6]

Note that the relative amount of bicarbonate changes, as would be expected, but the total amount of buffer base remains constant. This determination then satisfies the requirement of measuring only metabolic changes and also that of quantitating total base excess or deficit. The normal plasma buffer base is 41.6 mEq./L. The whole blood buffer base varies with the hemoglobin concentration, since hemoglobin contains large amounts of amino acids and serves as an excellent buffer. The normal blood buffer base then is 41.6 mEq./L. + 0.42 mEq./L./Gm. hemoglobin. To determine the excess amount of base or acid present in the blood, it is necessary to measure the hemoglobin, to calculate the

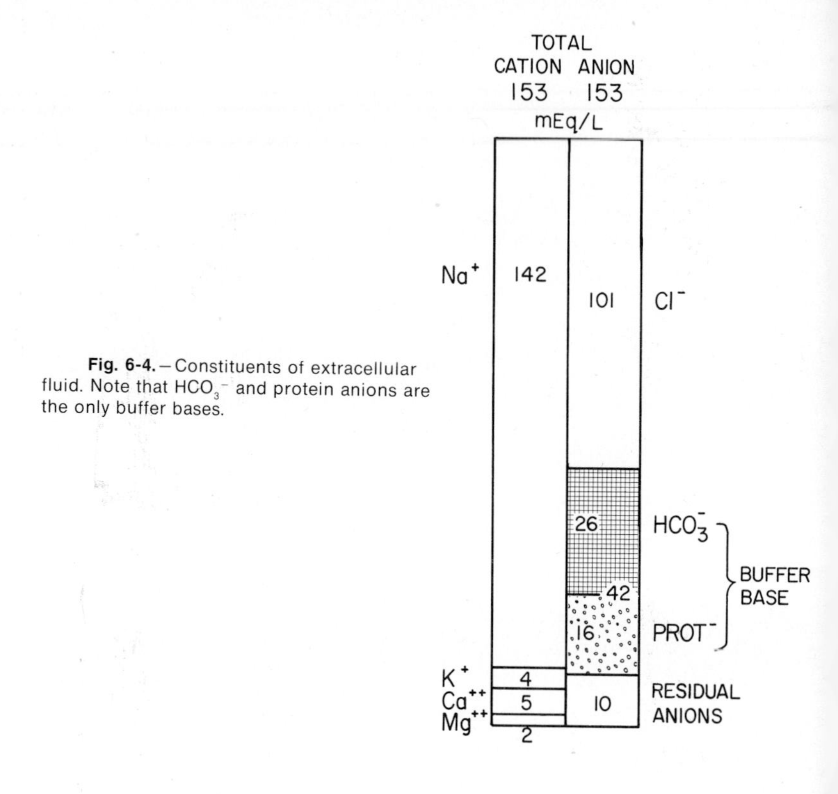

Fig. 6-4.—Constituents of extracellular fluid. Note that HCO_3^- and protein anions are the only buffer bases.

Fig. 6-5.—Effect of varying P_{CO_2} on bicarbonate and total buffer base.

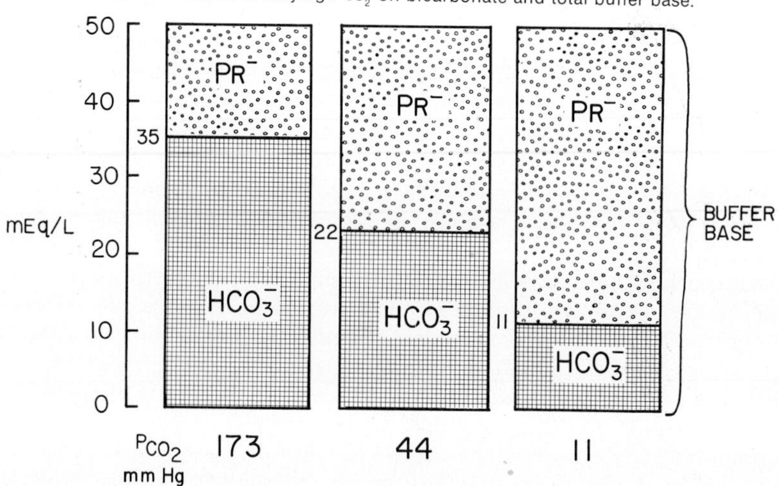

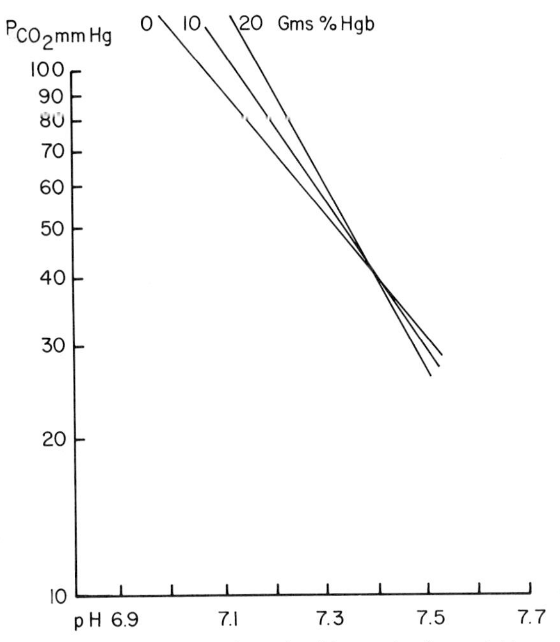

Fig. 6-6.—pH-log P_{CO_2} relationship determined for varying hemoglobin concentrations.

normal buffer base, and to subtract from this the patient's actual buffer base. The value obtained is expressed as base excess.

Base excess = normal buffer base − actual buffer base

BASE EXCESS.—Base excess can be determined in another way.[7,8] The pH-log P_{CO_2} equilibration line for normal blood is remarkably constant. If blood is anaerobically centrifuged to varying hemoglobin concentrations, and the pH-log P_{CO_2} relationship is determined on each sample, a family of lines is obtained which crosses at a constant point (Fig. 6-6).

Further, if fixed amounts of acid or base are added to the sample which is again centrifuged to varying hemoglobin concentrations, this family of lines shifts in a constant manner (Fig. 6-7). For example, in the diagram to the left, 10 mEq. acid/L. of blood was added, and to the right 10 mEq. of base/L. of blood was added. If this same technique is performed using varying amounts of fixed acid or base, a series of points can be drawn indicating the intersection of the family of lines at each of the different base excess or acid excess loci. If these points are connected, a nomogram is formed (Fig. 6-8).

If the pH-log P_{CO_2} relationship is determined on an unknown blood sample, the intersection of the straight line obtained with the nomo-

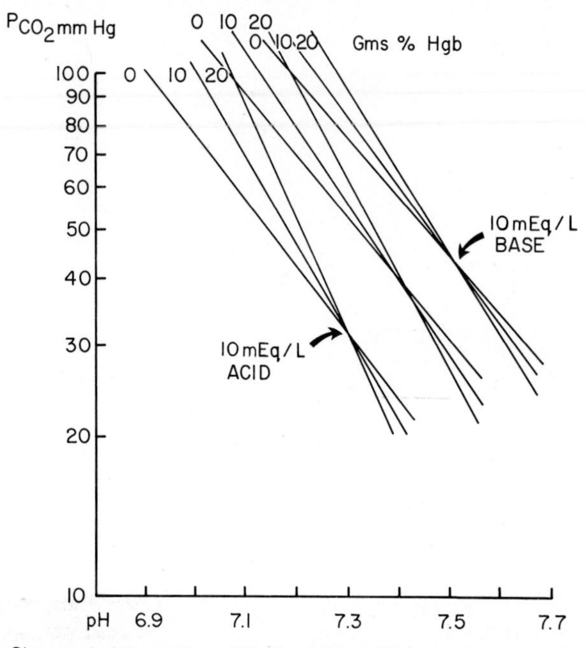

Fig. 6-7.—Changes in intersection of family of lines with base excess and acid excess.

gram can be read directly as the base excess or acid excess in milliequivalents/liter; this value is independent of the hemoglobin concentration. By convention, an acid excess is referred to as a negative base excess; thus, metabolic acidosis is diagnosed by a negative base excess and metabolic alkalosis by a positive base excess. This determination is simple, straightforward and reliable and is probably the determination of choice for the diagnosis of metabolic acid-base derangements. It has a major imperfection which will be discussed next.

EFFECTS OF CO_2 ON BASE EXCESS.—It was pointed out that the perfect test for metabolic acid-base derangement would be uninfluenced by the Pco_2. The base excess determination is actually an in vitro CO_2 titration, and it is apparent that Pco_2 changes in vitro will have no effect on the base excess. If, however, this titration is carried out in vivo, that is, if the whole-body Pco_2 is varied and the base excess determined, the relationship in Figure 6-9 is found.[9,10] This diagram is a plot of base excess versus Pco_2. One finds that in vitro wide changes in the Pco_2 cause no change in the base excess. However, in vivo, as the Pco_2 is increased, a negative base excess results. The shaded area on the diagram represents the 95% confidence limit for base excess as a function of Pco_2. For example, if a patient had an acute elevation of Pa_{CO_2} to 90 mm. Hg, he would be expected 95% of the time to have base excess

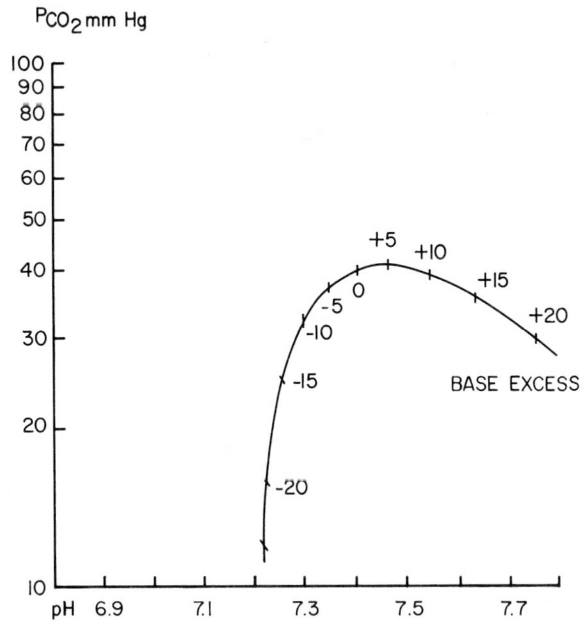

Fig. 6-8.—Nomogram for determination of base excess or acid excess in milliequivalents/liter.

between −4 and −7 mEq./L. An acutely elevated Pa_{CO_2}, as pointed out in the section on clinical acid-base balance, requires immediate improvement in the respiratory status, while a base deficit of −5 mEq./L. is not too worrisome. The above relationship, therefore, should be kept in mind, but it is not a serious detraction from the use of base excess as a means of quantitating metabolic acid-base derangement.

Fig. 6-9.—Relationship of base excess to changes in P_{CO_2} (see text).

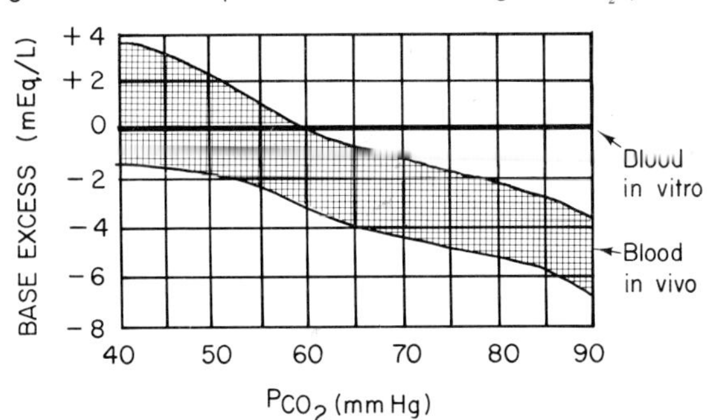

Obtaining and Storing Blood[13]

Accurate acid-base determinations may be performed on arterial, central venous and arterialized capillary blood.

ARTERIAL. – Many intensive care patients will have indwelling arterial cannulas. In others, the urgent need for a blood sample necessitates arterial puncture. The preferred sites for such a puncture are the femoral, brachial and radial arteries. A 2 or 5 ml. syringe with a 22 gauge needle is rinsed with heparin (1,000 units/ml.) and emptied. The selected area is shaved and prepared with iodine or a suitable substitute. The pulse is palpated in the vessel to be punctured, and the needle introduced so as to strike the vessel beneath the palpating fingers. The needle is introduced swiftly, often passing through the back wall of the artery, and then slowly withdrawn. When the blood is obtained, any air bubbles present are ejected and the syringe capped.

CENTRAL VENOUS. – Right atrial blood, obtained from a central venous pressure catheter, may be employed for acid-base determinations with minimal loss of accuracy. Peripheral venous blood is not acceptable because local ischemia may cause such a sample not to be representative of the whole body.

ARTERIALIZED CAPILLARY. – A heating pad applied to the forearm and hand for 20 minutes causes the capillary blood obtained by a finger stick to have acid-base and blood gas values nearly identical to arterial blood. By use of currently available microtechniques, complete analysis can be performed on 150 μl. of blood. The blood from the finger stick is collected in heparinized glass tubes and stirred by means of a small piece of wire placed within the tube and a magnet held outside the tube. This method is especially applicable to children, in whom the heel may be punctured instead of the finger.

STORAGE. – Blood may be stored for up to 3 hours with minimal change in acid-base values if it is stored at 0–4 C. This is readily done by placing the capped syringe or capillary tubes in a container and covering it with ice cubes. Blood should not be stored at room temperature for more than 15–20 minutes before completing the determinations.

REFERENCES

1. Astrup, P., *et al.*: The acid-base metabolism – a new approach, Lancet 1:1035–1039, 1960.
2. Davenport, H. W.: *The ABC of Acid-Base Balance* (4th ed.; Chicago: University of Chicago Press, 1958).
3. Mellemgaard, K., and Astrup, P.: The quantitative determination of surplus amounts of acid or base in the human body, Scandinav. J. Clin. & Lab. Invest. 12:187–199, 1960.
4. Mulhausen, R. O., and Blumentals, A.: Metabolic alkalosis, Arch. Int. Med. 116:729–738, 1965.
5. Nahas, G. G. (ed.): Current concepts of acid base measurement, Ann. New York Acad. Sc. 133:3–276, 1965.
6. Rooth, G.: *Introduction to Acid-Base and Electrolyte Balance* (London: Student Literature, 1966).

7. Schwartz, W. B.; Brackett, N. C., Jr., and Cohen, J. J.: Response of extracellular hydrogen ion concentration to graded degrees of chronic hypercapnia: Physiologic limits of defense of pH, J. Clin. Invest. 44:291–301, 1965.
8. Schwartz, W. B., and Relman, A.: A critique of the parameters used in the evaluation of acid-base disorders, New England J. Med. 268:1382–1388, 1963.
9. Severinghaus, J. W.: *Handbook of Physiology*, Vol. II, *Respiration* (Washington, D.C.: American Physiological Society, 1965).
10. Siggaard-Andersen, O.: *The Acid-Base Status of the Blood* (3rd ed.; Baltimore: Williams & Wilkins Company, 1965).
11. Siggaard-Andersen, O.: The pH-log pCO_2 blood acid-base nomogram revised, Scandinav. J. Clin. & Lab. Invest. 14:598–604, 1962.
12. Siggaard-Andersen, O., and Engel, K.: A new acid-base nomogram—improved method for calculation of the relevant blood acid-base data, Scandinav. J. Clin. & Lab. Invest. 12:177–186, 1960.
13. Siggaard-Andersen, O.: Sampling and storing of blood for determination of acid-base status, Scandinav. J. Clin. & Lab. Invest. 13:196–204, 1961.
14. Singer, R. B., and Hastings, B.: An improved clinical method for the estimation of disturbances of the acid-base balance of human blood, Medicine 27:223–242, 1948.
15. Van Ypersele de Strihou, C.; Brasseur, L., and DeConinck, J.: The carbon dioxide response curve for chronic hypercapnia in man, New England J. Med. 275:117–122, 1966.
16. Winters, R. W.: Terminology of acid-base disorders, Ann. Int. Med. 63:873–884, 1965.
17. Winters, R. W.: *Some Comments on the Validity of the Astrup Technique for the Measurement of Acid-Base Status of Blood* (Copenhagen: Radiometer).
18. Zimmermann, B.: Postoperative Management of Fluid Volumes and Electrolytes, in *Current Problems in Surgery* (Chicago: Year Book Medical Publishers, Inc., December, 1965).

7

Ocular Complications of Surgery

WILLIAM F. HUGHES, M.D.

Chairman, Department of Ophthalmology, Rush-Presbyterian-St. Luke's Medical Center; Professor of Ophthalmology, Rush Medical College

THIS CHAPTER will consider the ocular complications of anesthesia and those related to general surgery, especially cardiovascular and neurosurgery. It is the responsibility of those in direct charge of the patient in the intensive care unit to recognize the symptoms and signs of ocular complications so that more definitive examination with special instruments and ocular treatment can be continued by the ophthalmologist.

Corneal Abrasions and Foreign Bodies

Exposure and abrasion of the cornea during general anesthesia can be minimized by the instillation of an ophthalmic ointment, such as Neosporin, or by closing the eye with adhesive tape applied from the upper lid down to the skin below the eye.

If the patient complains of scratchy ocular pain on awakening, examination for a corneal or conjunctival foreign body is best made with focal illumination, for example, an ordinary flashlight, directed in from the side with magnification if possible (ordinary convex or plus lens, magnifying binocular loupe or slit lamp microscope). The upper lid should be everted by grasping the upper lashes, instructing the patient to look downward and applying pressure with a cotton applicator or the back of the thumbnail just above the tarsus. Foreign bodies often lodge on this conjunctival shelf at the upper border of the tarsus. Conjunctival and superficial corneal foreign bodies can be removed with a sterile cotton applicator. More deeply embedded corneal foreign bodies require the use of the slit lamp and a metal spud. This is usually done by an ophthalmologist and a follow-up examination is made to be certain that an infected corneal ulcer does not ensue.

Corneal abrasions may follow trauma of many types during general or local anesthesia. Contact with a toxic chemical, surgical drapes, anesthesia mask, or prolonged exposure can cause abrasion, especially in patients with exophthalmos. Diagnosis is easily made by staining the cornea with fluorescein, since any area denuded of epithelium stains green. Because fluorescein solutions are easily contaminated by pseudomonas organisms, use of commercially available, sterile, fluorescein-impregnated strips of filter paper is preferred; the filter paper is applied briefly to the inner surface of the lower lid.

Corneal abrasions usually heal rapidly after immobilizing the eyelids with a mild pressure bandage; for example, 2 eyepads or 1 eyepad reinforced with cotton may be used. However, most ophthalmologists prefer to instill a local antibiotic solution such as Neosporin in addition to patching. Instructions for the instillation of local anesthetics into the eye to obtain comfort are to be deprecated, because excess use of such agents retards regeneration of the corneal epithelium. Ordinarily, corneal abrasions heal within a day or two if there is no secondary infection. Rarely, however, a recurrent erosion of the corneal epithelium may follow macerating types of abrasions, for example, those caused by a fingernail, a piece of paper or other rough foreign body. Treatment of this stubborn complication lies with the ophthalmologist.

Glaucoma

ACUTE ANGLE-CLOSURE (CONGESTIVE) GLAUCOMA. – This relatively unusual but serious type of glaucoma, characterized by increased intraocular pressure and requiring immediate treatment, is caused by a mechanical blockage of the drainage of aqueous into the canal of Schlemm at the angle formed by the corneoscleral tissue and root of the iris (Fig. 7-1). This is most commonly seen in patients with relatively shallow anterior chambers (for example, hyperopes and older individuals). The depth of the anterior chamber can be estimated by oblique illumination of the anterior segment of the eye by the slit lamp or more accurately by gonioscopic examination of the angle of the anterior chamber using a special contact lens. Individuals susceptible to acute angle-closure glaucoma often give a history of seeing colored rings around lights (iridescent vision), or of mild aching of the eyes, especially in the dark. Semi-dilation of the pupil in such predisposed individuals can cause the pupillary block of aqueous flow from the posterior to the anterior chamber, resulting in forward bulging of the iris, occlusion of the drainage angle by the iris root and development of a high ocular tension (often 60–90 mm. Hg with the Schiøtz tonometer or "stony hard"). Instillation into the eye of any mydriatic which dilates the pupil of such an individual can initiate an attack of acute glaucoma. For example, anticholinergic drugs such as atropine, homatropine, scopolamine, cyclopentolate (Cyclogyl), tropicamide (Mydriacyl), or eucatropine (Euphthalmine); or sympathicomimetic drugs such as epinephrine,

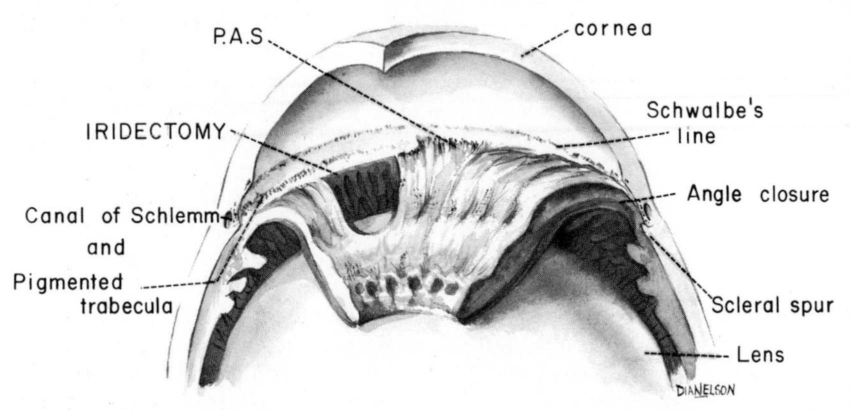

Fig. 7-1.—Cross-section and gonioscopic view of angle of anterior chamber, showing iris bombé or bulging of the iris (**right**), which closes the filtration angle in acute angle-closure glaucoma. A peripheral iridectomy (**left**) reopens the posterior-anterior chamber pathway for aqueous, eliminates the iris bombé and re-establishes normal drainage of aqueous through the trabecula into the canal of Schlemm. (Figs. 7-1–7-4 from Pushkin, E. A.: Etiology, diagnosis and management of glaucoma in adults, Presbyterian-St. Luke's Hosp. M. Bull. 4:110, 1965.)

or phenylephrine (Neo-Synephrine) can initiate acute glaucoma in predisposed individuals. The preoperative systemic administration of any of these or similar drugs will have correspondingly less effect in dilating the pupil, but they can initiate an attack of acute glaucoma. It is not uncommon that the stress of hospitalization and impending surgery per se can initiate such an attack. Mydriatics should be avoided, or miotics such as pilocarpine 2% can be instilled into the eyes of such individuals twice daily to avoid attacks during hospitalization or after surgery.

Symptoms of acute glaucoma usually develop within hours after the provocative mydriasis. These include pain directly in the eye which may be sufficiently severe to induce vomiting, external ocular congestion, haziness of the cornea, dilated pupil and rapid reduction of vision. The initial therapeutic attack consists in efforts to reduce the ocular tension, constrict the pupil and open up the drainage angle of the anterior chamber. Oral administration of a hyperosmotic agent such as glycerol (intravenous urea and mannitol are also effective but more difficult to administer) is given in dosage of about 0.5 ml./lb. body weight mixed with 2 teaspoonsful of concentrated lemon or lime juice for palatability. This dehydration of the intraocular fluids is more effective during the early congestive phases of acute glaucoma than the anti-secretory agent, Diamox. Vigorous attempts are made to constrict the pupil by instillation of 2% pilocarpine into the affected eye every minute for 5 minutes, then every 5 minutes for 30 minutes, then 3–4 times an hour until the angle opens. Stronger miotics are undesirable. Pilocarpine is also administered 2–3 times a day in the unaffected eye to prevent an attack. Severe or prolonged attacks of angle-closure glaucoma can produce necrosis of the iris with resultant poor constriction of the pupil, formation of adhesions of the iris root to the filtration angle (peripheral anterior synechias) and poor response to tension-lowering measures. This becomes a difficult problem for the ophthalmologist, usually requiring an emergency peripheral iridectomy in an attempt to re-establish normal posterior-anterior chamber flow of the aqueous. If the elevated tension does respond to medical therapy, the eye is allowed to "cool off" while on miotics and perhaps Diamox, and several days later a peripheral iridectomy is performed for permanent cure of the glaucoma. Usually, a week or so later, a prophylactic peripheral iridectomy is performed on the opposite, predisposed eye.

OPEN-ANGLE GLAUCOMA.—Chronic noncongestive or "simple" glaucoma occurs in 2% of all individuals over 40 years of age. The anterior chamber is of normal depth and the drainage angle between the root of the iris and corneoscleral trabecula is open, but the aqueous does not drain out properly through the trabecula-canal of Schlemm pathway (Fig. 7-2). This type of glaucoma is symptomless during the early stages and must be detected by routine measurement of the ocular tension or intraocular pressure with a tonometer (Fig. 7-3), usually less than 4 units on the 5.5 Gm. scale (22 mm. Hg). However, the definitive diagnosis of open-angle glaucoma rests on the development of early visual field changes corresponding to changes in the optic disc (Fig. 7-4). This type of chronic glaucoma usually is treated medically for the duration of the patient's life. Treatment consists of the use of miotics without or with epinephrine locally and, if necessary, Diamox or other carbonic anhydrase inhibitors systemically. Occasionally visual field loss with elevated tension progresses in spite of medical therapy. This requires

Fig. 7-2.—Diagram illustrating the normal flow of aqueous from the ciliary processes into the canal of Schlemm and then into the venous collector vessel on the surface of the eye. In chronic open-angle glaucoma, the drainage of aqueous is blocked in the region of the corneoscleral trabecula.

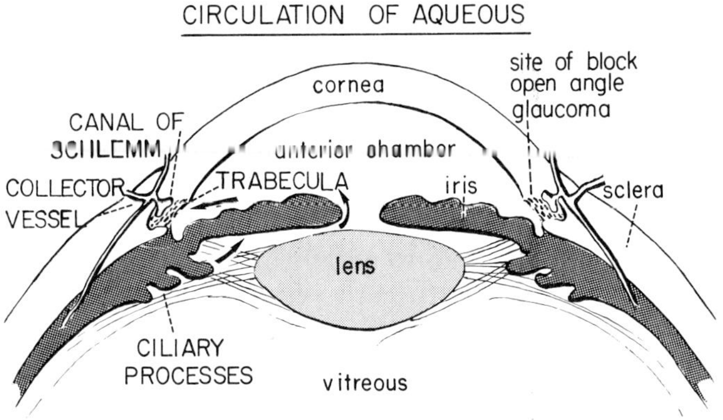

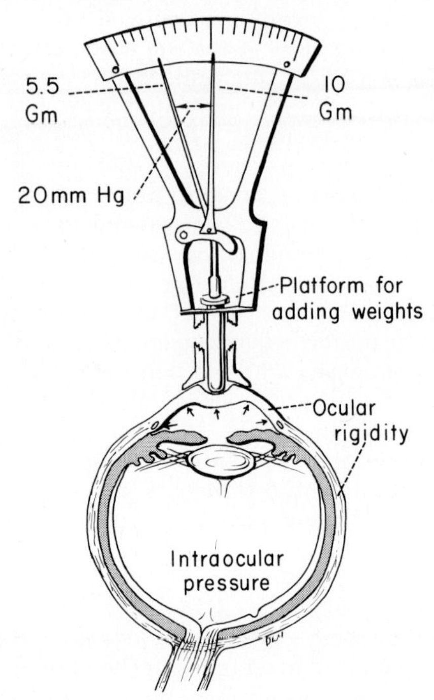

Fig. 7-3.—Determination of ocular tension using the Schiøtz tonometer. The 5.5 Gm. of the plunger indents the corneal surface, directly related to the intraocular pressure and the rigidity of the ocular coats plus vascularity of the choroid. Correlation of tensions with intraocular pressures on enucleated eyes permits correlation of the number of units of deflection of the pointer (indentation of the cornea) with intraocular pressure; normally this is 5 units with the 5.5 weight or 17–20 mm. Hg intraocular pressure.

some type of external filtering operation, such as a sclerectomy, to permit the aqueous to flow from the anterior chamber into the subconjunctival space instead of into the blocked trabecula-canal of Schlemm drainage mechanism.

There are a few special considerations in the general medical or surgical management of patients with open-angle glaucoma. Visual field loss is retarded by the presence of systemic hypertension, suggesting with some experimental evidence that an elevated intraocular pressure causes damage to the retinal or optic nerve fibers by compression of the nutrient capillaries, probably in the retina or possibly in the optic disc. Accordingly, rapid reduction of systemic hypertension by medical or surgical measures can result in serious deterioration of the visual field in patients with open-angle glaucoma. Mydriatics, anticholinergic agents and other stresses of hospitalization and surgery have little significant effect on the intraocular pressure. Such patients should be continued on previous anti-glaucoma medication. If this has been an

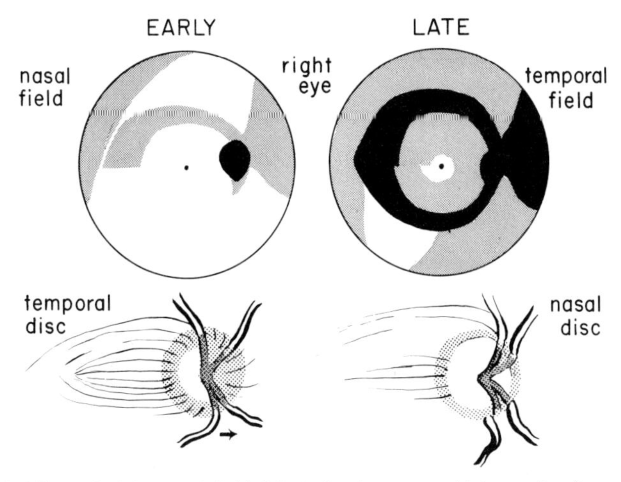

Fig. 7-4. – Characteristic visual field defects in glaucoma which are directly correlated with glaucomatous atrophy of the optic disc. An arcuate defect connected with the blind spot and arching over the area of central fixation is characteristic of the early stages of glaucoma, along with loss of the lower temporal rim of the disc. Late changes are associated with closing in of the peripheral field, often with retention of good central vision, further loss of the rim of the optic disc (enlargement of the cup) with nasal displacement of the retinal vessels and pallor of the disc.

anticholinesterase agent such as echothiophate (Phospholine iodide), demecarium (Humorsol), or isoflurophate (DFP or Floropryl), the serum cholinesterases and pseudocholinesterases are reduced. Accordingly, succinylcholine, which is widely used as a muscle relaxant during intubation and is destroyed by serum pseudocholinesterases, may produce unduly prolonged apnea in patients on anticholinesterase glaucoma therapy. Protopam appears to be a specific antidote for these drugs.

Retinal Complications

If, during general anesthesia, sufficient sustained pressure is applied to the eye to cause occlusion of the central retinal vein or artery and choroidal vessels, irreversible degenerative changes in the retina can occur. The duration of complete ischemia of the retina which will lead to permanent blindness is uncertain but probably lies within a 30–90 minute period. This complication is more likely when the patient is placed face down during operations, such as neurosurgical procedures. The characteristic clinical picture in occlusion of the central retinal artery is attenuation or absence of retinal arteries, boxcar blood segments in the veins, retinal edema with a cherry-red spot in the macula, gross loss of vision or light perception and, later, primary optic atrophy. Treatment is usually unavailing, but inhalation therapy of 5% carbon dioxide in oxygen might be tried.

EMBOLISM OF THE CENTRAL RETINAL ARTERY. – Unilateral attacks of cerebral ischemia and blurred vision, especially after cardiac and carotid surgery, suggest embolism. Thrombi or calcium from damaged heart valves or resulting after cardiac surgery may lodge in one of the larger retinal arteries, producing a localized white ischemia of the retina (cotton-wool exudate) and corresponding blind spot, which is usually permanent. Stenosis of an internal carotid artery is more apt to give off emboli of either cholesterol crystals or platelets. These may lodge in one or more of the smaller retinal arterioles, appearing as white or glistening plaques at the bifurcations of the retinal arteries. Most of these patients have transient visual disturbances without retinal opacity, the emboli being dislodged into smaller vessels and disappearing. Other, less common forms of retinal emboli include fat emboli following crush injuries or fractures and air emboli following operations on larger vessels and in caisson disease, some blood dyscrasias and malignancies.

Massage of the eye may facilitate dislodgment of retinal emboli. Carbon dioxide dilates the retinal arterioles, so a 5% concentration may be administered by inhalation. Although oxygen constricts retinal arterioles, it may be desirable in these cases to oxygenate the retina via the underlying choroidal circulation. Therefore, 5% carbon dioxide in 95% oxygen inhalation may be beneficial. Systemic administration of vasodilators does not improve the ocular blood flow or oxygenation because of the much greater effect on peripheral vasodilatation. Oral administration of glycerol will reduce the intraocular pressure and produce some retinal vasodilatation.

HEMORRHAGE.—Retinal hemorrhages can occur after angiography, usually without significant visual symptoms unless the macula is involved. Fortunately, most of these absorb without serious retinal damage.

Loss of Vision from Central Nervous System Complications

CEREBRAL EDEMA.—Ventricular puncture can result in cerebral edema with blindness due to involvement of the visual cortex. Pupillary reactions remain active. Fortunately, recovery from such blindness is usually complete within 24–48 hours.

CHRONIC PAPILLEDEMA.—This can result in slow contraction of the visual fields over the course of 6 months or more, with secondary optic atrophy. In such patients, neurosurgeons are aware of the risk of sudden and permanent loss of vision after craniotomy or decompression.

MASSIVE LOSS OF BLOOD.—This can rarely cause loss of vision, probably due to hypotension and ischemia of the visual cortex in the occipital lobe.

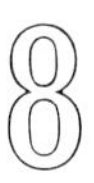

Postoperative Hemorrhage

WALTER FRIED, M.D.

Associate Attending Physician, Rush-Presbyterian-St. Luke's Medical Center; Associate Professor of Medicine, Rush Medical College

RICHARD J. SASSETTI, M.D.

Associate Attending Physician, Rush-Presbyterian-St. Luke's Medical Center; Assistant Professor of Medicine, Rush Medical College

AND

DAVID M. C. SUTTON, M.D.

Adjunct Attending Physician, Rush-Presbyterian-St. Luke's Medical Center; Instructor in Medicine, Rush Medical College

DIAGNOSIS AND MANAGEMENT OF SPECIFIC CAUSES

HEMOSTASIS IS OBTAINED during surgery through a combination of skill and judgment on the part of the surgeon and normal functioning of the patient's coagulation mechanism. When excess bleeding occurs, rapid diagnosis and treatment of the cause requires a basic understanding of the normal mechanism of coagulation and its disorders.

Normal Coagulation Mechanism

Normal coagulation involves the successful interaction of blood vessels, platelets and soluble factors required for deposition and lysis of fibrin. Following is a brief description of this process.

Trauma causes the involved blood vessels of all sizes to contract. This reaction is transient and is followed by vasodilation. The exposed collagen fibers of damaged vessels interact with circulating platelets in a manner that causes them to adhere to the site of injury.

Adhesion of platelets to collagen fibers results in the release of ADP from the platelet. This, in turn, promotes the aggregation of other platelets to form a platelet plug. The membranes of aggregated platelets undergo changes which tend to cement them together and to make available substances which are necessary for coagulation. The one is thrombasthenin, a contractile protein produced within the platelet, which is essential for clot retraction and thereby makes the clot a more dense barrier against extravasation. The other is platelet factor III, a phospholipid released during platelet aggregation, which is required for the conversion of prothrombin to thrombin. Thrombin, in addition to its role in the enzymatic degradation of fibrinogen to fibrin, enhances platelet aggregation and fusion of aggregated platelets into an amorphous plug.

To strengthen the platelet plug and prevent it from being washed out, fibrin must be deposited. Thrombin, the enzyme necessary for conversion of fibrinogen to fibrin, is not detectable in the plasma of normal subjects. The proenzyme prothrombin, formed in the liver, is converted to its active form, thrombin, in the presence of activated factor V and platelet factor III. The liberation of the latter from platelets has already been described. Factor V (proaccelerin) is synthesized in the liver and circulates in an inactive form which is activated in the presence of activated factor X (Stuart-Prower factor). Activation of factor X is accomplished by either of 2 mechanisms. The one (extrinsic) is initiated by the release of a substance found in most tissues (tissue thromboplastin), which in the presence of factor VII catalyzes the activation of factor X. The other pathway (intrinsic) for activation of factor X is initiated by activation of factor XII (Hageman factor). This occurs by contact with a coarse or rough surface, such as an injured blood vessel wall. Factor XII initiates a cascade of reactions which involves the sequential activation of factor XI (plasma thromboplastin antecedent or PTA), factor IX (plasma thromboplastin component or PTC), and factor VIII (antihemophilic globulin or AHG). The activated form of factor VIII can convert inert factor X to its active form. The relative roles of the intrinsic and extrinsic pathways for activation of factor X are not well known. Both are, however, essential for normal hemostasis, since lack of either factor VII or factor VIII results in defective clot formation.

Fibrinogen, a large protein formed in the liver, is enzymatically split by thrombin into a major and several minor peptides. A very small amount of the major peptide, fibrin monomer, combines with available fibrinogen to form a stable complex which is soluble at body temperature but precipitates in the cold (cryofibrinogen). Most of the fibrin monomer formed polymerizes by hydrogen bonding. Factor XIII (fibrin stabilizing factor) may promote the formation of disulfide bonds in fibrin polymers, and thereby make them more stable.

In addition to the mechanism for fibrin production, a system exists for lysis of fibrin. This consists of an enzyme, fibrinolysin (plasmin), whose primary substrate is fibrin but which reacts also with fibrinogen, factor VIII and factor V. As is the case for most activated clotting factors, fibrinolysin is not normally found in the plasma in significant quantities. An inactive precursor, plasminogen, is normally present in the plasma and in fibrin clots. Plasminogen is converted to fibrinolysin by activator substances which are found in most tissues. A plasminogen activator, urokinase, has also been isolated from the urine of normal persons, but its physiologic role remains to be determined. Release of plasminogen activators and the consequent formation of fibrinolysin occurs in response to injury, coagulation, ischemia, exercise and emotional upset; it is accelerated by catecholamines and probably by thrombin. Under normal circumstances plasminogen is activated primarily within fibrin clots, resulting in local fibrinolysis with little effect on circulating fibrinogen. However, during pathologic states, the release of excess plasminogen activator may cause the plasma fibrinolysin activity to rise to significant levels. This in turn leads to a decline in the plasma fibrinogen, as well as factor V and factor VIII. The reaction between fibrinolysin and fibrinogen results in the formation of fibrinogen split products, which retain binding sites for thrombin and thereby interfere with its action on fibrinogen. The physiologic role of fibrinolysin is not quite clear. However, normal functioning of the coagulation mechanism requires a proper balance between fibrin production on the one hand and lysis on the other. Imbalance in either may result in a bleeding diathesis.

Figure 8-1 illustrates, in diagrammatic form, a scheme for the interaction of coagulation factors which is consistent with most current concepts.

Fig. 8-1.—Normal coagulation. Asterisk refers to active form of the factor.

VASCULAR RESPONSE	Vascular damage → Vascular contraction and exposure of collagen Exposure of collagen + platelets → Adhesion of platelets + release of ADP	
PLATELET PLUG FORMATION	ADP + platelets → platelet aggregation Aggregated platelets + thrombin → platelet metamorphosis into a platelet plug Platelet plug → thrombasthenin release + release of platelet factor III Thrombasthenin + platelet plug → contraction of plug to form a dense barrier	
FORMATION OF STABLE FIBRIN	(Extrinsic) + (CA^{++}) + Tissue thromboplastin + VII + X →	(Intrinsic) XII* ← contact + XII XI* ← XI + XII* IX* ← IX + XI* VIII* ← VIII + IX* X* ← X + VIII*

X* + V + platelet factor III → V*
V* + prothrombin → thrombin
Thrombin + fibrinogen → fibrin monomer → fibrin polymer
Fibrin polymer + XIII → STABLE FIBRIN

Preoperative Workup

A thorough preoperative workup is apt to detect most of the underlying disorders which predispose toward excessive bleeding. The patient's history should specifically include information on the following: (1) excessive hemorrhage at the time of previous surgical procedures, dental procedures or accidents, (2) occurrence of hematemesis, hemoptysis, melena, epistaxis, hematuria, excessive menstrual bleeding, petechiae, "easy bruising" and bleeding from the gums and (3) bleeding complications in family members.

A thorough physical examination will usually detect evidence of existing systemic disorders which predispose to the occurrence of clotting abnormalities. Careful inspection of the skin and mucosa for petechiae, ecchymoses and hemorrhage is essential.

The following laboratory tests are recommended to screen for coagulation abnormalities which might significantly affect hemostasis during surgery.

BLEEDING TIME.—The Duke or the Ivy method measures the time required for a small superficial wound, in either the ear lobe or on the forearm, to stop bleeding. In order for bleeding to stop in the allotted time, contraction of the vessels must occur, and a platelet plug must form and retract properly. The bleeding time is not dependent on fibrin production. A hemophiliac, for instance, may have a normal bleeding time, unless thrombin production is impaired to such a degree that platelet metamorphosis is inhibited. However, the lack of fibrin deposition makes the platelet plug insecure. It may later be washed out, resulting in recurrence of bleeding from the test site. Vascular disease, thrombocytopenia and qualitative platelet disorders can prolong the bleeding time.

PLATELET COUNT.—Bleeding can rarely be attributed to thrombocytopenia alone if the platelet count is above 50,000.

ONE-STAGE PROTHROMBIN TIME.—A reagent containing tissue thromboplastin and calcium is added to decalcified plasma. The time required for fibrin formation to occur is measured. Since tissue thromboplastin is added, coagulation proceeds by the extrinsic pathway, which requires factors VII, V, X, prothrombin and fibrinogen.

PARTIAL THROMBOPLASTIN TIME.—In this test, a reagent containing platelet factor III activity (but not tissue thromboplastin) and calcium is added to decalcified plasma; the time required for fibrin formation is measured. Coagulation proceeds by the intrinsic pathway, requiring factors XII, XI, IX, VIII, V, X, prothrombin and fibrinogen.

THROMBIN TIME.—Thrombin is added to decalcified plasma and the time required for fibrin formation is measured. Since both pathways toward thrombin formation are bypassed, this test is affected only by the amount of fibrinogen available and by factors which interfere with the conversion of fibrinogen to fibrin. Excess heparin in the plasma and

TABLE 8-1.—DISORDERS PREDISPOSING TOWARD EXCESS SURGICAL BLEEDING AND THEIR EFFECTS ON SCREENING TESTS

Prolonged Prothrombin Time

FIBRINOGEN DEFICIENCY

1. Congenital causes
2. Severe hepatocellular disease
3. Fibrinolysis
4. Intravascular coagulation

VITAMIN K DEFICIENCY

1. Malabsorption
2. Obstructive liver disease
3. Blind loop syndromes
4. Broad spectrum antibiotic therapy
5. Coumadin therapy

HEPATOCELLULAR DISEASE NOT SEVERE ENOUGH TO PRODUCE FIBRINOGEN DEPLETION

CIRCULATING ANTICOAGULANTS

1. Spontaneous
2. Heparin
3. Paraproteins

CONGENITAL FACTOR DEFICIENCY

1. Fibrinogen
2. Prothrombin
3. Factor V
4. Factor X

Prolonged Partial Thromboplastin Time

FIBRINOGEN DEFICIENCY

VITAMIN K DEFICIENCY

HEPATOCELLULAR DISEASE

CIRCULATING ANTICOAGULANTS

CONGENITAL FACTOR DEFICIENCIES

1. Fibrinogen
2. Factor XI
3. Factor IX
4. Factor VIII
5. Factor V
6. Factor X
7. Prothrombin
8. Von Willebrand's disease

Prolonged Bleeding Time

THROMBOCYTOPENIA

QUALITATIVE PLATELET DEFECT

1. Uremia
2. Paraprotein
3. Myeloproliferative disorder
4. Aspirin ingestion
5. Thrombasthenia

VASCULAR DISORDER

1. Hereditary hemorrhagic telangiectasia
2. Pseudoxanthoma elasticum
3. Ehlers-Danlos syndrome

VON WILLEBRAND'S DISEASE

Thrombocytopenia

BONE MARROW SUPPRESSION

1. Toxic (alcohol, drug induced)
2. Secondary to carcinoma
3. Secondary to leukemia or lymphoma
4. Congenital
5. Irradiation

INCREASED DESTRUCTION

1. Drug induced
2. ITP
3. Lupus erythematosus
4. Lymphoma
5. Hypersplenism
6. Extracorporeal circulation
7. Septicemia
8. Intravascular coagulation

(Continued)

TABLE 8-1. – Disorders Predisposing Toward Excess Surgical Bleeding and Their Effects on Screening Tests (*Cont.*)

Prolonged Thrombin Time

Fibrinogen Deficiency	
1. Secondary to intravascular coagulation	3. Secondary to massive hepatocellular failure
2. Secondary to fibrinolysins	4. Congenital
Excess Plasma Heparin	
Circulating Fibrinogen Breakdown Products	
1. Secondary to intravascular coagulation	3. Secondary to hepatocellular disease
2. Secondary to fibrinolysins	

also some of the products of fibrinogen breakdown by fibrinolysin interfere with the action of thrombin and prolong the thrombin time.

Table 8-1 lists some of the disorders which predispose toward excessive bleeding during surgery.

Coagulation Disorders during or after Surgery

Continued heavy bleeding from an operative site may result from either faulty ligation of a vessel or from a clotting disorder. The distinction between these is of obvious importance and requires a rapid but accurate workup either to exclude or identify an existing coagulopathy before re-exploration is attempted. Spontaneous bleeding from sites outside the surgical field and continued bleeding from venipuncture sites should particularly arouse suspicion of an underlying clotting abnormality, although their absence does not exclude this possibility. Normal results on preoperative clotting studies decrease the likelihood of a pre-existing coagulopathy. Diagnostic consideration is then directed toward differentiation of 4 general types of disorders: intravascular coagulation, excessive plasma fibrinolysin activity, thrombocytopenia and circulating anticoagulants. Differentiation is made primarily on the basis of laboratory tests.

Intravascular coagulation. – Intravascular coagulation and occasionally massive local clot formation can cause severe depletion of circulating fibrinogen, factor V, factor VIII, prothrombin and platelets. The degree to which these factors are involved varies considerably from patient to patient. Coagulation, probably through the action of thrombin, results in a reactive rise in the amount of local fibrinolysis. The plasma fibrinolysin activity also increases, but rarely to levels commensurate with bleeding. Fibrinogen breakdown products resulting from excess fibrinolysin are, however, usually detectable in the plasma and provide the most sensitive indication of intravascular coagulation. Acute intravascular coagulation is manifested primarily by bleeding due to depletion of clotting factors. The fibrinogen breakdown products also contribute by their interference with the action of thrombin. The excess fibrin formed is adequately removed by reactive fibrinolysis unless the process is prolonged or fibrinolysis is interfered with. Under these circumstances, the pathologic effects of excess fibrin deposition may become manifest. These effects include renal cortical necrosis, pulmonary hypertension, infarction of the adrenal and pituitary glands and intravascular hemolysis. The last results from damage to erythrocytes passing through depositions of fibrin in the small blood vessels.

FIBRINOLYSIS.—Sometimes this occurs as a result of the excess release of plasminogen activator into the circulation. This is an uncommon cause of bleeding, characterized primarily by a high plasma fibrinolysin titer. Fibrinogen, factor V and to a lesser extent factor VIII levels may also be somewhat reduced, but rarely to the extent that occurs with intravascular coagulation. Fibrinogen split products are present in the plasma and contribute to the bleeding diathesis by interfering with the action of thrombin. Thrombocytopenia can rarely, if ever, be attributed to fibrinolysin.

THROMBOCYTOPENIA.—Occurring postoperatively, thrombocytopenia may result from intravascular coagulation. In some cases, however, thrombocytopenia develops without significant depletion of other clotting factors. This, for instance, occurs during the early phase of cardiopulmonary bypass procedures, as a result of alteration and sequestration of platelets in the pump. Selective sequestration of platelets may also complicate the course of septicemia. Presumably, this reflects damage to the platelet membrane by some bacterial factor.

Patients who have received 15 or more units of stored blood within a 24 hour period frequently have a dilutional thrombocytopenia. In addition, the titers of other clotting factors may decrease and fibrinogen breakdown products may become detectable in the plasma. Accordingly, it has been suggested that intravascular coagulation, triggered by transfusion of large quantities of stored blood, sometimes contributes to the resulting clotting abnormality.

Several types of drugs can cause thrombocytopenia by an immune mechanism. Most common among these are quinine, quinidine, thiazide diuretics, sedormid, penicillin and ampicillin. Antibodies to these drugs become attached to the platelet surface by one of several mechanisms, rendering the platelet vulnerable to destruction in the reticuloendothelial system.

ANTICOAGULANTS.—Naturally occurring anticoagulants are a rare cause of impaired coagulation. If present in significant titer, they would most likely be detected by the preoperative screening studies suggested previously. A complete discussion of their detection and therapy is beyond the scope of this chapter. Postoperative high plasma anticoagulant titers are most commonly the result of incompletely neutralized heparin which had been administered at the time of surgery. During cardiopulmonary bypass, blood in the extracorporeal circulation is anti-

TABLE 8-2.—CONDITIONS PREDISPOSING TO SURGICALLY RELATED COAGULOPATHIES

	INTRAVASCULAR COAGULATION	FIBRINOLYSIS	THROMBOCYTOPENIA*	HEPARIN EXCESS
Surgical causes				
Thoracic surgery (particularly sternum-splitting operations)	+	±		
Extracorporeal circulation	+	±	+	+
Prostatectomy	+	±		
Others (particularly surgery of pancreas or stomach)	+	±		
Obstetric causes				
Abruptio placentae	+			
Retained dead fetus	+			
Septic abortion	+			
Amniotic fluid embolus	+			
Carcinomatosis	+	±		
Hemolytic transfusion reaction	+			
Massive blood transfusion therapy	±		+	
Gram-negative septicemia	+		+	
Gram-positive septicemia	±		±	
Severe and prolonged shock—hepatocellular disease	±	+	±	

+ Indicates that conditions are commonly associated.
± Indicates that association occasionally occurs or is doubtful.
* Thrombocytopenia independent of that secondary intravascular coagulation.

coagulated by administering heparin to the patient and neutralizing it afterward with a protamine preparation. In hemodialysis, the blood is heparinized as it enters the bypass and neutralized prior to re-entering the body (regional heparinization). In either instance, the amount of protamine must be accurately titrated, since either an excess of heparin or of its antagonist may interfere with the action of thrombin. "Heparin rebound" may cause bleeding several hours after completion of cardiopulmonary bypass. This probably results from dissociation of the protamine-heparin complex, leaving some of the heparin, which had been neutralized, again free to bind thrombin.

Table 8-2 lists some of the conditions which predispose to the development of 1 or more of the 4 clotting disorders just described.

Management of Bleeding during or after Surgery

DIAGNOSIS

Since speed is often of great importance in the management of seriously bleeding patients, the initial laboratory studies should be selected to provide a working diagnosis upon which therapy can be instituted within a short time. The following tests are recommended for this purpose since their results should be available within an hour or less.

1. Platelet count
2. Prothrombin time
3. Partial thromboplastin time
4. Thrombin time
5. Fibrinogen assay
6. Euglobulin lysis time*
7. Bleeding time

Results of these tests will in most instances provide sufficient information to formulate a presumptive diagnosis on which therapy can be initiated.

If the bleeding episode occurs at a time when the tests are not available to the ward physician, then a presumptive diagnosis must be made from close observation of clot formation in a sample of whole blood. For this purpose 10 ml. of blood is drawn by a clean venipuncture, and 3 ml. is placed into each of 3 tubes which are then placed in a water bath at 37 C. At 1 minute intervals, the first tube is gently inverted until a clot forms. The second is then slowly inverted; if the clot is not firm enough to prevent the blood from flowing, the process is repeated until the clot is firm enough. The same procedure is followed for the third tube. When all 3 tubes are firmly clotted, the time is noted. This is the clotting time, and it should be less than 10 minutes. Prolongation or failure of a clot to form may occur with depletion of clotting factors, circulating anticoagulants or extremely high plasma fibrinolysin titers (such that the clot lyses as it forms). Once the clot forms, note is made of how large the clot is and how firmly it attaches to the side of the glass tube. This is judged by gently agitating the first tube horizontally until the clot is freed from the wall of the tube. A small, soft, friable clot suggests a decrease in the amount of fibrinogen, whereas a large firm clot excludes a significant fibrinogen deficiency even if its formation is delayed. After the clot forms, the other tubes are replaced in the water bath and observed for clot retraction, which is dependent on normal platelet function. To judge the size, texture and retraction of the clot, it may be helpful simultaneously to observe clot formation in normal blood for comparison. Normally, no significant lysis of the clot occurs within the first 24 hours. If lysis begins in less than 6 hours, a significant increase in fibrinolysin is present in the plasma. Lysis is indicated when red cells fall from the clot (which adheres to the tube above the serum after contraction) and sink to the bottom of the tube.†

A prolonged clotting time may be due to either depletion of clotting factors or to interference with their function by a circulating anticoagu-

---

*The euglobulin lysis time is determined by precipitating the euglobulin fraction from plasma. This includes the factors required for fibrin formation and also fibrinolysin. Some of the antifibrinolysins are, however, excluded, and consequently lysis of the fibrin clot normally occurs in only 3 hours or so. This test is extremely sensitive to small changes in fibrinolytic activity, which are often not clinically significant. For this reason, some laboratories prefer less sensitive tests which more reliably detect significant fibrinolysis. Modifications of the thrombin time and fibrinogen titer assay have been devised for this purpose.

†In whole blood of patients with polycythemia rubra vera, clot lysis is difficult to evaluate because of the red cell fallout which often occurs in the absence of significant lysis.

TABLE 8-3. – DIAGNOSIS OF SURGICAL BLEEDING

	PLATELET COUNT	BLEEDING TIME	PARTIAL THROMBOPLASTIN TIME	PROTHROMBIN TIME	EUGLOBULIN LYSIS TIME	FIBRINOGEN TITER	THROMBIN TIME	CLOT FORMATION
Intravascular coagulation	Low	Prolonged*	Prolonged	Prolonged	Normal or shortened	Low	Prolonged	Delayed formation of small friable clot
Fibrinolysis	Normal	Normal	Mildly prolonged	Mildly prolonged	Markedly shortened (<45 min.)	Often low	Prolonged	Lysis of clot begins within 6 hr.
Circulating heparin	Normal	Normal	Prolonged	Sometimes prolonged	Normal	Normal to decreased†	Prolonged	Delayed clot formation
Thrombocytopenia	Low	Prolonged	Normal	Normal	Normal	Normal	Normal	Poor clot retraction

*Dependent on platelet count.
†The fibrinogen assay is performed by converting fibrinogen to fibrin and measuring the latter. A large amount of heparin will interfere with fibrin formation.

lant such as heparin. Where the latter is suspected, protamine in doses varying from 5 to 30 μg. can be added to 5 tubes each containing 2 ml. of blood. In the presence of hyperheparinemia, protamine at one of these concentrations will correct the abnormal clotting time. If protamine is not available, 2 ml. of the patient's blood can be added to 2 ml. of blood from a normal subject with compatible type.† If the clotting time of the mixture is closer to that of the normal blood, then a factor deficiency is the probable diagnosis. On the other hand, if the clotting time of the mixture is closer to that of the patient's blood, then a circulating anticoagulant must be sought. When no clot forms and heparin is not a factor, a deficiency of fibrinogen and/or some other clotting factors is most likely at fault. Occasionally, extremely high fibrinolysin titers may cause this. The mixture of the patient's blood with an equal amount of normal compatible blood should distinguish between these 2 causes. In the presence of excessive fibrinolysin, the mixture will either clot and soon lyse or else will still fail to clot, depending on the magnitude of the fibrinolysin level.

Table 8-3 summarizes the results expected in these laboratory tests with each of the 4 coagulopathies under discussion.

Specific Therapy

Thrombocytopenia

If only the platelet count is abnormal and is below 50,000/mm.^{3}, then platelet packs, each containing platelets removed from 3 or 4 units of blood, or fresh whole blood may be given. Platelets stored by standard methods survive only a short time in vitro and should be used as soon after collection as possible. The amount necessary will be determined by the underlying cause of the thrombocytopenia. The platelets in fresh whole blood or in platelet packs under normal conditions survive up to 8 days after transfusion. However, during active bleeding, platelet sequestration due to septicemia or drug-induced immune thrombocytopenia, the platelet life-span may be shortened to several hours or less. The number of platelet packs necessary to stop bleeding can then be determined only by repeated assessments of the platelet count and by close inspection for recurrent bleeding. The cause of the thrombocytopenia should be vigorously sought and treated.

Hyperheparinemia

A prolonged thrombin time and an abnormally low fibrinogen assay can result from intravascular coagulation, fibrinolysis or hyperhepari-

†Since both bloods must be compatible and drawn nearly simultaneously, this procedure is somewhat impractical. It is, however, occasionally useful and consequently is described here. Both the mixing test and addition of protamine are difficult for untrained observers to evaluate and should be done by experienced personnel.

nemia. The existence of the last should first be excluded in all patients to whom heparin has been administered. This is best done by repeating the thrombin time using aliquots of the patient's plasma to which various amounts of protamine has been added. The thrombin time will be corrected by protamine if excess heparin is present. Protamine should then be administered to the patient in a dose calculated from the amount required to correct the thrombin time of an aliquot of the patient's plasma. The thrombin time repeated shortly after protamine administration will indicate whether or not the dose was adequate. When excess circulating heparin is strongly suspected and a protamine titration cannot readily be done, 0.25 mg. of protamine is given for each 100 units of heparin which had been administered. The thrombin time is then repeated. If only partial correction occurs, this dose or a smaller dose is repeated. If the thrombin time is unaffected, then it is unlikely that excess heparin was at fault. This test should be done cautiously and only when hyperheparinemia is strongly suspected, because in the absence of excess heparin protamine can bind thrombin and further aggravate bleeding.

Intravascular Coagulation

The differentiation between intravascular coagulation and primary fibrinolysis is one which commonly faces the clinician. In both conditions, the thrombin time is prolonged. Thrombocytopenia occurs frequently during intravascular coagulation but not with primary fibrinolysis. The fibrinogen titer is usually reduced in both conditions. However, decreases to levels below 100 mg./100 ml. occur less commonly as a result of fibrinolysis than with intravascular coagulation. The euglobulin lysis time is abnormally short in both conditions but is commonly reduced to levels compatible with hemorrhage (<45 minutes) with primary fibrinolysis and only rarely with intravascular coagulation.

The provisional diagnosis of either intravascular coagulation or of fibrinolysis, made on the basis of the tests described, can be further documented by a search for fibrinogen split products in the blood. Fibrinogen split products are formed by the enzymatic breakdown of fibrinogen by fibrinolysin and can be detected by immunologic techniques. The presence of fibrinogen split products in the circulation in the absence of a markedly shortened euglobulin lysis time (<45 minutes) strongly favors the existence of intravascular coagulation with reactive local fibrinolysis. (The soluble fibrinogen breakdown products are released into the circulation by the action of fibrinolysin on fibrinogen at the site of fibrin deposition.) At times the presence of fibrinogen breakdown products is the only indication of intravascular coagulation, since consumption of clotting factors may be compensated by their more rapid production. This is more likely to occur in the less acute varieties of the disorder. Specific assays of factors V and VIII are helpful, since these factors are more consistently and severely depressed by intravascular coagulation than by fibrinolysis. Also, the detection of increased cryofibrinogen in the plasma, although nonspecific, provides evidence for the occurrence of intravascular coagulation. The cryofibrinogen is likely to include fibrinogen-fibrin monomer complexes due to excess thrombin activity. Other tests to detect these soluble complexes are under development and promise to be useful in the early detection of intravascular coagulation. Inspection of the morphology of erythrocytes in the peripheral blood smear may reveal the presence of schistocytes and microspherocytes in patients with intravascular coagulation.

Treatment of bleeding resulting from intravascular coagulation or from fibrinolysis cannot be standardized but must be specially tailored to fit each clinical situation. With intravascular coagulation there is great variability in the degree of depletion of the various factors relative to each other as well as in the ease and speed with which the cause of intravascular coagulation is eliminated. Therapy of bleeding due to intravascular coagulation should be directed first toward eliminating the underlying cause of clot formation and simultaneously to replacing those factors which are most severely depleted. In circumstances in which clot formation is severe and the cause is unlikely to be removed within several hours, intravascular coagulation per se must be treated by heparin infusion.

When fibrinogen is severely depleted during clot formation, as evidenced by a plasma fibrinogen concentration below 100 mg./100 ml., replacement in the form of a fibrinogen concentrate should be given. The amount necessary to raise the plasma concentration to 300 mg./100 ml. can easily be calculated.* This amount is diluted in about 300 ml. of saline and infused over about 30 minutes. If possible, determination of the fibrinogen concentration should be repeated 15 minutes later and at 6-hour intervals thereafter to determine its rate of disappearance. This provides an indication of the extent of consumption and whether or not the process is subsiding. Normally 15–25% of the infused fibrinogen disappears daily. When fibrinogen continues to be consumed rapidly, heparin must be administered without delay. Continued administration of fibrinogen in the presence of intravascular coagulation may aggravate the condition.

Severe depletion of factors V and VIII can be corrected by giving fresh whole plasma. The diagnosis of significant factor V or VIII deficiency cannot be made from the prothrombin time or the partial thromboplastin time in the presence of a low fibrinogen level. Under these circumstances, specific assays for these factors should be per-

---

*Subtract the patient's fibrinogen concentration from 300 mg./100 ml. Multiply this by 0.4 times the patient's weight in kilograms to obtain the appropriate fibrinogen deficit in milligrams.

formed. Bleeding cannot be attributed to depletion of factors V and VIII unless their plasma levels fall to less than 20% of normal. The amount of fresh plasma necessary to raise the plasma titer to over 20% can be easily calculated assuming each milliliter of fresh plasma contains 1 unit of these factors. Accordingly, a volume of plasma equivalent to 20% of the plasma volume will be required to raise the titer of a patient with no detectable factor activity to the acceptable level.

When the cause of intravascular clotting can be rapidly removed, which is the case in many obstetric problems, such as abruptio placentae or septic abortion, heparin therapy is often not necessary unless the consumption of fibrinogen, platelets and factors V and VIII is too rapid to permit adequate replacement. Heparin therapy is also unnecessary when intravascular coagulation is due to a hemolytic transfusion reaction. Exchange transfusion will often remove the mismatched cells and thereby the source of thromboplastin, which is triggering coagulation. Intravascular coagulation induced by extracorporeal circulation is usually self-limited and of short duration after discontinuing the procedure. However, if intravascular coagulation continues uninterrupted (as evidenced by rapid clearance of fibrinogen or other clotting factors) for more than 5 or 6 hours, then the danger of complications due to fibrin emboli is increased by continued infusions of fibrinogen. Under these circumstances heparin should be injected in the usual therapeutic dose of about 100 units/kg. every 4–6 hours. When the cause of coagulation is one which cannot predictably be corrected rapidly, such as septicemia or carcinomatosis, heparin should be started as soon as the diagnosis is made. After intravascular coagulation is halted, the levels of plasma fibrinogen, factor V and VIII rapidly return to normal, often within 24 hours. The platelet count, however, may recover more slowly.

Fibrinolysis

Excess fibrinolysis can be treated with ϵ-aminocaproic acid, a compound which interferes with the activation of plasminogen. This agent should be used only if the euglobulin lysis time is markedly shortened. Less severe changes in results of this test occur frequently in response to various stimuli and are unlikely to indicate fibrinolysin titers, which are capable of causing hemorrhage. ϵ-aminocaproic acid is given by infusing a loading dose of 4–5 Gm. within the first half hour, followed by 1 Gm. hourly in a continuous intravenous drip. The effect is monitored by clinical observation. If bleeding continues for several hours after onset of therapy, the diagnosis of the cause of bleeding should be reconsidered and therapy stopped. After the cause of excess fibrinolysis is corrected, administration of ϵ-aminocaproic acid should be discontinued. The plasma fibrinolysin activity is then tested at frequent intervals and, if necessary, ϵ-aminocaproic acid infusion restarted. In chronic fibrinolysis, ε-aminocaproic acid can be administered orally.

Where there is doubt as to whether intravascular coagulation or fibrinolysis is responsible for bleeding or when both mechanisms coexist, ε-aminocaproic acid should only be used concurrently with heparin. ε-aminocaproic acid, by interfering with lysis of fibrin, can otherwise accelerate the appearance of thrombotic complications of intravascular coagulation.

Table 8-4 lists the various blood components used in the therapy of specific disorders.

TRANSFUSION THERAPY

Blood contains numerous components each with specialized and vital functions. The most important of these are: (1) red blood cells, whose chief function is to store oxygen and make it readily available to the tissues; (2) white blood cells, which have numerous functions, most related to the removal of foreign substances from the body; (3) platelets, which are necessary for normal blood coagulation; (4) albumin, which among other functions maintains the osmolarity of blood at a level that prevents excessive extravasation of fluid; (5) immunoglobulins, primarily involved in maintaining a normal immune response; (6) circulating clotting factors, including fibrinogen, which are necessary for blood coagulation, and (7) certain essential electrolytes, particularly calcium. Blood collected in acid citrate dextrose solution and stored for up to 3 weeks in a blood bank contains near normal amounts of all these components except for platelets, some labile clotting factors (factors V and VIII) and calcium. Under ideal circumstances each unit of blood collected in a blood bank would be separated into its various components. Replacement therapy would then consist of ordering only those components which patients specifically require (Table 8-4). This would afford maximum use of each unit of blood collected and tend to reduce the incidence of both transfusion reactions and hepatitis. Complete component therapy is currently beyond the scope of most blood banks, but should be utilized to the greatest extent that is practical.

Hemorrhage occurring during and after surgery results first in hypovolemia and later in hypoxia due to depletion of circulating erythrocytes. Hypocalcemia becomes clinically important only after the loss and replacement of 8 or 9 units of blood within a relatively short time. Depletion of clotting factors (platelets and labile factors) is rarely significant unless 15 or more units of blood are lost within a period of 24 hours or less.

Hypovolemia stimulates reflex vasoconstriction in blood vessels leading to the skin, the splanchnic bed and the kidneys as well as tachy-

TABLE 8-4. – BLOOD COMPONENTS USED IN THERAPY

BLOOD OR BLOOD COMPONENTS	SOME INDICATIONS FOR USE	TIME REQUIRED BY BLOOD BANK TO PREPARE	HEPATITIS RISK	REMARKS
Citrated whole blood (human), ACD preservative	Acute blood loss, symptoms of hypovolemia and hypoxia, some value in proconvertin (factor VII) or PTC (factor IX) deficiency	At least 60 min. for routine cross-match	Average	After 4 days' storage, all labile clotting factors and platelets are lacking. Good up to and including 21 days' storage at 4–6 C.
Fresh whole blood (human), less than 6 hr. old	Never use for symptoms of blood loss alone. For any plasmatic deficiency and moderate thrombocytopenia	Depending on available donors, time to procure and bleed a suitable donor plus laboratory time of at least 1 hr.	Average	Make arrangements with blood bank first; must be infused within 3 hr. of preparation
Packed red cells (human)	Preferred for chronic anemia from neoplasms, chronic nephritis, cirrhosis, cardiac disease, aplastic anemia, CO poisoning, exchange transfusion and severe burns	At least 60 min. for routine cross-match	Average	Usually low potassium and ammonia content; less cost to patient; good up to 21 days' storage at 4–6 C.
Washed cells (washed packed cells)	For multiple transfusions over a long period. Plasma and buffy layer eliminated	3 hr. additional time	Less than average	Available only on request to medical director; Should be infused within 1 hr. after preparation
Packed red cells (human), leukocyte poor	For patients with demonstrable leukoagglutinins	1 hr. additional time	Average	For patients who receive multiple transfusions and have reactions
Resuspended red cells (human)	For ease of administration; normal saline added	10–15 min. additional time	Average	Should be infused within 3 hr. after preparation
Albumin (human)	Hypovolemia and hemoconcentration	Available immediately	None	Available as 5% or 25% solution
Plasma, type specific, less than 21 days old	Hypovolemia, some value in proconvertin (factor VII) or PTC (factor IX) deficiency; burn cases	At least 2 hr. for separation of cells and cross-match	Average	All labile clotting factors and platelets lacking
Single-donor plasma (human), type specific, fresh frozen plasma	For all plasmatic clotting deficiencies, but primarily for hemophilia A where AHG is needed. Protein and stable factors present 5 years (see	30 min. to thaw and at least 50 min. for routine cross-match if desired	Average	Has twice clotting factors of fresh whole blood, but platelets are lacking

Platelet rich plasma, type specific	Same as fresh blood. Has twice plasmatic clotting factors and double number of platelets per unit	Depending on available donors, 4 hr. after procurement of donor	Average	Make arrangements with blood bank first; infuse patient as quickly as possible after delivery of components to hospital; better than fresh blood for thrombocytopenia
Platelet concentrate, fresh	Indicated mainly in children and infants with severe thrombocytopenia when smaller blood volume precludes giving 4 units of fresh platelet rich liquid plasma	Depending on available donors, at least 4 hr. laboratory time after procurement of donor	Average	Make arrangements with blood bank first; infuse patient as quickly as possible after delivery of components to hospital; viable platelets in small total volume, probably slightly damaged by mechanics of concentration; no plasma coagulation factors
AHF (factor VIII)	Primarily for hemophilia A where AHG is needed	Available immediately	None	Amount of AHF varies with type of preparation; dosage must be calculated for each usage
PTC (factor IX)	Primarily for hemophilia B (Christmas disease, factor IX deficiency)	Available immediately	None	Contains 500 units factor IX and some factor II, VII and X; dosage must be calculated for each usage
Fibrinogen (factor I)	Defibrination syndromes	Available immediately	Less than average	Individual dosage varies from 2 to 6 Gm. and must be calculated for each infusion

General Notes

1. Sample required by blood bank for cross-matching consists of 8 ml. clotted blood, properly labeled. Cross-match is optional for single-donor plasma, platelet rich plasma and platelet concentrate.
2. Hepatitis risk is indicated relative to that of a single unit of whole blood.
3. Bleeding partially or entirely due to circulating anticoagulants or pathologic activity requires special treatment. Refer to section, Coagulation Disorders during and after Surgery.
4. None of the listed materials is useful in correcting very low fibrinogen level.
5. Do not use whole blood over 5 days old for hemodialysis. Eighty percent of red cells have normal viability in patients although cells are 21 days old (washed red cells are preferable if available).

cardia to maintain adequate blood flow to the brain and heart. Accordingly, tachycardia, a decrease in urine output and peripheral pallor may be the first signs of internal bleeding. With decompensation of these defense mechanisms, decrease in mentation and hypotension result. Hypovolemia per se can be treated by infusion of albumin solutions or of dextran. In the otherwise normal adult, depletion of the red cell mass to 40% of normal is tolerated as long as hypovolemia is corrected. The patient with coronary or cerebrovascular insufficiency, of course, requires a greater red cell mass to avoid serious hypoxia to these vulnerable tissues. Theoretically, therefore, if the cause of hemorrhage could be definitely brought under control after the loss of 3 units or less of blood, volume replacement alone would be sufficient. This is not practical therapy for most patients with surgical bleeding, since the possibility of recurrent or continued bleeding makes it unsafe to maintain patients at a level of only borderline compensation. With extensive hemorrhage, replacement therapy requires whole blood or both albumin solution and packed red cells. To avoid hypocalcemia, an ampule of calcium gluconate or chloride should be given after each 6 units of blood. After transfusion of 10 units of stored blood within 24 hours, replacement of platelets and labile clotting factors is indicated by giving fresh whole blood or frozen plasma and platelet concentrates. The replacement of clotting factors, specifically depleted by surgically acquired coagulation disorders, was discussed in the previous section.

Satisfactory response to replacement therapy must be monitored by the urinary output, the hemoglobin concentration or the hematocrit reading, the pulse and the blood pressure. Overcorrection of hypovolemia should be particularly avoided in patients with limited cardiac reserve and in those with decreased renal function. This can usually be done by close observation of the jugular venous pressure, but is better performed by monitoring with a central venous catheter.

Complications of Transfusion Therapy and their Management

With increasingly more complicated surgical procedures, use of blood transfusion has increased considerably and has made the complications of such transfusion more common. Well over 5,000,000 transfusions are given annually in the United States; 80–90% of these are given to surgical patients. With a complication frequency of about 5%, we will probably face this problem while caring for postoperative patients.

The reasons for an incidence rate of about 5% become obvious when one considers the potential sources of difficulty. (1) We speak of transfusing with compatible blood, but by this mean only that when donor and recipient bloods are mixed, there is no visible reaction in the test tube. (2) To arrive at this compatibility, a number of technical manipulations must be performed and, despite elaborate efforts to protect against them, errors do occur. (3) Though donors are screened for a variety of diseases, infections and allergies, occasionally there is some undesirable component in the donor's blood. (4) Finally, in spite of elaborate precautions, there is occasionally bacterial or chemical contamination of the blood or equipment used to transfuse it.

In addition, it must be recognized that complications are more apt to arise in a patient having certain underlying conditions, such as blood dyscrasias, "autoimmune" diseases or a previous history of multiple transfusions. In fact, it is well known that many patients with a history of multiple transfusions will react adversely to every transfusion, and foreknowledge of this may be quite helpful in dealing with such a patient. This discussion serves to point up the fact that knowledge of the patient's transfusion history is an important aspect of a physician's effort to deal with the untoward effects of blood transfusion, and it should be given no less attention than the drug reaction history.

The complications surrounding transfusion of whole blood or blood components can be classified in a number of ways: (1) immediate—febrile reactions, (2) delayed—hepatitis, (3) major—acute anuria and (4) minor—urticaria. Although delayed complications such as hepatitis or malaria are of serious consequence, complications relating to the intensive care of surgical patients are those which occur at the time of or shortly after transfusion and are generally known as "transfusion reactions." For this reason we shall confine ourselves to a discussion of this group of complications. Table 8-5 lists the most frequently encountered symptoms and signs of transfusion reactions.

Since the patients under consideration are usually unconscious or at least partially so, most of the subjective components such as nausea, chills, back pain, pruritus, dyspnea, substernal pressure and headache will be missing. As a result, only the objective components and the more serious reactions will manifest themselves. This is an important consideration, because while subjective components often occur in reactions to compatible blood, they occur with twice the frequency in more serious reactions to incompatible blood where the risk of hemolysis is greater. In the conscious patient subjective components provide a forewarning of possible serious consequences; deprived of this forewarning, the physician caring for unconscious patients must be alert to the earliest signs of a transfusion reaction and be ready to institute appropriate therapy without delay.

TABLE 8-5.—FREQUENCY OF REPORTED SYMPTOMS AND SIGNS IN TRANSFUSION REACTIONS

	%		%
Chill	60	Nausea and vomiting	10
Temperature elevations	50	Lumbar pain	10
Pruritus and urticaria	40	Red urine	10
Increased pulse rate	30	Shock (decreased BP)	5
Tightness in chest	10	Rales	5
Dyspnea	10	Jaundice	5

Transfusion reactions can be broadly categorized as: (1) febrile, (2) allergic, (3) hemolytic and (4) those related to the quantity of blood transfused. As can be determined from Table 8-5, these 4 types are definitely not mutually exclusive and frequently occur together. However, this classification is useful since reactions occur roughly in that order of frequency, and each type requires a different modality of therapy.

Certain general principles of evaluation should be applied to all transfusion reactions, regardless of their nature, because there is no way to determine that the minor forms, such as febrile or urticarial reactions, will not be accompanied by the more severe, life-threatening, hemolytic reactions. These principles can be applied in the following stepwise fashion.

Evaluation of Reaction

1. Stop the transfusion! Compare the serial number on the unit of blood and the unit serial number recorded on the transfusion form to make sure the statement of compatibility applies to the unit in question. Check the name on the transfusion form to make sure that the blood being given was meant for that patient. In addition, comparison of the transfusion forms from previously administered blood with that of the unit in question may give you sufficient information to begin treatment for a hemolytic reaction in the case of gross incompatibility, for example, when type A blood is given to a type O recipient. While minor forms such as a febrile or urticarial reaction may not require termination of the transfusion, it is worthwhile pausing to assess the situation and if there is no evidence of a hemolytic reaction or other serious consequences, the transfusion may be resumed.
2. Return the unit of blood to the blood bank for re-cross-match with the recipient's pretransfusion specimen.
3. Draw a sample of clotted blood for restudy by the blood bank and a sample of anticoagulated blood for a plasma hemoglobin determination.
4. Obtain a fresh sample of urine for hemoglobin determination. It is important that the urine obtained be produced during the transfusion reaction period in order to obtain valid information about the quantity of hemoglobin cleared by the kidney as a result of the reaction.
5. Proceed with the appropriate therapy.

Febrile Reactions

Febrile reactions are manifest by a chill, which may vary from a slight chilly sensation followed by a fever of 100 F. to a severe chill with rigor accompanied by a rise in temperature to 104 F.

Febrile reactions are due to a variety of factors. The problem of pyrogenic contaminants of solutions and administration apparatus, formerly a major cause of febrile reactions, has been reduced considerably by improvements in manufacturing and processing techniques and the use of disposable equipment. The causative agents in these circumstances are high molecular weight polysaccharides, which are products of bacterial growth and are unaffected by standard sterilization techniques.

Demonstration of the existence of leukoagglutinins in some patients experiencing febrile reactions has led to the recognition that in multiply-transfused patients there is an association of febrile reaction and leukoagglutinins in about 80% of the cases. However, in studies of febrile reactions, which include patients receiving single transfusions as well, only about 10–15% have demonstrable leukoagglutinins. This suggests that while leukoagglutinins are one cause for febrile reactions, they are not the most frequent cause, and there may be others which are poorly understood. As noted before, this may be the only reaction to the transfusion and as such will be overlooked in the unconscious or semi-conscious patient, unless it is of a more severe form. The temperature elevation is most frequently abrupt and short lived; it commences during the transfusion and lasts 6–8 hours, with return to normal without sequelae. The majority of febrile reactions are not accompanied by hemolysis and, as such, are not serious and do not require any specific therapy. Rarely a reaction of severe hyperpyrexia will occur and will require more aggressive therapy, such as termination of the transfusion and/or the use of hypothermia. If the patient is conscious, subjective complaints can be severe enough to require some relief. This can be accomplished with an intravenous or intramuscular injection of 15–30 mg. codeine or 8–15 mg. morphine.

Allergic Reactions

Allergic manifestations as isolated reactions to transfusions are relatively frequent and, conversely, are only rarely serious. These reactions are characterized by urticaria, pruritus and occasionally facial edema. The urticaria may be widespread or it may be extremely localized and may well be missed unless the patient is inspected closely. On occasion, external wheals may be accompanied by edema of the larynx or soft palate, resulting in catastrophic airway obstruction. These, along with the more rarely occurring angioneurotic edema and bronchial asthma, are the most serious aspects of the allergic reaction.

Allergic reactions may result from either of the following mechanisms: (1) Transfusion with the donor blood of reagins, which have a specificity for circulating antigens in the recipient, for example, anti-penicillin antibodies transfused into a patient receiving penicillin. (2) Transfusion of antigens in the donor plasma to which the recipient has been sensitized.

The first of these mechanisms is circumvented to some extent by careful screening of donors for an allergic history. The second mechanism reflects an abnormality in the recipient and cannot be avoided. However, it has been shown that the frequency of reactions due to the second mechanism is much greater (75%) in recipients with a known history of atopy than in nonallergic individuals. This fact, too, points up the importance of the patient's history in the treatment of transfusion reactions.

The vigor with which treatment of allergic reactions is undertaken should be proportional to their severity. If the hives are localized, or few in number, no treatment is necessary. If they are widespread, the transfusion should be stopped and antihistamines administered parenterally. Administration of 10 mg. chlorpheniramine maleate (Chlor-Trimeton) intravenously or intramuscularly should suffice for moderately severe reactions and diphenhydramine hydrochloride (Benadryl), 50 mg. intravenously, should be adequate for the more severe forms. Though the information brochures provided with these drugs suggest adding them to the unit of blood, this practice is to be strongly discouraged because it is dangerous and unwarranted. The occurrence of angioneurotic edema, bronchial asthma or laryngeal edema requires use of aminophylline, 250 or 500 mg. slowly intravenously; epinephrine, 0.5 to 1.0 ml. of 1:500 suspension in oil intramuscularly; or steroids, 100 mg. hydrocortisone intravenously over a 2–4 hour period.

Hemolytic Reactions

Hemolysis is the most frequently serious transfusion reaction and is fully a medical emergency. Its consequences are life threatening and require immediate recognition and institution of appropriate therapy without delay. For reasons not clearly understood, hemolytic reactions can vary from a mild reaction with a large volume of blood to a fatal reaction with as little as 10 ml. blood, but in general the severity is proportional to the amount of blood transfused. Thus it bears repeating that patients, especially unconscious patients, should be observed closely by a physician during the early phase of transfusion for each new unit of blood.

Generally, the severity of the reaction is related also to the nature of the incompatibility. Two types of hemolysis occur and produce different types of reactions. Extravascular hemolysis occurs when sensitized red cells (that is, those coated by antibody) are removed from circulation by the reticuloendothelial system. This seldom results in dramatic symptoms or life-threatening physiologic sequelae. Hemolysis usually manifests itself by failure of the hemoglobin to rise as expected, the production of a transiently positive Coombs' test and subsequent difficulty cross-matching blood for the patient. This produces clinical problems only when the rate of removal of cells by the reticuloendothelial system is such that frequent transfusions are necessary to maintain an adequate hemoglobin level. Frequent transfusion and rapid destruction leads eventually to a hyperbilirubinemia, which may produce jaundice and further obscure the patient's postoperative course. This type of reaction usually occurs in patients having received transfusions weeks or years before and is due to development of antibodies not detectable in vitro to a common, minor, red blood cell antigen.

The rapidity with which red blood cells are destroyed depends on whether or not the transfused cells are agglutinated within the vascular bed. If red cells become coated with antibody but do not agglutinate, they are removed by the spleen relatively slowly, and this form of extravascular hemolysis proceeds at a rate such that some sensitized cells may continue to circulate for 24 hours or longer. If, however, red cells are sensitized by antibodies capable of producing in vivo agglutination, the agglutinins will be cleared immediately by the reticuloendothelial system of the liver until its capacity is exceeded, then the agglutinins which escape the liver are cleared from the circulation by the lungs, resulting in total destruction of all cells administered. The clinical manifestations of this are the previously mentioned failure of the hemoglobin to increase, a more accelerated development of hyperbilirubinemia and difficulty in cross-matching units of blood.

The most severe form of reaction is associated with intravascular hemolysis, which is the result of sensitization of red cells by antibodies, usually complement dependent, which lyse them within the vascular bed. This reaction, which is immediate, results in liberation of hemoglobin and red cell stroma into the circulation and is responsible for physiologic changes which can produce shock, acute renal failure, hemorrhage and death. The mechanisms by which these effects occur may be potentiated by the underlying reasons for the transfusion, that is, oligemia, hypotension and hemorrhagic diathesis.

The pathogenesis of these effects is not fully understood, but it appears that precipitation of hemoglobin in acid urine and its deposition in the tubules may initiate renal failure in a kidney made ischemic and hypoxic by oligemia, dehydration and shock.

The onset of hypotension and shock is related, at least in part, to the physiologic response to circulating antigen-antibody complexes and diffuse intravascular coagulation resulting from activation of the clotting mechanism by these complexes—the generalized Shwartzman reaction.

Coagulation is initiated by the potent thromboplastic phospholipids contained in the stroma of lysed red cells. It has been estimated that 5 ml. of red cells or 10 ml. of whole blood contain enough thromboplastic substance to deplete 5,000 ml. of blood (all of the blood in a 70 kg. man) of clotting factors. Hemorrhage is due to such depletion of clotting factors and platelets as a result of the intense intravascular coagulation coupled with simultaneous activation of the fibrinolytic system.

The occurrence of a severe hemolytic transfusion reaction in a conscious patient is heralded by symptoms such as chills, fever, nausea, vomiting, headache, dyspnea, tachypnea, chest pain and flank pain. These are followed by hypotension, shock, purpura and generalized oozing from surgical wounds. This particular combination of symptoms and signs is fairly specific and points directly to the transfusion, which has usually been running but a few minutes. However, in the unconscious patient only the hypotension will manifest itself early and may at first be thought to be due to other causes, such as cardiac arrhythmia, pulmonary embolus or internal hemorrhage. In the postanesthesia recovery room, unless looked for, oozing from wounds will not be noticed until the blood has soaked the dressing. The occurrence of purpura with hypotension may then be the only signs of the transfusion reaction.

It is of the utmost importance that the possibility of a transfusion reaction in a patient be kept in mind by the physicians in attendance. Among the first questions asked with the occurrence of any adverse change in the patient's status should be, "Is this due to a transfusion reaction?" Further, with each unit that is infused, the patient should be watched minute by minute during the first 15–20 minutes of infusion. It bears repeating—with *each* unit.

The occurrence of a hemolytic transfusion reaction can be established by the detection of free hemoglobin in the plasma and urine. This can be exactly quantitated by a variety of means in the laboratory, but a rule of thumb for the bedside is helpful. Hemoglobin in the plasma cannot be detected by the naked eye until it exceeds 25 mg./100 ml. At this point the plasma is pink. At levels of 100 mg./100 ml. the plasma is red. A level of 25 mg./100 ml. will be reached by hemolyzing only 8–10 ml. of blood. Thus, the existence of any significant degree of hemolysis will be readily detected with the naked eye.

Also, as a result of binding to serum haptoglobin, hemoglobin will not appear in the urine until it exceeds 150 mg./100 ml. in plasma (hemoglobin from 50–60 ml. blood). The quantitation of urine hemoglobin and/or plasma hemoglobin permits a rough estimation of the amount of hemolysis which has taken place. As soon as a hemolytic reaction is suspected, the transfusion should be stopped, because it is well known that the severity of sequelae is proportional to the amount of blood infused.

Therapy is directed at specific expected sequelae. Hypovolemia should be corrected with 5% albumin. Osmotic diuresis can be achieved with administration of mannitol, 12.5–25 Gm. every 2 hours, to maintain a urine output of 50–100 ml./hour. Do not exceed 100 Gm. in a 24-hour period. Judicious use of sodium bicarbonate may be made to induce an alkaline urine which will prevent precipitation of hemoglobin. However, the additional sodium load is undesirable if anuria develops.

Hemorrhagic manifestations are usually due to a consumption coagulopathy and/or fibrinolysis, but in a massively transfused patient they may be complicated by dilutional effects. The nature of such hemorrhage should be determined and treated in the manner outlined earlier.

Reactions Related to Quantity of Blood Transfused

Patients receiving large amounts of stored blood face the possibility of dilution of platelets and labile plasma clotting factors (factors V and VIII) as well as handling large amounts of citrate anticoagulant and potassium, which has leaked from the red cell into the plasma during storage.

These may in their turn produce a hemorrhagic diathesis, a decrease in myocardial irritability and acidosis. Dilutional hemorrhagic diathesis can be corrected with fresh whole blood or platelets and fresh frozen plasma. Decrease in myocardial irritability may be treated by administered calcium gluconate. Increase in potassium may be treated with Kayexalate enemas or IV insulin and dextrose. Because of normal hepatic reserve, acidosis secondary to large amounts of citrate is likely only in patients with severe liver disease. In these patients the problem can be prevented or ameliorated with transfusions of heparinized blood.

Finally, the problem of circulatory overload can be minimized by using only packed red blood cells, restricting infused ancillary fluids and maintaining a high urine output. If hypertransfusion substantiated by blood volume determinations inadvertently occurs and results in congestive heart failure, the standard therapy for this is indicated. In addition, phlebotomy with or without plasmapheresis can be used to dramatically reduce the circulatory load.

9

Renal Failure

FRANKLIN D. SCHWARTZ, M.D.*

Associate Attending Physician, Rush-Presbyterian-St. Luke's Medical Center; Associate Professor of Medicine, University of Illinois Abraham Lincoln School of Medicine

ALTHOUGH ACUTE RENAL FAILURE can result from many diverse causes, it presents a distinct clinical syndrome with a characteristic histologic pattern, follows a well-defined clinical course and is amenable to certain specific forms of therapy. Sudden profound impairment or cessation of renal urinary function encompasses a number of pathologic conditions, including acute vasculitis, glomerular or interstitial nephritis and obstructive uropathy. However, the major emphasis in this chapter will be placed on the syndrome of post-traumatic renal failure seen in the surgical patient (acute tubular necrosis).

General anesthesia and surgery are frequently associated with an acute depression of renal function and are occasionally followed by oliguric renal failure. More appropriately, the acute oliguria and depression of renal function postoperatively should be categorized with other forms of post-traumatic renal failure, a syndrome first recognized during the early stages of World War II. Occurrence of renal failure following trauma or surgery is a catastrophic event. Renal insufficiency in these patients is coincident with an accelerated catabolic rate and rapid development of uremia. Whereas uremia itself is amenable to specific therapy, for example, peritoneal or hemodialysis, these patients are particularly susceptible to other postoperative complications, such as infection, delayed wound healing and bleeding tendencies. Ultimately, prognosis depends primarily on the underlying disease and concurrent complications. Despite refinements in treatment, which include more rapid resuscitation, increased attention to precise fluid, electrolyte and caloric requirements and increased use of dialysis, the overall mortality rate remains 50–60%. In recent years, because of the unfavora-

*Supported in part by United States Public Health Service Grants Nos. HE09851, HE02253, TIAM5525.

ble prognosis, more emphasis has been placed on prevention of acute renal failure in the surgical patient.

Renal Circulation and Function in Health

Physiologic variations in renal sodium and water handling can be explained by examination of the unique architecture and structure of the kidneys. Actually, the kidney is a compound organ made up of a large number of functioning components or nephrons, operating in parallel. Each nephron consists of a glomerulus and its tubule which includes a proximal convolution, loop of Henle and a distal convolution connecting to the collecting ducts. Each kidney contains approximately 1,000,000 nephrons, and the nephron population of the kidney may be divided into 2 groups (Fig. 9-1). First, the *cortical nephrons* whose glomeruli lie within the outer 2/3 of the cortex have a relatively simple

Fig. 9-1.—Diagrammatic representation of intrarenal circulation and nephron population. Note differences in both blood supply and structure of the tubules between cortical and juxtamedullary nephrons. (From Gordon, B. L., *et al.* [eds.]: *Clinical Cardiopulmonary Physiology* [3d ed.; New York: Grune & Stratton, Inc., 1969].)

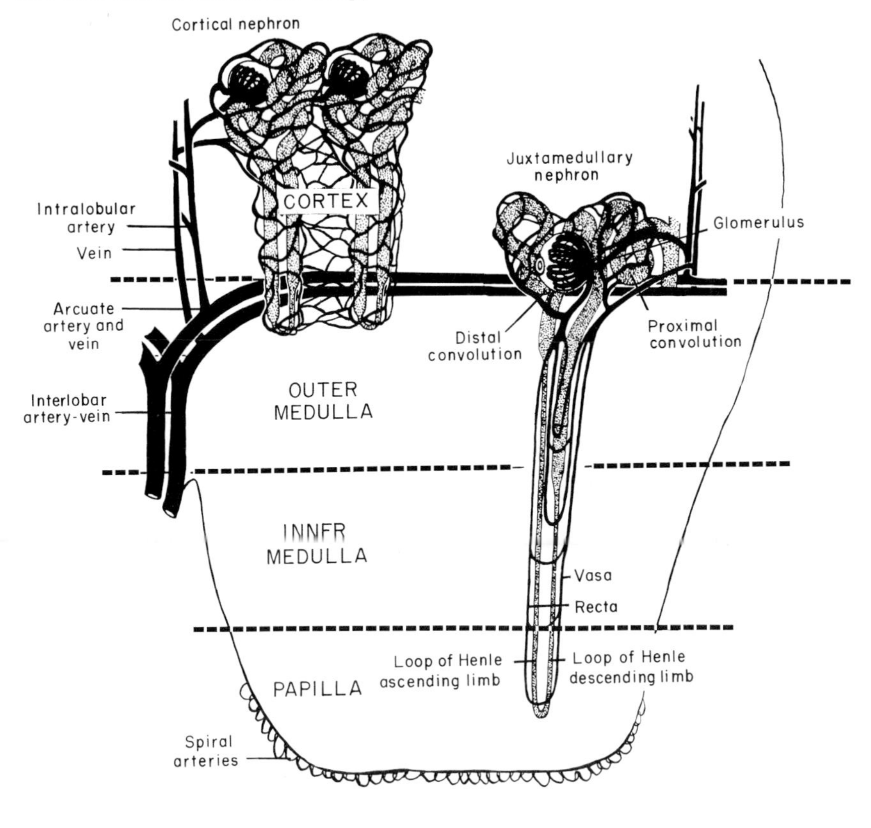

blood supply composed of capillary networks which communicate freely from glomerulus to glomerulus. In addition, these nephrons have relatively short loops of Henle. On the other hand, the *juxtamedullary nephrons*, whose glomeruli lie within the inner 1/3 of the cortex, have an individual blood supply and have relatively long loops of Henle which

Fig. 9-2. – Representative scintillation curves following injection of xenon-133 into the renal artery of a dog. The upper curve is from a normal animal, the lower following renal artery constriction. The values for components I and II, cortical and outer medullary flow, are calculated. Components III and IV represent flow to the papilla and to hilar and perirenal fat; these are of small magnitude. (From Gordon, B. L., *et al.*[eds.]: *Clinical Cardiopulmonary Physiology* [3d ed.; New York: Grune & Stratton, Inc., 1969].)

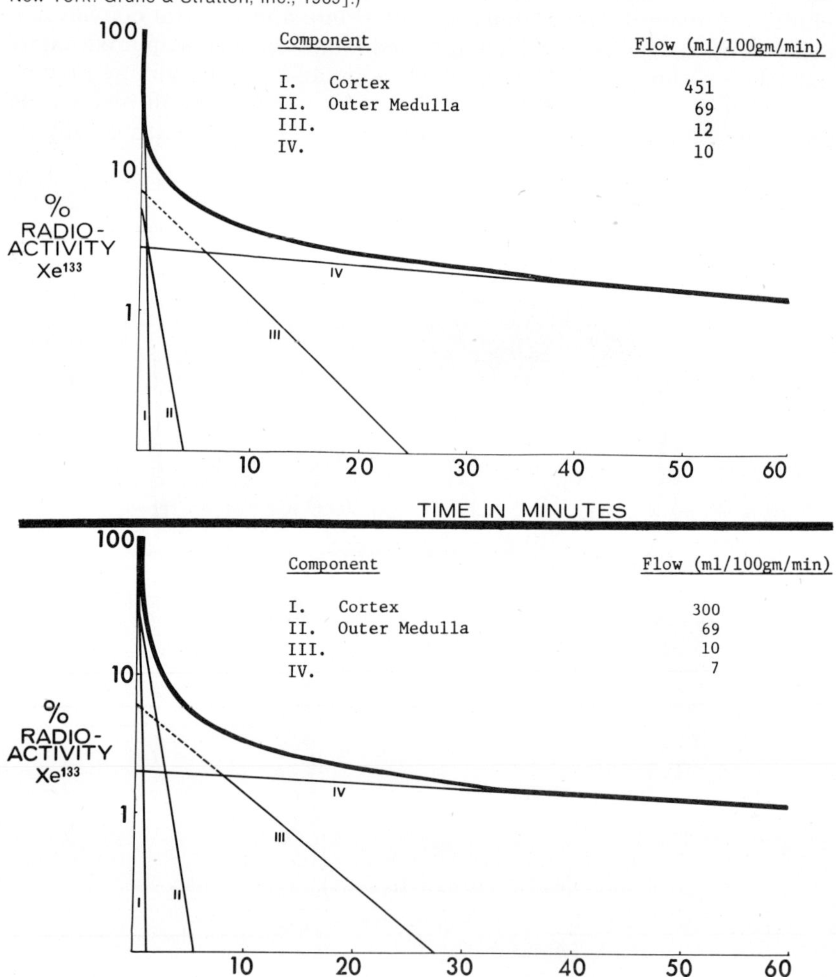

dip deeply into the renal medulla and papilla. Thus, one may expect that a simple redistribution of intrarenal blood flow away from the cortex to juxtamedullary nephrons might result in a more concentrated urine and enhanced retention of sodium. On the other hand, a shunting of blood supply to the outer cortex, whose nephrons have relatively short loops of Henle, should lead to diuresis and increased sodium excretion.

Normally, the total renal blood flow is approximately 1,200 ml./minute or 20–25% of the resting cardiac output (5–6 L./minute). Of this, approximately 80% of total flow supplies the renal cortex and about 20% supplies the medulla. The renal papilla, pelvis and perirenal structures have a relatively small blood supply. Recently, studies utilizing isotopically labeled inert gases, krypton-85 and xenon-133, along with external scintillation counting have allowed more precise determinations of intrarenal blood flow in health and disease (Fig. 9-2).[1] These techniques were developed in the experimental animal and have proved valuable in studying the renal circulation in man.

Renal Circulation in Disease

The general pattern of vascular response within the kidney suggests that the renal vasculature responds to a variety of stresses in a similar fashion. A common pattern of redistribution of intrarenal blood flow has been noted following hemorrhage, renal sympathetic nerve stimulation, carotid sinus stimulation, congestive heart failure and more recently has been noted in early and advanced stages of acute tubular necrosis.[14] In general, the initial effects include an increase in outer medullary blood flow resulting in relative cortical ischemia. Later, total renal blood flow is reduced. Further, this redistribution of intrarenal blood flow and relative cortical ischemia is closely associated with varying degrees of oliguria and sodium retention.

Etiology of Acute Renal Failure

The pathophysiology of acute tubular necrosis has been the subject of controversy for over 2 decades. Recent micropuncture studies have allowed determination of precise fluid and electrolyte handling of isolated segments of tubules from single nephrons. A major drawback to this method is that in mammals only cortical nephrons are readily accessible to micropuncture. Nevertheless, results after administration of nephrotoxic agents (for example, mercury) have suggested that the initial defect in these forms of acute renal failure is cessation of glomerular filtration, perhaps indicating a primary vascular injury. Also, this may represent an imbalance between the tone of the afferent and efferent arterioles entering and leaving the glomerulus, leading to slowing down or cessation of the circulation (sludging) to the innermost region of the medulla. On the other hand, similar studies during experimental hemorrhagic hypotension show initially a loss of integrity of the proximal tubular epithelium, leading to total reabsorption of glomerular filtrate, although filtration may continue for varying periods. Other studies, particularly with mismatched blood transfusions, have suggested actual tubular obstruction due to cast formation following reduction of glomerular filtration or tubular collapse secondary to increased renal interstitial fluid pressure. Undoubtedly, depending on the initiating process, several mechanisms are involved and more study is needed to thoroughly elucidate these.

Nevertheless, in all studies, general anesthesia has been shown to cause an acute depression of renal hemodynamics. These renal functional changes are initiated following premedication and are intensified by induction of anesthesia.[17] In studies done during the course of anesthesia, no influence was observed by the effects of surgery per se, regardless of the operative procedure. Multiple factors have been implicated in attempting to explain these observed effects of general anesthesia.[12,20] These factors include secretion of antidiuretic hormone (ADH), or of aldosterone or catecholamines; decreased cardiac output; decreased systemic and renal arterial pressure; decreased peripheral resistance; peripheral shunting of systemic blood flow with renal vascular constriction and changes in body temperature and acid-base balance. Though a number of factors are operating in the surgical patient, one may assume that the final common pathway leading to operative and postoperative oliguria, sodium retention and its more severe form, acute renal failure, is probably related to alterations of intrarenal blood flow.

Clinical Course of Acute Renal Failure

The Initiating Episode

In the beginning, the condition primarily responsible for the development of renal failure predominates, that is, trauma, septicemia, hypotension, hemorrhage, etc. The onset of oliguria may often be overlooked in the face of the more alarming manifestations of the presenting condition. It is important that the physician and nurse be aware and be alert to those conditions that predispose a patient to acute renal failure, particularly if the primary concern is prevention.

The period of acute renal failure usually begins with the onset of circulatory shock and is manifested by complete to varying degrees of anuria and/or oliguria. Oliguria we define arbitrarily as a urine volume of less than 300 ml./24 hours. Complete anuria occasionally occurs in acute tubular necrosis, but is more commonly seen in complete renal cortical necrosis or obstructive uropathy. In occasional patients, progressive uremia develops despite a relatively normal urine volume—"high output" renal failure. This condition most commonly resembles the early diuretic phase of acute renal failure and, in most cases, a transient period of oliguria or anuria can be documented.

The Period of Anuria or Oliguria

This period is manifested by a gradual to rapid rise in serum concentrations of substances normally excreted by the kidney. As the kidney is normally responsible for maintenance of the internal environment of the body—including water content, acid-base balance and also for excretion of end products of protein metabolism—the concentrations of these substances rise. Fats and carbohydrates are completely metabolized to carbon dioxide and water. However, the end products of protein metabolism are seen in increased concentrations in the serum of patients with renal insufficiency. These include urea (the major end product of protein metabolism), creatinine (the end product of muscle protein metabolism), uric acid (the end product of nucleoprotein metabolism), organic acids (particularly phosphate and sulphate), the intercellular cations (potassium and magnesium) and numerous other fragments of protein metabolism such as indoles, phenoles, indicans, peptides, polypeptides, amino acids, etc.

The average daily rise in blood urea nitrogen concentration varies greatly from patient to patient and is dependent on a number of factors other than renal function.[9] For assessment of renal function, the serum creatinine is much more reliable, because the increased serum concentration depends on decreased excretion alone. On the other hand, blood urea nitrogen concentration depends not only on the rate of excretion but also on dietary intake, rate of protein synthesis and on the rate of tissue catabolism. The absolute level of blood urea nitrogen in the surgical patient is dependent primarily on the rate of tissue catabolism. For example, in the uncomplicated patient with acute tubular necrosis secondary to ingestion of a nephrotoxic agent or hemolytic transfusion reaction, the average rise of blood urea nitrogen is about 20 mg./100 ml./day. In many postoperative patients, particularly when renal failure is precipitated by extensive trauma, heat stroke or burn, the daily rise in blood urea nitrogen may reach 100 to 150 mg./100 ml./day. These patients have been classified as hypercatabolic and carry, in general, a very poor prognosis. Based on experience during the Korean War,[23,24] it was suggested that rapid increments in serum phosphorus concentrations are also indicative of extensive tissue breakdown.

The substance originally thought responsible for production of the "uremic syndrome" was, of course, urea. However, studies have shown that the symptoms of uremia can be completely independent of the levels of blood urea. In fact, in chronic renal failure, uremic symptoms and clinical deterioration are usually well related to the level of the serum creatinine. The uremic syndrome is probably caused by retention of a variety of toxic substances, many of which remain to be identified.

Nevertheless, the substance or substances responsible for symptoms are of small molecular weight and they are probably freely dialyzable, in that anephric patients can be maintained in reasonable health by chronic hemodialysis.

The systemic manifestations of uremia are outlined in Table 9-1. At the cellular level, numerous specific defects in membrane transport, enzyme systems and intermediary metabolism have now been described. The uremic syndrome is manifest by deranged function of every organ system.

CENTRAL NERVOUS SYSTEM.—Early manifestations are agitation, shortening of attention span and some loss of memory. Later, these are followed by apathy, delirium and eventually coma. The electroencephalogram is commonly abnormal in the patient with uremia. These abnormalities are probably due to a combination of overhydration; electrolyte imbalance, particularly hyponatremia, and also direct effects of uremic toxins. Uremic convulsions are usually preterminal and are often preceded by increasing agitation and muscle twitching. More commonly, they are of the grand mal type, although sometimes there are jacksonian features.

PERIPHERAL NERVOUS SYSTEM.—Peripheral neuropathy is quite common in chronic renal failure and appears to be related to duration rather than severity of uremia. Sensory nerves are primarily involved, resulting in paresthesias and the typical "burning foot" syndrome characteristic of uremic neuropathy. Here, the patient complains of severe burning involving the dorsum of the foot. The functional impairment is usually bilateral and symmetrical. Even in the absence of subjective symptoms or signs, nerve conduction times are prolonged in almost all patients with advanced renal insufficiency. In severe cases, motor neuropathy may develop and is frequently manifested as a foot drop; in these cases this may progress to produce a syndrome resembling transverse myelitis.

TABLE 9-1.—ACUTE RENAL FAILURE—SYSTEMIC MANIFESTATIONS

System	Manifestations
Neurologic:	Central—apathy, delirium, coma, convulsions Peripheral—paresthesia, "burning feet," foot drop
Hematologic:	Anemia, bleeding diathesis
Cardiovascular:	Pericarditis, myocarditis, hypertension
Respiratory:	Uremic pneumonitis, pleuritis
Gastrointestinal:	Anorexia, nausea, vomiting, gastritis, colitis, parotitis
Cutaneous:	Pruritus, uremic frost
Musculoskeletal:	Osteoporosis, secondary hyperparathyroidism, pseudo-gout, metastatic calcification
Ocular:	Conjunctivitis, retinal detachment
Systemic:	Acidosis, glucose intolerance, susceptibility to infection

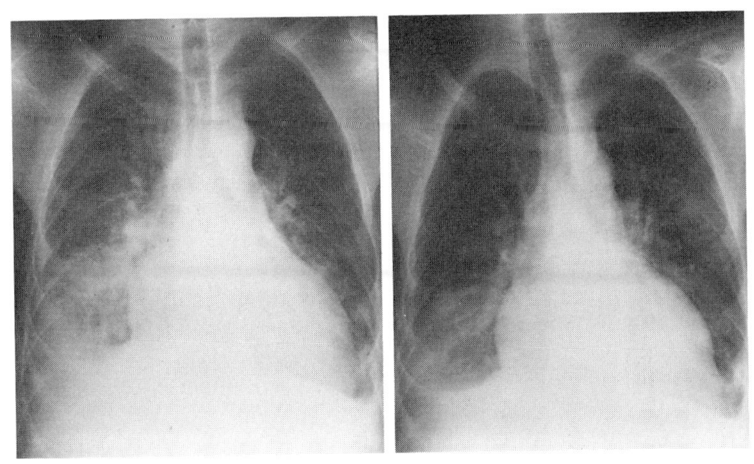

Fig. 9-3.—Chest x-rays of a patient with acute renal failure before, **left**, and after, **right**, 4 hours of peritoneal dialysis with extraction of approximately 3 L. fluid. The characteristic "butterfly" infiltrate of uremic pneumonitis clears rapidly with dehydration. There is no significant change in cardiac contour.

Hematologic system.—Anemia and increased bleeding tendency are common in acute renal failure. Leukocytosis is common in the absence of overt infection. The anemia is caused by a combination of factors. These include decreased red cell survival and hemolysis due to abnormal erythrocyte metabolism, deficiency of erythropoietin production and a direct depressant effect of uremic toxins on the bone marrow. One specific abnormality in platelet function has been identified—a deficiency in platelet factor III, which is normally responsible for adhesiveness of platelets in early formation of the clot. In part, the bleeding diathesis may be due to increased vascular permeability.

Cardiovascular system.—At one time, uremic pericarditis was felt to be an irreversible and terminal event. However, this entity can be seen early and responds reasonably well to frequent repeated dialysis. Hemopericardium with tamponade is not uncommon and should be suspected in the patient whose pericardial rub has disappeared, and who has developed increasing signs of acute congestive heart failure. Uremia and systemic acidosis contribute to diminished myocardial function, producing a toxic myocardiopathy.

Hypertension is common in acute renal failure and can be a devastating component of chronic renal insufficiency. Severe hypertension may be partially due to increased renin production by the ischemic kidney, although overhydration plays a significant role.

Respiratory system.—Classic uremic pneumonitis (Fig. 9-3) probably represents no more than pulmonary edema. Most pathologists agree that it cannot be distinguished histologically from pulmonary edema. Also, this picture responds readily to dialysis and correction of overhydration. The etiology is probably a combination of congestive heart failure with increased pulmonary vascular permeability. Uremic pleuritis is also common, particularly in patients with long-standing renal failure, and may lead to organization with chronic pleuritis and some degree of respiratory insufficiency.

GASTROINTESTINAL SYSTEM.—The earliest symptom is anorexia accompanied by varying degrees of weight loss, followed by nausea and vomiting, particularly upon arising. Characteristically, the small bowel is uninvolved in uremia and major manifestations are confined to the stomach and colon. These areas, particularly the colon, normally have some secretory function, particularly for urea and heavy metals. In the absence of renal excretion, increased gastrointestinal secretion of these substances takes place, resulting in local irritation. Uremic gastritis and colitis can be severe and healing may be delayed despite intensive conservative measures and dialysis. One patient had to undergo a total colectomy because of intractable bleeding some time after he had recovered from acute renal failure. In the same manner, the salivary glands also secrete urea and heavy metals in significant amounts, so parotitis and stomatitis are commonly observed. In fact, parotitis with secondary septicemia is an occasional cause of death that can be prevented by strict attention to oral hygiene.

INTEGUMENTARY SYSTEM.—Pruritus is a common symptom in patients with chronic disease and can become debilitating. Recent investigations have suggested that pruritus is more common in patients with severe secondary hyperparathyroidism, and pruritus in some patients has responded to subtotal or total parathyroidectomy. Whether the pruritus is a direct effect of parathormone or is due to increased calcium content of the skin is still unknown. Classic uremic frost is merely the deposition of urea crystals on the skin due to enhanced urea elimination in sweat. The sauna bath has proved to be an interesting and effective adjunct to hemodialysis in the therapy of terminal renal failure. This accomplishes two functions: (1) correction of overhydration and (2) increased cutaneous excretion of urea.

MUSCULOSKELETAL SYSTEM.—All patients with renal insufficiency have some degree of hyperparathyroidism as determined by immunoassay of parathormone. In addition, most are in negative calcium balance due to failure of the kidney to compensate for decreased intestinal absorption of calcium. Diminished intestinal absorption is due to a vitamin D resistance, probably representing abnormal metabolism of the active metabolites. The bone disease seen in uremia varies from osteoporosis or osteomalacia to a full-blown osteitis fibrosis cystica. The precise mechanism for bone disease in any particular patient is still unknown. Many with long-standing disease develop a goutlike picture which is actually "pseudogout" due to deposition of calcium phosphate in soft tissue, particularly in tendons.

OCULAR SYSTEM.—A severe conjunctivitis—the "red eye" of uremia – is caused by precipitation of calcium phosphate crystals in the conjunctiva and responds quickly to dialysis. Extensive retinal edema may be observed due to overhydration, hypertension and other factors and can result in retinal detachment.

SYSTEMIC MANIFESTATIONS. – Metabolic acidosis is due to failure of the kidney to excrete hydrogen ion and organic acid. Some degree of glucose intolerance is observed in all patients due to diminished peripheral utilization because of altered cell membrane permeability and interference with the actions of insulin.

There is a strong tendency, unfortunately, to blame uremia for any clinical deterioration of the patient with acute renal failure. It should be reemphasized that, clinically, uremia is rarely observed before the fifth day of oliguria.[23,24] This is particularly important in the postoperative patient, and a search should be made for other pathologic processes such as muscle necrosis, shock or generalized sepsis, which may be responsible for the observed symptoms. Further, each patient must be treated individually and the degree of susceptibility to biochemical abnormalities varies greatly. We have, for example, observed patients who are clinically uremic with a blood urea nitrogen of 90 mg./100 ml., in whom symptoms respond readily to dialysis. In others, the blood urea nitrogen may reach 200 – 250 mg./100 ml. in the absence of overt symptoms.

PERIOD OF DIURESIS

Classically, the period of oliguria or anuria lasts from 7 to 21 days. As mentioned, it may be extremely brief, lasting only a number of hours. At times this interval may last for 30 days or more with subsequent recovery of renal function.

At the conclusion of the oliguric period, diuresis may set in gradually, or abruptly, over a period of several days. During this time the patient's clinical condition may actually deteriorate, and confusion, vomiting, abdominal cramping and hyperreflexia associated with increasing azotemia may appear for the first time. In general, the blood urea nitrogen will continue to rise for 3 or 4 days after the onset of diuresis; it will then level off and gradually decrease. Not uncommonly, dialysis is required for relief of symptoms of uremia at this time despite the onset of diuresis. Further, while salt losing may not begin for 24 – 48 hours after the onset of diuresis, potassium loss is usually seen early, and hyperkalemia is no longer a problem. Onset of diuresis is associated with an outpouring of casts in the urine sediment.

In general, the magnitude of the diuresis depends on the prior state of hydration of the patient. In former years, when patients were generally overhydrated, it was not uncommon to see urine volumes of 8 – 10 L./day during this period. Now, urine volumes of more than 6 L./day are rarely seen. Nevertheless, these patients can become rapidly dehydrated and salt depleted, and strict attention must be accorded to fluid and electrolyte replacement. Most conveniently, urine output should be measured at 4–6 hour intervals. This should be replaced with an equal volume of one-half normal saline, plus 500 ml./day or 5% glucose and water to cover insensible losses. Supplemental potassium may be required, and serum electrolyte concentrations should be determined twice daily.

Renal function may not return completely for 3–6 months following an acute insult, and as expected, urinary concentrating ability is the last parameter to return to normal. Some individuals may have a degree of permanent functional impairment, as measured by a decreased glomerular filtration rate and renal blood flow with normal tubular function, suggesting loss of part of the total nephron population.

In general, the degree of return of renal function is related to the duration of the period of oliguria and/or anuria. In other words, the more benign the precipitating insult and the shorter the degree of oliguria, the more likely the patient is to regain totally normal renal function. More recent studies of renal biopsies in patients who originally presented with acute renal failure suggest that renal function and histology return completely to normal in the majority of cases.

Treatment of Acute Renal Failure

General Management

The postoperative patient in whom acute renal failure develops is gravely ill. While successful management requires intimate knowledge of the physiologic and therapeutic principles involved, careful attention to the more traditional aspects of supporting and nursing care is vital. Rarely, patients can be managed on the general surgical ward, but there is a definite advantage in having them in surgical intensive care or specialized renal failure units. In general, protective isolation is not required and, when possible, early ambulation and return to activity should be encouraged.

In former years, overhydration, acute potassium intoxication and uremia ranked as the leading causes of death in acute renal failure. These diseases have been largely circumvented by means of careful fluid restriction, development and use of effective cationic exchange resins and early dialysis. At present, the leading causes of death are infection, hemorrhage and complications of the underlying disease.

Overhydration can be prevented by limiting total fluid intake to 500 ml./day plus visible output. (Although average and insensible fluid losses average 800–900 ml./day, water of oxidation and water released from cells during starvation accounts for 300–400 ml.) The patient ideally should be weighed twice daily. When fluid restriction is adequate, approximately 1 lb./day should be lost due to catabolism of body tissue. If tolerated, fluids can be administered orally and can be supplemented by various modifications of the Giordano-Giovanetti diet.[11] The diet used is low protein (20–22 Gm. of high biologic activity) and supplies all essential amino acids with approximately 1,700 cal./day. There is evidence to show that even patients who have a significant rate of tissue breakdown can be kept in relatively normal nitrogen balance with this diet. In fact, via the liver-ammonia cycle, blood urea nitrogen can be reutilized for protein anabolism as a nonspecific nitrogen source. If oral alimentation is not possible, 500 ml. of 20% dextrose is administered daily to supply adequate carbohydrate for protein sparing. Caloric intake should be administered throughout the 24 hours because there may be a tendency toward hypoglycemia due to depleted glycogen stores. Any gastrointestinal losses due to drainage or other means may be replaced with one-half normal saline.

Perhaps the most outstanding and yet the least appreciated contribution of the Korean War medical experience with post-traumatic renal failure was the recognition that adequate debridement of devitalized tissue played an important role in the ultimate prognosis.[23,24] Experimentally, acute renal failure can be induced by trauma and production of devitalized tissue. Though difficult to prove clinically, patients in whom the oliguric and/or anuric phase of renal failure cleared shortly after amputation of a devitalized limb or debridement of necrotic tissue have been seen, for example, hysterectomy during acute renal failure secondary to septic abortion. Thus, all efforts should be made to restrain tissue breakdown and hypercatabolism.

Once the diagnosis of acute renal failure has been established, a Foley catheter should be avoided. Anoxia of any duration must be prevented, and use of an airway or tracheostomy should be considered early. Even mild anoxia can precipitate an acute hyperkalemic crisis and cardiac arrest, because intracellular potassium is released during acute acidosis in the presence of inadequate renal compensation.

Emergency Treatment

Hyperkalemia.—This is a common complication, particularly in the hypercatabolic surgical patient, and remains the commonest cause of sudden death in uremia. Specific measures to counteract hyperkalemia are outlined in Table 9-2. Administration of the various electrolyte and carbohydrate solutions can reverse myocardial toxicity in minutes. Acute correction of extracellular acidosis with sodium bicarbonate causes intracellular shift of potassium in exchange for hydrogen ion. Since potassium is also directly involved in glucose transport into the cell, this can be exploited by the administration of hypertonic glucose with insulin. Finally, the calcium ion exerts a direct antagonistic effect on myocardial conduction.

TABLE 9-2.—ACUTE RENAL FAILURE—MANAGEMENT OF HYPERKALEMIA

SUBSTANCE	DOSE	ONSET OF EFFECT	DURATION OF EFFECT
Prophylactic			
Kayexalate	10–20 Gm. oral or rectal	1–2 hr.	4–6 hr.
Acute hyperkalemia			
Calcium gluconate	2–10 Gm. I.V.	min.	30–60 min.
Sodium bicarbonate	45–90 mEq. I.V.	min.	1–2 hr.
Hypertonic glucose and insulin	25–50 Gm. I.V. 10–20 units	min.	2–4 hr.
Kayexalate	50–60 Gm. retention enema	30 min.	4–6 hr.

A somewhat delayed but more prolonged effect is obtained with the various cationic exchange resins, for example, Kayexalate, which have a greater affinity for potassium than other cations. Since the colon is the major site of potassium exchange, administration of these resins by a retention enema is effective most rapidly. Routinely, if tolerated, patients may be given these resins orally at the first signs of elevated serum potassium concentrations. Studies, particularly in hypercatabolic patients, suggest that ideally the serum potassium should be routinely maintained in the range of 3–4 mEq./L.

PULMONARY EDEMA.—In most cases, acute pulmonary edema is precipitated by excessive administration of parenteral fluids. However, severe hypertension and/or altered vascular permeability associated with uremia can contribute. Digitalis should be administered cautiously, if at all, due to limited excretion in patients with renal insufficiency. In addition, there is a hazard from arrhythmia in patients receiving digitalis following acute reductions of serum potassium by dialysis or other means. If conservative measures are unsuccessful, pulmonary edema represents a definite indication for early dialysis.

HYPERTENSIVE CRISES.—Accelerated hypertension is a frequent and prominent finding in acute renal failure. While this frequently subsides following removal of excess fluids by dialysis, specific drug treatment may be required. Most patients respond readily to parenteral administration of reserpine or ganglionic blocking agents such as pentolinium. The effects of drugs may be augmented by reduction of extracellular fluid and salt content by a combination of dialysis and restricted intake.

CONVULSIONS.—Uremic convulsions are most frequently grand mal in type but may have some jacksonian features. They are frequently preceded by increased irritability and muscle twitching. These signs are not related to hypocalcemia and do not respond to calcium infusion. The muscle twitching and seizures do respond to small doses of barbiturates. Secobarbital or amobarbital should be administered slowly intravenously. Usually 30–50 mg. of either drug is rapidly effective. Also diphenylhydantoin can be used in doses of 100 mg. either orally or intramuscularly 3–4 times daily.

Use of Drugs

All medications should be used with caution, because many drugs are excreted by the kidney, and toxic blood levels can be obtained using routine dosages. In some cases, renal and extrarenal excretion as well as removal by dialysis is known. Caution, however, should be exercised when this information is not available. In general, the dose of drugs normally excreted by the kidney should be significantly reduced. For example, the standard digitalizing dose of any digitalis preparation can usually be reduced 20–50%. In addition, maintenance doses of digitalis need be administered only every third to fourth day. Many of the commonly used antibiotics also require adjustment of dosage. Some drugs, however, do not rely on renal excretion primarily for elimination or detoxification, but are metabolized elsewhere, principally by the liver. These may be administered in standard dosage. As a general rule, most

TABLE 9-3.—Acute Renal Failure—Drug Administration

Class of Drugs	Drugs Requiring Reduced Dosage	Drugs Requiring No Modification of Dosage
Antibiotics	Streptomycin Kanamycin Colistin Tetracycline Chlortetracycline Nitrofurantoin Amphotericin Vancomycin	Penicillins Cephalothin Erythromycin Chloramphenicol Novobiocin
Cardiovascular drugs	Digitalis Procaine Procaine amide Guanethidine* Alpha-methyldopa* Reserpine*	Quinidine
Barbiturates	Phenobarbital Barbital	Secobarbital Amobarbital Pentobarbital Thiopental
Sedatives and tranquilizers	Chlorpromazine Prochlorperazine	Chloral hydrate Paraldehyde Meprobamate
Anticonvulsives	Phenobarbital	Diphenylhydantoin Trimethadione
Narcotics and analgesics	Morphine* Salicylates	Meperidine

*Probable requirement based on available data.

drugs are not removed by dialysis, and the interjection of peritoneal or hemodialysis should not alter the regimen for patients with renal failure. Caution must be used when administering such potentially nephrotoxic agents as colistin, kanamycin, etc. Table 9-3 gives a general outline for dosage of drugs in patients with acute renal failure.

Role of Dialysis in Acute Renal Failure

In general, dialysis is instituted for relief of signs and symptoms of impending uremia. Early hemodialysis may prevent many complications of acute renal failure and actually increase survival in post-traumatic cases.[19] Further, it is difficult at times to assess curious clinical findings as indicative of impending deterioration. Once deterioration begins, however, the course is frequently fulminating. Many patients are mildly obtunded and neuromuscular hyperirritability and anorexia may appear shortly before development of more severe clinical abnormalities. These symptoms can be controlled by early dialysis. On the other hand, there are patients in whom acute renal failure can be managed conservatively as outlined above. Most important, the use of dialysis should be used to supplement—not supersede—good medical and nursing management. Specific indications for dialysis are outlined in Table 9-4.

Peritoneal and hemodialysis are equally effective in reversing the symptoms of uremia and in correcting abnormal fluid-electrolyte and acid-base balance. Peritoneal dialysis is safe and relatively simple but carries some risk of infection. Though this procedure is less efficient for extraction of urea, creatinine and other nitrogenous substances, it is more efficient for removal of excessive fluid. At one time, presence of recent laparotomy, abdominal drains, fecal contamination and severe hypercatabolism were considered contraindications to peritoneal dialysis. In my experience, this procedure has been effective despite the presence of these conditions, and in many patients, it has been life saving.[16] Experimentally, peritoneal dialysis or lavage has been beneficial in the treatment of peritoneal fecal contamination and peritonitis, and these actually may be considered indications for, rather than contraindi-

TABLE 9-4.—ACUTE RENAL FAILURE—SPECIFIC INDICATIONS FOR DIALYSIS

CLINICAL INDICATIONS

1. *Uremia:* Early signs of deterioration—anorexia, nausea, changes in mental status, neuromuscular hyperirritability, etc.—may be indications for early dialysis.
2. *Overhydration:* Pulmonary edema or "uremic pneumonitis," refractory edema

BIOCHEMICAL INDICATIONS

1. BUN > 150 mg./100 ml.
2. Serum creatinine > 15 mg./100 ml.
3. Serum carbon dioxide < 15 mEq./L.
4. Hyperkalemia unresponsive to conservative management

cations to, peritoneal dialysis. Further, this treatment is effective in increasing caloric intake due to concomitant glucose administration.

On the other hand, hemodialysis is more rapidly effective than peritoneal dialysis, resulting in a lower blood urea nitrogen and serum creatinine level. Hemodialysis permits a greater flexibility in general management of uremia, particularly for early ambulation. Extracorporeal dialysis is more dangerous in inexperienced hands and requires general or regional heparinization as well as access to blood vessels. It may be unduly hazardous to patients with bleeding tendencies or unstable blood pressure.[3,21]

In general, either method of dialysis should benefit most patients with uremia due to acute renal failure. They are not mutually exclusive; both have been used in the same patient at different times for specific indications. The choice of therapy is often a matter of available facilities and personal preference.

Prevention of Acute Renal Failure

Prognosis

As mentioned previously, the syndrome of acute tubular necrosis was first recognized as a distinct clinical syndrome during World War II. Most cases reported at this time were traumatic in origin and the overall mortality rate was 94%.[15] By the time of the Korean War, considerable knowledge had been gained as to precise fluid, electrolyte and caloric requirements. Further, hemodialysis was available and a well-trained and staffed renal failure team supervised the care of these patients. Despite these innovations, the mortality rate was over 67% in patients with post-traumatic renal failure.[9,12] In 1957 a national study group in the United States reviewed over 1,000 patients with acute renal failure and reported similar results. Mortality statistics in several large series have shown no significant change since that time. Thus, precipitation of acute renal failure in the critically ill patient is ominous. For this reason, more stress and investigation in recent years has been placed on measures directed toward prevention.

It should be re-emphasized that intensive care patients do not succumb to uremia, because this can be effectively managed by conservative measures and dialysis as required. Death is a result of complications of the underlying disease, and the incidence of these complications is enhanced by the development of renal failure.

Prevention of Postoperative Oliguria

As previously mentioned, general anesthesia in man is frequently associated with acute depression of renal function and is occasionally followed by oliguric renal failure. In the past, attempts have been made to minimize these effects by giving fluid and electrolyte infusions varying in quantity and electrolyte composition and administered at varying times prior to the operative procedure. No method was completely successful.[7,10] Further, precipitation of water intoxication and congestive heart failure in some patients offered the rationale for routine fluid restriction applied by most physicians.[18]

A high incidence of acute renal failure following surgical removal of aneurysms of the abdominal aorta led to reinvestigation of renal function during and after this procedure. In the experimental animal, it was found that adequate hydration prior to the surgical procedure offered some protection against acute renal failure postoperatively.[8] Initially, many vascular surgeons employed routine infusion of 1,000–1,500 ml. of dextrose/water prior to anesthesia for aneurysmectomy.[13] Later, Barry[2] demonstrated that infusion of hypertonic mannitol was more effective in maintaining renal plasma flow, glomerular filtration rate and diuresis during the operative period. Further studies[5] in renal hemodynamics during anesthesia and surgery showed that preoperative hydration alone prevented much of the deterioration seen in patients treated routinely by preoperative dehydration. In a group of poor risk patients undergoing surgery on the genitourinary tract, preoperative hydration plus osmotic diuresis completely prevented the expected depression of renal function.[22] Subsequent investigations have tended to support this concept that adequate preoperative hydration and circulatory support effectively decrease the incidence of postoperative oliguria and renal failure. Further, there is some evidence that the incidence of acute tubular necrosis in a renal homograft can be reduced by prior treatment of the donor with hydration and osmotic diuresis.

Treatment of Postoperative Oliguria

The physician must be aware of those clinical settings which may result in precipitation of acute renal failure. Usually at this time, his primary concern is directed toward the presenting signs and complaints of a gravely ill patient (the initiating episode). Thus, the patient who is seen with gram-negative sepsis, extensive trauma or prolonged hypotension for any reason is a potential candidate for development of acute renal failure. A patient with an acute hemolytic transfusion reaction or one who develops a complication of pregnancy, such as eclampsia or premature separation of the placenta, is likewise at risk. Too often in the past, acute renal failure went unrecognized until symptoms of significant overhydration were present. These include hyponatremia, edema, nausea and vomiting, diarrhea and excessive tearing and salivation. Prompt resuscitation, restoration of blood volume and improvement in cardiac output can help prevent this complication.

Barry first outlined a model for development of acute tubular necrosis.[4] The initial episode is characterized as acute, functional, reversible renal failure, which gradually or more precipitously, depending on the severity of the renal insult, progresses to true organic or irreversible renal failure. Since that time, other investigators have supported the use of adequate hydration or osmotic diuresis to improve effective renal blood flow and to alter the natural course of the disease. Initially, the benefits of such therapy were somewhat obscure, but recent advances in renal physiology have shown that there is distinct rationale for diuresis in improving renal hemodynamics and preventing ischemia.

A reversible or treatable cause of acute renal failure is to be sought in every case with oliguria, and an anatomic and a histologic diagnosis is desirable. One approach to the patient with oliguria is:

1. After initial assessment of the patient an attempt is made to induce diuresis and improve renal blood flow by infusion of 1,000 ml. of normal saline intravenously in 60–90 minutes, 25 Gm. mannitol intravenously, 200 mg. ethacrynic acid or 160 mg. furosemide intravenously. The rationale for this procedure is fairly well established. First, in the absence of obvious cardiopulmonary overload or peripheral edema, rapid infusion of normal saline results in an acute increase in plasma volume, resulting in increased renal blood flow and glomerular filtration rate. These changes are observed only after rapid plasma volume expansion, and there is no advantage to saline infusion over a 3–4 hour period. Second, there is now significant experimental evidence to suggest that hypertonic mannitol infusion causes an acute reduction in intrarenal vascular resistance, resulting in improved total renal blood flow. The precise mechanism is still unknown but a direct myotrophic effect on the smooth muscle of renal arterioles has been postulated. Finally, the potent diuretic agents, ethacrynic acid and furosemide, in addition to having specific effects on the renal tubule also have marked effects on redistribution of intrarenal blood flow. These agents have been shown to initiate diuresis simultaneously with shunting of blood flow from the outer medulla to the cortex. Thus, blood flow is improved to the area of ischemia as described previously.

2. The response to these agents is observed by following hourly urine volumes. If necessary, an indwelling urethral catheter is inserted. Once renal failure is established definitely, the indwelling catheter is to be avoided because of the hazard of urinary tract infection. The patient with established oliguria is ordinarily able to void small urine volumes several times daily. If diuresis is established within 3 hours (urine volume of 60–100 ml./hour), it is sustained by hourly replacing the measured urine volume with an equivalent volume of half normal saline. Hypotonic saline is the ideal replacement solution for 2 reasons. First, this solution approximately represents the electrolyte concentrations of urine produced by the failing kidney. Second, the diuretic response to such agents as mannitol and ethacrynic acid produces urine of this composition. If diuresis is established, it should be maintained for at least 24–36 hours until the danger of precipitation of irreversible renal failure is passed. If during this time, urine flow diminishes (below 30

ml./hour), additional doses of the diuretic agents can be administered at 6–8 hour intervals. If diuresis fails to ensue (less than 60 ml. urine/hour) within 3 hours, the diagnosis of acute organic renal failure is established and appropriate general measures and fluid restrictions, as described previously, are then instituted.

3. In the absence of a clear precipitating cause, urinary tract obstruction must be excluded, particularly following urologic or gynecologic surgery. Infusion (high dosage contrast media) pyelography has been helpful, particularly with the use of delayed films. Renal blood flow is markedly reduced and sufficient radiographic dye may not accumulate in renal parenchyma for a number of hours; thus adequate visualization is rare before 4–6 hours. We usually rely on a 6-hour film. If this is unsuccessful, a 24-hour examination with tomography is usually adequate. In some patients, cystoscopy and retrograde ureteral catheterization is required. Most texts suggest that catheterization of one ureter is adequate to exclude obstruction. However, there are patients with a unilateral nonfunctioning kidney due to other causes, and we would recommend bilateral catheterization. Renal biopsy has been helpful in disclosing unrecognized acute vasculitis or glomerulonephritis, indicating need for steroid or immunosuppressive therapy. Because most patients with acute renal failure are quite ill postoperatively, and since these procedures are somewhat taxing, dialysis is often instituted prior to investigation in order to restore proper fluid and electrolyte balance and to avert symptoms of uremia.

The Surgical Patient with Renal Insufficiency

Clinical Course of Chronic Renal Failure

As mentioned previously, it is frequently impossible in individual patients to correlate abnormal blood chemistries with clinical symptoms of uremia. Unlike acute renal failure, the level of blood urea nitrogen in chronic renal insufficiency is rarely indicative of the patient's physical, physiologic and functional status. In this case, symptoms of uremia are correlated better with the level of serum creatinine. Again, there is extreme variability, and there are exceptional patients who are completely asymptomatic and lead an active vocational and social life with serum creatinine levels of 25 mg./100 ml. or higher. On the other hand, most patients will have some symptoms, particularly fatigue, when the serum creatinine reaches 3–5 mg./100 ml.

Since the production of creatinine is related to body muscle mass, one would expect to see higher serum levels without overt symptoms in a well-developed, muscular individual. In contrast, severe uremic symptoms are often noted in female patients at a lower concentration of serum creatinine.

Patients with moderate renal insufficiency (serum creatinine less than 5 mg./100 ml.) usually require no medication and no restriction of diet and activity. Early impairment of the renal concentrating mechanism leads to polyuria and nocturia. At this stage, excessive urine output is readily compensated for by a normal thirst mechanism.

As renal failure becomes more progressive, easy fatigability is usually an early symptom, and this is accompanied by a moderate to progressive anemia. Although the severity of the anemia is usually directly related to decreased renal function, there may be at times a striking disproportion. The reason is obvious, since the erythropoietic and excretory functions of the kidney are not necessarily related. Paradoxically, several types of renal disease (for example, polycystic renal disease, renal artery disease with ischemia, etc.) are associated with increased production of erythropoietin.

Commonly, the next symptoms of renal failure include some cerebral impairment, such as loss of concentration span and memory defects. Also, such gastrointestinal disturbances as anorexia and nausea are quite distressing to the patient. The nausea and vomiting of chronic renal failure patients are most commonly present on arising in the morning. In addition, at this time a moderate metabolic acidosis is present. Therapy at this time consists of increased salt and water intake. In general, urine volumes should reach 3–4 L./daily. Supplemental sodium chloride is given per mouth in the range of 6 Gm./daily. If acidosis is significant, half of this can be administered as sodium bicarbonate, 3 Gm./daily.

As renal function continues to deteriorate, protein restriction is necessary. Protein intake is stepwise diminished to 60, 40 and finally 20 Gm./day, depending on symptomatology. In all of these diets, fluid and electrolyte content are unrestricted so long as urine volume is adequate and there is no edema or rapid weight gain. Most individuals cannot maintain nitrogen balance on protein intakes of less than 0.75 Gm./kg., and some muscle wasting is inevitable. Some muscle wasting can be prevented by providing adequate caloric intake with increased carbohydrate and fat. There is some clinical evidence that increased urine volume and perhaps some improvement in renal blood flow can be achieved by long-term use of potent diuretic agents, such as furosemide and ethacrynic acid. Again, these must be administered in relatively high doses to achieve any effect in patients being treated for renal failure.

The course of progressive renal insufficiency may be prolonged (particularly in patients with polycystic renal disease and such renal medullary diseases as chronic pyelonephritis). The neurologic and skeletal manifestations of uremia are ultimately the most disabling. At present, there is no satisfactory treatment for the bone disease of chronic renal failure. The most rational approach is directed toward correction of the metabolic acidosis, elevation of serum calcium toward normal values and prevention of the hyperphosphatemia. The first two are accomplished by administration of calcium carbonate with or without supplemental vitamin D. The latter can be prevented by gastrointestinal binding of phosphorus by one of the various aluminum hydroxide gels. (Magnesium preparations are contraindicated, as significant absorption and possible symptomatic hypermagnesemia have been demonstrated following long-term use of these preparations.)

Ultimately, renal failure becomes terminal and life cannot be sustained with a creatinine clearance of less than 3 ml./minute. Clinically, this is manifest by failure to achieve a urine output of 2 L./24 hours under maximal stress of water, salt and diuretic administration. At this point, of course, the only available treatments today are chronic intermittent dialysis and/or transplantation. It is interesting, however, that some patients who can adhere to the strict renal failure diet, described previously, can be maintained in reasonably good health for a number of months with serum creatinine concentrations of 40 mg./100 ml. or higher.

Surgery in the Patient with Renal Failure

Despite some trepidation, major surgical procedures of various types have been routinely performed in patients with moderate to severe chronic renal impairment and are usually tolerated surprisingly well. Obviously, patients with terminal renal failure tolerate such procedures as subtotal or total parathyroidectomy, bilateral nephrectomy and, of course, renal transplantation. Thus, advanced renal insufficiency is not an absolute contraindication to surgical procedures of any type. I have had the opportunity of following several patients through open heart surgery who have had serum creatinine concentrations as high as 10 mg./100 ml. In general, no special difficulties have been encountered, but there is a more urgent need for careful hemostasis.

In the patient with acute renal failure, efforts should be made to perform the procedure under local or spinal anesthesia to avoid further embarrassment of the renal circulation. Dialysis in the oliguric patient shortly prior to surgery and frequently in the postoperative period is clearly indicated. Frequent dialysis improves wound healing in addition to alleviating the postoperative complications of bleeding and hyperkalemia.

In the patient with chronic renal failure, renal functional capacity should be preserved by appropriate preoperative preparation, which includes prevention of dehydration and institution of sustained osmotic diuresis. The choice of the anesthetic is based primarily on the consideration that diminished or absent renal function requires some limitation of fluid. Thiopental and halothane-nitrous-oxide-oxygen sequence have most frequently been used with succinylcholine administered for muscle relaxation as needed. Further, accessory agents that are primarily eliminated by the kidney should be avoided.

In the absence of hypertension, patients with renal failure rapidly adjust to significant degrees of anemia without overt cardiovascular effects. With moderate renal impairment, the serum hematocrit usually stabilizes at 25–30% and is only transiently elevated following blood transfusion. Without transfusion, patients with terminal renal failure frequently stabilize with hematocrits of 18–22%. There is some experimental and clinical evidence that hypertransfusion (to normal values) results in further embarrassment of renal blood flow. For this reason, preoperative transfusion is generally contraindicated and patients with serum hematocrits of 25–30% tolerate extensive surgery quite well.

Summary

Surgical patients have comprised, perhaps, the majority of admissions to dialysis centers scattered throughout the world.[6] Acute renal failure is a serious complication in the postoperative patient. Oliguria or anuria with progressive development of uremia results in markedly increased morbidity and mortality.

Whereas the precise pathogenesis of acute renal failure or acute tubular necrosis is still unknown, increasing evidence incriminates a primary disturbance in the renal blood flow, probably redistribution of intrarenal blood flow. Clinically, the final common pathway is hypotension, regardless of the basic etiology. A marked depression in renal hemodynamics and renal function is common to all patients undergoing general anesthesia, and superimposition of the surgical trauma obviously plays an important role in some patients.

Regardless of the etiology or precipitating event, the symptoms, clinical course and biochemical abnormalities of uremia are similar. Despite refinements in conservative management and use of more frequent dialysis, the mortality rate remains high. Death is usually a result of complications of the underlying disease, and the incidence of postoperative complications is increased in patients with renal failure.

There is increasing evidence, both in the experimental animal and in man, that renal hemodynamic depression and postoperative oliguria can be prevented by adequate support of the renal circulation preoperatively and during surgery. Acute "functional" renal failure in the postoperative period can be reversed by appropriate measures prior to precipitation of irreversible "organic" renal failure. Acute renal failure is no longer as common a complication of such procedures as open heart surgery and valve replacement, but we now see patients with this complication following cardiac transplantation. Interestingly, while surgical procedures have become more complex, the incidence of postoperative renal failure has remained relatively constant. Further elucidation of basic circulatory changes during anesthesia and surgery should lead to better methods of eliminating renal failure as a complication of more radical procedures.

On the other hand, patients with chronic renal disease and varying degrees of renal insufficiency tolerate anesthesia and extensive surgical procedures remarkably well. Because of the prolongation of life in patients with chronic renal disease due to the growth of chronic dialysis and renal transplantation programs, the general surgeon will gain more experience with various operative procedures in these patients. Experience to date suggests again that careful preoperative management and strict attention to premedication and anesthetic agents permits perfectly satisfactory results in patients with chronic renal disease.

REFERENCES

1. Barger, A. C., and Herd, J. A.: Study of renal circulation in the unanesthetized dog with inert gases: External counting, Proc. 3d Internat. Cong. Nephrol. 1:174, 1967.
2. Barry, K. G., *et al.*: Mannitol infusion: II. Prevention of acute functional renal failure during resection of an aneurysm of the abdominal aorta, New England J. Med. 264:967, 1961.
3. Barry, K. G., *et al.*: Peritoneal dialysis: Current applications and recent developments, Proc. 3d Internat. Cong. Nephrol. 3:288, 1967.
4. Barry, K. G., and Malloy, J. P.: Oliguric renal failure: Evaluation and therapy by the intravenous infusion of mannitol, J.A.M.A. 179:510, 1962.
5. Barry, K. G.; Mazze, R. I., and Schwartz, F. D.: Prevention of surgical oliguria and renal-hemodynamic suppression by sustained hydration, New England J. Med. 270:1371, 1964.
6. Cohn, H. E., and Capelli, J. P.: The diagnosis and management of oliguria in the postoperative period, S. Clin. North America 47:1187, 1967.
7. Coller, F. A., *et al.*: Effects of ether and cyclopropane anesthesia on renal function in man, Ann. Surg. 118:717, 1943.
8. Doolan, P. D., *et al.*: Acute renal insufficiency following aortic surgery: A discussion of the pathogenesis and a consideration of gangrene of an extremity as a complication, Am. J. Med. 28:895, 1960.
9. Dossetor, J. B.: Creatininemia versus uremia: The relative significance of blood urea nitrogen and serum creatinine concentrations in azotemia, Ann. Int. Med. 65:1287, 1966.
10. Dudley, H. F., *et al.*: Studies on antidiuresis in surgery: Effects of anesthesia, surgery and posterior pituitary antidiuretic hormone on water metabolism in man, Ann. Surg. 140:354, 1954.
11. Giovannetti, S., and Maggiore, Q.: A low-nitrogen diet with proteins of high biological value for severe chronic uraemia, Lancet 1:1000, 1964.
12. Habif, D. V., *et al.*: Renal and hepatic blood flow, glomerular filtration rate and urinary output of electrolytes during cyclopropane, ether and thiopental anesthesia, operation and immediate postoperative period, Surgery 30:241, 1951.
13. Hatcher, C. R., Jr.; Gagnon, J. A. and Clarke, R. W.: Effects of hydration on ephedrine induced renal shutdown in dogs, S. Forum 9:106, 1958.
14. Hollenberg, N. K., *et al.*: Acute oliguric renal failure in man: Evidence for preferential renal cortical ischemia, Medicine 47:455, 1968.
15. Lucke, B.: lower nephron nephrosis: The renal lesions of the crush syndrome of burns, transfusions and other conditions affecting the lower segments of the nephrons, Mil. Surgeon 99:371, 1946.
16. Maxwell, M. H., *et al.*: Peritoneal dialysis: 1. Technique and applications, J.A.M.A. 170: 917, 1959.
17. Mazze, R. I., *et al.*: Renal function during anesthesia and surgery: I. The effects of halothane anesthesia, Anesthesiology 24:279, 1963.
18. Moyer, C. A.: Acute temporary changes in renal function associated with major surgical procedures, Surgery 27:198, 1950.
19. O'Brien, T. F.; Baxter, C. R., and Teschar, P. E.: Tr. Am. Soc. Artificial Internal Organs 5:577, 1959.

20. Papper, E. M., and Ngai, S. H.: Kidney function during anesthesia, Ann. Rev. Med. 7: 213, 1956.
21. Schwartz, F. D., *et al.*: Peritoneal dialysis: An appraisal of its value in acute renal failure, Med. Ann. Dist. of Columbia 35:181, 1966.
22. Seitzman, D. M., *et al.*: Mannitol diuresis: A method of renal protection during surgery, J. Urol. 90:139, 1963.
23. Smith, L. H., Jr., *et al.*: Post-traumatic renal insufficiency in military casualties: 2. Management, use of artificial kidney, prognosis, Am. J. Med. 18:187, 1955.
24. Teschan, P. E., *et al.*: Post-traumatic renal insufficiency in military casualties: 1. Clinical characteristics, Am. J. Med. 18:172, 1955.

10

Acute Surgical Infections

STUART LEVIN, M.D.

Associate Attending Physician and Director, Section of Infectious Diseases, Rush-Presbyterian-St. Luke's Medical Center; Assistant Professor of Medicine, Rush Medical College

THE PATIENTS in the intensive care unit are by definition seriously ill. The emphasis of this chapter will be directed to two major areas: (1) diagnosis and therapy of acute infections, which must be accomplished as soon as possible because of the compromised host and (2) prevention of infection. A reduction in the infection rate can be accomplished not only by often emphasized careful surgical techniques, but by attention to those areas in which postoperative infections commonly occur. Most hospital-acquired infections are bacterial and can be classified according to major sites, as follows: (1) intravenous catheter, (2) wound, (3) genitourinary and (4) pulmonary.

Use of a check list (Table 10-1) should be considered when a postoperative patient becomes febrile or is "toxic looking" in the absence of fever. Fever without systemic symptoms is common in the postoperative period, and in its benign form may not allow a specific diagnosis to be made. However, the association of fever and progressive systemic symptoms has a tangible cause in most cases. Institution of antibiotic therapy prior to elaboration of the cause of fever cannot be condemned too strongly.

Diagnosis and Management of Postoperative Infection

Intravenous Catheter Infections

All venous catheters or needles in place for more than 48 hours should be removed. The tip of the catheter should be aseptically removed and placed into bacterial culture media. Cultures should also be made for fungi, particularly Candida species. Venous catheter infec-

TABLE 10-1.—CHECK LIST FOR POSTOPERATIVE FEVER

First 48 Hours: In all patients with fever over 101 F. or appearing toxic, draw blood for cultures.

1. Atelectasis and pneumonia: Cough or tracheal aspiration to obtain sputum for Gram's stain and culture.
2. Wound infection (streptococcal or clostridial): Inspect wound, do Gram's stain, culture and sensitivity tests.
3. Drug reactions: Stop all drugs except those absolutely necessary.
4. Urinary tract: Do microscopic urinalysis, culture, sensitivity tests, compare results of prior culture. Recent instrumentation or a catheter in place makes GU tract likely source of infection.

After 48 Hours: In all patients with fever over 101 F. or appearing toxic, draw blood for cultures.

1. Wound infection (usually staphylococcal): Inspect wound, do Gram's stain, culture and sensitivity tests.
2. Pneumonia (bacterial): Aspirate trachea, do Gram's stain, culture and sensitivity tests.
3. Intravenous catheter infection: Remove catheter and culture the tip.

Less Common Infections

1. Endometritis (usually anaerobic): Gram's stain and culture.
2. Decubitus ulcer: Gram's stain and culture.
3. Perirectal abscess: Do rectal examination!
4. Acute suppurative parotitis: Milk Stensen's duct and do Gram's stain and culture.
5. Acute cholecystitis: Treat with ampicillin or tetracycline.
6. Acute enterocolitis: Gram's stain of stool and culture; if all staphylococci—Rx.
7. Meningitis: Lethargy an important indication even if no stiff neck.
8. Acute sinusitus, otitis media: Culture and sensitivity tests of exudate.
9. Sterile abscess of buttock following intramuscular injection.
10. Spontaneous septicemia: Hidden source often in gastrointestinal tract (diverticulitis).

Noninfectious Causes of Fever

1. Fat emboli (bone trauma)
2. Thromboembolic phenomena
3. Drug hypersensitivity
4. Thyroid storm
5. Brain damage, brain stem injury
6. Pelvic thrombophlebitis after genitourinary or gynecologic surgery
7. Postpericardiotomy syndrome

tions are common, serious and almost entirely preventable. Surgical cutdowns lead to infections more often than percutaneous cannulas, which in turn appear to impose greater risk than short needles. The incidence of infection rises daily after the first 48 hours. The staphylococcus has been the most important pathogen, but gram-negative rods frequently assume major significance and even candida organisms can lead to fatal fungemia in patients receiving broad spectrum antibiotics and long-term intravenous therapy.

WOUND INFECTIONS

Inspection of the wound becomes urgent if fever and/or deterioration of the patient occur at any time, particularly during the first 48 hours after surgery. The presence of a cast or heavy dressings should not be a deterrent to immediate inspection of the wound.

Predisposing factors in wound infection include prolonged surgery,

TABLE 10-2.—DRUGS OF CHOICE FOR HOSPITAL-ACQUIRED INFECTIONS OF KNOWN OR STRONGLY SUSPECT ETIOLOGY

ORGANISM	DRUG OF CHOICE	DOSE	ALTERNATE
Streptococcus (group A)	Penicillin	0.6–1.2 million units/24 hr.	If sensitive or allergic, erythromycin 1–2 Gm./24 hr. I.V. lincomycin 1–4 Gm./24 hr. I.V.
Nongroup A or D streptococcus	Penicillin	1.2–2.4 million units/24 hr.	Erythromycin, lincomycin
Enterococcus (group D)	Penicillin or ampicillin	10–20 million units/24 hr. I.V. 8–12 Gm./24 hr. I.V.	Vancomycin 1–2 Gm./24 hr. I.V.
Pneumococcus	Penicillin	0.3–0.6 million units/24 hr.	Erythromycin
Staphylococcus (coagulase-positive or negative)	Methicillin	8–16 Gm./24 hr.	Lincomycin 3-6 Gm./24 hr. I.V. If serious infection, prefer vancomycin 1–2 Gm./24 hrs. I.V.
Staphylococcus (coagulase-positive or negative)	Vancomycin	1–2 Gm./24 hr. I.V.	Kanamycin-cephalothin combination
Escherichia coli	Kanamycin or gentamicin	1.5 mg./kg./24 hr. I.M. 3-8 mg./kg./24 hr. I.M.	Chloramphenicol, ampicillin, cephalothin, tetracycline (Furadantin or nalidixic acid can be used if genitourinary tract only)
Klebsiella	Kanamycin or gentamicin	as above	Chloramphenicol, cephalothin
Enterobacter	Kanamycin or gentamicin	as above	(Enterobacter always resistant to penicillin, ampicillin or cephalothin)
Proteus mirabilis	Ampicillin or cephalothin	4–16 Gm./24 hr. 4–16 Gm./24 hr.	Kanamycin, chloramphenicol, gentamicin
Other proteus (indole +)	Kanamycin or gentamicin		Chloramphenicol 1-3 Gm./24 hr. I.V. or carbenicillin 12-24 Gm./24 hr. I.V.
Pseudomonas	Gentamicin	3-8 mg./kg./24 hr. I.M.	Carbenicillin 24-32 Gm./24 hr. I.V.
Salmonella	Chloramphenicol or ampicillin	2-4 Gm./24 hr. I.V. 8–12 Gm./24 hr. I.V.	
Coliforms	Kanamycin or gentamicin		Polymyxin or chloramphenicol
Serratia	Gentamicin		Chloramphenicol 3-6 Gm./24 hr. I.V.
Bacteroides	Lincomycin	3–4 Gm./24 hr. I.V.	Chloramphenicol 3-6 Gm./24 hr. I.V.
Staphylococcus (enterocolitis)	Vancomycin	1–2 Gm./24 hr. P.O.	Add methicillin or oxacillin 6–12 Gm./24 hr. (I.V.) if septicemic
Candida (local)	Nystatin (tablets and solutions)	6–24 million units/24 hr. P.O.	
Candida (systemic)	Amphotericin B	Begin with test dose 5–10 mg. and continue at 10–20 mg./24 hr. I.V. (maximum 75–100 mg./24 hr. I.V.)	
Clostridia	Penicillin	2.4–10 million units/24 hrs. I.M. or I.V.	

previously contaminated tissue, old age, obesity and prior therapy with antibiotics (Table 10-3) and steroids. Gram-positive bacteria are more commonly pathogenic in this situation.

EARLY WOUND INFECTIONS (first 48 hours).—There are three important syndromes associated with wound infections to consider in the immediate postoperative period. These can be detected by an emergency Gram stain of the wound drainage.

Clostridial wound infections (gram-positive rods).—If the temperature is subnormal, the pulse rapid and the patient apathetic, clostridia must be strongly suspected. Clostridial infections are usually associated with edema and whitish to brownish discoloration of the skin. A frothy, malodorous brownish discharge and subcutaneous emphysema are late manifestations. Recognition of clostridia in the wound, by Gram's stain and anaerobic culture in the absence of invasion of normal tissue, is usually of no great significance. However, most clinicians prefer to eradicate the organism with an antibiotic (penicillin) in order to decrease the likelihood of later invasion and to prevent transfer to other patients in the unit. If active gas gangrene is present, radical debridement, penicillin therapy, hyperbaric oxygen therapy and occasionally gas gangrene antitoxins are employed, although each of these measures is of successively decreasing importance. It is to be stressed that no therapy has as yet supplanted surgical debridement. If gas gangrene is strongly suspected, the patient should be removed from the intensive care unit and isolated. Emphasis on hand washing and isolation techniques is essential for ward personnel.

Group A streptococcal cellulitis (gram-positive cocci in chains).—High fever and toxicity associated with cellulitis or erysipelas within the first 24 hours are usually secondary to a group A beta hemolytic streptococcal infection, and immediate treatment with penicillin is mandatory. Broad spectrum agents are not necessary and may be ineffective for this organism. Characteristics to be noticed are color, odor, drainage, viability of muscle, presence of edema, necrotic material, vesicles and subcutaneous emphysema. Vesicles and bullae are es-

TABLE 10-3.—PROPHYLACTIC ANTIBIOTICS AND COMMON SUPERINFECTING ORGANISMS

Antibiotic	Superinfecting organisms
Penicillin:	Penicillinase-producing staphylococci and coliforms
Ampicillin:	Klebsiella, penicillinase-producing staphylococci (coagulase positive or negative)
Cephalothin, cephaloridine:	Pseudomonas, also aerobacter, indole-positive proteus; the indole test on proteus helps differentiate the cephalothin-ampicillin-sensitive indole-negative strains from the indole-positive strains that are resistant to those antibiotics
Tetracyclines:	Proteus, staphylococci
Polymyxins:	Staphylococci and proteus
Methicillin, oxacillin:	Gram-negative rods
Carbenicillin:	Klebsiella

pecially characteristic. Penicillin 600,000–1,200,000 units/24 hours intramuscularly is important. Debridement in group A streptococcal infections, unlike the previous group of infections, is not usually as necessary.

Necrotizing fasciitis (gram-positive cocci in clusters or chains).—This can be recognized by subcutaneous necrosis and marked undermining of the skin edges. It is caused by hemolytic staphylococci and/or hemolytic streptococci. It can be rapidly progressive and very dangerous. Here, as in clostridial infections, antibiotics are useful, and penicillin or methicillin 4–8 Gm./24 hours intravenously is the drug of choice. However, extensive debridement is again the most important therapy.

LATER WOUND INFECTIONS (over 96 hours).—*Common organisms.*—Other types of gram-negative and gram-positive organisms can cause wound infections. However, these are not usually manifest until the fourth to seventh postoperative day. In previous years, the staphylococcus was the most common organism causing wound infections after the first several postoperative days. There is growing evidence that gram-negative rods of all types also cause infections. A Gram stain of drainage from the wound can be extremely useful to the clinician. This simple procedure is not utilized often enough. Gram-positive cocci in chains (streptococci), large gram-positive cocci in clusters (staphylococci), large gram-positive rods (clostridia) and gram-negative rods (predominant) are the major categories observed. In each instance, a different course, prognosis and therapy will follow. It should be stressed that discovery of gram-positive cocci or rods and/or gram-negative rods in the wound does not guarantee that those organisms are responsible for the clinical syndrome.

In both gram-negative and staphylococcal wound infections, local care includes incision and drainage, irrigation and frequent dressing changes. This treatment is often sufficient for eradication of the infection. A decision as to the use of systemic antibiotics is dependent upon the extent of invasion of the infection into skin, subcutaneous tissue and muscle, as well as on the presence or absence of systemic manifestations of infection.

Pseudomonas.—This is a special problem in wounds, but is seen usually in specific clinical situations. Factors leading to pseudomonas infections are: burns, leukopenia, diabetic acidosis, leukemia, aerosol therapy, tracheostomy, cephalothin therapy, combined kanamycin-penicillin or methicillin therapy. When indicated, therapy is carbenicillin 20–32 Gm./24 hours intravenously, or gentamicin, 4–8 mg./kg./24 hours in 3–4 divided doses. Ultraviolet light (Wood's light) may show a green fluorescence in a wound, suggesting the presence of pseudomonas.

Anaerobic streptococci.—There are two other well known classical skin and subcutaneous infections in the postoperative period, Meleney's bacterial synergistic gangrene and Meleney's undermining ulcer, but these are usually more indolent and are problems that become manifest in the second and third weeks after surgery. Both usually require extensive debridement and antibiotics after obtaining aerobic and anaerobic cultures. The anaerobic streptococcus is the most important etiologic agent in both these infections.

Perineal infections.—Infections of the perineum are usually secondary to pressure sores, diarrhea, pilonidal cysts or intramuscular infections. They are usually foul smelling and are often due to anaerobic organisms. Any malodorous abscess at any site should be considered anaerobic and cultured in appropriate media. Most of these organisms are penicillin sensitive, but if bacteroides (small gram-negative rods) predominate, Lincomycin (3–4 Gm./24 hours intravenously) would be the drug of choice. If multiple spontaneous or unusual sites of thrombophlebitis are found associated with a potential source of anaerobic infection (mouth, gastrointestinal tract, pelvis, perineum), bacteroides septicemia should be suspected and therapy begun immediately. An unusual but important organism to look for in perineal ulcers is Entamoeba histolytica, which is best diagnosed by a smear or biopsy. A rectal examination, though essential, is often neglected, particularly after the admission physical, leading therefore to a failure to diagnose periprostatic and perirectal abscesses.

PREVENTION OF WOUND INFECTIONS.—This is to a great extent related to surgical technique, but careful postoperative wound care is also important. The use of gloves and masks when changing dressings provides an important barrier to wound contamination. Many discussions, often contradictory, have been written about the usefulness of prophylactic antibiotics in prevention of wound infections. It is generally agreed that prophylaxis is best achieved when there is an antibiotic effective against a specific potential invader, whose sensitivity to the drug remains constant. Therefore, prophylaxis against Clostridium tetani, Diplococcus pneumoniae and group A streptococci is possible because these bacteria consistently remain sensitive to penicillin. Prophylactic therapy of endocarditis in preoperative patients with pre-existing valvular heart disease is indicated in an attempt to reduce the inoculum of oral streptococci invading the bloodstream. Antibiotic prophylaxis for all organisms causing pneumonia, genitourinary tract infections and wound infections has been ineffective. Multiple organisms with different antibiotic sensitivities are potentially invasive in these situations. It would appear that the use of prophylactic antibiotics only selects the pathogen that will eventually cause the infection. Most studies do not justify the routine use of prophylactic antibiotics in surgical patients. In addition, the physician must weigh the dangers to the patient and to the hospital environment of using this antibiotic therapy. Superinfections, drug reactions and the production of antibiotic-resistant bacterial strains are just a few of the obvious hazards of antibiotic administration even when this therapy is justified.

Genitourinary Infections

Diagnosis and treatment.—The genitourinary tract is easily checked by a microscopic urinalysis, which is best performed by the physician. Results of prior urine cultures and an awareness regarding recent genitourinary tract instrumentation are essential. The genitourinary tract is the major source of early postoperative (first 48 hours) febrile toxic states in patients in whom instrumentation has been performed.

If, however, genitourinary instrumentation or pelvic examination has not recently been performed, and if prior urine cultures were negative, the urinary tract will rarely be implicated. Aside from prostatic abscesses, gram-negative rods are almost exclusively the pathogens in urinary tract infections. It should be stressed that an unspun fresh urine showing about 10–20 rods per high-power field (Gram's stain not necessary) is equivalent to a quantitative urine culture containing 10^5 organisms/ml. of urine and, therefore, is indicative of a urinary tract infection. If these features are not present, the genitourinary tract is not likely to be the source of infection, and the need for gram-negative antibiotic "coverage" is statistically much less important. Under ideal conditions, therapy is guided by bacterial culture and sensitivities (24–48 hours).

Prevention.—Careful studies verify that the single most common hospital-acquired infection occurs in the urinary tract. Urinary retention catheters are associated with a high rate of infection, which approaches 100% between the third to tenth day following insertion, depending upon the care given the catheter system. Prevention starts with adequate hydration and catheter drainage only when necessary. The following suggestions for catheter care have been stressed by different groups of investigators, but unfortunately the relative importance of each measure has never been adequately determined.

A triple lumen catheter will permit periodic or continuous instillation of an antiseptic solution such as 0.25% acetic acid or the use of a neomycin-polymyxin bladder solution (20 mg. polymyxin and 40 mg. neomycin/1,000 ml. fluid). A closed bladder drainage system with an air-trap valve system and collecting bag containing an antiseptic solution such as formaldehyde has also been suggested. Careful and repeated cleansing of the urethral meatus with 0.05% chlorhexidine and glycerin is another potential aid. As in other areas where multiple organisms are present, systemic antibiotics have little place in routine prophylaxis of patients having genitourinary instrumentation of any kind. There can be no defense for their routine use. When one recognizes the wide spectrum of gram-negative rods present in hospital-acquired urinary tract infections, it is obvious why most studies have indicated the futility of systemic antibiotic prophylaxis.

Pulmonary Infections

Diagnosis and treatment.—Pulmonary infections are often difficult to prevent and may present diagnostic dilemmas. Coma, obesity, bronchitis, esophagitis, chronic cigarette smoking and congestive heart failure are some of the factors predisposing to the development of pneumonia in the postoperative patient. Classically, a pulmonary density, decreased lung volume, rales, rhonchi and fever are indicative of atelectasis. This occurs within the first 24–48 hours after surgery and is usually reversible without antibiotics. Cyanosis, tachycardia, tachypnea and tracheal deviation are common only with massive atelectasis. Extension of the pulmonary infiltrate is most likely due to a progressive bacterial infection and requires appropriate antibiotic therapy. If an adequate sputum cannot be obtained for smear, nasotracheal aspiration or even transtracheal needle aspiration should be performed in order to obtain sputum for Gram's stain and culture. Appropriate therapy is instituted on the basis of the Gram stain and modified according to the results of the culture.

Several advantages of a sputum Gram stain should be stressed:

1. Information is available immediately instead of 24–48 hours later when culture reports would become available. In postoperative pneumonia, either gram-positive or gram-negative bacteria may predominate.
2. If either staphylococci or gram-negative rods are predominant, an appropriate drug can be started.
3. If the stain contains primarily gram-positive diplococci, penicillin 300,000–600,000 units/24 hours intramuscularly is sufficient therapy.
4. Discovery of gram-positive diplococci in a sputum specimen is not an indication for antibiotic therapy unless clinical findings support the diagnosis of pneumonia. Alpha streptococci, a component of the normal flora, have a similar morphologic appearance.

The diagnosis of pulmonary infarction should be strongly considered each time the physician considers the diagnosis of pneumonia. If the patient has been receiving aerosol therapy, the diagnosis of pseudomonas pneumonia becomes more likely and should be documented by stain and culture. The drugs of choice for pseudomonas infections are carbenicillin 20–32 Gm./24 hours intravenously, or gentamicin, 4–8 mg./kg./24 hours intramuscularly in 4 divided doses. The polymyxin agents are often effective even when sensitivity tests indicate that contrary results may be expected. In general, all other antibiotics are ineffective against pseudomonas, irrespective of the results of in vitro disk sensitivities.

Prevention.—Vigorous coughing and nasotracheal suction should prevent the majority of postoperative pneumonias.

Aerosol therapy includes the hazard of instilling pseudomonas organisms and other gram-negative rods into the alveoli. Effective nebulizers (ultrasonic) are capable of delivering large numbers of bacteria into the alveoli. In this situation, the most important preventive measure is complete sterilization of all respiratory equipment after each use.

A new sterile catheter should be used each time a tracheostomy is suctioned. Sterile disposable gloves are a necessity. The practice of keeping a catheter in a container filled with sterile water is to be condemned. Water supports growth of pseudomonas organisms, which reach great numbers within hours. Thus, each time the catheter is used to suction the trachea, an inoculum of pseudomonas will be instilled deep into the tracheobronchial tree.

SEPTICEMIA

There is one particular situation in which "shotgun" therapy may be indicated. This is the "etiology unknown" septicemia syndrome. This situation arises occasionally, but not nearly so often as the dangerous and nonselective overuse of antibiotics in the postoperative period. As mentioned previously, in the vast majority of situations a clue to the offending organism will be forthcoming if the involved organ system is identified and a Gram stain of the appropriate material is obtained.

The septic patient is identified by gross observation. Findings include tachycardia, pinched facies, lethargy and mild to moderate confusion. The respirations are rapid, but unless pneumonia is present, are not labored or associated with dyspnea. The more toxic the patient appears, the more urgent therapy becomes and the less information will be available for an educated guess. At the same time, because of the usual combination of toxic cardiomyopathy, dehydration and a decreased effective circulating plasma volume, the renal and hepatic circulation become compromised and the multiple toxic drugs necessary to "cover all possibilities" are potentially even more dangerous. The usual regimen is to combine full doses of several effective bactericidal agents. Methicillin or oxacillin (12–24 Gm./24 hours intravenously) is usually combined with either kanamycin (15 mg./kg./24 hours intramuscularly) or gentamicin (4–8 mg./kg./24 hours intramuscularly). Gentamicin is particularly useful if pseudomonas bacteremia is suspected (Table 10-2). Antibiotic levels should be checked when available.

Combinations of bacteriostatic agents, such as the tetracyclines or chloramphenicol, with the above-mentioned agents are rarely useful and potentially detrimental to this group of patients.

SEPTIC SHOCK.—Central venous pressure monitoring is essential in the septic shock syndrome. After careful attention to ventilation, oxygen supply, arrhythmias, blood loss and acid-base balance, the physician should follow the following regimen in the face of decreased tissue perfusion (shock).

If the venous pressure is low or even normal, the plasma volume should be rapidly expanded with saline, plasma, whole blood or dextran, depending upon the indication. By continuous monitoring of the electrocardiogram, urine output, mental status and venous pressure, the most effective arterial pressure can be attained without causing acute pulmonary edema. If there is no response to massive fluid infusion, careful administration of vasopressors can be attempted, remembering that a pressure somewhat lower than the normal pressure is usually optimal with vasopressor therapy. In my experience, isoproterenol is contraindicated in the patient with septic shock and low venous pressure.

If the venous pressure is high, rapid digitalization (Chapter 21) and isoproterenol, 0.001–0.01 mg./minute intravenously, should be given (1–2 mg. in 1,000 ml. of 5% D/W 10–50 gtt./minute). Peripheral blocking agents, such as dibenzyline or chlorpromazine (5–10 mg. intravenously) are also useful. Saline and plasma expanders are contraindicated in those patients with high venous pressure.

Consideration of intravascular coagulation is appropriate in decreased perfusion states. The septic shock syndrome can be suspected upon noting peripheral gangrene, a petechial or ecchymotic rash or bleeding from unusual or nontraumatized sites. In these cases, the clot should be observed and a blood smear should be obtained for estimation of platelets. The fibrinogen level (measured directly or by thrombin time) and a one-stage prothrombin time should be determined. If available, a partial thromboplastin regeneration time is also very helpful. Specific determinations of factor V or VIII and fibrin degradation products will confirm the diagnosis, but these may not be available on an emergency basis. An initially fair to good clot that disintegrates within a short time gives circumstantial evidence for excess fibrinolysis. Once the diagnosis is made, appropriate therapy is instituted (Chapter 8).

Less Common Complications

Acute enterocolitis.—Sudden development of a toxic state which includes tachycardia, hypotension and a tender distended abdomen suggests the diagnosis of acute staphylococcal enterocolitis. This diagnosis must be considered even in the occasional absence of diarrhea. An immediate Gram stain of the stool is mandatory; if staphylococci are dominant, the diagnosis of staphylococcal enterocolitis is quite likely. This syndrome usually occurs after the use of oral prophylactic antibiotic therapy, such as neomycin. Systemic antibiotic therapy can also cause this syndrome. A successful therapy has been oral administration of vancomycin 1–2 Gm./24 hours in divided doses. In the extremely ill patient, methicillin 8–16 Gm./24 hours intravenously should be added.

Acute salmonella enteritis.—Salmonella is an important cause of postoperative diarrhea, septicemia and wound infection. The infection may be related to a hospital carrier or to a previously asymptomatic patient carrier state. An acute infection would then be secondary to gastrointestinal surgery or to the use of "prophylactic" antibiotics. In these patients the antibiotics would likely suppress normal flora, permitting the salmonella to become invasive. The therapy of choice for a salmonella infection is somewhat dependent upon the results of sensitivity studies, particularly in a situation in which multiple resistant transfer factors are present in the gram-negative bacteria of the community. The most effective agent is ampicillin 3–12 Gm./24 hours intravenously. Chloramphenicol (Chloromycetin) 2–3 Gm./24 hours may also be used when indicated.

ACUTE CHOLECYSTITIS.—Acute cholecystitis is a potential complication of any operation, particularly when dehydration is present and anticholinergic drugs are used. In addition to the clinical examination, diagnostic studies may require intravenous or oral cholangiograms on an emergency basis. This illness can be confused with acute pancreatitis. Escherichia coli, anaerobic streptococci, other coliforms and bacteroides are common pathogens in biliary tract infections. Intravenous administration of ampicillin or tetracycline is the most useful therapy in this situation.

ACUTE PAROTITIS.—This is an important postoperative complication in elderly dehydrated patients, particularly those with poor dental hygiene or parotid duct stones. The responsible organism is usually a coagulase-positive staphylococcus. Unless a Gram stain of the discharge from Stensen's duct shows predominantly gram-negative rods, methicillin or oxacillin in doses of 12–24 Gm./day intravenously is the therapy of choice. This may be a particularly serious complication after any oral surgery. Prevention requires careful oral hygiene with mouth washes and mechanical care of the teeth and gums.

HEAD AND NECK INFECTIONS.—Staphylococci and streptococci are common to the flora of the head and neck. Laryngectomy, intraoral resections and radical neck operations are not uncommonly complicated by open wound infections due to staphylococci, and these usually require incision and drainage. Group A streptococcal infections can be catastrophic in this area. Penicillin is the drug of choice for the latter group.

CENTRAL NERVOUS SYSTEM.—The most important sign of a central nervous system infection is deterioration of the mental status. Fever and meningeal signs may be absent. A spinal tap and Gram stain, culture, cell count, as well as sugar and protein determinations are obligatory to rule out active bacterial meningitis. This may be secondary to hematogenous spread in the usual manner or may be a complication of craniotomy, vertebral disk surgery, mastoidectomy, hypophysectomy, skull trauma, ventricular shunt for hydrocephalus and, rarely, may even follow spinal anesthesia. In these situations, the usual pathogens—pneumococci and meningococci—are rarely seen. Antibiotic-resistant organisms such as the staphylococcus, pseudomonas and aerobacter are most commonly the causative organisms.

A particularly perplexing clinical situation may occur following surgery of the central nervous system or occasionally following the injection of diagnostic dyes or radioactive substances into the spinal canal. The symptoms include fever, nuchal rigidity, lethargy and headache. The laboratory findings consist of elevation of the cerebrospinal fluid pressure, protein and polymorphonuclear cell count in addition to a decreased cerebrospinal fluid sugar. All of these may be caused by the surgical procedure itself without the presence of active infection. The decision regarding the institution of therapy is dependent upon the Gram stain, the clinical course of the patient, particularly the mental status and especially the results of serial lumbar punctures. In general, if therapy is considered, it is well to remember that gram-negative rods generally multiply more rapidly than do many of the gram-positive coccal organisms which cause meningitis. Gram-negative rods are therefore less likely to be associated with a negative Gram stain and a clinically active bacterial meningitis.

It is important to emphasize that an early postoperative change (48–72 hours) in the mental status will be most often due to other organ system failures, such as pulmonary insufficiency with hypoxia and/or hypercapnia, hepatic coma and cardiovascular collapse. Drug reactions are quite common and difficult to diagnose. Anesthetics, tranquilizers, anticonvulsants and pain medications may all contribute to mental depression, since the excretion and/or conjugation of various drugs may be markedly compromised in the postoperative period.

Cardiovascular system.—Patients undergoing open heart surgery and prosthetic valve replacement have many potential sites of infection. Most of these complications present with fever after the first 5–7 postoperative days. Streptococcal or pneumococcal septicemias can be particularly virulent in the first 72 hours, but rarely occur because of the common use of high doses of prophylactic antibiotics.

Purulent pericarditis, mediastinitis, postpericardiotomy syndrome, osteomyelitis of the ribs or sternum, abscess of vascular cutdown sites, phlebitis of the vein used for diagnostic cardiac catheterization, acute hemolytic anemias, transfusion reactions, infectious mononucleosis syndromes (secondary to cytomegalovirus or E.B. virus), drug reactions (particularly quinidine and penicillin), peripheral and pulmonary emboli, empyema, atelectasis, pneumonia and endocarditis are some of the many possibilities to consider. If a specific diagnosis cannot be made, additional antibiotic therapy is not indicated unless the patient is quite septic or toxic.

The presence of fever alone is not an indication to add or change antibiotic therapy. Endocarditis is one of the most feared complications of valve replacement. Such infections are very difficult to diagnose and treat. They may be due to so many different organisms that "shot-gun" therapy, even in view of a reasonably compatible syndrome, is rarely indicated without positive blood cultures. The diagnosis of endocarditis on an artificial valve requires ultimate replacement with a new valve in most cases.

It is appropriate to mention the use of prophylactic antibiotics in both open heart and peripheral vascular surgery in which prosthetic materials are used. High doses of penicillinase-resistant penicillins may be successful in diminishing acute gram-positive septicemias and perhaps also in decreasing the incidence of coagulase-negative and coagulase-positive staphylococcal endocarditis. Drug reactions and the inducement of resistant staphylococci are potential hazards of prophylactic therapy. Insufficient controlled data are available to determine the "correct" regimen.

NONINFECTIOUS CAUSES OF FEVER.—These include fat embolism following bone trauma (petechial hemorrhage and fat globules in the urine, retinal vessels and saliva), thyroid storm, pulmonary emboli, hypothalamic damage, drug reactions, postpericardiotomy syndromes and, most commonly in my opinion, superficial or deep thrombophlebitis.

It is important to remember that the longer a patient has been in the hospital and the higher the dose and wider the spectrum of antibiotics administered, the more likely the new infection will be of a resistant strain. Appropriate therapy then requires careful deliberation.

If a specific bacterial infection suddenly becomes frequent, intensive epidemiologic investigation is necessary to define the source and to prevent further spread.

11

Psychiatric Complications

RAYMOND N. MILLER, M.D.

Adjunct Attending Psychiatrist, Rush-Presbyterian-St. Luke's Medical Center; Assistant Professor of Psychiatry, Rush Medical College

AND

IRA S. HALPER, M.D.

Associate Attending Psychiatrist, Rush-Presbyterian-St. Luke's Medical Center; Assistant Professor of Psychiatry, Rush Medical College

IT HAS BEEN POPULAR in recent years to emphasize treatment of the whole patient. There is some virtue in this, particularly in the case of general practitioners and specialists who are primary physicians. However, "treat the whole patient" is sometimes simplistic and unrealistic advice when applied to surgical specialties. We assume that surgeons go into their specialties because they are particularly interested in treating patients by means of surgery. In addition to this, perhaps some surgeons should not be involved in the emotional aspect of medical care. We are thinking particularly of surgeons who specialize in operations which have a high mortality rate or those which are necessarily mutilating, such as radical surgery for cancer. We should also take into account individual differences in physicians. Some physicians are by the nature of their personalities more sensitive in picking up psychiatric problems. Some are more effective than others in giving their patients emotional support. We believe it is naive to expect all physicians to be sophisticated about unconscious processes and nuances of psychiatric diagnosis and treatment.

What then is a realistic approach for surgeons to take? First, they should understand that all people are motivated by unconscious as well as conscious processes. This means that each of us has a rational, here-

and-now oriented side, and each of us has an irrational side of which we are often unaware. The irrational side is related to old psychic scars, conflicting emotions and childhood wishes and fears. Ordinarily, it is not necessary to pay attention to this side of patients' personalities. However, first, when psychiatric symptoms or maladaptive behavior complicate recovery from surgery, one should recall that there is more to patients and their behavior than is seen on the surface. Second, surgeons should realize that preoperative laboratory studies, surgical procedures and other things that happen to patients while they are in the hospital are frightening, even to patients who are psychologically normal. Third, surgeons should know something about their own interest and skill in handling emotional problems in their patients. All physicians can learn something about the early diagnosis of these problems. Some physicians in surgical specialties do a good job of managing these problems themselves, either on an intuitive basis or by conscious plan. Others have less interest in this area, and prefer to refer these cases to psychiatrists.

Problem Patients

Whereas formulas cannot be applied neatly to the management of psychiatric problems, some generalizations are helpful. Below, some common, troublesome personality types are discussed. Actually, one often sees combinations of these and other types.

THE OVERLY DEPENDENT, DEMANDING PATIENT.—This patient urgently asks for attention from physicians and nurses. He is resentful if his wishes are not gratified promptly. Illness tempts him to return to an infantile state. He equates food, medication and special consideration with love. He fears that he will be left abandoned and helpless like an infant who has been deserted by his mother. Some of these patients become depressed and withdrawn. Another variation on this theme is the hyperindependent patient, who is frightened by being in a dependent position and resists appropriate care.

The demands of overly dependent patients can sometimes be reduced by nurses checking on them from time to time without being called. In other cases it is necessary to explain the limits of the kind and amount of care that is available.

THE OVERLY CONTROLLED, ORDERLY PATIENT.—This patient desires as much knowledge about himself as possible to handle his anxieties. He substitutes thinking for action. Like a child trying to be clean and good, he is preoccupied with tidiness, punctuality and right and wrong.

It is often helpful to take a scientific approach with such patients; giving them detailed information about their illness can lead to intellectual mastery over their anxieties. This can be done without describing all of the upsetting possibilities.

THE DRAMATIC, CAPTIVATING PATIENT.—This patient charms and challenges his or her physician. Her manner is warm and personal, and she expects the people around her to respond the same way. She has a need to be attractive and outstanding and sees sickness as a defeat. She feels weak, unattractive and unsuccessful. Her dramatic bids for attention remind one of the little girl who has a strong attachment to her father and competes with her mother for his love. She feels guilty about hostile feelings toward her mother and fears punishment.

Too much warmth and involvement on the part of the physician add to these patients' anxieties and aggravate management problems. A calm, firm, interested, but uninvolved approach is most effective.

THE LONG-SUFFERING, SELF-SACRIFICING PATIENT.—This patient overemphasizes unpleasant aspects of his illness and exhibits his suffering. His history often reveals repeated illnesses and adversities. Close examination discloses a predilection on the part of the patient to put himself in difficult situations and precipitate misfortune. It is hard to understand a person who seeks pain, but we know that this occurs. In the childhood of such a patient, pain has become connected psychologically with pleasure. In some cases, childhood illnesses become connected with love and attention from parents.

Comfort has a paradoxical effect on these patients. They reject encouragement and work against recovery. They respond better to acknowledgment of their pain and suffering. Their sickness can be described as a burden they must carry, and their recovery can be talked about in terms of benefiting others rather than themselves.

THE SUSPICIOUS, QUERULOUS PATIENT.—This patient blames the disabilities and discomforts of his illness on physicians and nurses. He feels let down and taken advantage of; he feels weak and vulnerable. He is angry about old hurts, real and imagined. He projects his anger to other people and claims that they treat him badly.

To avoid distortions of reality, these patients should be told explicitly about the diagnosis and treatment of their illnesses. One should avoid being too friendly to such patients. They tend to develop a feeling of closeness which is followed by a sense of disappointment and a feeling of being abused. One should also avoid power struggles. This makes them feel more weak and mistrustful. Irrational beliefs may persist despite explanations by the physician.

THE SUPERIOR, "SPECIAL" PATIENT.—The superior, "special" patient has a need to see himself as powerful and important. He wants only the most eminent or senior physician to treat him. He tries to outdo his doctors and searches for weaknesses in them. He rejects medical opinions on the basis of his own conclusions. Actually, this patient fears he is weak and unimportant. Illness threatens his image of perfection.

One should acknowledge the achievements of such patients; however, the physician should not minimize his own expertise. At the same time that these patients tear down their doctors, they fear that they are in the hands of incompetent physicians.

Pain

All pain is real. At the same time, all pain is psychologic. To say that a pain is purely physical denies the fact that the patient is aware of hurting. To say that a pain is purely mental denies the fact that a part of his body hurts. This is not merely an exercise in semantics, for narrow thinking about this symptom often leads to diagnostic errors and inadequate relief of pain.

Pain is a phenomenon which has several facets: neurologic, physiologic, interpersonal and intrapersonal. Actual or impending tissue damage stimulates free nerve endings. Responses are transmitted to the dorsal horn of the spinal cord and then to thalamic nuclei. Pain signals may be dampened or potentiated by cells of the substantia gelatinosa and the cerebral cortex and other cephalic structures. Physiologic changes with pain include inhibition of gastrointestinal motility and increased muscle tension, pulse rate and blood pressure.

Pain is also a means of relating to and communicating with other people. Pain responses can mean: "Look how much I suffer," "See how brave I am," "Look what you do to me," "Help me (but you'll fail!)." These are often unconscious, automatic responses of which the patient is unaware.

When people are sick their feelings and actions commonly return to childhood. Old associations between pain and punishment by an angry parent are reawakened. An old wish for a parent to make the hurt go away casts the patient in the role of an unloved child and the physician in the role of a parent.

In childhood, pain is frequently linked with anxiety. It is experienced in situations which evoke anxiety about damage to the body or anxiety about losing the love of a parent. Pain and anxiety can become confused, so that one can produce responses appropriate to the other. Thus, pain in adult life can lead to responses like those of a child faced with bodily harm or withdrawal of parental love. Anxiety in adult life about bodily integrity and/or loss of a loved person can lead to pain sensations and responses. These psychosomatic phenomena are not restricted to patients with psychiatric problems; they are common in normal patients as well.

Depression

Depressive reactions to surgery include adjustment reactions, depressive neuroses and psychotic depressive reactions.

An adjustment reaction is a transient reaction to stress in an individual who has no apparent psychiatric disorder. Symptoms recede as the stress diminishes.

The patient with a depressive neurosis complains of feeling sad, hopeless, lonely and guilty. Self-esteem is low, and he has a sense of inadequacy and inferiority. Anxiety may be present. He craves affection, reassurance, sympathy and attention. However, his hostile complaints and his demands may irritate and alienate people around him. He may have trouble falling asleep, or he may escape into long hours of sleep. Some patients with neurotic depressions believe that life is not worth living, and may attempt suicide. The patient with a depressive neurosis looks unhappy and discouraged; there is a lack of color in his speech and manner.

The patient with a psychotic depressive reaction shares some signs and symptoms with the neurotic depressive; however, the depression is much more severe, and his behavior is much more disorganized. There is much more deterioration in his relationship with reality. When challenged, the neurotic is aware that he is exaggerating and distorting. The psychotic depressed patient may have delusions of sinfulness or guilt. He may believe others are talking about him in a derogatory way or trying to harm him. Hypochondriac complaints may assume a delusional character, and the patient may be convinced he has heart disease, cancer or a brain tumor. Hallucinations are rare; when present, they are usually auditory and condemnatory in nature. When retardation is present, it is much more severe than in the neurotic patient. Speech, thinking and movement are slowed. Some patients are immobile for long periods. Others are agitated or irritable. The psychotic depressive characteristically awakens early in the morning between 2:00 and 6:00 A.M. and is unable to go back to sleep.

Childhood experiences predispose patients to develop depressions in reaction to stress in adult life. These experiences include separation from parents or loss of parents, insufficient acceptance and affection from parents, excessive frustration in early social and educational activities and illnesses in childhood. Many depressions respond to psychotherapy and psychotropic drugs. Medication for depressions is discussed in the section on psychotropic drugs.

The Suicidal Patient

Many depressed people think about killing themselves, but most of them do not act on these thoughts. It is natural for a patient who believes his physical condition is hopeless and who imagines an uncomfortable or painful death to consider ending his life. Again, most of these patients do not commit suicide. How can one identify the patient whose depressive feelings are so terribly painful that he prefers death and will attempt to kill himself?

The risk of suicide should be assessed in all patients with severe or moderately severe depressions. Some patients will volunteer thoughts about suicide; others must be asked. One need not be a psychiatrist to question patients about suicidal thoughts. They are not offended if they are tactfully asked questions such as: "Do you sometimes think about ending it all?" and "How close have you come to acting on these thoughts?"

Some patients hide depressive feelings behind masks of emotional flatness or pseudocheerfulness. One should also not be reassured by the patient who denies suicidal thoughts, but who indicates in indirect ways that there is a danger of his killing himself. One should look honestly at the illness and the circumstances of the patient's life. How would an average person react to the stresses that confront him? In addition to the illness and the surgery, does he have an unhappy marriage? Are there difficulties at work or financial problems? Does he lack emotional support from friends and family? Is there anything that makes the patient feel his life is worth living? Talking to family members can be helpful in assessing the risk of suicide.

There is a greater danger of suicide when retardation and psychosocial inhibitions begin to lift than there is when a patient is in the depths of a depression. This makes sense in the light of evidence that depression can serve a defensive function. During periods of depressive equilibrium, an individual can avoid confronting and dealing with the pain of loss and mourning. During times of acute psychotic turmoil, the individual deals with the loss that precipitated the depression and experiences the effects of grief and anxiety. Some patients may be overcome by painful emotions during unstable periods when they seem to be recovering from depressions.

If a seriously suicidal patient must remain in the intensive care unit, restraints may be indicated. They must be securely applied if they are to be effective.

Delirium

Delirium is a syndrome of cerebral insufficiency. It is potentially reversible if etiologic factors are eliminated before cell death occurs. The term "delirium" includes the diagnosis "toxic psychosis" and is related to the diagnosis "acute brain syndrome" in another classification of organic brain disorders. At least in the light of our present knowledge about brain function, organic factors determine the clinical picture in a relatively nonspecific way. The disturbances in psychic functioning are similar regardless of the etiologic agent. The manifestations of delirium reflect an interaction of organic and psychologic factors. Reduction in the level of awareness and cognitive defects are direct consequences of brain damage. Anxiety, the content of hallucinations, etc., are determined by past psychologic development, current conflicts and individual patterns of defense and coping. Some of the behavior observed in delirium is a result of efforts to avoid the anxiety and depression which the patient experiences when he cannot cope with cognitive tasks. The hospital environment also contributes to the clinical picture.

Delirium is caused by cerebral metabolic insufficiency. Etiologic agents include: pulmonary disease, anemia, febrile states, decreased cardiac output, hypertensive encephalopathy, hypoglycemia, liver disease, kidney disease, hyper- or hypofunction of endocrine organs, drugs and electrolyte abnormalities. The basic disturbance in delirium is a reduction in the level of awareness and cognitive defects. Reduction in the level of awareness includes fluctuating attention, inattention and somnolence. Cognitive defects include deficits in orientation, memory, comprehension, calculation, learning and judgment. With milder degrees of delirium, the patient may be able to compensate for defects with increased effort. The electroencephalogram in delirium shows diffuse slowing, sometimes with paroxysmal bursts of slow activity superimposed on a background of mildly slow activity. The degree of delirium can be measured by the level of awareness; this correlates with the electroencephalogram because greater reduction of awareness is associated with more electroencephalographic slowing. The extent of bizarre thought content or disturbed behavior does not seem to reflect the degree of cerebral damage and does not correlate with the electroencephalogram. Some patients go from a subtle decline in cognitive performance to coma without grossly disturbed behavior. Others, with relatively mild basic defects, manifest gross anxiety, hallucinations, delusions, irrational speech or outbursts of rage.

There are several typical patterns of delirium:

1. The quiet, lethargic patient. This patient does not have obvious defects; however, observation of his behavior shows such things as an inability to recognize hospital personnel or a failure to cope with tasks such as eating. This patient denies difficulties or attempts to conceal them, often by saying he is weak or tired.

2. The blandly confused patient. This patient responds in a friendly, smiling manner and claims to feel well. However, further questions elicit slow, uncertain answers and a puzzled expression. He tends to avoid questions by means of humor or irritability. He may become upset if he is pressed too hard.

3. The anxious patient. This patient is greatly disturbed by his cognitive defects and responds with severe anxiety. Restlessness, tremor, tachycardia, hyperventilation and sweating may be present. Disorientation and misinterpretation of events around him may be seen.

4. The hallucinating patient. He is often misinterpreting sensory stimuli. Sounds are mistaken for familiar voices, and shadows and shapes are confused with familiar persons or objects. True hallucinations may also occur.

5. The muttering, incoherent patient. This patient is usually experiencing a more advanced degree of delirium. Disorientation is gross, as are other cognitive defects.

In many cases the diagnosis of delirium can be made without a formal mental status examination. One can unobtrusively evaluate cognitive functions by asking questions about the onset and course of illnesses. During physical examinations, one can observe such things as confusion about directions, difficulty initiating or persevering in requested acts and persevering in the same act in response to a new request.

The differential diagnosis of delirium includes chronic brain syndrome (dementia). Chronic brain syndromes frequently become worse during a serious systemic illness or with drugs that depress cerebral functioning. Such patients may be said to have a superimposed delirium. Hysterical states such as fugues and amnesia may be differentiated by inconsistent cognitive performance at a given time, excellent in some areas and markedly deficient in others. For example, the disorientation to time or place of the dissociated hysteric is not consistent with his alertness and his ability to assimilate new information.

Patients in a state of delirium may fall out of bed or wander off the ward. They may become seriously suicidal. A light should be kept burning at night, for darkness accentuates disorientation and hallucinations. Physicians and nurses should introduce themselves at each contact and remind the patient where he is. Procedures should be carefully and, often, repetitiously explained in simple terms. Nonessential drugs should be discontinued, including sedatives, narcotics and tranquilizers which may aggravate delirium. For some agitated patients, however, chlordiazepoxide or a phenothiazine is indicated.

Careful attention should be paid to other disorders which can increase delirium. Oxygen should be given to mildly hypoxic patients, and transfusions may be indicated for patients with anemia. Mild electrolyte disorders such as hyponatremia and hypokalemia should be corrected. Such measures often improve delirium significantly, even if the primary cause is not eliminated. Vital signs and the level of consciousness should be checked frequently to ensure that sudden worsening does not go undetected.

Delirium may be aggravated by experiences the patient has in the intensive care unit. He is in pain and is unable to move freely. He is deprived of familiar sights and sounds and is bombarbed with strange stimuli from respirators, monitoring devices, etc. This set of factors is discussed in more detail in the following section on the open heart patient.

The Open Heart Patient

Patients who have open heart surgery are particularly prone to have psychiatric symptoms postoperatively. Often these symptoms are of psychotic severity.

There is evidence that a substantial number of open heart patients have cerebral dysfunctions. Hemiplegia, visual field defects and generalized convulsions have been observed, and anoxic damage to the brain has been found on postmortem examination. Psychiatric symptoms, disorientation, memory disturbances, restlessness and visual hallucinations have been correlated with neurologic findings.

Several psychiatric syndromes have been described following open heart surgery. One is a delirium which begins several days after surgery. Illusions are early symptoms, stimulated by sounds from air conditioner vents, reflections of light from oxygen tents, etc. This syndrome includes disorientation, delusions and hallucinations. A "catastrophe reaction" during the first week has been reported by several investigators. These patients are oriented but appear dazed. They are tired and apathetic. They lie immobile, and their monosyllabic responses lack emotion. The vacant expressions on their faces remind one of the photographed faces of survivors of civil disasters. This syndrome usually disappears after a few days and is followed by a mild depression which gradually lifts. Sometimes, however, the catastrophe reaction is followed by a psychosis.

Several kinds of factors are probably responsible for these postoperative syndromes. Possible organic factors include cerebral anoxia and fluid and electrolyte disturbances. The preoperative psychologic state of the patient, including feelings about his illness and the life-threatening surgery, no doubt contribute to these problems. There is also good evidence that the intensive care unit is psychologically stressful. These units provide excellent and sometimes life-saving care, and it is easy to overlook the emotional impact of this care. One can make a long list of uncomfortable, painful and disturbing experiences an open heart patient has in the intensive care unit. The list includes the placement of an endotracheal tube or tracheostomy, a urinary catheter, a nasogastric tube and chest tubes. Vital signs are taken frequently; sleep is interrupted, and day merges into night. There are strange noises, and crises occur with patients in neighboring beds. The room is unfamiliar and sterile in appearance. The patient lies immobile, looking up at a white ceiling through an oxygen tent. It is interesting that in one study, visual hallucinations began as faces protruding from the small holes in the ceiling tiles. There is a mixture of deprivation of normal sensory cues and bombardment with strange and frightening stimuli.

The incidence of psychiatric reactions to the intensive care unit can be reduced substantially by relatively simple measures. Nurses should check repeatedly on the patient's orientation to time and place. They should carefully explain procedures and equipment. Interrupting sleep should be avoided unless necessary. At Rush-Presbyterian-St. Luke's Medical Center, a nurse talks with patients before open heart surgery. She answers their questions and prepares them for the operation and the intensive care unit. She is with them when they awaken from the anesthesia. This program is both practical and very sound from a psychiatric standpoint.

If a delirium does develop, the patient may pull out tubes, exhaust himself and disturb other patients. Such patients have been successfully treated with phenothiazines, orally or intramuscularly. Trifluoperazine (Stelazine) 2 mg. three or four times daily is often effective. Chlorpromazine (Thorazine) is more likely to cause hypotension and aggravate confusion. In some cases, however, the sedation produced by chlorpromazine may be desirable. The initial intramuscular dose of chlorpromazine should not exceed 25 mg., and the pulse and blood pressure should be watched carefully. If the patient tolerates this, additional or larger doses may be given every 4–6 hours. General rules for managing delirium should be followed: ensure adequate pulmonary function and cardiac output, maintain electrolyte balance, avoid drugs such as barbiturates which lead to confusion and avoid digitalis toxicity.

Psychotropic Drugs

Drugs for Psychosis

The phenothiazines are the most widely used group of drugs in this category. The indications for phenothiazines include schizophrenia, mania, paranoid disorders, psychoses associated with organic brain syndromes, borderline psychotic states and agitated depressions. It was thought that depressions were aggravated by phenothiazines, and this may be so in the case of retarded depressions. There is evidence, however, that phenothiazines are superior to tricyclic antidepressants in the treatment of depressions in which anxiety is prominent. Symptoms which respond to phenothiazines include anxiety, delusions, hallucinations, destructive behavior and schizophrenic withdrawal. The effectiveness of these drugs in neurotic patients is less impressive, although good results have been reported with severe neurotic disorders.

The incidence of certain side effects varies within the phenothiazine group of drugs. There is a higher incidence of jaundice and agranulocytosis with chlorpromazine. Extrapyramidal side effects are more likely to occur with trifluoperazine. Changes in the electrocardiogram and arrhythmias seem to be more common with thioridazine. Drowsiness is seen more frequently with chlorpromazine than with trifluoperazine or thioridazine.

Chlorpromazine (Thorazine) is prescribed in doses ranging from 25 mg. three times daily to 1,500 mg./day. Disturbed psychotic patients commonly require 200–800 mg./day. The first intramuscular dose should not exceed 25 mg. to minimize the danger of hypotension.

Trifluoperazine (Stelazine) is prescribed in doses of 2 mg. twice daily to 40 mg./day. Prophylactic anti-parkinsonism medication such as benztropine mesylate (Cogentin) may be indicated in some cases, particularly when the daily dose of trifluoperazine is 10 mg. or more. Thioridazine (Mellaril) is prescribed in doses ranging from 25 mg. three times daily to 800 mg./day.

Some patients with schizophrenia can safely discontinue phenothiazines after recovering from an acute episode. Others should remain on a maintenance dose for long periods of time or indefinitely to avoid a relapse. Intermittent phenothiazine therapy seems to be adequate in some of these cases. Changes in skin color and melanin-like deposits in the lens and cornea have been noted in patients taking phenothiazines for a period of 2 years. Most of these patients have not had a reduction in visual acuity; however, we recommend periodic slit lamp examinations in the long-term use of these drugs.

Drugs for Anxiety

Chlordiazepoxide, diazepam and tybamate are helpful in neuroses, adjustment reactions, psychosomatic disorders and anxiety associated with organic brain syndromes. They are not effective in psychoses. Chlordiazepoxide and diazepam are in the benzodiazepine family; tybamate is chemically and pharmacologically related to meprobamate. Serious side effects with these drugs are uncommon. Chlordiazepoxide (Librium) is prescribed in doses ranging from 15 to 100 mg./day. The dose of diazepam (Valium) is 4–40 mg./day. Tybamate (Solacen) is prescribed in doses of 750–2,000 mg./day.

Drugs for Depression

The tricyclic antidepressants are the most important group of drugs in this category. The indications for tricyclic antidepressants include involutional melancholia; manic-depressive illness, depressed type; psychotic-depressive reaction; and the schizo-affective type of schizophrenia (sometimes in combination with a phenothiazine). Antidepressants appear to be more effective in psychotic than in neurotic depressions, but they seem to have a place in the treatment of severe neurotic depressions as well. Electric convulsive treatment remains the therapy of choice for some patients, particularly when there is a high risk of suicide. The drugs for anxiety may be helpful in mild depressions.

The tricyclic antidepressants are chemically related to phenothiazines, and similar side effects are seen. Amitriptyline may have more of a sedative effect than imipramine. Anticholinergic side effects are more likely to be a problem in patients who receive a combination of an antidepressant, a phenothiazine and an anti-parkinson drug, all of which have anticholinergic actions. Desipramine, a demethylated derivative of imipramine, seems to be less potent than the parent compound; however, it has the advantage of being less likely to produce atropine-like side effects. Hypertensive episodes have been observed during surgery in patients on desipramine.

The dose of imipramine (Tofranil) and amitriptyline (Elavil) is 25 mg. three times daily to 250 mg. daily. The best results seem to be obtained with doses of 150–250 mg./day, a level which can be reached over a period of several days. Desipramine (Norpramin and Pertofrane) is given in doses of 25 mg. three times daily to 200 mg./day.

In psychotic-depressed patients, an effect is usually seen within 10 days. But some patients do not respond for 3 weeks. It is necessary to prescribe a relatively high dose for 3 weeks to consider the trial of therapy an adequate one.

To reduce the likelihood of a relapse, it is safer to continue a high dose for 2–3 months after recovery from the depression. If there is no recurrence, the drug can be withdrawn at the rate of 50 mg. every 2 weeks. If a relapse occurs, the dose can be raised again and maintained at a high level for 4–6 weeks before withdrawal is attempted again. Some patients may require antidepressants for long periods of time or indefinitely.

REFERENCES

1. Abram, H. S.: Adaptation to open heart surgery: A psychiatric study of response to the threat of death, Am. J. Psychiat. 122:659–667, 1965.
2. Blachly, P. H., and Starr, A.: Treatment of delirium with phenothiazine drugs following open heart surgery, Dis. Nerv. System 27:107–110, 1966.
3. Cole, J. O., and Davis, J. M.: Antidepressant Drugs, in Freedman, A. M., and Kaplan, H. I. (eds.): *Comprehensive Textbook of Psychiatry* (Baltimore: Williams & Wilkins Company, 1967).
4. Denber, H. C. B.: Tranquilizers in Psychiatry, in Freedman, A. M., and Kaplan, H. I. (eds.): *Comprehensive Textbook of Psychiatry* (Baltimore: Williams & Wilkins Company, 1967).
5. Posner, J. B.: Delirium and Exogenous Metabolic Brain Disease, in Beeson, P. B., and McDermott, W. (eds.): *Cecil-Loeb Textbook of Medicine* (12th ed.; Philadelphia: W. B. Saunders Company, 1967).
6. Sternbach, R. A.: *Pain, A Psychophysiological Analysis* (New York: Academic Press, Inc., 1968).

12

Gastrointestinal Intubation

MARSHALL D. GOLDIN, M.D.*

Fellow in Cardiovascular-Thoracic Surgery, Rush-Presbyterian-St. Luke's Medical Center; Instructor in Surgery, Rush Medical College

Complications of Gastrointestinal Intubation

GASTROINTESTINAL INTUBATION is an essential in the armamentarium of the surgeon. It may be used for pre- and postoperative decompression, nonoperative decompression and for alimentation. The associated complications, however, must be kept in mind to aid in their prevention or to permit their early detection. For these reasons a detailed list of complications of gastrointestinal intubation is included.

NOSE.—Pressure necrosis of the ala or columella is most often caused by improper positioning of nasal tubes. This may occur when the tube is taped to the forehead or when it is pulled upward by the tape onto the dorsum of the nose (Fig. 12-1, *A* and *B*). Continuous tugging by peristaltic action against balloon-tipped tubes may also cause pressure necrosis at points of friction. Obstruction of the middle meatus may cause maxillary sinusitis.

A convenient method of securing nasal tubes to minimize pressure on the nares and to permit adjustment is depicted in Figure 12-1, *C*. Entwining the tube with tape makes adjustment difficult and is uncomfortable for the patient.

ORAL CAVITY.—Most patients with indwelling tubes are forced to breathe through the mouth. Oral breathing results in dehydration of the mucous membranes of the mouth, pharynx, larynx and tracheobronchial tree. Long-term intubation, particularly in the debilitated patient, predisposes him to suppurative parotitis. Prevention is best accomplished by adequate hydration and careful attention to mouth care. Frequent use of mouth wash or sialagogues such as sour candy are additional helpful measures.

*Supported in part by United States Public Health Service Grant No. 1T12HE05808.

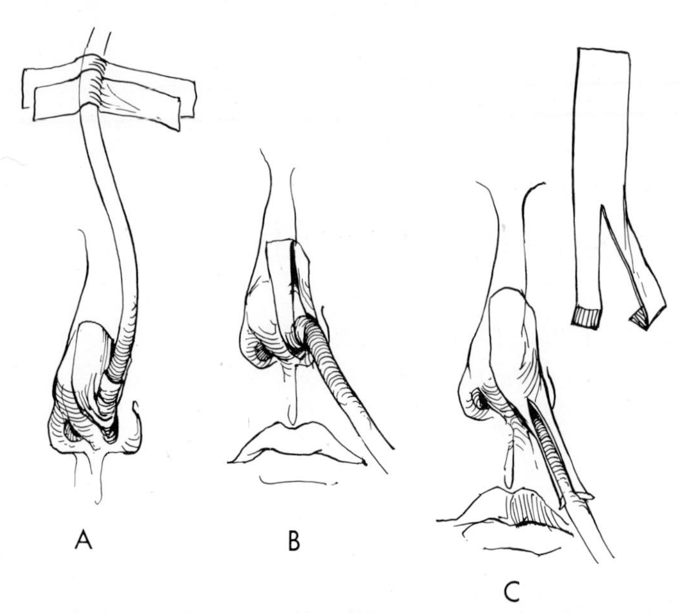

Fig. 12-1. – **A** and **B**, incorrect fixation of nasal tube. Pressure necrosis of the tip of the nose may occur if the tube is fixed to the forehead in a tight loop **(A)** or pulled upward by tape **(B)** over the tip of the nose. **C**, correct fixation of nasal tube. A longitudinal tear is made halfway through a 2–3 in. strip of 1 in. tape, and the tips of the 2 ends are folded over each other. The tape is placed on the nose and the ends applied longitudinally to facilitate repositioning of the tube.

OTITIS MEDIA. – Pain referred to the neck or ear can result from otitis media, secondary to local irritation and swelling of the eustachian ostia. This condition is best treated by removal of the tube, but if this is not possible, a change in position of the tube will usually relieve the symptoms. A vasoconstrictor spray will afford temporary relief.

PHARYNX AND LARYNX. – Local trauma by an indwelling tube may cause painful ulceration of the pharyngeal wall or the cricoid cartilage. A late complication of the latter may be manifest as laryngeal stenosis. The adhesive used on tape is irritating to mucosa. Adhesive, therefore, should not remain when advancing the tube. If the adhesive present on the tube is removed with a solvent, any residue of solvent should be carefully removed.

ESOPHAGUS. – Erosion of the wall of the esophagus occurs with some degree of frequency, particularly with use of large or nonflexible tubes. Erosion also may occur at the gastroesophageal junction. Incompetence of the gastroesophageal sphincter, especially in older patients, may be produced or increased by means of an indwelling tube. Those patients with hiatus hernia are even more likely to suffer from this complication. Ulceration of esophageal varices can compound an already serious situation.

STOMACH.—Local effects of indwelling tubes on the stomach include erosion by the tip of the tube and occasionally multiple small areas of ecchymosis resulting from vigorous attempts at aspiration of the tube.

INTESTINE.—Long gastrointestinal tubes are prone to kink or twist, and occasionally they double back through a gastroenterostomy, making retrieval difficult. All of the preceding should be suspected when irrigation becomes difficult. The most common cause of obstruction is clogging of the lumen by food and debris.

Necrosis of the wall of the intestine may occur if the tube crosses an area of acute angulation. Pressure from an inflated balloon or from the tip of the tube distal to the balloon may also be a cause of tissue damage. Excess suction can result in mucosal damage or even retard passage through the intestine.

PULMONARY EFFECTS.—Indwelling nasal tubes may cause or compound pulmonary complications. Coughing causes the tube to rub against the pharynx and thus make the patient gag. The patient guards against this by coughing feebly—already necessary because of incisional pain. Ineffective coughing results in retained secretions and possible atelectasis and pneumonia. Mouth breathing impairs maintenance of airway humidity and further contributes to pulmonary complications.

FEEDING.—Symptoms and signs of the dumping syndrome—mainly nausea, hypotension and diaphoresis—may occur in patients given hypertonic feedings into the upper small bowel. The best alternative is to give less concentrated feedings. Hypertonic feedings may also result in dehydration, since inadequate fluid is administered to provide for solute excretion.

Hypertonic feedings may cause diarrhea. Persistence of the diarrhea results in a chronically moist perineum, which predisposes to the formation of decubitus ulcers. The addition of 5–10 ml. paregoric to each feeding or of 5 ml. Lomotil may modify the diarrhea.

It is essential to ensure gastric emptying in the elderly or debilitated patient. Gastroesophageal reflux is particularly prone to occur in the supine patient. For this reason it is advisable to elevate the head of the bed. Continuous feeding by gravity drainage or peristaltic pumps can cause distention, nausea, vomiting and aspiration. Such a routine often precludes intermittent aspiration and the detection of incomplete gastric or intestinal emptying.

Nasogastric Tube

INDICATIONS

Diagnostic uses include aspiration to determine: (1) the site of bleeding, (2) the volume of secretion, (3) acid concentration and (4) cellular morphology. Therapeutic indications are decompression, mainly of the stomach, and alimentation.

DECOMPRESSION.—Emptying of the stomach preoperatively is particularly important in the unprepared patient who is about to have surgery under emergency conditions. All patients about to undergo major abdominal surgery should have gastric decompression. The decompression serves to prevent gastric distention, vomiting and pulmonary aspiration during the operative and postoperative period. Acute gastric dilatation (manifested by nausea, vomiting, hypotension and tachycardia) most often occurs in patients without nasogastric tubes, but may also be seen in patients in whom the tube has not been functioning.

Preoperative decompression is used to empty the stomach, preventing the progression of air and fluid into the small bowel. This procedure is helpful in cases of bowel obstruction, whether due to mechanical or adynamic causes. Decompression also facilitates exposure during major abdominal procedures.

Intraoperative decompression reduces the likelihood of aspiration, particularly during upper abdominal manipulation. Especially important is intubation and gastric emptying in the patient with a gastroenterostomy, pyloroplasty or gastroesophageal anastomosis in whom there is no sphincter mechanism to prevent reflux into the pharynx.

Postoperative decompression prevents abdominal distention and its undesirable accompaniment of an elevated diaphragm, tension on the wound and poor ventilation. The ever-present danger of aspiration, particularly in the obtunded individual, is also minimized.

ALIMENTATION.—Nasogastric and Mead Johnson tubes may also be used for alimentation. Careful monitoring of gastric emptying must be guaranteed in order to prevent overdistention and subsequent aspiration, particularly in the lethargic or elderly patient. Further protection can be afforded these patients by elevating the head of the bed. A convenient method is to raise the head of the bed with 4–6 in. blocks. This minimizes the likelihood of aspiration should the head of the bed be rolled down inadvertently.

Tube feedings may be administered on a continuous or intermittent routine. It is extremely important to aspirate the stomach on a regular schedule, in order to detect any impairment of gastric emptying or reverse peristalsis.

For the average patient (70 kg.), a program of 200 ml. of a blenderized general diet followed by 40 ml. of water or saline to irrigate the tube every 2 hours will provide 2,400 calories and the daily fluid requirement. It is essential to flush the tube with water or saline after each feeding to minimize obstruction of the lumen. This volume may be given continuously by infusion pump, gravity drainage or intermittently using the barrel of a bulb syringe as a funnel. Instillations into the gastrointestinal tract should not be given under pressure. For this reason, use of infusion pumps may be dangerous, since great pressures may be achieved. Indeed, large volumes of air may be introduced into the gastrointestinal tract if the reservoir is empty. A further disadvantage of the continuous method of alimentation is that there is a greater tendency to omit the frequent aspirations needed to evaluate gastric emptying.

INTERMITTENT INSTILLATION.—This method, along with intermittent gentle aspiration, is most reliable. If the volume in the stomach is 75 ml. or less and the tube is properly positioned, this volume can be returned and the next feeding given. If the volume is greater than 75 ml., most of it can be returned to the stomach, provided gastric distention will not result. The scheduled feeding is then delayed and the entire process repeated after 1 hour. It is often helpful, particularly in the patient with poor peristalsis, to turn the patient on the right side to promote drainage toward the pylorus.

INSERTION

Placing the nasogastric tube in ice makes it a stiff object which is difficult to pass without causing nasopharyngeal trauma. Warming the tube under the faucet makes it soft and easier to pass in an atraumatic manner. It is essential to use a water-soluble lubricant when inserting the tube. Lipoid pneumonia can occur following aspiration of oily lubricants.

Insertion with the patient in the erect position minimizes the likelihood of aspiration and permits the patient to swallow water during the procedure. The patient is most likely to aspirate when supine, especially if the tube is partially through the gastroesophageal junction.

Once in place, the position of the tube is verified by injecting air into it while listening over the stomach. For nasogastric decompression in the average-sized patient, the second mark on the tube should be at the level of the external nares.

1st mark: 45 cm. from tip to nares (level of cardia)
2d mark: 55 cm. from tip to nares (level of antrum)
3d mark: 65 cm. from tip to nares (level of pylorus)

Plastic tubes are preferred for insertion because they are less irritating, do not collapse, and permit evaluation of the character of the aspirate and the rate of flow.

MAINTENANCE POSTOPERATIVELY

In the recovery room, confirm that the tube is patent and functioning. Check the suction of the machine: (1) Disconnect the nasogastric tube and listen for rushing of air. (2) If there is no suction, there may be a leak in the system; occasionally this is caused by a loose-fitting cap or connection. (3) Observe the motion of aspirate in the tube.

Irrigate the nasogastric tube with 30 ml. of water or saline every 2 hours and resume the suction. If the tube is functioning, it is not always necessary to aspirate with a syringe, especially since inexperienced personnel may produce excess negative pressure and cause gastric hemorrhage by sucking mucosa into the holes. If the tube cannot be irrigated, it is kinked at the level of the esophagus or stomach.

Removal

Before the nasogastric tube is removed, the patient should exhibit good bowel sounds and pass stool or flatus. If no stool has been passed and hyperactive sounds are present, check for impaction. If diarrhea occurs, also check for impaction. When listening for bowel sounds, detach the tube or other sumps from the suction machine to avoid misleading extraneous noise. A patient with a patent nasogastric tube or gastrostomy should not vomit or become distended. If nausea or vomiting occurs with a functioning tube, a review of the medications will often uncover the cause.

Tube testing is performed when indicated. The usual procedure is to aspirate the stomach, instill 100 ml. water and clamp the tube for 1 hour. This is repeated twice more (total, 300 ml. water) and at the end of the 3d hour aspiration is again performed. If the residual volume is less than 100 ml., the tube is removed and a liquid diet is begun and slowly advanced. The suction is maintained during removal to aspirate nasopharyngeal secretions which collect around the tube.

Complications

The hazard of complications should not preclude the use of nasal tubes. Awareness of complications will provide a basis for their early recognition and prevention. Ulceration of the external nares and necrosis of the alar cartilages are painful and may be disfiguring. Proper fixation and occasional change in position will prevent this complication. Prolonged intubation can cause necrosis of the anterior wall of the upper esophagus and perichondritis of the cricoid cartilage.

Perforation may occur proximal to a carcinoma or benign stricture or through a diverticulum or ulcer of the esophagus. The tube may follow an abnormal route in the patient with a gastroenterostomy. It is important to remember that long gastrointestinal tubes do not effectively remove gastric secretions. Gastric distention, tracheobronchial aspiration or gastric ulceration may occur if an abnormal state prevents gastric emptying. The nasogastric tube may be in too far, removing biliary secretions and resulting in fluid and electrolyte imbalance.

Gastrostomy

Tube gastrostomy is mainly used for postoperative decompression. It is indicated primarily in the patient with pre-existing pulmonary disease in whom nasogastric intubation would significantly impair ventilation and expectoration of secretions. It also is often used as a route for alimentation.

Several types of tubes may be employed, the Foley catheter and the straight French catheter being among the most common. When the balloon of the former is inflated, it can be pulled up against the ventral wall of the stomach and parietal peritoneum and the tube then secured to the skin with a stitch. In this way a more effective seal is obtained against leakage of gastric content through the stoma. Pezzar and mushroom catheters may also be utilized in similar fashion, but their removal and replacement are more difficult and hazardous.

IMMEDIATE POSTOPERATIVE CARE.—Following major abdominal surgery, the gastrostomy tube should be attached to intermittent low pressure suction (90 mm. Hg). Irrigation and aspiration are performed every 2 hours to assure patency. Sterile water or saline (30 ml.) is used for tube irrigation. Preparations of antacid solution are substituted for water or saline in patients who are prone to develop stress ulcers or who have a history of ulcer.

Aspiration must be performed gently. Traumatic aspiration pulls the mucosa into the holes of the catheter and can incite gastric bleeding.

FURTHER MANAGEMENT.—After peristalsis has returned, the need for decompression is past. Tube testing is performed as described previously.

REMOVAL.—The tube may be clamped after peristalsis has returned and decompression is no longer necessary. It is wise to irrigate the tube with 30 ml. water or saline every 6–8 hours to keep the lumen patent, should it be necessary to use it again. The tube is ordinarily removed after the eighth postoperative day, since by this time there is a good seal between the serosa of the stomach and the abdominal wall.

Following removal, the wound is covered with a small dressing and the patient is instructed to lay supine following meals and to ingest a minimum amount of liquid with meals for 24–48 hours. This minimizes leakage and prevents soiling. An effective closure of the stoma occurs within 24–48 hours in most instances.

REPLACEMENT.—When a gastrostomy is to be maintained over a long period, Foley and French catheters are usually used. Application of small amounts of lubricant to the tube and stoma serves to make introduction less traumatic.

The catheter should be secured to the abdominal wall to prevent inadvertent removal or advancement into the gut. If the latter occurs with a Foley catheter, there may be gastric distention and vomiting due to obstruction of the pylorus by the inflated balloon.

Jejunostomy

The jejunostomy is used primarily for supplementary feedings. Occasionally a long jejunostomy (Baker) tube may be used for intraoperative decompression and then for continued postoperative decompression. However, the use of a jejunostomy is usually for alimentation during gastric ileus and pyloric obstruction. Jejunostomy is also beneficial in the debilitated patient with esophagogastric carcinoma who requires nutrition prior to resection.

In general, small-diameter tubes are used as jejunostomies. For this reason French catheters or Levine tubes are often used. The presence of a balloon-tipped catheter is obviously apt to produce obstruction to food and secretions coming from above. Depending on the size of the lumen, the diet may vary from a blenderized general diet to commercial supplements.

Irrigation of the tube with water or saline is performed on a regular basis. Ordinarily, suction is not required. Fixation of the tube to the skin by tape or stitch safeguards against accidental removal. If removed, immediate reintroduction is mandatory, since the stoma closes rapidly. A stiff catheter should never be used, since pressure erosion may occur. For the same reason, once the stoma is stable, in or out movement of the tube for a short distance once daily may prevent pressure ulceration.

Feedings may be instituted when peristalsis has returned. Initially, the patient is tested with water, dextrose/water or normal saline in a manner similar to tube testing. If there is no distal obstruction, rarely will much fluid be obtained on aspiration.

Hypertonic feedings may cause symptoms and signs of the dumping syndrome. Should this occur, the osmolar content of the feedings must be decreased. Intravenous fluids with glucose decrease the appetite in the patient who is about to eat; therefore, the intravenous fluids must be stopped 1–2 hours prior to beginning oral alimentation. High protein diets may produce diarrhea. This can be ameliorated by administration of 5 ml. paregoric with each feeding.

Long Gastrointestinal Tubes

Common indications for use of long gastrointestinal tubes include: (1) gastrointestinal decompression of fluid and air in patients with bowel obstruction, (2) preoperative decompression to facilitate exposure in major abdominal procedures, (3) postoperative internal splinting to minimize angulation and postoperative obstruction, (4) aid in the determination of the site of a bowel fistula or obstruction and (5) administration of intestinal feedings in patients with postoperative gastric fistulae or uncontrollable vomiting.

INSERTION.—In general these tubes, even those with attached balloons, are only slightly more difficult to insert than the standard nasogastric tube. Above all, it is essential to apply a liberal amount of water-soluble lubricant to the tube once the patient is positioned (erect with hyperextension of head) and the balloon is folded and held ready for insertion (Fig. 12-2, *A*). Forming a point by twisting or folding the balloon over a cotton swab can help facilitate insertion into the nasophar-

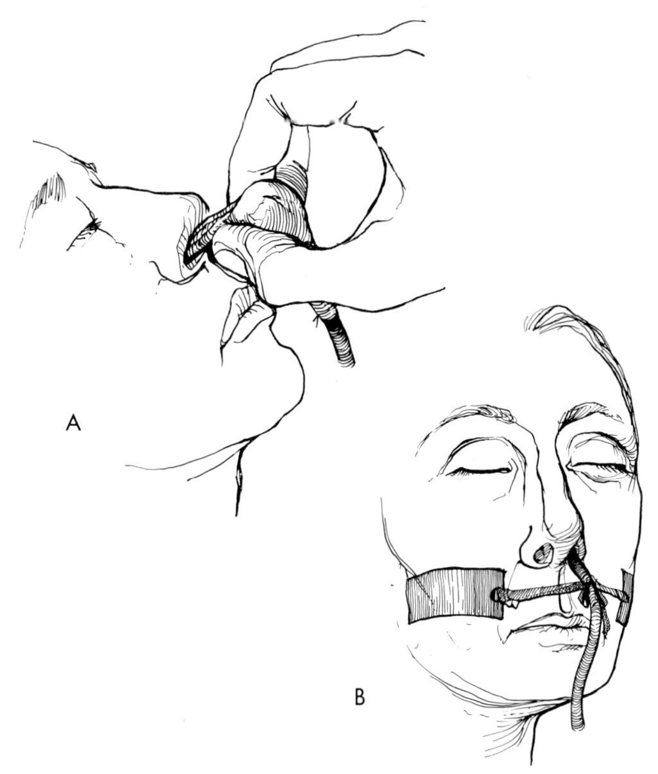

Fig. 12-2. – **A**, insertion of long gastrointestinal tube. The optimal position is hyperextension of the neck with the patient erect. Folding the balloon over a cotton swab facilitates insertion through the nasopharynx in difficult cases. **B**, mustache for temporary fixation of long gastrointestinal tube during advancement.

ynx. With balloons containing mercury, the weight serves to advance the tube into the stomach without need for swallowing. In those tubes in which mercury or air is to be inserted into the balloon after it is placed in the stomach, some swallowing is necessary to convey the tube to the stomach.

In most instances, particularly with bowel obstructions in which active peristalsis may soon disappear, fluoroscopic guidance is extremely helpful to advance the tip to or through the pylorus. Gastric emptying is often incomplete when a long tube progresses well into the small bowel. When hyperacidity is suspected or nausea and vomiting occur despite a functioning long tube, gastric decompression is in order.

Maintenance. – Once abdominal x-rays have comfirmed passage beyond the duodenum, the long gastrointestinal tube is advanced 4–6 in./hour. A temporary "mustache" (Fig. 12-2, *B*) prevents expulsion of the tube, yet permits loosening and facilitates advancement. This arrangement also prevents irritation of the nasopharyngeal mucosa by remnants of adhesive on the tube. Application of a small amount of anesthetic cream on the tube prior to each advancement replenishes the anesthetic on the nasopharyngeal mucosa and makes each manipulation virtually painless.

An abdominal x-ray is generally taken 6–8 hours after insertion to verify the position of the tube in the small bowel. Improvement in the abdominal x-ray picture and the clinical state of the patient serve as indicators of progress.

Irrigation with 30 ml. water or saline is performed at 2-hour intervals to ensure tube patency. Difficult or impossible irrigation signifies kinking or intraluminal obstruction. X-ray confirms kinking, and gentle traction usually relieves this problem. Intraluminal obstruction can sometimes be overcome by forceful irrigation.

COMPLICATIONS.—The complications associated with tubes passing through the upper tract have been described. Several problems unique to long tubes include looping through a gastroenterostomy, kinking and small bowel ulceration and necrosis. If the tube advances past the ileocecal valve, it then is incapable of small bowel decompression. Accidental loss of the proximal end is not an indication for operative removal. In general, if there is no longer a significant obstruction, the distal end will present at the rectum within several days.

REMOVAL.—Slow, firm tension (6–12 in. in 30–60 minutes) is used to remove the tube. Rapid removal or pulling against resistance can cause intussusception and necrosis at points of pressure and/or angulation.

INDICATIONS FOR SURGERY.—If peristalsis is poor and progress into the small bowel cannot be accomplished, decompression is unlikely and operative intervention becomes imminent. Other indications for operation include aspiration of dark bloody fluid, systemic signs of infarction or strangulation and progressive abdominal distention. Continued obstruction for 48–72 hours is often a further indication for definitive therapy.

DOUBLE-LUMEN LONG TUBES

MILLER-ABBOTT TUBE.—This tube (Fig. 12-3, *A*) has markings at 3 levels to designate the cardia, antrum and pylorus and at 1 ft. levels thereafter for a total length of 8 ft. This tube is least desirable because for the equivalent external diameter there is less suction lumen; therefore plugging is more likely.

Its major use is for intestinal decompression. It has 2 lumens; the smaller lumen serves as an inlet for inflation of the balloon after it has been inserted, and the larger lumen is used for decompression. Presence of a second lumen for inflation allows for less traumatic passage of the balloon through the nasopharynx. When air is used for inflation,

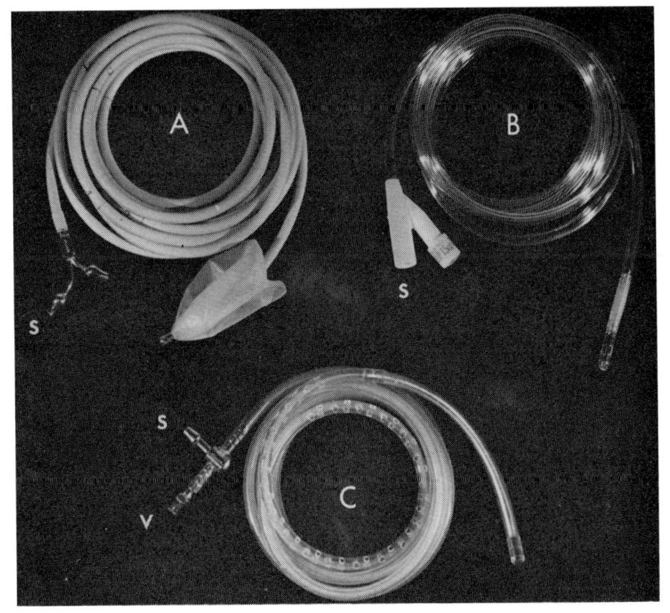

Fig. 12-3.—Double-lumen long tubes. **A,** Miller-Abbott; **B,** Baker; **C,** Devine. *s*, suction and *v*, vent.

it can usually be removed once the balloon has reached the site of obstruction. However, if mercury is used to weight the balloon, it cannot be removed.

The presence of a hole at the tip provides for decompression distal to the balloon. Small amounts of soluble contrast material may be injected to aid in diagnosis of the site of bowel obstruction or enteric fistula.

BAKER TUBE.—Similar to a Foley catheter but made of vinyl plastic, 6 ft. long and with an internal diameter of 4 mm., this tube (Fig. 12-3, *B*) is most useful in decompression of the small bowel during and after operation. Inflation of the balloon provides a bolus which can be easily advanced during operation. Presence of the tube in the lumen of the bowel postoperatively serves as a splint to reduce the incidence of postoperative obstruction.

This tube may be used via a gastrostomy or jejunostomy at the time of surgery or via the nasopharynx in nonoperative or preoperative decompression. Passage of the balloon through the pylorus is not accomplished as easily as with the weighted tubes.

The disadvantages of the Baker tube include the possibility of ischemic necrosis if the balloon is not deflated shortly after surgery and the danger of perforation by the firm tip distal to the balloon if it rests against a "fixed" bowel. The danger of perforation may be minimized by advancing the tube several inches each day. Of further note is the relatively small lumen available for suction; however, in the postoperative period the volume of aspirate is neither great nor is obstruction of the lumen apt to occur.

MAINTENANCE AND REMOVAL.—(1) Deflate balloon shortly after surgery. (2) Irrigate with 30 ml. water or air every 2–4 hours, depending upon the viscosity of the aspirate. (3) Drainage by gravity is adequate when the tube is used for postoperative decompression and splinting. Intermittent low pressure suction may be used if large volumes of aspirate are anticipated. (4) Removal may be accomplished by slow, gentle traction over 5–10 minutes or by advancing the tube 6–12 in. every 30–60 minutes. Rapid removal may cause intussusception.

DEVINE TUBE.—This tube (Fig. 12-3, *C*) is also used for small bowel decompression, but works on the principle of a sump. Two concentric tubes communicate near the tip, the inner tube serving to conduct gastrointestinal content to the suction source while the outer lumen allows entrance of outside air to prevent adjacent tissues from obstructing the holes at the end of the tube. Slow, gentle traction is the best method of removal.

SINGLE-LUMEN LONG TUBES

CANTOR TUBE.—This tube (Fig. 12-4, *A*) is 10 ft. long. Markings are present to designate the stomach, pylorus and duodenum and at 1 ft. intervals thereafter, beginning at 4 ft. There are 8 holes proximal to the balloon for aspiration.

Of the long gastrointestinal tubes, the Cantor tube has the largest internal diameter. Absence of a lumen for inflation and deflation provides a larger diameter for intestinal decompression. A balloon containing mercury serves as a bolus which is propelled through the intestine by peristalsis. From 3 to 5 ml. of mercury is usually injected into the balloon before insertion. All air is aspirated from the balloon following injection of the mercury.

Insertion is most easily accomplished with the patient in the erect position with the neck extended. Water-soluble lubricant should be used to facilitate insertion. In most cases it is helpful to fold the balloon over the end of the tube and to lubricate it after the patient is positioned, since manipulation of a well-lubricated balloon is awkward. The tube is pointed directly posterior and, once into the nasopharynx, the weight of the balloon carries it down to the stomach, usually without need for swallowing.

The tube is advanced to the level of the pylorus and positioning of the tip is best confirmed under fluoroscopic control. Maintenance is as described for other long intestinal tubes.

HARRIS TUBE.—This tube (Fig. 12-4, *B*) is 6 ft. long. Markings are

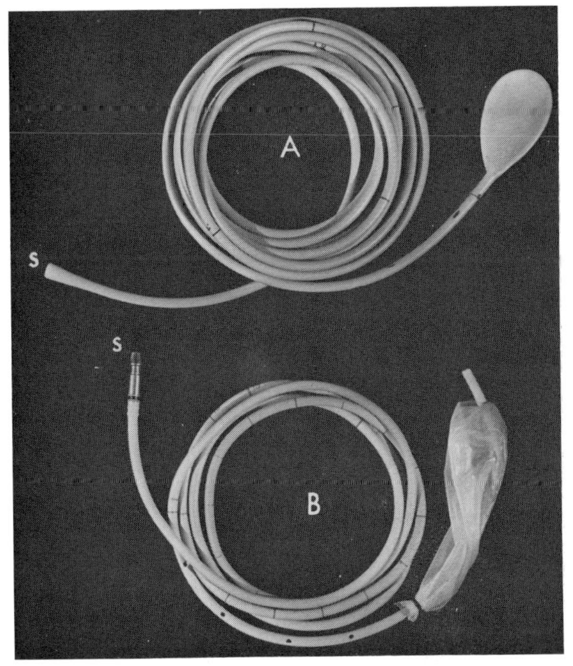

Fig. 12-4.—Single-lumen long tubes. **A,** Cantor and **B,** Harris. *s,* suction.

present at 1 ft. intervals. Mercury (2–5 ml.) is injected into the balloon prior to insertion. There are 9 holes proximal to the balloon plus a single hole at the tip for aspiration. Insertion is performed as above.

Short Gastrointestinal Tubes

Double-Lumen Short Tubes

Abbott-Rawson and Puestow-Olander tubes.—These tubes (Fig. 12-5) make it possible to decompress the stomach through one lumen while simultaneously feeding through the second lumen, which is in the jejunum. These tubes are particularly useful in major abdominal surgery such as pancreaticoduodenectomy and selective vagotomy, in which prolonged ileus may occur.

The major disadvantage lies in the small diameter of the lumens, which predisposes to clogging. For this reason these tubes are best managed by frequent irrigations (20 ml. water or saline every 1–2 hours). When feeding is begun, commercially manufactured mixtures such as Sustagen are preferred, since the particulate material in blenderized diets predisposes to tube obstruction.

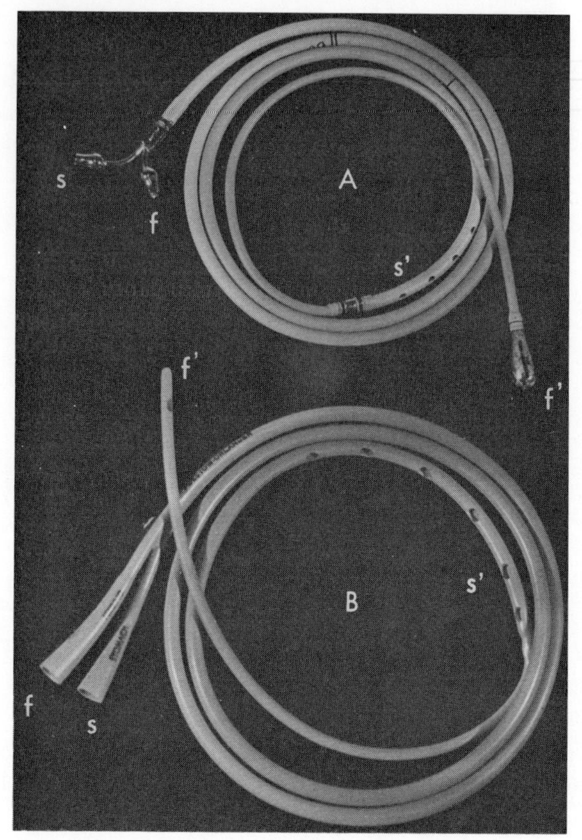

Fig. 12-5.—Double-lumen short tubes. **A,** Abbott-Rawson and **B,** Puestow-Olander. *s*, suction; *f*, feeding; *s'*, gastric suction lumens; *f'*, intestinal feeding lumen.

Sengstaken-Blakemore Tube

This tube (Fig. 12-6) is 50 cm. long and has 3 lumens. The largest lumen communicates with the hole in the gastric portion for irrigation and aspiration of the stomach. The other lumens serve as routes for inflation of the esophageal and gastric balloons.

The Sengstaken-Blakemore tube is used to produce tamponade of the esophagogastric junction and lower esophagus in patients with bleeding esophageal varices. The immediate objective is control of hemorrhage. An added benefit is that, by controlling hemorrhage, there is decreased protein absorption from the gut with a lowering of the blood urea nitrogen and nitrogenous load to the liver and kidneys.

Diagnosis of the site of hemorrhage may also be aided by use of the tube. If the tamponade of the esophagus and the esophagogastric junction is effective, it can be assumed that one of these sites is the proba-

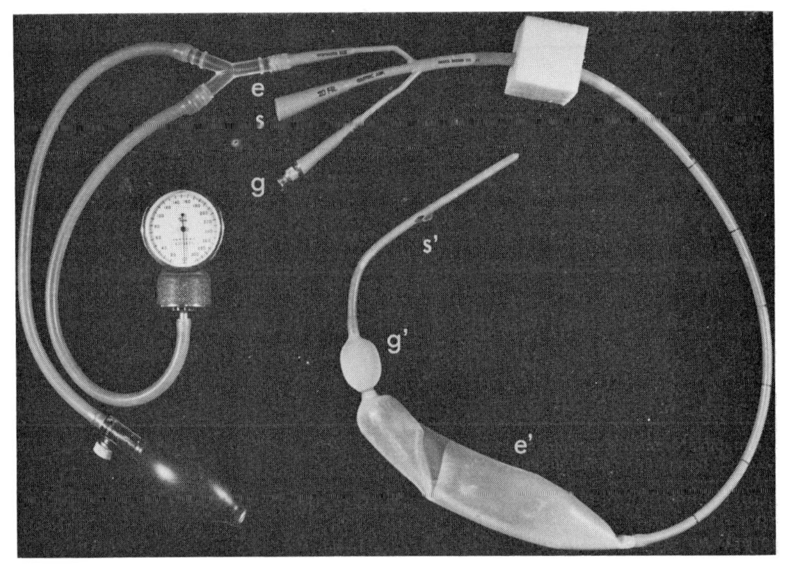

Fig. 12-6.—Sengstaken-Blakemore tube. *e*, inlet for inflation of esophageal balloon (*e'*); *s*, outlet for gastric suction orifice (*s'*); *g*, inlet for inflation of gastric balloon (*g'*).

ble source of bleeding. If, however, blood continues to emit from the gastric position of the tube, one can be relatively sure that the bleeding is from the stomach or duodenum rather than from the esophagus or esophagogastric junction.

INSERTION AND MANAGEMENT

1. Test balloons prior to insertion. Inflate the gastric balloon with 150–300 ml. air. Note the approximate size for a later comparison with the appearance on x-ray. Inflate the esophageal balloon to 20–40 mm. Hg pressure and note the size.
2. Keep patient in an erect or semi-erect position. Because patients in intensive care are often obtunded and the indication for use of the Sengstaken-Blakemore tube is upper gastrointestinal hemorrhage, the danger of aspiration is great. Equipment for nasotracheal suction should be available.
3. Use local anesthesia for passage of the tube. Because the tube is large, passage without local anesthesia is quite uncomfortable. Spraying the nasopharynx with 2% Pontocaine or directly applying it with cotton swabs may be carried out at the bedside.
4. After insertion of the tube, inflate the gastric balloon first. Do not begin inflation until the tube is well into the stomach.
5. Pull the tube so that the balloon is snug against the esophagogastric junction. If it is not snug, continued esophageal bleeding with trap-

ping of blood from the esophageal tamponade can lead to an internal tourniquet; this may actually increase hemorrhage from vessels at the esophagogastric junction.

6. Inflate the esophageal ballon to 20–40 mm. Hg.
7. Secure tube to the nose. A 1 lb. weight suspended over a pulley at the foot of the bed is often advised for securing the tube, but this is cumbersome and dangerous. A safer method is to pass the tube through a foam rubber cube which is positioned just distal to the nose and secured at that point (Fig. 12-7).
8. Irrigate the stomach with cold saline to determine the effect of the tube on hemorrhage as well as to maintain patency. Antacids are helpful as a preventive measure, especially in those patients with ulcer or gastritis.
9. Obtain a portable x-ray film to check proper placement of the balloon. If indicated (particularly with ineffective tamponade), dye may be injected into the gastric portion.

COMPLICATIONS OF ESOPHAGOGASTRIC TAMPONADE.—*Airway obstruction.*—One of the major dangers of esophagogastric tamponade is

Fig. 12-7.—Fixation of Sengstaken-Blakemore tube by attachment to foam rubber cube. Note position of gastric balloon against esophagogastric junction.

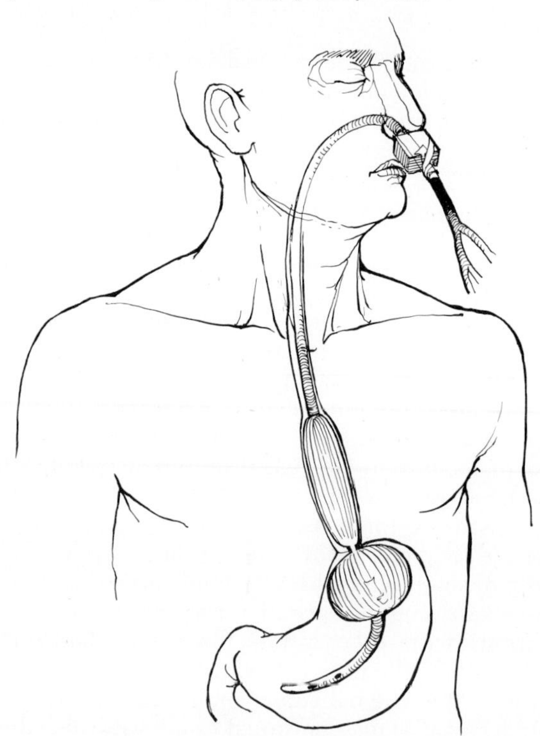

airway obstruction secondary to malposition of the tube. Causes of this calamity include: (1) inadvertent traction by a patient who is obtunded or in delirium tremens, (2) spontaneous deflation of the gastric balloon and advancement of the esophageal balloon into the nasopharynx, (3) spontaneous advancement and nasopharyngeal obstruction in patients with associated hiatus hernia and (4) increase in traction secondary to bumping or entanglement with suspension apparatus by an attendant.

The best treatment is prevention, which includes use of restraints and sedation in agitated patients with delirium tremens. Competence of the balloons and of the entire system must be checked carefully prior to use. Reuse of the tube is not recommended. Daily x-ray to ascertain the site of the tube and the state of the lungs is recommended. Because the Sengstaken-Blakemore tube is often ineffective in patients with hiatus hernia, the presence of this anatomic disorder is likely a contraindication to its use. Balanced traction systems are cumbersome; entanglement and resultant dislodgment are prone to occur, especially when many persons are involved in the care. For this reason, traction by means of a foam rubber cube attached to the nose and tube is safer and more efficient.

Continued hemorrhage.—Only after the Sengstaken-Blakemore tube has been inserted does the work begin. Intermittent irrigation must be performed on a regular schedule to verify the effectiveness of the tube. As mentioned, improper positioning of the tube may actually increase the rate of hemorrhage.

Bleeding gastric and duodenal ulcers and hemorrhagic gastritis are not affected by tamponade. These lesions occur with such a significant degree of frequency in patients with cirrhosis that, if tamponade is ineffective, a careful search for these causes of hemorrhage is mandatory.

Aspiration pneumonia.—Frequent oropharyngeal aspiration is essential in the patient with an esophagogastric tamponade. Since the inflated esophageal balloon precludes swallowing of salivary secretions, overflow into the tracheobronchial tree can easily result. Further, because of the difficulty encountered during swallowing, even with the balloon deflated, patients should have nothing by mouth during the entire period of intubation.

Since aspiration pneumonia is often fatal, frequent clinical and radiologic evaluation of the lungs is necessary. Bronchoscopy should be performed immediately if aspiration occurs. If there is any indication that aspiration will recur, tracheostomy is indicated.

Pressure effects.—Erosion of the mucosa of the esophagus or esophagogastric junction is directly related to the mechanical effect of a foreign object under both pressure and tension. The incidence of pressure ulcers increases with time. Clinical findings of esophageal rupture include subcutaneous crepitus, fever, substernal pain and pleural effusion. The diagnosis of esophageal rupture is confirmed by oral ingestion of a soluble contrast medium and immediate fluoroscopy.

Overdistention of the esophagus may cause discomfort and even agitation in the patient who is unable to communicate. Rupture of the esophagus may be secondary to overdistention or may follow rapid removal of the tube without deflation.

Sump Drains

Many different types of sump drains are available. In all, an inlet for air is present. In this way low-pressure suction will always be present within the system, promoting removal of collections of liquid in the area adjacent to the tube. Obstruction of the air inlet may result in suction sufficient to cause the orifices near the tip of the tube to be obliterated by the tissue surrounding them. The immediate result is complete loss of tube function.

It is essential to prevent obstruction of the air inlet(s) by tape, dressings, fluid, tissue, etc. Common causes of obstruction include overzealous fixation of the tube with tape and dressings which occlude the air inlet. Saturation of dressings and subsequent crusting and caking often produce the same effect. Intraoperative fixation of the tube with the inlet beneath the skin or subsequent retraction to this level are additional causes. Stagnant blood during brief periods of obstruction may clot and obstruct the lumen. Inspection will occasionally reveal tape placed directly over the orifices by nursing personnel in an attempt to diminish the noise of the rushing air. Indeed, the nursing personnel should be made aware that cessation of the noise is a situation which requires attention.

Drainage of fluid from the air vent signifies loss of function. This is an indication that temporary or permanent obstruction of the system has occurred.

For these reasons it is important to maintain constant suction and to change the connecting tubing at necessary intervals. Prevention of kinks or collapse of the tube by excess suction increases the useful span of sump drains.

ARGYLE (SARATOGA).—This version (Fig. 12-8, *A*) consists of 2 concentric tubes with multiple lumens near the tip. Free communication between the tubes with an air vent (*v*) near the proximal end allows air to enter. The holes in the inner tube are quite small and occlude easily if stagnation occurs even for brief periods.

CHAFFIN.—In this version (Fig. 12-8, *B*), 2 tubes with separate lumens are joined at the side. Both lumens are large. The tube is moderately stiff, and the holes in the ends are large and do not readily become occluded. The opening at each end is large and allows much air to pass through the inner portion with resultant danger of bacterial contamination. A convenient method of eliminating the possibility of contamination is to bend over one end, stabilize it with a rubber band and insert a

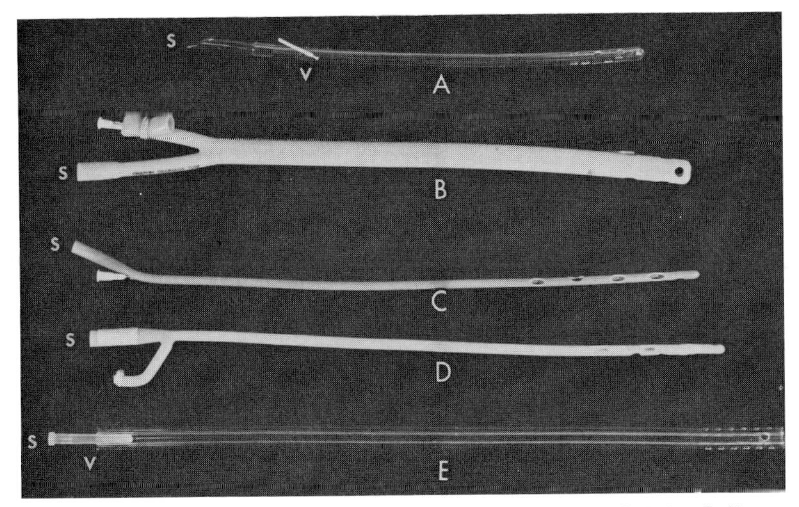

Fig. 12-8.—Sump tubes. **A,** Argyle (Saratoga); **B,** Chaffin; **C,** homemade; **D,** Foley; **E,** Abramson.

large-gauge needle to act as a vent. Large needles are more apt to stay open and do not clot as would gauze or cotton used as a filter over the orifice.

HOMEMADE TUBE.—A French catheter and a polyethylene tube or needle can be used to make an efficient, simple sump drain (Fig. 12-8, *C*). Extra holes are made near the tip of a standard urethral catheter and a polyethylene tube or needle is inserted through the wall into the lumen to work as an air vent. Suction is then applied to the larger catheter.

FOLEY.—Extra holes which include both lumens are placed in the distal portion of a Foley catheter (Fig. 12-8, *D*). This permits the tube to act as a sump if the side arm is left open. Suction is connected to the larger lumen.

ABRAMSON.—This version (Fig. 12-8, *E*) consists of a pliable tube with 3 parallel lumens which communicate at the distal end. Suction is applied to the large lumen in the center; the smaller lumens act as vents.

13

Useful Pharmacologic Agents

PAUL J. SCHECHTER, M.D., Ph.D.

Intern 1968–69, Presbyterian-St. Luke's Hospital; Research Associate in Pharmacology, National Institutes of Health, Bethesda, Maryland

AND

BARBARA R. SCHECHTER, Ph.D.

Assistant Professor of Pharmacology, George Washington University School of Medicine, Washington, D.C.

PHARMACOLOGIC AGENTS contribute greatly to the comfort, recovery and, indeed, survival of the pre- and postoperative patient. A comprehensive understanding of the basic pharmacology of various drugs used in intensive care is essential for many reasons:

1. The altered physiology of the intensive therapy patient requires careful attention to dose-effect relationships.
2. The coexistence of secondary conditions or diseases which pose definite contraindications to drug use is more likely.
3. The intensive care patient generally is given more than one class of pharmacologic agents, increasing the potential for drug antagonism, synergism and potentiation.
4. The possibility of iatrogenically induced complications is increased in the debilitated postoperative patient.

The routes of drug administration available for the intensive care patient differ somewhat from those usually used for the hospital inpatient. Immediately after surgery the patient is certain to have one or several intravenous infusions, and more likely than not will also have nasogastric decompression. Consequently, oral administration of drugs may not be possible. The usual route of administration is parenteral. Special caution is indicated in those patients in whom peripheral vasomotor changes are apt to occur. In such patients the intramuscular and subcutaneous route of administration should be avoided because of the delayed uptake or the danger of a sudden vasomotor alteration and altered tissue perfusion causing the sudden delivery of a large bolus of drug into the systemic circulation. Thus, in the majority of patients the intramuscular route is preferred, but the intravenous route is essential in any situation of vasomotor collapse or peripheral vasoconstriction.

The intensive therapy setting, with the extensive monitoring of each patient, provides an excellent and unique opportunity for the physician to observe the specific effect of various pharmacologic agents on a variety of organ systems. Experience in the use and observations of the action of these agents should increase the clinician's appreciation and understanding of the pharmacodynamics of the drugs used and should add to his ability as a therapist.

Analgesics

MORPHINE AND POSTOPERATIVE PAIN.—The single drug which probably has the most widespread use in the intensive care of the surgical patient is morphine sulfate. Morphine and related narcotics can be considered indispensable in the postoperative control of pain and discomfort. Indiscriminate use, however, of narcotic analgesics may mask early complications of surgery and may retard the course of recovery.

An almost universal result of surgery is incisional pain. Studies have shown that upper abdominal incisions appear to be more painful than lower abdominal incisions, and a majority of patients having extra-abdominal operations require little or no postoperative analgesia. Postoperative pain, of course, is best treated by elimination of contributing factors, for example, tension, inflammation, pressure, ischemia of the wound, hematoma formation, etc. Another complication of the immediate postanesthetic period is hypoxia, which may be incorrectly interpreted as pain.

Once it has been established that the complaints of the patient emerging from anesthesia are not due to correctable causes of incisional pain, and once hypoxia has been ruled out, narcotic analgesia is indicated to afford the patient maximal comfort. At this point, since the patient is in the twilight zone between anesthesia and wakefulness, approximately half the normal dose of analgesic to relieve pain should be given, that is 3–5 mg. morphine intravenously or intramuscularly. The remaining half dose should be given 30 minutes to 1 hour later if pain is not relieved. Thereafter, most pain can be controlled, apprehension allayed and sedation accomplished with 6–10 mg. of morphine intravenously or intramuscularly, the route of administration dependent on whether vasomotor stability has been established. When given by the intravenous route, the analgesic effect starts immediately, reaches its peak in about 20 minutes and has a duration of action of several hours. The dose may be repeated every 3–4 hours as needed for the first 48–72 hours postoperatively. Pain of sufficient intensity to require narcotics is usually maximal between 12 and 36 hours postoperatively and usually disappears by 48–72 hours. Any prolongation of this type of pain beyond 72 hours may signal complications. In the average person receiving the outlined dosage regimen, there is no danger of drug addiction from morphine.

CAUTIONS AND CONTRAINDICATIONS TO USE OF OPIATE NARCOTICS.—*Ventilation and coughing.*—The opiates depress respiration in a dose-dependent fashion, that is, part of this effect is due to a rise in the threshold of the central respiratory center to respond to a rise in P_{CO_2}. Also by direct central action the opiates act as cough suppressants, being among the most effective agents for this purpose. On the other hand, the effect of morphine to decrease the pain encountered on movement of the chest wall can increase the ability of the postoperative patient to breathe deeply, to cough voluntarily and to facilitate early ambulation. Morphine is usually contraindicated in the patient with asthma.

Hypotension.—Morphine acts directly on the vasculature as well as centrally to produce a peripheral vasodilatation. In addition, the release of histamine by morphine and other narcotics contributes to the hypotension observed after morphine administration. Patients with reduced blood volume are considered more susceptible to the hypotensive effects of morphine and related drugs than are normovolemic patients.

Elevated cerebrospinal fluid pressure.—Morphine has a tendency to increase the cerebrospinal fluid pressure. In the presence of an elevated cerebrospinal fluid pressure, the respiratory depressant effects of morphine are exaggerated. In addition, miosis, emesis and lethargy produced by morphine may obscure important parameters of neurologic functions. Hence, morphine is absolutely contraindicated in head injury or after brain surgery.

Effects on antidiuretic hormone.—Morphine increases the release of antidiuretic hormone from the posterior pituitary with a resultant decrease in urinary output. Furthermore, morphine acts to increase the tone of the bladder sphincters. Therefore, morphine should be used with caution in any condition of relative oliguria or obstructive uropathy.

Myxedema, hypopituitarism, Addison's disease and hepatic failure.—Persons with myxedema have an exaggerated response to the depressant effects of small doses of morphine. Morphine also inhibits the release of adrenocorticotropic hormone and of pituitary gonadotropic hormones. Therefore, cautious use of morphine is necessary in patients with myxedema, Addison's disease and hypopituitarism. The major pathway for the detoxification of morphine is via conjugation with glucuronic acid in the liver. Hence, in the presence of hepatic insufficiency one may expect the duration of action of a dose of morphinc to be prolonged.

Although morphine sulfate remains the standard in treatment of pain, large numbers of other potent analgesics are available (Table 13-1).

TABLE 13-1.—POTENT ANALGESICS

	DOSE,* MG.	DURATION OF ACTION, HR.	ROUTES OF ADMINISTRATION					COMMENTS
			Oral	SC	IM	IV	Rectal	
Natural alkaloids of opium								
Morphine	10	4–7	X	X	X	X		Oral administration 1/6 to 1/15 as effective as parenteral
Codeine	60–120	3–5	X	X	X			Weak analgesia, oral 1/3 as effective as parenteral
Semisynthetic opium alkaloids								
Dihydromorphinone (Dilaudid)	1–4	2–5	X	X	X	X	X	
Oxymorphone (Numorphan)	1–3	4–6	X	X	X	X	X	Oral dose 10 mg., little or no cough suppression
Methyl dihydromorphinone (Metopon)	3.5 oral only	4–5	X					↓ Respiratory depression ↓ Emetic properties
Synthetic compounds								
Meperidine (Demerol)	80–100	2–4	X		X	X rare		Subcutaneous injection irritating; equianalgesic doses depress respiration to same degree as morphine
Methadone (Dolophine)	5–15	3–5	X		X	X		Subcutaneous injection irritating; good oral effectiveness
Levorphanol (Levo-Dromoran)	2–3	4–8	X	X	X	X		↑ Oral effectiveness
Pentazocine (Talwin)	10–30	2–5	X	X	X	X		Oral dose 50–100 mg. non-narcotic; narcotic antagonist
Propoxyphene (Darvon	32–65 oral only	4–6	X					Non-narcotic, analgesia potentiated by A.S.A.

*Average adult dose by intramuscular route unless otherwise specified.

NARCOTIC ANTAGONISTS.—Both available narcotic antagonists, nalorphine (Nalline) and levallorphan (Lorfan), are potent antagonists of all opiate narcotics as well as the synthetic morphine substitutes. Consequently, they are indicated in counteracting respiratory depression, hypotension and other undesirable side effects of the narcotic analgesics. They are ineffective in reversing the actions of barbiturates, anesthetics and other non-narcotic agents.

Nalorphine is a synthetic congener of morphine. The dose to treat respiratory depression and/or hypotension secondary to the use of narcotics is 5–10 mg. given slowly intravenously. Within 1–2 minutes after intravenous administration of nalorphine, increase in respiratory rate and respiratory volume should be apparent, and blood pressure should return to normal. Nalorphine antagonism of narcotic-induced respiratory depression lasts 1–4 hours.

Levallorphan is not a congener of morphine. It is effective in antagonizing the effects of narcotics in a dose of 1 mg. intravenously. Onset and duration of action are similar to that of nalorphine.

Both nalorphine and levallorphan are respiratory depressants. If given alone in excessive doses they will mimic most of the pharmacologic effects of morphine.

Diuretics

Diuretics are useful in a wide variety of conditions and diseases which may be encountered during the intensive care of the surgical patient. The common denominator indicating diuretic therapy is the abnormal retention of water and salt.

FUROSEMIDE AND ETHACRYNIC ACID. —The introduction of furosemide (Lasix) and ethacrynic acid (Edecrin) into the diuretic regimen provides the 2 most potent diuretic agents available. Both are effective orally and parenterally; both have a rapid onset of action with a relatively short duration. When used together, furosemide and ethacrynic acid do not have an additive effect, suggesting that both act at the same site within the kidney. The principal action of these diuretics is to increase the excretion of sodium and chloride, with the loss of chloride exceeding that of sodium. In addition, these drugs increase excretion of hydrogen and potassium ions; hence, a metabolic alkalosis and hypokalemia should be anticipated. A wide variation in the response of individual patients to these agents has been observed.

Furosemide (Lasix) is an anthranilic acid derivative. The onset of action is within 30 minutes of either oral or parenteral administration; diuresis lasts 4–6 hours. The usual dose required to produce a satisfactory diuresis is 20–80 mg. either orally, intravenously or intramuscularly. However, due to its relative potency and the variability in response, furosemide therapy should be initiated using the smaller dose. The dosage should be increased only after evaluation of the response to each dose.

Ethacrynic acid (Edecrin) is a phenoxyacetic acid derivative. Diuresis begins within 30 minutes and a maximum effect is reached within 60–90 minutes of oral or intravenous administration. The usual dose by either route is 25–50 mg., although much larger doses have been safely given to severely edematous and refractory patients. As with furosemide, a small dose should be used to begin therapy and the dose then progressively increased depending on the response.

Furosemide and ethacrynic acid are indicated in the treatment of edema associated with congestive heart failure, anasarca due to cirrhosis or nephrosis, acute pulmonary edema (because of the rapid onset of action) and in patients refractory to other diuretics. Furosemide and ethacrynic acid remain effective in patients with a low glomerular filtration rate, with azotemia and with severe electrolyte disturbances.

During use of these agents, careful observation is necessary to guard against hyponatremia, hypochloremia, hypokalemia and acute alkalosis. Because of the tendency for hypokalemia and hypochloremic alkalosis to develop, as a general rule potassium chloride supplements should be used with these diuretics. Potassium chloride may be given intravenously or orally. Use of concentrations greater than 40–60 mEq./L. causes localized phlebitis and pain. However, higher concentrations may be given via a central venous catheter. Potassium chloride is administered orally as a 20% solution in cherry syrup or other palatable medium.

Mercurial diuretics.—Although the use of the mercurial diuretics has declined since the introduction of new, more potent diuretics, the mercurials remain among the most effective and useful diuretic agents available. They depress tubular reabsorption of sodium and chloride, and they increase the excretion of potassium, probably by a mechanism which involves sulfhydryl enzyme inhibition. The preferred route of administration is intramuscular. Diuresis should occur within 1–2 hours, reach a maximum in 6–9 hours and be complete within 12–24 hours.

The most commonly used mercurial diuretic is meralluride (Mercuhydrin). It is marketed in combination with theophylline, which aids in rapid absorption and reduces local tissue irritation. The usual intramuscular dose is 1–2 ml. given every 2–3 days, after a positive response has been established.

The mercurials tend to produce a hypochloremic alkalosis. In the presence of serum alkalosis, the diuretic response to these agents is markedly reduced. On the other hand, acidifying salts, for example, ammonium chloride and lysine monohydrochloride, tend to potentiate the effects of the mercurials.

Mercurial diuretics are excreted almost exclusively by the kidney; hence, their use is contraindicated in moderate to severe renal insufficiency from any cause.

Mannitol.—This is the reduced form of the 6-carbon sugar, mannose. Mannitol is not metabolized. Following intravenous infusion its distribution is limited to the extracellular space. It is freely filtered across the glomerulus and is not reabsorbed from the renal tubule. By an osmotic effect, it obligates a large volume of fluid to enter the tubule. Maintenance of intratubular volume and pressure, therefore, produces an osmotic diuresis.

Mannitol, administered in doses of 12.5–25 Gm. as a 25% solution, is useful in the treatment of the early phases of acute oliguria, which may occur following major surgical procedures, shock, massive hemorrhage, burns and reactions to transfusions. In hypovolemic patients, hydration should be instituted concomitantly or prior to mannitol therapy.

Mannitol has also been used in neurosurgery to reduce cerebrospinal fluid pressure by increasing the osmolarity of extracellular fluid. Its osmotic gradient effect will reduce edema of the brain, which in turn lowers intracranial pressure. By the same mechanism mannitol will also cause a rapid reduction in intraocular pressure in some glaucomatous patients refractory to other measures.

Mannitol must be used cautiously since the expansion of the extracellular fluid following its administration can result in circulatory overload and congestive heart failure.

BENZOTHIADIAZIDE (THIAZIDE) DIURETICS.—The benzothiadiazides represent a class of oral diuretics with both diuretic and antihypertensive efficacy. They act as diuretics by inhibiting the proximal tubular reabsorption of sodium and chloride and possess a variable degree of inhibitory action on carbonic anhydrase. Because the benzothiadiazides also produce a significant kaluresis, the serum potassium levels should be routinely monitored and supplemental potassium given as needed. A variety of oral thiazide preparations are available (Table 13-2).

Side effects of the benzothiadiazides are minimal and consist of skin rashes, hyperglycemia, gastric irritation and hyperuricemia. The thiazide diuretics should be used with caution in patients with hepatic insufficiency, since ammonia excretion is impaired by these agents.

SPIRONOLACTONE (ALDACTONE).—This diuretic is a steroid com-

TABLE 13-2.—BENZOTHIADIAZIDE DIURETICS

	DOSE/DAY,* MG.	DURATION OF ACTION, HR.
Chlorothiazide (Diuril)	500–2,000†	6–10
Hydrochlorothiazide (Hydrodiuril, Esidrix)	50–200	8–12
Bendroflumethiazide (Naturetin)	2–5	18–24
Cyclothiazide (Anhydron)	1–4	18–24
Trichlormethiazide (Naqua)	2–8	24–36
Chlorthalidone (Hygroton)	25–100	48–72

*Average adult daily oral maintenance dosage.
†Available also for intravenous use.

pound which acts as a competitive antagonist of aldosterone. This drug is administered orally in doses of 100 mg./day and is usually used in conjunction with other diuretics, for example, thiazides. The hyperkalemia induced by spironolactone is counteracted by the kaluresis of the thiazide diuretics.

Sedatives and Hypnotics

Sedative-hypnotic drugs have a wide variety of indications in the postoperative surgical patient. They are useful as adjuncts in the treatment of pain, in allaying anxiety, in hypertension and as anticonvulsants. Generally, these agents are cortical depressants and as such alter or diminish the awareness of pain. They are not analgesics.

Any discussion about sedatives and hypnotic drugs can only be meaningful if the reader appreciates the fact that there is no clear pharmacologic difference between those drugs that are used as sedatives and those that are used as hypnotics. Generally, the effect obtained is a dose-dependent phenomenon rather than drug specific. Sedation can be defined as a state of relief without deleterious effects on mental capacity in times of mental stress. Hypnosis, on the other hand, is induction of sleep without loss of consciousness, alteration of sensory sensitivity or muscular responsiveness.

BARBITURATES.—These are general tissue depressants, with their depressant actions most notable on the central nervous system. Derivatives of barbituric acid provide the entire spectrum of durations of action, varying from that of the ultrashort to the very long.

The ultrashort-acting barbiturates, for example, thiopental and methohexital, are used exclusively for parenteral administration as intravenous anesthetics or in the preinduction stage of anesthesia.

The short- to intermediate-acting barbiturates, such as amobarbital, pentobarbital and secobarbital, have an onset of action within minutes after parenteral administration and a duration of action of 3–6 hours. The hypnotic dose of these agents is 100–200 mg., either orally or parenterally while the sedative dose is one-fourth to one-half of the hypnotic dose. The short- to intermediate-acting barbiturates are primarily degraded by the liver; hence, they must be used with caution and in smaller doses in persons with hepatic insufficiency.

The long-acting barbiturates, for example, phenobarbital (hypnotic dose 100–200 mg.), have an onset of action 15–30 minutes after parenteral administration, and the effects last 4–8 hours. These are excreted largely unchanged by the kidney. The problem of "hangover" appears to be greater with the long-acting barbiturates than with the others.

In the presence of pain and in older patients, the barbiturates may cause a paradoxical effect, that is, an excitement-like state of delirium, unless adequate pain relief is given simultaneously. Tolerance as well as dependence can be developed for the barbiturates; however, this is seldom of consequence in short-term use.

Anticonvulsant action of barbiturates.—For the control of convulsions, short- to intermediate-acting barbiturates are usually chosen due to the rapid onset of action. Care should be taken to use only that amount of barbiturate necessary to control the seizure, since the postictal depression may be additive with the drug-induced depression. For this reason 300–500 mg. of pentobarbital or amobarbital is given slowly intravenously until the seizure stops, with careful attention taken to avoid apnea.

CHLORAL HYDRATE.—This halogenated hydrocarbon acts as an effective sedative in doses of 250–500 mg. and hypnotic in doses of 1–2 Gm. Onset of action after oral administration occurs within 30 minutes and its effects last 5–8 hours. Chloral hydrate is available also as suppositories (650–1,300 mg.) or as a retention enema in olive oil.

Chloral hydrate is irritating to the skin and mucous membranes, and this local irritation accounts for its main side effects of gastric distress, nausea and vomiting. Since chloral hydrate is largely metabolized in the liver, hepatic insufficiency is a relative contraindication to its use.

CHLORODIAZEPOXIDE AND DIAZEPAM.—Chlorodiazepoxide and diazepam are both benzodiazepine derivatives. They have sedative, muscle relaxant and anti-anxiety as well as hypnotic properties.

Chlorodiazepoxide (Librium) is used in doses of 5–25 mg. orally or parenterally 3–4 times daily. When given by the oral route, peak action is reached in about 8 hours with a duration of several days.

Diazepam (Valium) is given in doses of 2–5 mg. orally or parenterally. Owing to some anticholinergic action, it is advisable not to use this drug in the presence of glaucoma.

Both of these agents have been reported to cause confusion, especially in the elderly. Additive and supra-additive effects have been observed in combination with alcohol, barbiturates, phenothiazine and monoamine oxidase inhibitors and combinations of these agents should be used cautiously.

Diazepam is also of use in status epilepticus or in continuous focal seizures. Doses of 5–20 mg. intravenously can cause abrupt cessation of seizure activity in 80% of patients with status. Diazepam has not been shown to be of any use, however, in the long-term control of seizure activity.

PARALDEHYDE.—This is a rapidly acting hypnotic with maximal brain concentrations occurring within 30 minutes of oral administration. One can expect hypnosis within minutes. Paraldehyde has no analgesic properties and, like the barbiturates, may produce stimulation and delirium in the presence of pain. Paraldehyde is unstable with long storage, decomposing to acetaldehyde and acetic acid; therefore, fresh solutions should always be used.

The oral dose is 3–8 ml. well diluted with a pleasant tasting vehicle, such as fruit juice, milk or tea. Like chloral hydrate, paraldehyde tends to produce local irritation. In addition, it has a disagreeable taste and a characteristic pungent odor; 10–20 ml. may be given in olive oil as a retention enema.

Drugs Useful in Treatment of Shock

The term "shock" is applied to a number of pathologic hemodynamic dislocations with many etiologic factors. The basic aims in the treatment of shock are (1) to maintain effective blood volume and (2) to increase cardiac output without causing an undue increase in peripheral resistance. The treatment of shock varies considerably depending on the cause, on the laboratory data being quoted and on the clinician's experience. No attempt will be made at this point to recommend a specific course of therapy for shock; however, a number of drugs which have been applied to the treatment of shock will be discussed with regard to their pharmacologic actions.

CONCEPT OF α AND β ADRENERGIC RECEPTORS.—The concept of α and β adrenergic receptors provides a convenient tool to classify sympathomimetic agents. The order of potency of these drugs on different structures of the body divides them into 2 distinctly different groups, the α-adrenergic stimulators and the β-adrenergic stimulators. All responses that are classified as α can be blocked by specific α blockers, for example, ergotamine and dibenzyline. All β responses, on the other hand, can be blocked by β blockers, for example, propranolol. Thus, all adrenergic effects and sympathomimetic actions are classified with respect to their potency on α and β receptors.

All sympathomimetic drugs known, however, have a mixed action, that is, they affect structures of both types of receptors to various degrees. Their clinical use is determined by their dominant action.

By the use of the principles just outlined, the α-adrenergic responses are:

contraction of vascular smooth muscle
contraction of gastrointestinal tract sphincters
contraction of the splenic capsule
contraction of the uterine smooth muscle
contraction of radial fibers of the iris
contraction of radial fibers of the ciliary body
contraction of pilomotor muscles
relaxation of intestinal smooth muscle

The β-adrenergic responses are:

positive inotropic response of the heart
positive chronotropic response of the heart
relaxation of the vascular smooth muscle
relaxation of the uterus
relaxation of bronchioles
relaxation of intestinal smooth muscle

Originally it was thought that α receptors mediated excitatory effects, and β receptors mediated exclusively inhibitory effects. As can be seen from the preceding list, such division is not entirely correct. The metabolic effects of catecholamines (glycogenolysis and hyperglycemia) are not included in the list, because it is not clear into which category they belong.

EPINEPHRINE.—The pharmacologic effects of epinephrine in general duplicate the effects of stimulation of adrenergic nerves, that is, both α and β receptors. The effect of epinephrine on blood pressure depends on the ratio of α to β activity in the various vascular beds. The blood vessels to the skin, mucosa and kidney are constricted, that is, α-receptor stimulation dominates, whereas the vessels to skeletal muscles are dilated due to predominantly β-receptor stimulation. The sensitivity of β receptors to epinephrine is greater than that of the α receptors. Therefore, small doses of epinephrine can be expected to cause a relative vasodilatation and a fall in blood pressure, whereas larger doses will cause an increase in peripheral resistance and consequently a rise in blood pressure. On the heart, epinephrine causes an increase in both rate and force of contraction, and at therapeutic doses the rise in blood pressure is largely due to an increase in cardiac output. Epinephrine may be administered subcutaneously (0.1–0.5 ml. of a 1:1,000 solution) or intramuscularly in oil suspension for prolonged use (0.4–1 ml. of a 1:500 solution every 8–16 hours). Epinephrine is useful in bronchospasm, in hypersensitivity reactions and as a cardiotonic in cardiac arrest.

ISOPROTERENOL (ISUPREL).—This may be considered to be almost exclusively a β-adrenergic stimulator. As such it has a positive inotropic and positive chronotropic action on the heart and thereby increases cardiac output. Isoproterenol also causes peripheral vasodilatation, resulting in a fall in peripheral resistance. Usually, however, the effects on the myocardium are sufficient to cause a net increase in cardiac output and to maintain or raise systolic blood pressure with a reduction in mean pressure.

Isoproterenol is useful in the treatment of heart block, in shock and as a bronchodilator in respiratory disorders. It may be administered sublingually, intramuscularly, subcutaneously, by inhalation, as an intravenous drip (using 1–2 mg. diluted in 250–500 ml. of 5% dextrose) or by intravenous push (0.4–1 mg. diluted to 10 ml. with saline or 5% dextrose) to treat cardiac standstill.

LEVARTERENOL (LEVOPHED, NOREPINEPHRINE).—This drug acts predominantly on α-receptors with minimal β stimulation, except on the heart where positive inotropic and chronotropic effects are apparent. Levarterenol increases peripheral resistance and raises systolic and diastolic blood pressures. The effect on cardiac output is variable and usually depends on the degree of compensatory vagal reflex activity which actually may slow the heart rate and decrease cardiac output.

The main use of levarterenol is in the treatment of hypotension secondary to circulatory collapse and/or decreased cardiac output as an intravenous drip of 4–10 mg. in 500–1,000 ml. of parenteral diluent with careful titration of drug versus blood pressure. Subcutaneous extravasation of norepinephrine carries the danger of tissue slough.

METARAMINOL (ARAMINE).—This acts by releasing norepinephrine from adrenergic nerve endings. As can be expected, its effects are similar to those of norepinephrine. It is used almost exclusively to treat hypotension and may be administered subcutaneously, intramuscularly or intravenously in doses of 2–10 mg. or as an intravenous infusion, 50–100 mg. in 1,000 ml. diluent. With prolonged use of metaraminol, norepinephrine is depleted from its storage sites at the adrenergic nerve endings. The hypertensive effects of metaraminol will be then diminished, that is, by development of a tachyphylaxis or tolerance to metaraminol. The so-called "Aramine-fast" patient must then be switched to levarterenol to maintain the blood pressure.

PHENYLEPHRINE (NEO-SYNEPHRINE).—This drug acts as an α-adrenergic stimulator with little β effect. It increases blood pressure by peripheral vasoconstriction followed by reflex bradycardia. Phenylephrine is used exclusively to treat hypotension, and due to its reflex vagotonic effect, it is especially useful in treating hypotension and shock secondary to supraventricular tachycardia. The dose is 5–10 mg. intramuscularly or as an intravenous infusion (50 mg. in 250–500 ml. 5% D/W).

ANGIOTENSIN (HYPERTENSIN).—This is not a catecholamine but a polypeptide. It is the most potent pressor substance known. Its action is rapid, producing a rise in blood pressure within 1 minute with a duration of 5 minutes after a single intravenous injection with no secondary fall in blood pressure. Angiotensin has little or no effect on the heart except for a reflex bradycardia. It causes a sharp reduction in both renal blood flow and in glomerular filtration rate due to a vasoconstriction of the renal vasculature, even at very low doses. Since it also releases aldosterone from the adrenal cortex, one should expect a decreased urine flow as well as a decreased natriuresis when using this agent. Angiotensin is administered by intravenous infusion, 2.5 mg. in 250–1,000 ml. of diluent.

Antihypertensives

One of the principal uses of antihypertensive agents in surgical intensive care is in the management of dissecting aortic aneurysms. The literature provides ample discussion and debate as to the relative merits of "medical" management, that is, antihypertensive therapy, versus surgical intervention. Even when the surgical approach is used, antihypertensive agents are indicated to reduce blood pressure to normal levels preoperatively. (Up to 80–90% of patients with dissecting aneurysms exhibit elevated blood pressure.) Acute and chronic postoperative hypertension is most apt to occur in patients with pre-existent hypertension and after renal artery surgery.

TRIMETHAPHAN (ARFONAD).—This antihypertensive drug is a monosulfonium ganglionic blocking agent. As such, it interrupts adrenergic control of the arterioles, causing vasodilatation and a fall in blood pressure. Trimethaphan is the drug of choice in the acute hypertensive crisis and for short-term hypotensive control.

On intravenous administration it lowers blood pressure immediately, and its hypotensive action is quickly dissipated when the drug is discontinued. Trimethaphan is used as an intravenous infusion, 500 mg. in 500 ml. of 5% D/W with an infusion rate of about 5 mg./minute, to reduce systolic blood pressure to 100–120 mm. Hg. Blood pressure must be carefully monitored every 2–5 minutes during use of trimethaphan. Patients become refractory to the action of trimethaphan within 24–48 hours; therefore, other antihypertensive agents, for example, reserpine and guanethidine, should also be initiated at the onset of therapy.

In addition to frequent blood pressure recordings and electrocardiograms, careful monitoring of urinary output and neurologic status is necessary when trimethaphan is used. The blood pressure may be reduced to such a low level that renal failure, myocardial infarction or cerebral ischemia may occur. As with all ganglionic blocking agents, the actions of trimethaphan are nonspecific, so that all autonomic ganglia are effectively blocked. As expected, this results in many undesirable side effects. Visual disturbances (mydriasis, difficulty in accommodation), paralytic ileus, constipation and urinary retention are all found. In addition, trimethaphan causes liberation of histamine.

PENTOLINIUM (ANSOLYSEN).—This diquaternary amine compound is, like trimethaphan, a ganglionic blocking agent. It is usually administered intramuscularly into the distal muscle groups of the upper extremities so that if severe hypotension develops, a tourniquet can be applied proximal to the injection site. The initial dose should not exceed 2.5 mg., with 1 mg. increments at 6 hour intervals until the desired blood pressure is attained. Maximum response occurs in about 2 hours. Pentolinium is also available for oral administration; however, absorption from the gastrointestinal tract is poor. The side effects of pentolinium are similar to those of trimethaphan.

RESERPINE.—This antihypertensive drug is a naturally occurring alkaloid of Rauwolfia serpentina. Although several natural and semisynthetic alkaloids of rauwolfia are available, there are only minor qualitative and quantitative differences between them. Consequently, reserpine is considered the prototype of the rauwolfia alkaloids. Reserpine acts as an antihypertensive agent by depleting the catecholamines from binding sites within sympathetic postganglionic nerve endings. This results in a block of impulse transmission at the sympathetic neuroeffector junctions and, therefore, a decreased sympathetic influence on the effector cells. This decrease in sympathetic tone also decreases myocardial contractility, produces a bradycardia and lowers cardiac output. In treating acute hypertension reserpine is given intramuscularly in doses of 1–2.5 mg. every 4–8 hours. By this route reserpine has a slow onset of action, 1–3 hours, and has a variable and prolonged duration of action which may last for days. A cumulative effect, therefore, should be expected and subsequent doses omitted if blood pressure levels as low as 180/100 are found.

Reserpine is also effective orally with limited antihypertensive potency. The oral dose is 0.1–0.25 mg. daily. By the oral route the onset of action is about 1 week, with full effectiveness occurring in 3–4 weeks.

The side effects of reserpine include psychic depression, nasal stuffiness, fluid retention, Parkinson-like symptoms and diarrhea. Reserpine is also a potent stimulator of gastric secretion so that there is a threat of acute peptic ulceration. Therefore, especially when large doses of reserpine are used, a bland diet should be prescribed.

When surgical intervention appears necessary in a patient on reserpine therapy, the anesthesiologist must be forewarned. The sympatholysis produced by reserpine renders adrenergic effector organs supersensitive to the effects of endogenous epinephrine and norepinephrine. Hence, reserpine is contraindicated in the presence of pheochromocytoma.

METHYLDOPA (ALDOMET).—This is the methylated derivative of dihydroxyphenylalanine, a natural precursor in the synthesis of epinephrine and norepinephrine. α-Methyldopa is metabolized to form α-methyl norepinephrine which replaces norepinephrine at nerve endings and exhibits only a fraction of the pressor activity of norepinephrine at the neuroeffector sites, that is, methyldopa leads to the formation of a "false transmitter." Furthermore, methyldopa inhibits decarboxylase, the enzyme necessary for the formation of dopamine, a precursor of norepinephrine. Either or both of these actions contribute to the hypotensive properties of methyldopa.

Methyldopa is administered by intravenous infusion in the treatment of the acute hypertensive crisis, 250–500 mg. in 100 ml. of 5% D/W over 30 minutes and repeated as needed every 6 hours. By this route the onset of action is 4–6 hours with a duration of 10–16 hours.

Methyldopa is also effective orally in doses of 500–2,000 mg. Orally its onset of action occurs in 6–10 hours with hypotensive effects lasting 18–24 hours.

By either route of administration the side effects of methyldopa include dry mouth, sedation, vertigo, gastrointestinal upset (diarrhea or constipation), fluid retention and, less commonly, impairment of liver function and hemolytic anemia. It is therefore contraindicated if liver damage is suspected.

HYDRALAZINE (APRESOLINE).—A phthalazine derivative, this antihypertensive drug acts directly on arteriolar smooth muscle to decrease peripheral resistance. It is effective orally as well as parenterally. By intravenous administration, an effective dose of hydralazine lowers blood pressure in 15–20 minutes and has a duration of action of 4–6 hours. The dose by the intravenous or intramuscular routes is 10–40 mg. (50 mg. in 200 ml. of 5% D/W intravenously.) The oral dose is 100–400 mg. daily, with maximal effects occurring in 3–4 hours.

Hydralazine causes an increase in renal blood flow in association with an increase in cardiac output; hence, it is considered by some to be the drug of choice when hypertension is complicated by impaired renal function. Chronic administration of daily doses of 400 mg. or greater of hydralazine produces a lupus-like syndrome in 10% of patients. This includes arthralgias, fever, skin rash, positive L.E. preparations, anemia, thrombocytopenia, etc., indistinguishable from classical systemic lupus erythematosus. Smaller doses of hydralazine may produce headache, flushing, palpitations and can provoke anginal pain in susceptible individuals due to a tachycardia and increased cardiac work. Hydralazine therefore should be used with caution in patients with coronary artery disease.

GUANETHIDINE (ISMELIN).—This is the most potent oral antihypertensive available. It selectively depletes catecholamines from adrenergic postganglionic nerve fibers at the neuroeffector junctions. Unlike the ganglionic blocking agents, it has no parasympatholytic effects. Guanethidine does not cross the blood-brain barrier and has no central nervous system effects.

Guanethidine is usually reserved for moderate to severe hypertension. Following oral administration the onset of action is delayed for 5–7 days; hence, the usual oral dose is 10 mg./day initially with an increase weekly until a desired effect is obtained.

Guanethidine causes a bradycardia via blockade of sympathetic impulses to the sinoauricular node, and its antihypertensive effects are due to a decreased cardiac output with little effect on peripheral resistance.

The principal side effect of guanethidine is orthostatic and exercise hypotension, since the cardiac acceleratory nerves are not functioning normally. The decreased cardiac output produced by guanethidine also decreases the glomerular filtration rate and renal blood flow. It should therefore be used with caution in patients with incipient congestive heart failure, renal insufficiency or cerebral insufficiency. Other side effects are diarrhea and impotence.

The depletion of catecholamines at nerve endings induced by guanethidine produces a supersensitivity to endogenous and exogenous epinephrine and norepinephrine. Therefore, if guanethidine has been used within 1 week prior to surgery, the anesthesiologist should be informed of this fact. Furthermore, guanethidine is contraindicated in hypertension secondary to pheochromocytoma.

BENZOTHIADIAZIDES.—These diuretics are effective as mild antihypertensive agents by a direct action on peripheral vascular resistance.

Owing to their relatively low potency, the thiazides are of little use in the intensive care surgical patient.

DRUGS USEFUL IN THE TREATMENT OF PHEOCHROMOCYTOMA

The preoperative and operative management of hypertension in the patient with pheochromocytoma provides special problems because of the possibility of wide fluctuations in blood pressure as well as arrhythmias produced by sudden release of large concentrations of sympathomimetic amines from the tumor. The control of blood pressure may be accomplished by the use of α-adrenergic blockers, while the effects of catecholamines on the heart rate and rhythm may be controlled with β-adrenergic blockade.

α-ADRENERGIC BLOCKING AGENTS.—*Phenoxybenzamine* (Dibenzyline) is a haloalkylamine which acts as a potent competitive blocking agent of α-adrenergic actions of sympathomimetic amines. At present, phenoxybenzamine is only available for oral administration. Absorption from the gastrointestinal tract is incomplete and variable. The oral dose varies between 20 and 200 mg./day, and dosage is adjusted by increasing it slowly until the desired effects are obtained. The duration of action is 12–24 hours; however, a cumulative effect over 3–4 days should be anticipated.

Phenoxybenzamine is given for 3–4 days before surgery for removal of a pheochromocytoma. This should achieve complete antagonism of α-receptors and fully dilate the vascular compartment. Blood pressure will now depend solely on cardiac output and blood volume.

Phentolamine (Regitine) is an imidazoline competitive α-adrenergic blocker. It is usually administered intravenously in doses of 2.5–5 mg. It has an immediate blocking effect, but this effect persists for only 5–10 minutes. Therefore, repeated doses are necessary, and wide swings in blood pressure may occur. Phentolamine has the disadvantage of causing a tachycardia by a direct stimulatory effect on the myocardium.

Since both phenoxybenzamine and phentolamine are competitive α-adrenergic blockers, their action can be reversed by large doses of norepinephrine.

β-ADRENERGIC BLOCKING AGENTS.—*Propanolol* (Inderal) is a specific β-adrenergic blocking agent. It acts by competitive antagonism of sympathomimetic amines at the β-adrenergic receptor sites to block the positive inotropic and chronotropic effects of these amines on the heart.

In the preoperative management of pheochromocytoma, propanolol is given in daily oral doses of 60 mg. for 2–3 days prior to surgery in conjunction with α-adrenergic blocking agents. Propanolol will control the tachycardia and arrhythmias produced by α-blockade and by endogenous catecholamines. It should not be used in the absence of α-receptor blockade, since the vasoconstrictor α-effects of epinephrine will be unopposed by β-antagonism and cause a dangerous rise in blood pressure.

Propanolol is also used in the long-term management of hypertension in dissecting aneurysms. Propanolol is contraindicated in bronchial asthma, bradycardia or congestive heart failure unless the failure is secondary to arrhythmias. The effects of propanolol can be reversed by large doses of isoproterenol.

Other Useful Drugs: The Phenothiazines

The phenothiazine derivatives are a group of drugs with diverse pharmacologic actions. Because of the indications for their use in a variety of conditions, they are useful adjuncts to the therapeutic armamentarium of the intensive therapy physician.

The phenothiazines act as sedatives, antihistamines, anticholinergics, antipsychotics, antinauseants and antiemetics, local anesthetics, peripheral adrenergic blocking agents, mild diuretics and antiserotonin agents. Alterations in chemical structure of the phenothiazines have produced congeners with a predominance of one or several of these actions which determine the therapeutic applications.

The phenothiazines are rapidly absorbed from the gastrointestinal tract within 30–60 minutes. Onset of action occurs 5–10 minutes after intramuscular administration. From 60 to 70% of a given dose is rapidly removed from the portal circulation by the liver and conjugated with glucuronide. There is, however, an active enterohepatic circulation and, following discontinuance of drug therapy, the phenothiazines remain in the body tissues for several months. Most phenothiazines may be administered orally, rectally or intramuscularly in equivalent doses. They are infrequently given intravenously in smaller doses. The potential uses of phenothiazines in the intensive therapy unit include:

1. Sedation (chlorpromazine 10–25 mg.). Sedation with chlorpromazine, unlike that with the barbiturates, causes little ataxia or incoordination.

2. Treatment of functional and organic psychoses, neuroses and personality disorders. The dose of phenothiazine will differ, depending on the patient, his condition and the effects desired (Chapter 11).

3. Control of nausea and emesis secondary to uremia, carcinomatosis, gastroenteritis, irradiation, pregnancy, alcoholism and drugs (prochlorperazine 5–10 mg.). The phenothiazines have no effect, however, in nausea and vomiting caused by digitalis intoxication or labyrinthitis.

4. Relief of peripheral vasoconstriction often encountered after cardiopulmonary bypass (chlorpromazine 5–10 mg. intravenously and repeat every 10–15 minutes as needed).

TABLE 13-3.—PHENOTHIAZINES

MAJOR CONSTITUENT GROUPS	EXTRAPYRAMIDAL EFFECTS	SEDATION	ANTIEMETIC EFFECTS	HYPOTENSION
Aminoalkyls	++	++	++	++
Chlorpromazine (Thorazine)				
Promazine (Sparine)				
Triflupromazine (Vesprin)				
Piperazines	+++	+	+++	−
Prochlorperazine (Compazine)				
Trifluoperazine (Stelazine)				
Perphenazine (Trilafon)				
Piperidyls	−	++	−	++
Thioridazine (Mellaril)				

5. Control of hiccups, which may be secondary to uremia (chlorpromazine 25–50 mg.).

6. Potentiation of the effects of narcotic analgesics and barbiturates (promethazine 25–50 mg.). Phenothiazines will potentiate the effects of a given dose of narcotic and other central nervous system depressants by 25–50%.

The specific phenothiazine derivative chosen (Table 13-3) and the dose employed will depend on the condition being treated and on the judgment of the physician. In general, sedation can be accomplished with smaller doses than are necessary to control nausea and vomiting. Slightly higher doses are needed to control intractable hiccups. The largest doses of the phenothiazines are used in treating psychiatric problems.

Side effects.—The most serious side effects of the phenothiazines result from hypersensitivity reactions. These include blood dyscrasias (leukopenia, eosinophilia, leukocytosis), cholestatic jaundice and dermatologic reactions. The incidence of these reactions is low. More commonly, extrapyramidal effects such as parkinsonism, dyskinesia and akathisia (motor restlessness) occur, especially with high doses of phenothiazines. Other side effects include tachycardia, dryness of the mouth and orthostatic hypotension. The phenothiazines potentiate the actions of many drugs. Chlorpromazine causes an increase in barbiturate sleeping time, potentiates the effect of alcohol, increases the sedative effect of morphine and enhances the respiratory depression produced by meperidine.

REFERENCES

1. Cannon, P. J., and Kilcoyne, M. M.: Ethacrynic acid and furosemide: Renal pharmacology and clinical use, Prog. Cardiovasc. Dis. 12:99, 1969.
2. Earley, L. E., and Orloff, J.: Thiazide diuretics, Ann. Rev. Med. 15:149, 1964.
3. Gaffney, T. E., *et al.*: The clinical pharmacology of antihypertensive drugs, Prog. Cardiovasc. Dis. 12:52, 1969.

4. Gildea, J.: The relief of postoperative pain, M. Clin. North America 52:81, 1968.
5. Goodman, L. S., and Gilman, A.: *The Pharmacological Basis of Therapeutics* (3rd ed.; New York: The Macmillan Company, 1965).
6. Hodge, R. L., and Dornhorst, A. C.: The clinical pharmacology of vasoconstrictors, Clin. Pharmacol. & Therap. 7:639, 1966.
7. Hollister, L. H.: Clinical use of psychotherapeutic drugs: Current status, Clin. Pharmacol. & Therap. 10:170, 1969.
8. Martin, W. R.: Opioid antagonists, Pharmacol. Rev. 19:463, 1967.
9. McQuarrie, D. G., and Humphrey, E. W.: Vasopressors and vasodilators in surgery, S. Clin. North America 48:877, 1968.
10. Mendlowitz, M.: Hypertension, in Conn, H. F. (ed.): *Current Therapy* (Philadelphia: W. B. Saunders Co., 1969).
11. Perlroth, M. G., and Harrison, D. C.: Cardiogenic shock: A review, Clin. Pharmacol. & Therap. 10:449, 1969.
12. Ross, E. J., *et al.*: Preoperative and operative management of patients with phaeochromocytoma, Brit. M. J. 1:191, 1967.
13. Wheat, M. W., Jr., and Palmer, R. F.: Dissecting aneurysms of the aorta: Present status of drug versus surgical therapy, Prog. Cardiovasc. Dis. 11:198, 1968.

14

Interpretation of Postoperative Chest X-Ray

HAROLD N. WALGREN, M.D.

Former Associate Attending Radiologist, Rush-Presbyterian-St. Luke's Medical Center; Attending Radiologist, Oak Park Hospital, Oak Park, Illinois

COMPREHENSIVE KNOWLEDGE of normal anatomy and expected postoperative changes provides a foundation on which to evaluate postoperative chest x-ray films of critically ill patients. For this reason frequent consultations between surgeons and radiologists are beneficial in that, in collaboration, both groups can improve their acumen and thereby improve patient care.

In order to facilitate interpretation of postoperative chest x-ray films, it is good practice to provide copies of the films and to maintain a folder in the intensive care unit for each patient during the critical phase of his illness. Optimally, a multi-panel, well-illuminated, electrically operated film viewer allows frequent comparison and ready accessibility of all films stored on the unit.

There are several variables that must be controlled when taking postoperative chest x-ray films. Those related to the equipment include: (1) kilovoltage (energy of the x-rays), (2) milliamperes (quantity of x-rays per unit time), and (3) time (measured in seconds or fractions thereof). In performing postoperative chest roentgenography, optimal results are obtained with the high-kilovoltage technique. Additional factors that must be controlled include the position of the patient and the distance from the x-ray tube. These factors are best controlled by affixing a piece of tape on which is recorded the information mentioned above to the patient's bed to serve as a guide for further exposures. The x-ray film speed for portable roentgenograms usually remains constant within a given institution. Such variations in technique must be kept to a minimum in order to provide a sound basis on which to compare x-ray films.

There is considerable difference between the P-A and the A-P projections in an otherwise normal chest x-ray film. Ordinarily, in critically ill patients, chest roentgenography is most efficiently and safely performed with the cassette behind or under the patient (A-P). In evaluating postoperative films, one must be aware of the basic differences between the preoperative P-A and the postoperative A-P projections. The addition of postoperative changes further complicates interpretation of these films.

Comparison of serial films is essential in x-ray interpretation. Further, an orderly routine is necessary in the evaluation of a given film. Initially, consideration of all foreign objects introduced into the chest (chest drainage and endotracheal tubes, CVP catheters) is a good beginning. Frequent comparison of one side with the other will aid in the detection of many abnormalities. Familiarity with "normal" postoperative findings provides a firm base on which to evaluate portable x-ray films in the intensive care unit.

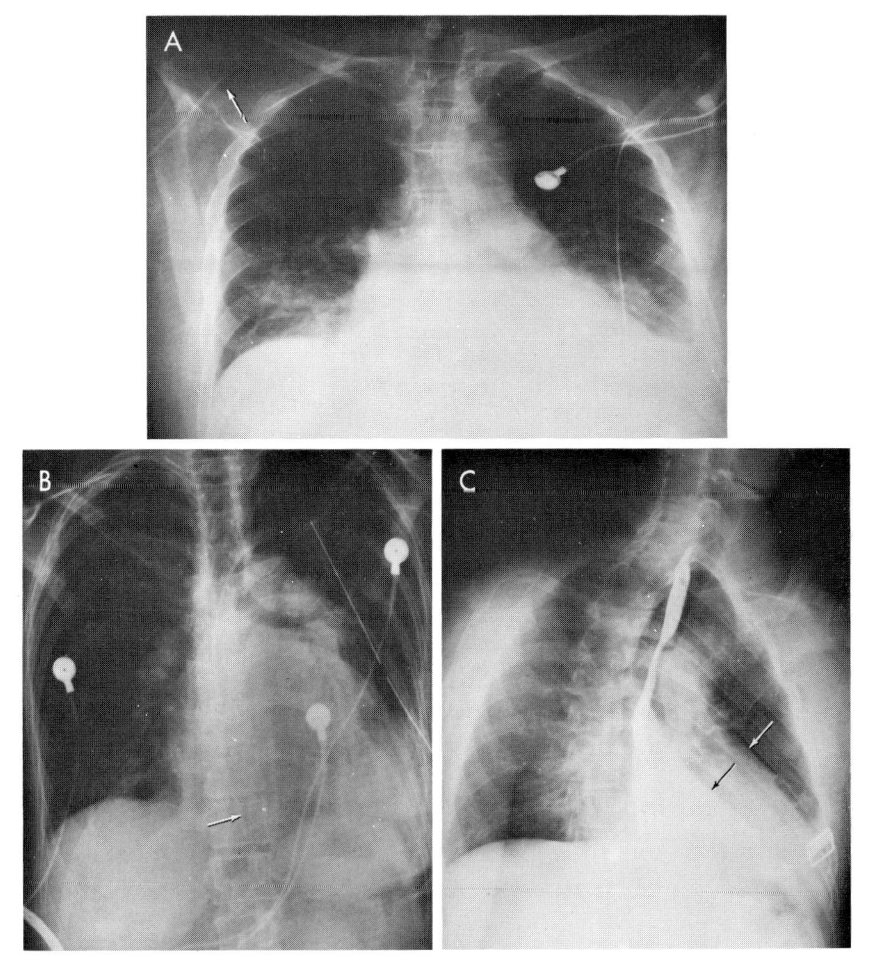

Fig. 14-1.—Atelectasis, intracardiac central venous pressure catheter. **A,** portable chest film of an obese patient with an elevated diaphragm and poor excursion. Bilateral basilar atelectasis is present. Note also the peripheral location of the central venous pressure catheter (*arrow*). The catheter may coil back up on itself, pass into the neck veins, the vena cava or into the right ventricle. **B,** location of the catheter within the right ventricle (*arrow*) is occasionally a cause of ventricular arrhythmias. **C,** lobar atelectasis, particularly of the left lower lobe (*bottom arrow*), is frequently difficult to diagnose because the shadow may be concealed behind the heart border (*top arrow*) or blend with the mediastinum.

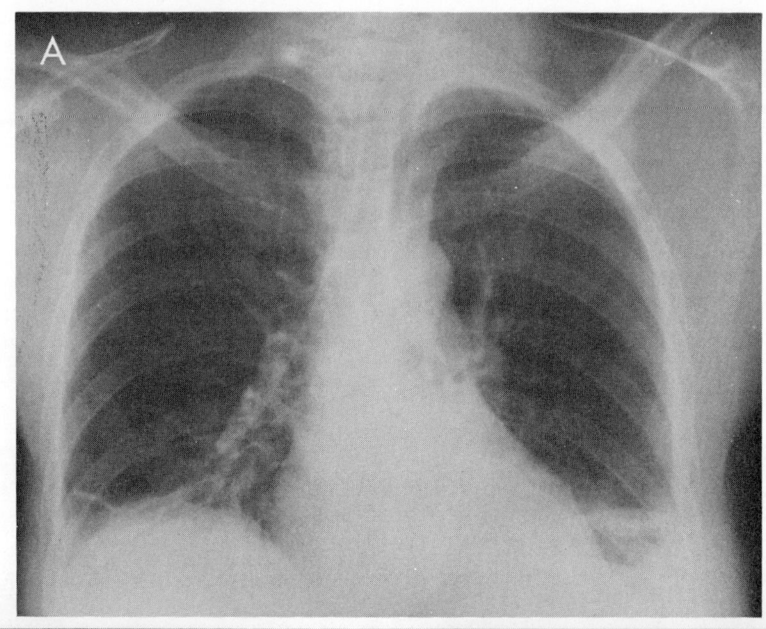

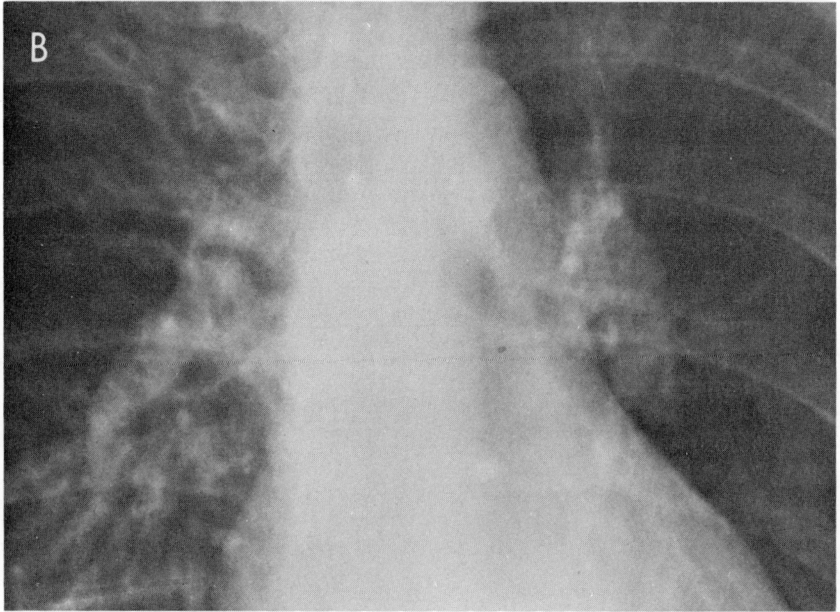

Fig. 14-2.—Pulmonary embolus. **A,** this view shows prominence of the main pulmonary arteries, a basilar infiltrate and pleural effusion. **B,** another view of the same patient demonstrates marked prominence of the pulmonary arteries.

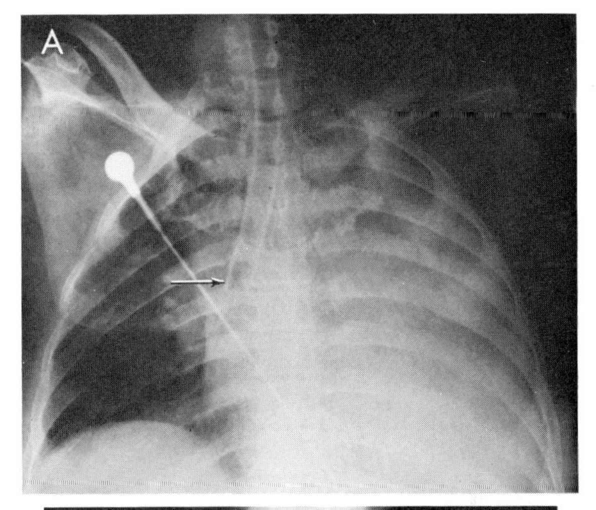

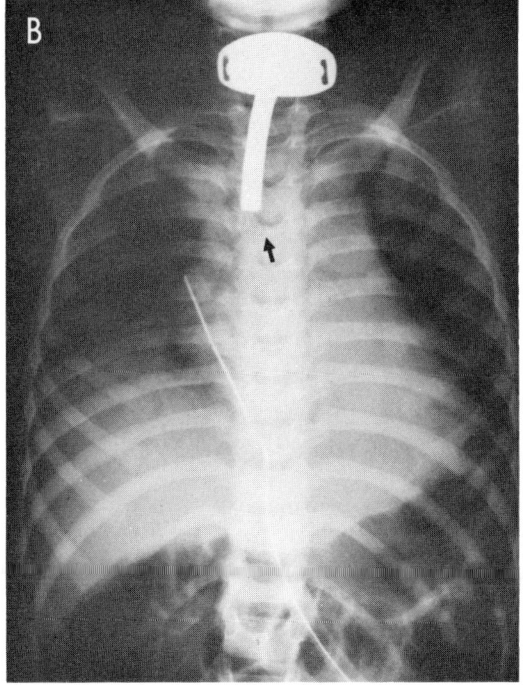

Fig. 14-3.—Iatrogenic bronchial obstruction. **A,** an occasional cause of atelectasis of the left lung in the postoperative patient is improper positioning of the endotracheal tube. The right upper lobe can also be involved if the tube extends distal to the right upper lobe orifice. This example shows the tip of the endotracheal tube beyond the carina (*arrow*) causing total atelectasis of the left lung. **B,** a long tracheostomy tube in a low stoma may enter the right main stem bronchus and cause atelectasis of the left lung. In this case the tip of the tracheostomy tube lies just above the carina (*arrow*).

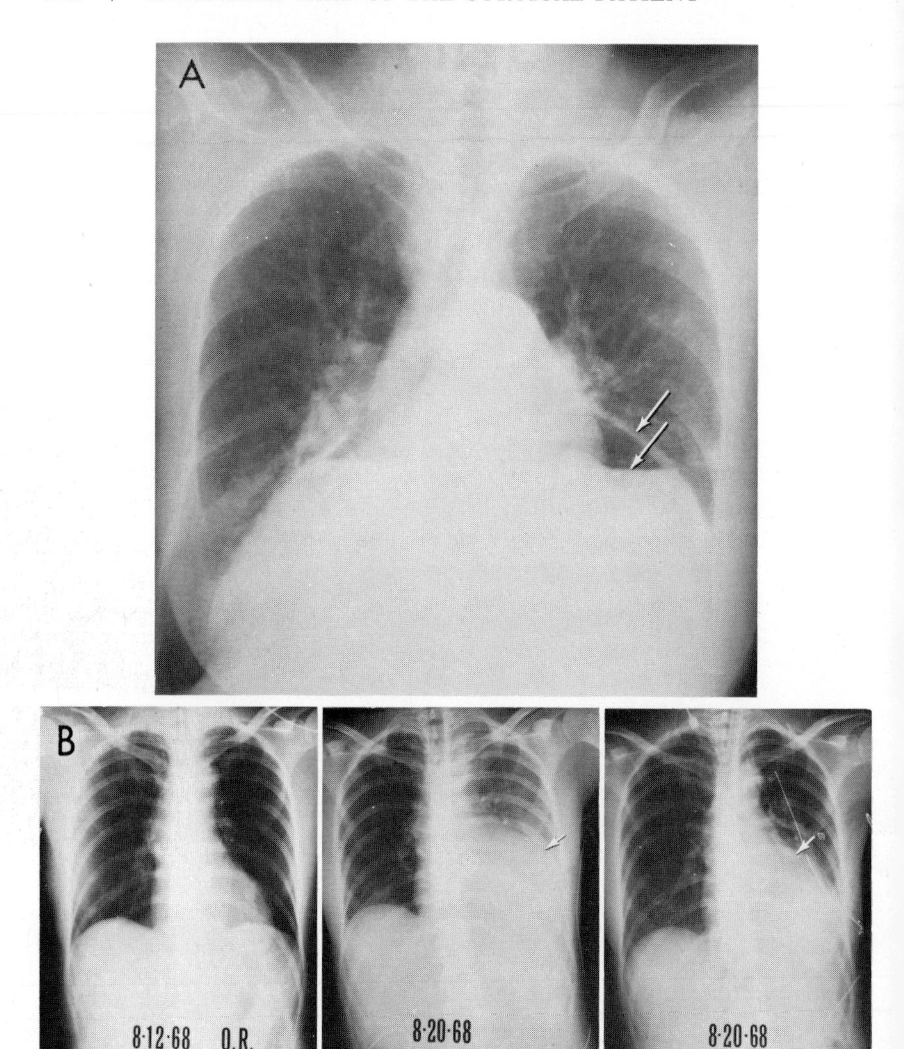

Fig. 14-4. – Pericardial effusion and tamponade. **A,** enlargement of the cardiac silhouette may be due to pericardial effusion. Postoperative and post-thoracentesis air-fluid levels aid in evaluation of the heart, fluid (*bottom arrow*) and the pericardium (*top arrow*). In some operative cases the pericardium is left open to provide decompression into the pleural cavity. **B,** enlargement of the silhouette following cardiac surgery is often secondary to congestive failure. An occasional cause of cardiomegaly and low cardiac output is occult cardiac tamponade. This may occur gradually over an interval of days or weeks, as shown in the first 2 frames. The third frame reveals a decrease in size following pericardial drainage.

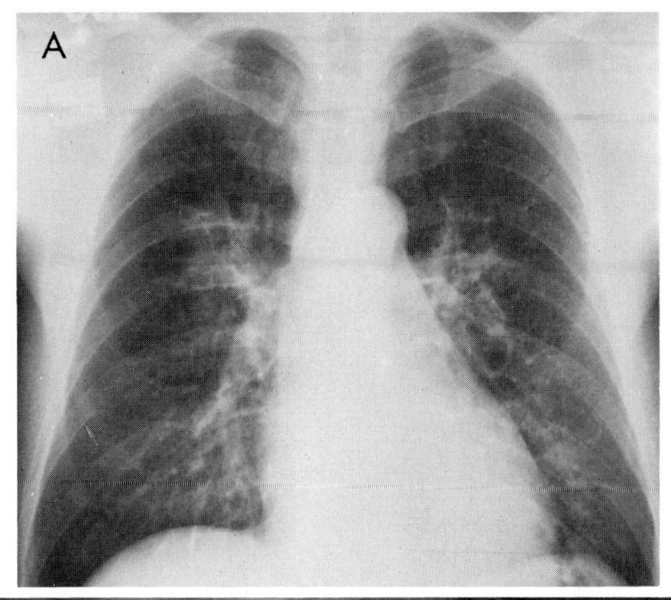

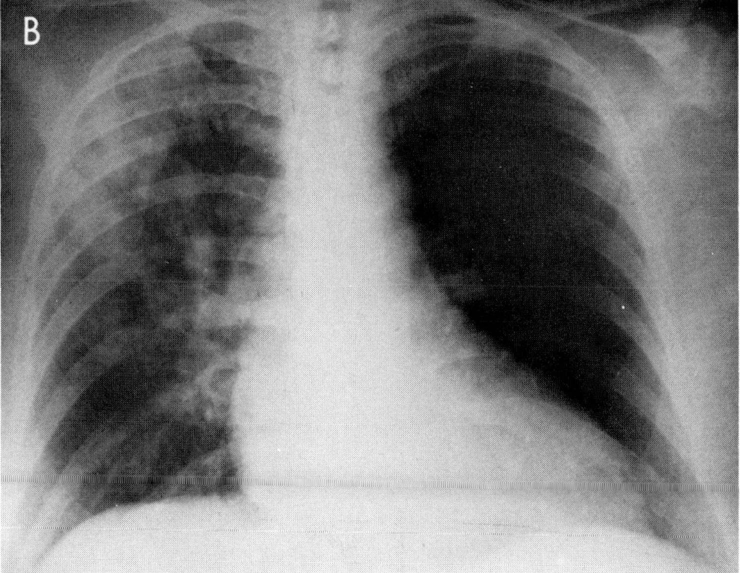

Fig. 14-5.—Congestive heart failure. **A,** the early radiographic signs of congestive failure with pulmonary edema can be subtle. The earliest finding consists of an "angel wing" enlargement of the hilar areas. **B,** unilateral pulmonary edema due to overhydration in a patient with known ischemic heart disease.

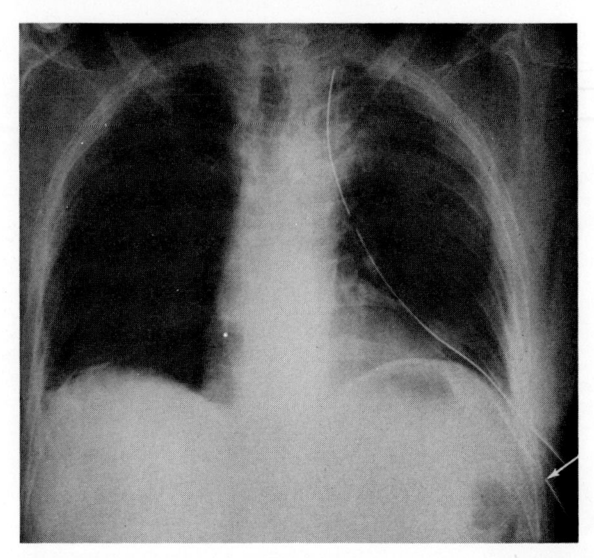

Fig. 14-6.—Malposition of chest tube. Postoperative x-ray following left thoracotomy shows 2 drainage catheters in place. Usually, immediate attention is directed to note the presence or absence of hemothorax or pneumothorax. In this instance neither is present, but the lowest hole (*arrow*) in the inferior chest tube extends outside the bony thorax. It is kept from producing pneumothorax only by the overlying soft tissues.

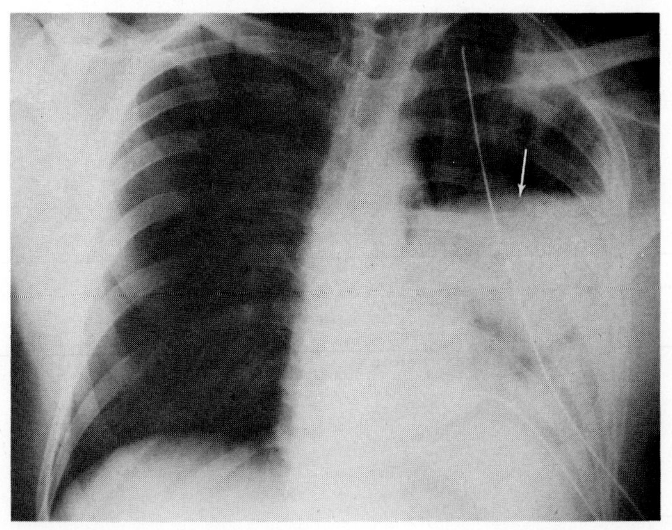

Fig. 14-7.—Hemothorax. Rapid accumulation of fluid in a chest postoperatively indicates hemorrhage, as shown by the air-fluid level (*arrow*). In this patient the air and blood collection is due to malfunctioning chest tubes.

Accumulation of blood in the thoracic cavity can cause tension hemothorax and result in mediastinal shift. The shift can in turn cause vena caval obstruction and cardiac arrest.

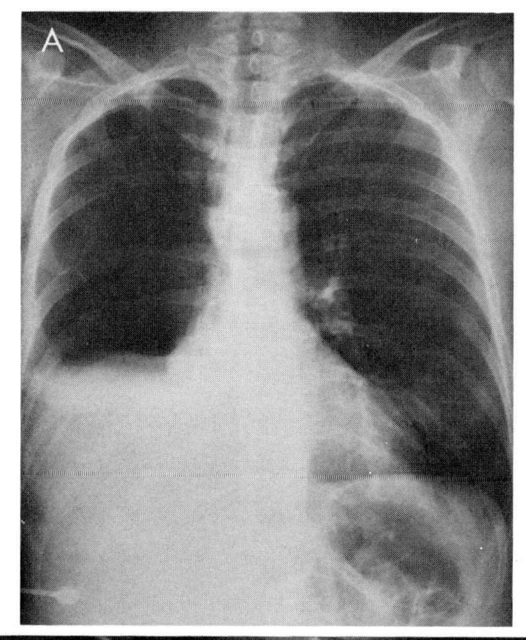

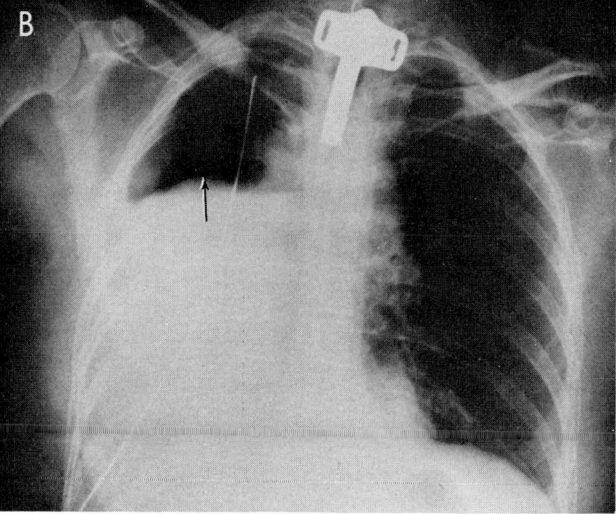

Fig. 14-8. – Pneumonectomy. **A,** following pneumonectomy, serosanguineous fluid accumulates in the empty pleural cavity. Usually, the fluid rises to the level of the eighth or ninth rib (posteriorly) on the first postoperative day and to the level of the sixth or seventh rib on the following day. The entire space gradually fills during the subsequent days to weeks. **B,** a rare, usually fatal complication of radical pneumonectomy is herniation of the heart through a surgical defect in the pericardium. There are air and fluid in the right hemithorax, a chest tube (clamped) and a tracheostomy tube. The left heart border is markedly shifted to the right, but the degree of mediastinal shift is not commensurate. The heart border is evident just above the air-fluid level (*arrow*).

15

Pre- and Postoperative Cardiovascular Nursing

ANNETTE ROBERTS, R.N.

Clinical Specialist in Cardiovascular Nursing, Rush-Presbyterian-St. Luke's Medical Center

AND

WILLIAM E. OSTERMILLER, JR., M.D.*

Former Fellow in Cardiovascular-Thoracic Surgery, Presbyterian-St. Luke's Hospital; Attending Surgeon, St. Joseph Hospital, Santa Ana, California; Assistant Professor of Surgery, University of California College of Medicine (Irvine)

ADVANCES IN CARDIOVASCULAR SURGERY during the past 10 years can mainly be attributed to laboratory and clinical investigation, improved operative techniques, advanced electronic monitoring devices, new therapeutic adjuncts and a better understanding of cardiac physiopathology. Because of these advances, cardiovascular nursing has assumed a new and specialized role. The professional nurse, in addition to gaining specialized technical skill, must also be able to calm the fears and anxieties of the patient and his family.

Preoperative Instruction

In preparing a patient for surgery, the nurse approaches him as an individual. By being a good listener she becomes aware of his physical and psychologic needs, and is able to gain rapport which will be needed throughout the course of the hospital stay. Some important points to be ascertained in the preoperative nurse-patient conversation are: (1) the patient's relationship with his family, and how they can help in the pre-

*Supported in part by United States Public Health Service Grant No. IT12HE05808.

and postoperative periods; (2) the various fears and misinformation of the patient, so they can be discussed; (3) the patient's knowledge of his disease – will more information regarding his illness and its therapy be of value? (4) what reassurance the patient should have and what his psychologic needs will be before and after the surgical procedure.

Because of the varied duties that exist on a busy cardiovascular service, a sense of the patient's identity as an individual can be lost. This is when the clinical specialist in cardiovascular nursing assumes a most important and satisfying role.

In many institutions the field of cardiovascular surgery encompasses both cardiac and peripheral vascular surgery. It is not uncommon to have several patients with multiple types of cardiovascular problems in the intensive care unit at one time. Patients with repair of congenital heart defects or acquired heart lesions, myocardial revascularization procedures or peripheral vascular surgery usually require the services of this special unit. What is discussed with the patient preoperatively depends upon his degree of intelligence and level of anxiety. Socioeconomic factors must be considered in correlating the preoperative instructions to be given. The clinical nursing specialist perceives this and instructs the patient according to his ability to accept the information.

Generally, the candidate for cardiovascular surgery wants to be informed about the various phases in the therapeutic regimen which he is about to enter. It will help him to learn about the environment in which he will be placed, to be told about the procedures to be performed and then to have his role in the pre- and postoperative management verbalized. Family participation in the discussion will reinforce various aspects of the instruction as it is given. This instruction is usually best given when the physician and nurse work as a team. The amount of technical information that the patient is given depends upon research information obtained about the patient and upon his ability to accept the information. The guiding principle that the professional nurse should follow is to consider the patient as an individual and to deal with him with interest and sincerity.

TIMING. – The timing of preoperative instruction depends upon the factors which initiate the ultimate decision for surgery. Urgent or emergency surgery may be required. The amount of preoperative information and instruction given will vary according to the urgency of the procedure. Often the patient who requires emergency surgery has little capability of receiving preoperative instruction. However, when possible, time should be allocated prior to surgery to explain the procedure and what is expected of the patient. This will relieve his anxieties and will help to obtain optimal patient cooperation following surgery.

EXPLAINING PREOPERATIVE PROCEDURES. – In the usual situation, the patient is initially admitted to the hospital on the medical service for diagnosis. He may be subjected to a multitude of physicians and an array of laboratory tests which could bewilder even the most emotionally stable patient. Often cardiac catheterization follows, a procedure which in itself should be done only subsequent to precatheterization instruction. Following the diagnostic evaluation, the patient may be discharged to be readmitted to the hospital at a later time for elective surgery. During the initial hospitalization the patient gains some information regarding his disease and may know a considerable amount about the procedure he will undergo at a subsequent date. During the interval at home he often discusses the impending surgery with members of the family, neighbors or other patients who have had similar procedures. Information may be misconstrued, due to the manner in which it is presented, or it may be entirely erroneous. Fear and anxiety are often created, initiating an emotional climate which may be difficult to reverse.

The patient is admitted to the hospital several days before the scheduled operation so that certain preoperative data may be obtained. Usually a chest x-ray, an electrocardiogram and blood tests are included. The cardiovascular nursing specialist who is to prepare the patient for surgery meets the patient soon after admission. Preoperative instruction is correlated with the physician, and preoperative examinations and procedures are explained to the patient. Details of this instruction include the explanation for hexachlorophene showers twice daily and the reason why certain examinations are performed. For instance, culture of specimens from the nose, throat and perineum could cause apprehension if the patient is unaware of the purpose.

Early confidence and trust can be gained by listening to and placing an interest in the patient. The environment in the hospital can directly affect the psychologic preparation for surgery. If a recent postoperative heart patient is placed next to the patient who is about to have heart surgery, the effect will be related to the patient's postoperative course. In general, it is better not to place a preoperative heart patient with one who has had recent cardiac surgery. Also, the attitudes of various ward personnel will affect the patient's response to the impending surgery. There is nothing more destructive to a preoperative heart patient than to hear ward personnel talking about the outcome of an operated patient who did poorly. Educational sessions with ward staff personnel will help to alleviate this problem.

Part of the educational program for the preoperative heart patient includes presenting him with diagrams and charts explaining his disease and the anatomy of the affected organ. Examples of valve prostheses or other prosthetic devices used in cardiovascular surgery will help to indoctrinate him. An album of pictures of patients successfully operated on can be utilized by the nurse to exhibit results of this type of surgery and what the patient may expect following discharge from the hospital.

Several days before surgery the patient is introduced to a respirator and given instruction in its use. He should be given an opportunity to practice with it several times before surgery. In this way he can learn to use it proficiently and will know that it will be of help to him in the postoperative period. He is also taught deep breathing and effective coughing exercises, often by a physical therapist. It is important that he practice coughing with the nurse who will be caring for him in the postoperative period. It should be explained that he will have a tendency to refrain from coughing because of the postoperative pain.

The patient takes surgical soap showers several times daily; this is continued until surgery. On the day before surgery the patient is started on a regimen of parenteral antibiotics if a prosthetic device is to be used. The antibiotics are given through an intravenous catheter inserted the evening before surgery, but this should not limit the ambulatory patient. He is given the usual evening meal. It is important that enemas and preps be done after the visiting hours. Adequate sedation is given to ensure a restful night's sleep. If the patient is apprehensive, further time should be set aside for discussion, preferably by both the nursing specialist and the physician. The family is instructed as to the time the surgery is expected to take and where to wait during the procedure so the physician can talk with them following surgery. They are informed that the patient's clothing and valuables will either be taken to the intensive care unit or given to them for safe keeping. The location of the intensive care unit is described and the visiting hours explained.

On the morning of surgery the patient is awakened early to prepare for the trip to the operating room. Preparation includes the shaving of prescribed areas and the removal of dentures, hairpins, nail polish or valuables. The patient is advised to wash his face and brush his teeth. Premedication is given, and he is taken to the operating room.

Preoperative orientation should include some details concerning the operating room, such as its appearance and the personnel administering care, as well as information about preanesthetic procedures. These include the placement of the cardiac monitor and the electroencephalographic monitor, and the introduction of the central venous pressure catheters, arterial catheters and Foley catheters. The induction of anesthesia is best explained by the anesthesiologist.

Postoperative Management

The cardiovascular system is stabilized in the operating room prior to moving the patient to the intensive care unit. The endotracheal tube is left in place for the period of time that it is needed and removed only after the patient is able to ventilate adequately spontaneously. Indoctrination of the patient to the endotracheal tube in the preoperative period will alleviate many problems in its use. Apprehension occurs particularly when the patient is placed on assisted ventilation. Anxiety is also associated with sleeping with the endotracheal tube in place, not being able to talk and periodic tracheobronchial suctioning. Basic sign language, taught preoperatively, will improve communication. Pointing to the lips if thirsty or to the chest for chest pain illustrates this technique.

Often a nasogastric tube is utilized postoperatively, and its purpose is explained to the patient. In the intensive care unit the tube is irrigated every 2 hours with sterile water and gently aspirated. Any unusual nasogastric return is promptly reported to the physician. Other tubes or connections to the patient should be explained in detail prior to surgery. Chest tubes placed in the pleural or mediastinal spaces during surgery should be demonstrated to the patient. Their purpose is described with an explanation that their presence causes little discomfort. Apprehension is apt to occur if the patient has not been informed of the routine in emptying the chest tubes or the frequent inspection of underwater-seal bottles. The temporary pacing wires which are attached to the myocardium are explained. If cardiac pacing becomes necessary, its use as a safety factor instead of as an indication of a deterioration in condition is stressed. It is important for the nurse to be able to evaluate the condition of the patient in relation to the possible need for cardiac pacing.

Clinical nursing specialist's responsibilities.—In the management of the patient arriving in the intensive care unit, the clinical specialist is responsible for the availability of necessary equipment and personnel.

The room in the intensive care unit must be in readiness for the patient. This includes a well-padded bed, adequate intravenous stands, ventilatory equipment including extra endotracheal tubes, oxygen tubing, respirator equipment, endotracheal suctioning apparatus and an Ambu bag. In the transfer from the operating room to the intensive care unit, portable equipment may be necessary, including an oxygen tank and an Ambu bag. Suction devices for the chest tubes should be readily available. Monitoring equipment is balanced and ready for placement on the patient. A sheepskin placed on the bed will help prevent skin breakdown.

At least two nurses should be available for care of the patient on his return. Also, an inhalation therapist and a technician who is familiar with the monitoring equipment must be available for attachment of monitoring equipment and initial adjustment of the respirator. It is important that the nursing specialist who has counseled the patient preoperatively be present in the intensive care unit when the patient arrives. The familiar voice of this nurse, along with the calm, organized work of the team, will do much to allay apprehension.

The prevention of anoxemia is important, and an adequate oxygen supply must be assured. The patient is placed on the ventilator if necessary. Auscultation of the lungs and the chest x-ray will help determine if the endotracheal tube is in the bronchus or trachea. Adequacy of ventilation can be judged by movement of the chest and color of the lips and nail beds. If the endotracheal tube has migrated to a position distal to the carina, it should be repositioned immediately.

Monitoring devices.—The patient is attached to monitoring devices, including the electrocardiograph and arterial and venous pressure catheters. The clinical nursing specialist should be familiar with the monitoring equipment, and in particular should be able to recognize when the equipment is malfunctioning. She is responsible for maintaining patent arterial and venous lines. In checking the patency of the arterial catheter, the pressure curve should demonstrate a prompt response. Ease in obtaining blood samples and in irrigating the catheter will confirm its patency. The central venous pressure catheter, inserted in the operating suite, is attached to a water manometer or a pressure transducer. It is leveled at the anterior axillary line at the fourth intercostal space (right atrium). Fluctuation in the column should be checked so that it corresponds with the respiration and not the heartbeat. If the central venous pressure is inordinately elevated or fluctuates with the heartbeat, the catheter is probably in the right ventricle. The most important aspect of the measurement is the correlation of the initial reading with other physiologic parameters and progress of the measurement through the postoperative period. The central venous pressure catheter is kept open with a small amount of solution amounting to approximately 400 ml./24 hours. It can be utilized for the sampling of blood specimens when the arterial catheter is not functioning.

The electrocardiogram is utilized directly after the return of the patient from the operating room. Serious arrhythmias often occur in the early hours following surgery. It is important for the clinical specialist to have knowledge of abnormal rhythms and basic electrocardiographic patterns. Recognition of arrhythmias and proper treatment have been instrumental in saving many lives.

Other tubes and catheters.—Chest tubes are attached to underwater drainage bottles in the operating room. En route to the intensive care unit the tubes may be clamped unless large pulmonary air leaks preclude this routine. The chest tubes are periodically stripped to help remove blood from the chest cavity or tubes. If the drainage is moderately heavy, suction can be applied to the chest bottles to facilitate the removal of fluid.

The Foley catheter is attached to sterile connecting tubes and allowed to drain by gravity. The color, specific gravity and amount of urine is noted and recorded hourly. A urinalysis is performed in the early postoperative period. If either polyuria (more than 150 ml./hour) or oliguria (less than 25 ml./hour) is present, the physician is immediately notified. Electrolyte depletion can occur if the volume is excessive. Likewise, oliguria may signify the need for increased fluid replacement or diuretic management.

The nasogastric tube must be checked for proper location and patency. This can be done by instillation of air into the tube with auscultation over the left upper abdominal quadrant. Air can be heard to enter the stomach. The tube is then irrigated and the stomach thoroughly aspirated of its contents. The amount and type of drainage are important observations that should be recorded. The tube is irrigated every two hours or as often as needed with 30 ml. of water. It is taped in place so that no pressure is exerted on the nose and attached to low suction.

Management of the endotracheal tube is of prime importance. Sterile technique should be utilized in its care. Instillation of small amounts of sterile saline into the tube, followed by tracheobronchial suctioning, is done as often as needed. The head is positioned in both lateral positions and the midline with each aspiration so that the catheter enters both major bronchi. Suction is applied only when withdrawing the catheter. The period of suctioning should not be prolonged, as deprivation of oxygen may cause cardiac arrhythmias. The patient should be hyperventilated every hour to decrease the possibility of atelectasis.

Other observations of importance are the patient's color, temperature, peripheral pulses, level of consciousness and saturation of the dressings. Any change in these parameters throughout the postoperative period may alert the clinician to impending problems.

THE EARLY POSTOPERATIVE PERIOD.—At this time the patient should be reassured. He should know that his surgery has been completed, that he is doing well in the recovery room or intensive care area and that his family has been notified of his progress.

During the early postoperative period several problems may occur which can be anticipated by the nursing staff. A change in vital signs (taken every 15–30 minutes) may precede more serious cardiopulmonary problems. Drainage from the chest tubes may be excessive, or drainage may abruptly cease with a deterioration of the patient's condition. These changes should raise the suspicion of hemorrhage or pericardial tamponade. Persistent coolness of the extremities may occur. A high rectal temperature, shivering and peripheral vasoconstriction are often associated. Augmentation of intravenous volume and/or administration of a vasodilator may alleviate this problem. Persistent elevation of the temperature should be treated with antipyretics and cooling measures. Insufficient ventilation or difficulty in managing the patient on the respirator often signifies basic abnormalities of the cardiovascular system or defects in acid-base balance. This should be correlated with other physiologic parameters and the blood gases. Cardiac electrical instability is detected by arrhythmias occurring on the electrocardiogram. Premature ventricular contractions may signify irritability and precede more serious rhythm problems. The physician should be notified immediately when electrical abnormalities occur.

The family is encouraged to visit the patient after he has become stable and the intensive care specialists have performed all initial duties. Family members should be reassured that the monitoring devices do not signify deterioration in the patient's condition. They should not display undue concern during the visit, as this might have an effect on the patient. Prior to the visit the patient's appearance and his ability to respond are explained. The nurse should stay with the family during the short visiting period.

The patient is gradually taken off the respirator for short periods of time, depending upon his ability to ventilate. Clinical correlation in conjunction with the blood gases will help in determining this. As soon as the patient can do well without assisted ventilation, the endotracheal tube is removed. Prior to tube removal, the tracheobronchial tree is thoroughly irrigated with sterile saline and aspirated. The patient is placed in a high-humidity oxygen tent. If possible, the patient should be placed in the sitting position and assisted in coughing every 1 or 2 hours. If the patient has difficulty in removing secretions, the nursing specialist who has been trained in the technique of nasotracheal aspiration proceeds with this therapeutic modality.

The nasogastric tube is removed as soon in the postoperative period as possible. When oral intake is tolerated, the peripheral intravenous fluids are discontinued. Central venous catheters left in place more than 72 hours are associated with an increase in infection and thrombophlebitis and should be removed prior to that time. If dressings around arterial and central venous catheters become saturated, they should be changed, using sterile technique. Antibiotic ointment applied to the dressings may help decrease the incidence of infection. The arterial catheter can usually be removed 12–24 hours following surgery, depending on the patient's condition and the need for further arterial monitoring.

The patient should be mobilized early in the postoperative period. At first, turning from side to side will ease the discomfort of prolonged immobilization. As soon as possible the patient should be placed in a sitting position, particularly when he is being urged to cough. Dentures can be returned and oral hygiene instituted. Dressings should be changed and cardiac electrodes replaced. Pain medications should be given as necessary, but not in such excessive amounts as to dull the patient's consciousness.

By the second postoperative day the patient's cardiovascular status is usually quite stable. He is more aware of the aches and pains which he has, and because of the difficulty in sleeping for the two previous nights, he will probably be tired and irritable. Although it is important for him to have increasing physical activity, he should be sedated at intervals to obtain rest. Vital signs can be taken less frequently, concurrent with his improving status. Usually by this period various tubes can be removed, including the nasogastric tube, the Foley catheter, one of the intravenous catheters, the arterial catheter and often the chest tubes. The patient begins to see himself as an individual who has recovered from surgery and has a good chance for survival. At every stage of management he should be given encouragement and complimented on his ability to perform. He may feel that his progress has been too rapid and become overdependent upon the nursing staff.

As soon as possible the patient is moved to a closely supervised private room. This area offers the advantages of cardiovascular monitoring, less direct nursing supervision, privacy and an opportunity to sleep and rest while increasing ambulation and normal activities. This unit is staffed by cardiovascular nursing specialists who can recognize and treat those problems which can occur in the postoperative cardiac patient. During this period in the postoperative course, the patient has a tendency to mental depression. The physician and cardiovascular nursing specialist should give needed encouragement, and the family can assume an increasing role in the patient's recovery.

The role of the nurse in cardiovascular procedures not requiring cardiopulmonary bypass is similar to that which has been described for open heart surgery. Usually the patient does not require such intensive management as those having open heart surgery; however, this is not always true. Patients having a closed mitral commissurotomy, myocardial revascularization without cardiopulmonary bypass, pericardiectomy or pacemaker insertion are monitored in the intensive care or adjacent area, according to their need. Principles outlined earlier in the management of patients undergoing open heart surgery apply also to this group of patients.

Peripheral Vascular Surgery

Preoperative instruction and postoperative management for the patient who is to have major vascular surgery is similar to that described for open heart procedures. Peripheral vascular procedures most commonly involve the abdomen, lower extremities and neck. The incisions in the abdomen and legs are painful and interfere with coughing and ambulation. Preoperatively the patient about to undergo abdominal surgery is taught to cough effectively with the use of a support over his abdomen. Methods of ambulation are taught for patients with abdominal or leg incisions.

In patients who have *distal aortic or lower limb vascular reconstruction* certain postoperative observations are important. The arterial pulses distal to the reconstruction should be checked periodically if expected to be present. Any changes in the quality of these pulses should be immediately transmitted to the physician. The temperature and color of the revascularized extremity should be frequently checked and compared with that of the other extremity. When a sympathectomy has been performed, the extremity is generally warm and dry.

The involved extremity must be protected. A foot cradle should be placed over the extremity to keep it from being abraded by the bed covers. The heel should be protected, particularly in the early postoperative period when continuous pressure on the heel may cause skin necrosis. Constrictive devices or heat in excess of body temperature should not be placed on limbs where vascular compromise has been present. Care should also be taken that the bed is free of objects which may cause pressure necrosis. If the patient has inordinate pain in the foot or lower leg, ischemia should be suspected and the physician notified.

Following resection of an abdominal aortic aneurysm, postoperative distention is common. This is even more prominent after surgery for ruptured abdominal aortic aneurysm. Retroperitoneal hematoma and ileus are responsible for the distention. If the girth of the abdomen is periodically measured, rate of distention may be helpful in determining inordinate retroperitoneal or intraperitoneal hemorrhage.

Carotid artery surgery usually imposes little postoperative morbidity on the patient. However, when complications occur, they may be catastrophic. The state of consciousness should be noted immediately after surgery, and any deterioration should be immediately reported. Convulsions, coma and sensory or motor changes may indicate cerebral thrombosis or hemorrhage. Blood pressure changes should be carefully noted. Hypotension and hypertension are not uncommon and may be responsible for cerebrovascular complications. Sustained elevation or depression of the blood pressure should be avoided. The incision in the neck should be periodically inspected. Continuing bleeding through the drain site or progressive hematoma collection may require re-exploration of the wound.

The patient may have some difficulty in swallowing related to retraction of the hypoglossal nerve. If dysfunction occurs, the tongue will deviate toward the side of the operation. This is particularly important because the nurse will be able to tell whether the patient will be able to take liquid or food satisfactorily. Patients who have difficulty in this regard have a tendency to aspirate.

Summary

The degrees of preoperative and postsurgical intensive therapy vary with the magnitude of the surgical procedure, the amount of physiologic depletion and the patient's ability to cooperate in the postoperative management. The principles of intensive care have been useful in lowering the mortality and morbidity of extremely ill patients requiring major surgery. These principles can be individualized to fit the needs of the institution and the patient.

16

The Neurosurgical Patient

WALTER W. WHISLER, M.D., Ph.D.

Attending Surgeon and Chairman, Department of Neurosurgery, Rush-Presbyterian-St. Luke's Medical Center; Professor of Neurological Surgery, Rush Medical College

THE NEUROSURGICAL PATIENT is uniquely different from most other surgical patients. The unconscious patient is unable to act as a witness to inform his physicians of changes in his physiologic processes. Vital signs and other more obvious clues that are used for evaluation of the status of most surgical patients must be supplanted by neurologic signs, the interpretation of which cannot be entrusted to untrained personnel. The postoperative treatment is also different in that a considerable amount of emphasis must be placed on protecting and performing functions that are normally reflex in nature but are transiently absent in the unconscious patient.

Evaluation of the Patient in Coma

The early discovery of a neurologic deficit and the subsequent treatment of a postoperative hematoma or cerebral edema is dependent upon the early recognition of a change in neurologic status and not on the alterations of vital signs or a gross change in the patient which finally alerts the unskilled observer.

Although a complete and thorough neurologic examination is helpful, most of the necessary information can be obtained by a limited examination, such as the following.

LEVEL OF CONSCIOUSNESS.—Instead of classifying the patient's level of consciousness by a term such as "semicomatose" or "stuporous," which may mean different things to different observers, it is more appropriate to describe the actual state. This description should note whether the patient is irritable or restless; whether he is oriented to time, place and person; whether the patient is able to follow commands or answer questions and whether the patient responds to verbal stimuli or must be aroused by painful stimuli.

VITAL SIGNS. — Note is made of the pulse, blood pressure and respirations. The chest should be uncovered and respiration noted as being regular, irregular, shallow or rapid. If there is a high increase in the intracranial pressure as the result of a rapidly expanding intracranial mass, the pulse will slow (as low as 50/minute), the blood pressure will increase and the respirations will become irregular.

MOTOR POWER. — The patient is asked to move all four extremities and the degree of weakness is assessed. If the patient is not responsive to verbal commands, a painful stimulus is applied to each extremity and the response to pain noted. One method of applying a painful stimulus to an extremity is to apply pressure to the nail bed with the back of a key. When the painful stimulus is applied, the nonparalyzed side will move, the face will grimace and an attempt will be made to withdraw from the pain unless the extremity is anesthetic. If there is no response, then more than one area should be stimulated. In the decorticate state, with a painful stimulus, the legs will stiffen and the arms will be rigidly flexed. When the lesion is in the brain stem, a painful stimulus will elicit decerebrate rigidity, in which the legs and arms are rigidly extended and pronated.

EYES. — The pupil size is measured in millimeters. The response, both direct and consensual, to a bright light is noted. Often it is necessary to use a bright flashlight in a slightly darkened room before it is possible to say that a light reflex is definitely absent. In certain instances it is necessary to check both the "doll's head eye movement" (oculocephalic reflex) and caloric stimulation (oculovestibular reflex) (Table 16-1). The "doll's head eye movement" is the preservation of the conjugate lateral eye movements which are produced by rapidly turning the patient's head (the eyelids are held open). Upon rapid turning of the head, the eyes will conjugately tend to lag behind the rotation of the head.

In the caloric test, the patient's head is elevated and the wax-free external auditory canal slowly irrigated with ice water until there is a response or until 200 ml. of the ice water has been utilized. In a normal patient who is awake, nystagmus is produced with the quick component away from the irrigated ear. In an unconscious patient with an intact brain stem, the eyes will conjugately deviate toward the side of the irrigation. With the ciliospinal reflex, mydriasis is produced by pinching the skin of the neck (Table 16-1).

CLOUDING OF CONSCIOUSNESS. — As either edema or hemorrhage progresses in a supratentorial process, there will be a clouding of consciousness which may be joined by focal hemispheric findings, signs of uncal herniation and finally brain stem dysfunction. The progression of clouding of consciousness begins with drowsiness, which becomes more marked to the point of sleeping in spite of mild discomfort and

TABLE 16-1.—LEVELS OF BRAIN STEM DYSFUNCTION*

Diencephalic stage (decorticate)
Respiration: Cheyne-Stokes
Eyes: small and reactive; ciliospinal reflex present
Oculocephalic and oculovestibular reflexes present
Response to painful stimuli: decorticate rigidity

Midbrain stage
Respiration: hyperventilation
Eyes: midposition fixed, ciliospinal reflex absent
Oculocephalic and oculovestibular reflexes: dysconjugate and sluggish
Response to painful stimuli: decerebrate response

Pontine stage
Respiration: tachypnea or eupnea
Eyes: midposition fixed, ciliospinal reflex absent
Oculocephalic and oculovestibular reflexes absent
Response to painful stimuli: lessened decerebrate response

Medullary stage
Respiration: slow and irregular
Eyes: midposition fixed or fixed and dilated, ciliospinal reflex absent
Oculocephalic and oculovestibular reflexes absent
Response to painful stimuli: patient is flaccid

*Modified from McNealy, D. E., and Plum, F.; Arch. Neurol. 1:10-32, 1962.

falling asleep during conversation. As the process continues, the patient becomes confused and disoriented to time, place and person. More and more stimuli become necessary to arouse the patient, and the answers become more inappropriate until the patient cannot be aroused by painful stimuli. If the lesion is in the dominant hemisphere, the patient may not respond appropriately because of an aphasia.

Focal hemispheric findings may present as a hemiparesis which may be more marked in the upper or the lower extremity and may involve the face. If the frontal eye-field area of the brain is involved, then the eyes will be conjugately deviated to the affected hemisphere.

Syndrome of Uncal Herniation

THE PRIMARY LESION.—The primary expanding lesion will begin to make itself known in accordance with the special areas of the brain affected. Signs of this lesion usually are progressive mental obtundation associated with a hemiparesis and a Babinski sign.

THIRD NERVE CHANGES.—In the initial stages of injury to the third nerve by the herniating uncal cortex, there is moderate dilatation of the pupil ipsilateral to the primary lesion in the hemisphere. The pupil gives a sluggish response to light and has a sluggish ciliospinal response. The oculocephalic reflex is present, but with ice water there is dysconjugate movement of the eyes due to failure of medial deviation by the affected third nerve. As the herniation injury to the third nerve progresses, the pupil becomes widely dilated and fixed to light, both direct and consensual. The ciliospinal reflex is also lost. The affected eye fails to give either the oculocephalic or oculovestibular reflex.

THE LATERAL BRAIN STEM SYNDROME.—As the uncal lobe continues to herniate against the brain stem, the opposite cerebral peduncle is compressed against the tentorial edge with an associated hemiparesis ipsilateral to the mass lesion; finally the other pupil may become widely dilated. As the herniation continues, there is progressive lateral compression of the brain stem. The brain stem dysfunction (Table 16-1) is then seen, with the pupils assuming the midrange fixed position.

Evaluation of the Spinal Cord

Following either surgery or trauma to the spinal cord, the presence of a hematoma can only be determined by neurologic examination.

The neurologic examination essentially consists of a motor, sensory and reflex examination. In evaluating the function of the spinal cord, each muscle does not have to be tested, only selected muscle groups as representative of each neural segment (Table 16-2). The representative deep tendon reflexes listed in Table 16-2, as well as the abdominal reflex, the cremasteric reflex and the presence of a Babinski sign, should also be recorded.

The presence or absence of a spinal subarachnoid block is determined by means of the Queckenstedt test. After a lumbar puncture the patient is asked first to cough and then to strain as if to defecate. In

TABLE 16-2.—NEURAL SEGMENTS REPRESENTED BY TENDON REFLEXES AND MUSCLE GROUPS

	LOCALIZATION
Reflex	
Biceps reflex	C_5-C_6
Triceps reflex	C_6-C_7
Cremasteric reflex	L_1-L_2
Knee jerk	L_2-L_3-L_4
Ankle jerk	L_5-S_1-S_2
Plantar reflex	S_1-S_2
Motor innervation	
Diaphragm (phrenic)	C_3-C_4
[illegible]	[illegible]
Deltoid	C_5-C_6
Biceps	C_5-C_6
Triceps	C_7-C_8
Muscles of hand (radial)	C_6-C_7-C_8
Muscles of hand (median and ulnar)	C_7-C_8-T_1
Iliopsoas	L_1-L_2-L_3
Quadriceps femoris	L_2-L_3-L_4
Adductors of thigh	L_2-L_3-L_4
Hamstring muscles	L_5-S_1-S_2
Gastrocnemius	L_5-S_1-S_2
Extensor hallucis longus	L_4-L_5-S_1

both instances the pressure should increase and then decrease at about the same rate. The Queckenstedt maneuver is then performed by compressing the jugular veins in the neck. The pressure should increase to 300 mm. within 10 seconds and then return to normal within 10 seconds of release of the jugular pressure if there is no spinal subarachnoid obstruction.

The sensory level to pinprick should be tested, as should the position sense in all four extremities. The sensory level should be obtained fairly rapidly as the patient will quickly fatigue if the examination is pursued in a tedious and drawn-out manner. The presence or absence of a level of sweating as well as the presence or absence of bladder function should also be noted.

Management of the Craniotomy Patient

One of the most difficult postoperative evaluation problems that the surgeon encounters is deciding whether the craniotomy patient has had postoperative bleeding. This bleeding may be intraparenchymal, subdural, intraventricular, epidural or within the cavity remaining after tumor removal. Such bleeding may be difficult to differentiate from vascular thrombosis or cerebral edema. Most of the problems of postoperative bleeding are avoided by the use of drains and by attention paid to detail at the time of surgery. Still, the diagnosis of postoperative bleeding is suspected when the patient does not respond as expected or when his neurologic condition deteriorates. If a clot is suspected, then the craniotomy wound must be reopened in the operating room and not in the patient's bed.

If problems secondary to cerebral edema develop, then the use of hypertonic solutions as well as steroids may be considered.

The velocity of many biologic reactions roughly doubles for each 10 C. rise in temperature (13% increase in the metabolic rate for each 1 C. of fever). Bearing this in mind, it is easy to see that despite the fact that oxygenation is decreased by vessels in spasm and the edematous brain cells have a decreased efficiency, the metabolic activity of the cells may still be normal. When the metabolic demands are increased by a higher temperature, the system does not have its normal reserve and cannot therefore keep up with the metabolic demands of the cell. This cellular metabolic anoxia is just as lethal to the cell, although not nearly so rapidly, as anoxia secondary to vascular occlusion. It therefore becomes necessary to keep the patient normothermic during the postoperative period. This may necessitate the use of aspirin, alcohol sponge baths or the ice water mattress. It should also be kept in mind that if the patient has been in coma for considerable time, he may actually be dehydrated. In that case he may have a fever, but the skin will not be warm. Along with methods to lower the temperature to normal, the cause of the fever should be sought and specific therapy instituted. Hyperpyrexia of central origin will often be less responsive to salicylates than will a fever which is secondary to infection.

Except for the patient with diabetes insipidus, the neurosurgical patient, unlike most surgical patients, does not require a large amount of fluids, as he is in a semidormant state of very low activity and is not losing fluids through external drainage. In fact, it is wise to keep the patient slightly underhydrated to help combat cerebral edema. This is accomplished by restricting the intravenous fluids to 1,500–2,000 ml. for the first 24 hours. As the patient is followed, the fluid intake and output, as well as electrolytes, should be recorded. In surgery for lesions in the area of the pituitary or hypothalamus, the urinary specific gravity should be recorded. If after a period of time the patient should slowly worsen or never improve, special attention should be paid to the electrolytes as well as to the blood sugar. An associated loss of sodium and chloride will be seen as marked weakness, lethargy and even coma, while a low potassium will present as confusion and decreased responsiveness.

In some patients who have undergone surgery in the area of the diencephalon or for an anterior communicating artery aneurysm and are apparently recovering, a worsening of the mental status may be due to hypernatremia. Serum sodium levels as high as 180 mEq./L. are seen. This process is produced either by a disturbance of the thirst mechanism in combination with excretion of massive amounts of urinary nitrogen or by a defect in the osmoregulatory mechanism. Rather than trying to correct the water balance defect in a 24 hour period, which may result in cerebral edema, it is best to lower the serum electrolytes gradually over a period of several days. This is done by the use of 10% dextrose in water. If possible, fat should also be given, along with protein restriction to lessen endogenous catabolism of nitrogen and the excretion of urinary nitrogen with the subsequent osmal diuresis.

Probably the most frequent problems in the postoperative neurosurgical patient involve the respiratory tract. Placing deeply comatose patients in any but the head-down coma position is inviting aspiration and a definite respiratory complication. The comatose patient should be placed in a slightly head-down position on his side with the arms extended around a pillow and the uppermost leg flexed over a pillow. Every 2 hours the patient is turned to the opposite side. In the immediate postoperative period the patient is placed in the coma position to prevent aspiration of mucus or emesis until the effect of the anesthetic has worn off. If the level of consciousness improves, then the head may be elevated 12 in. to aid venous drainage from the brain; otherwise, as long as the patient remains in coma, he should remain in the coma position. If the level of consciousness is markedly depressed, tracheopharyngeal aspirations are necessary—at least hourly, more frequently if necessary. A rather severe atelectasis may require bronchoscopy, and if the patient is in coma, it is often wise to perform a tracheostomy to be able to suction him adequately and to prevent a recurrence of secretion retention and the resulting atelectasis. Naturally a tracheostomy should be performed on any patient in imminent danger of airway obstruction. Surgery in the posterior fossa is often associated not only with problems of respiration but also with impairment of the swallowing and cough reflexes, resulting in difficulty in handling secretions. In this type of patient a tracheostomy is almost mandatory. A conscious patient who responds poorly to direction can be made to cough by having him take 10 deep breaths of 100% CO_2 administered from a catheter held 5 in. from his face. The CO_2 will make him cough. This is repeated hourly or more often if needed.

The comatose patient will need either an indwelling catheter, or an external catheter if he is a male. When an external catheter is used, it is necessary to be certain that the patient has no evidence of urinary retention. A dry bed is necessary in the comatose patient to prevent maceration of the skin. For the immediate postoperative period it is usually most efficient to use an indwelling catheter, not only to keep the patient dry but also to permit an accurate method of measuring intake and output. An indwelling catheter is a necessity if hypertonic solutions are required to combat edema.

The patient with intracranial disease is especially sensitive to respiratory impairment by narcotics, and therefore their use in the immediate postoperative period is unwise. Any discomfort the patient has can usually be readily relieved by either oral or rectal aspirin. If the obtunded patient is restless, the discomfort is usually due to an airway problem or a distended bladder or meningeal irritation caused by bloody cerebrospinal fluid. Correction of these problems will quiet the patient. These problems are frequently seen secondary to head injury.

POSTOPERATIVE ORDERS – CRANIOTOMY

The usual postoperative orders for a craniotomy patient in the first 24 hours are as follows:

1. Vital signs until stable, then every hour.
2. Neurologic signs (level of consciousness, pupil size and reaction to light, hand grasp, leg strength) every 15 minutes for 1 hour, then every 30 minutes for 2 hours, then every hour.
3. Notify service of any change in neurologic or vital signs.
4. Coma position until patient is alert, then elevate the head of the bed 12 in.
5. Turn patient every 2 hours.
6. Aspirate every hour as necessary; keep airway open.
7. N.P.O.
8. Intake and output – indwelling catheter.
9. 1,500 ml. of 5% dextrose in water for the first 24 hours.
10. Dilantin 500 mg. intramuscularly stat, and then 100 mg. intramuscularly or orally 3 times daily.

11. ASA 1,800 mg. every 3 hours as necessary for pain per rectum—no narcotics.
12. Decadron 4 mg. every 8 hours for 3 days.
13. Hemoglobin and hematocrit in A.M.

If the patient is to have surgery upon the pituitary gland, then special attention must also be paid to endocrine status.

PREOPERATIVE ORDERS—HYPOPHYSECTOMY

1. Cortisone acetate 100 mg. intramuscularly 12 hours before surgery (12 hour peak of action).
2. Cortisone acetate 100 mg. orally 1 hour prior to surgery—in spite of N.P.O. order (4 hour peak of action).
3. During surgery begin a 1,000 ml. bottle of 5% dextrose/water containing 100 mg. hydrocortisone and run for 6–8 hours.

POSTOPERATIVE ORDERS—HYPOPHYSECTOMY

1. Restrict intravenous fluids to 2,000 ml. for the first 24 hours postoperatively.
2. Each 1,000 ml. of intravenous fluids should contain 50 mg. hydrocortisone.
3. Immediately postoperatively start cortisone acetate, 75 mg. intramuscularly every 8 hours.
4. On the second day, depending on the clinical state, give cortisone acetate 50 mg. intramuscularly every 8 hours.
5. Gradually reduce to oral maintenance dose of cortisone acetate, 37.5 mg./day (give in divided dose 3 to 4 times/day).
6. After 48 hours patient should be evaluated for diabetes insipidus. (See section on Diabetes Insipidus.)
7. For transphenoidal hypophysectomy surgery the patient is placed on Keflin, 2 Gm./day, starting the day before surgery and continued for 5 days or until the wound is healed. The patient is then placed on penicillin, 400,000 units orally twice daily for 2 weeks.
8. Thyroid replacement may be started after the patient is able to take oral medication. Begin with desiccated thyroid, 30 mg./day, and gradually increase to 100 mg./day over several months as required.
9. Sex hormones may be given for their general anabolic effect and for improvement of libido.

Management of the Patient with Head Trauma

There is considerable disagreement in neurosurgery as to the type and timing of surgery in cerebral trauma and cord trauma. In general, the patient who reaches the intensive care unit will have already had surgery or will be there primarily for observation, with the plan that, should he deteriorate, diagnostic studies or surgery will be performed. It is therefore of paramount importance that both types of patients have continuous observation. Changes must be promptly reported. Every unconscious patient (of unknown cause) who has a scalp laceration should not be assumed to be in coma because of a head injury. He may have a head injury, but other associated, as well as contributing, conditions should be considered. Did the patient receive head trauma and then lose consciousness, or did he lose consciousness first? Many of these questions can be answered by a factual eyewitness account of the injury. There may not be any evidence that the patient sustained head trauma. He may be in diabetic or barbiturate coma. He may have lost consciousness and then fallen because of a myocardial infarct, ruptured intracranial aneurysm or epileptic seizure. The patient's pockets may contain vials of medicine which may solve the problem. It is important to remember that the force of injury may also have produced internal injuries or a fracture dislocation of the cervical spine. In many severe head injuries there is also a fracture of the cervical spine. If any doubt exists, cervical spine films should be taken before the patient is moved.

CARE OF PATIENT WITH CEREBRAL TRAUMA

1. Establish and maintain an adequate respiratory exchange. This may require the use of an oral airway or tracheostomy, or, if a chest injury is present, a chest tube may be required.
2. Vital signs. Patients do not go into shock from a head injury. If the patient is in shock, look elsewhere for signs of internal bleeding. Rarely a patient may lose enough blood from an extensive scalp laceration to go into shock.
3. Neurologic signs. These include level of consciousness, pupil size and reaction to light, hand grasp and leg movement. Any deterioration should be promptly reported.
4. If the patient is in coma, he should be placed in the coma position, turned every 2 hours and aspirated every hour as needed.
5. Fluid intake should be restricted to 2,000 ml. of 5% dextrose and 0.2N saline for the first 24 hours. Accurate intake and output should be recorded.
6. No narcotics. If the patient is restless, the cause of the restlessness should be found. Under no circumstances give narcotics. The patient may be restless because of a distended bladder, inadequate airway with air hunger, internal injuries, fractured ribs, a fractured long bone, blood in the cerebrospinal fluid or headache. Aspirin is usually adequate to relieve the discomfort of headache. In exceptional circumstances when headache alone is the cause of the discomfort and the patient is fully responsive, a small amount of codeine may be used. Removal of the bloody cerebrospinal fluid may also improve headache secondary to meningeal irritation.
7. If the patient has a cerebrospinal fluid rhinorrhea, he is immediately placed on oral penicillin, 400,000 units twice daily. This is contin-

ued for 2 weeks beyond the time when all signs of the leakage have stopped. This low dosage of penicillin should not be increased, as theoretically it will only kill the pathogenic pneumococcus and not change the flora. Cerebrospinal fluid can be readily differentiated from mucus since the cerebrospinal fluid contains glucose. A drop of the fluid can be collected on a Dextrostix (used for measuring blood sugar); if it turns the indicator blue, sugar is present. Any patient with a rhinorrhea should have repeat skull films on several occasions to make sure pneumocephalus is not developing.

Care of the Spinal Cord Injury Patient

Although there is considerable disagreement as to which cord injury patients are surgical candidates, most patients undergo a decompressive laminectomy if there is a progressive loss of neurologic function or evidence of a spinal subarachnoid block. In both the operated and unoperated patient the neurologic status of the cord must be carefully evaluated. Evidence of neurologic deterioration may indicate cord edema or postoperative hematoma in the postsurgical patient or may signal the need for surgery in the unoperated patient.

Along with the neurologic examination, a lumbar puncture and manometric studies should be performed. So that the patient may remain immobilized, he is turned into the prone position in a frame or Circ-O-lectric bed and a #18 spinal needle is inserted into the L_2-L_3 interspace. The manometer is then attached directly to the hub of the needle without the use of a stopcock. The manometer will be pointing directly upward, perpendicular to the patient's back. The pressure will have to be corrected by adding the distance from the patient's back to the start of the manometer. In this way, the lumbar puncture and Queckenstedt maneuver can be performed without turning the patient onto his side.

Aside from the important neurologic observations which may indicate the need for surgery or signal a postoperative complication, the main direction of the care of the patient will be to protect his body until spinal shock remits and the system has recovered from the traumatic insult. Rehabilitation can then begin, and what at first may appear to be an insurmountable deficit can be modified by proper training to produce a wholly or partially self-sufficient patient.

Injuries of the back may present as paraplegia and are treated differently from injuries of the cervical spine. Traction is unnecessary but the patient must be placed on a firm bed with bed boards. To aid in care and to speed mobilization, it may be necessary to fuse an unstable spine. All of the fracture-dislocation injuries, whether they occur in the cervical area or the back, will fuse if the patient is immobilized for a long enough period. The retroperitoneal hemorrhage present with fracture of the low back frequently produces a paralytic ileus. General care of the skin, bowels and bladder is similar for patients with cervical spine or back injuries.

Fracture-dislocation of the cervical spine requires immediate immobilization. The patient should be met in the emergency room with tongs and a special bed. After insertion of the skeletal traction tongs the patient may be safely moved. The closer the dislocation is to the skull, the less weight is needed to obtain reduction. As much as 25–30 lb. may be required for the lower cervical fracture-dislocations. Once the dislocation is reduced, reduction can usually be maintained by 5 lb. of weight. When the larger weights are being used, it is often necessary to elevate the head of the bed about 15 degrees so that the body itself may act as a counterweight and thus prevent the patient from being pulled to the top of his bed. Occasionally a patient will worsen after traction is instituted. The worsening may be due to a completely extruded disk or to an increasing angulation of the spine because of locked facets. I feel that when the inferior surface of the lower facet is locked above the superior surface of the higher facet, the spine should be reduced at surgery. Occasionally, when enough traction is applied, especially if the tongs are placed more posteriorly on the skull, there will be minimal angulation and no increase in neurologic deficit, and the facets will unlock to permit the fracture to be reduced.

The paralyzed patient should be placed on a special frame or bed to aid in turning. If one is not available, then an alternating pressure mattress should be used. Although the Stryker frame and Foster frame have proved adequate for care and turning of the patient, the Circ-O-lectric bed is far superior. This bed will accommodate a taller individual than the others and is wider and therefore more comfortable. Since the bed is electrically operated and turns the patient in a head-over-heels fashion, it is of paramount importance that turning of the patient, once started, must continue rapidly without stopping until the patient is again in the horizontal position. The cord paralyzed patient is without vasomotor tone in the lower extremities and will become hypotensive when placed in the upright position. To prevent the skin from breaking down, the patient must be turned at least every 2 hours without fail.

When the Crutchfield type of tongs are used, they must be tightened every day as they slowly cut through the bone. The weights must hang freely with the patient toward the foot of the bed so that the tongs are not against the pulley at the head of the bed.

If the patient is paralyzed and unable to void, an indwelling Foley catheter must be inserted before the bladder becomes overdistended and permanently damaged. Once a day the bladder is irrigated with 4% boric acid solution or 10% Renacidin, and the catheter is changed every 5 days. After the stage of spinal shock has elapsed and the patient is being rehabilitated, bladder re-education should begin. Before this is started the patient should have bladder manometry studies and the ice water test for reflex bladder activity. Instead of Munro tidal drainage, an indwelling catheter with a clamp is used. At every 2–3 hour interval the clamp is opened so that the bladder volume does not exceed 400–500 ml.

Attention is paid to diet so that constipation will be avoided. In addition, the patient is given a stool softener, such as Colace, Doss or Doxinate, every day. In the morning a Dulcolax (contact laxative) suppository is inserted. Once spinal shock has subsided, the bowel can be trained by use of the above agents and enemas can be avoided.

The skin must be frequently inspected for evidence of decubitus ulcers and when they are found, pressure must be avoided in these areas. Once a decubitus ulcer forms, it should be exposed to the air, debrided and kept clean and free from further pressure. "Donut" supports usually make the problem worse. The artificial fat pad manufactured by Stryker is helpful to redistribute weight over problem areas and permit healing.

Frequent neurologic examination is necessary to be able to gauge progress and prognosticate. If the patient has deep tendon reflexes present from the time of injury, there is minimal cord shock and the prognosis is more favorable. Once the patient is stabilized, it may be desirable to perform an anterior cervical fusion to aid in mobilization. If the patient is kept in tongs alone, it will then take at least 12 weeks before adequate stabilization is obtained.

Cerebral Edema

The use of hypertonic solutions in the treatment of cerebral edema is based on the assumption that the edema problem is a transient one and is not chronic. Since agents such as urea produce a marked rebound, it is not unusual to see obtunded patients perk up when intravenous urea is given, only to lose ground 6 hours later and be worse off than before the urea was given. The use of hypertonic solutions is contraindicated in active intracranial bleeding.

The use of large doses of steroids is excellent adjunct treatment in cerebral edema. The steroids are especially effective in the prevention of edema and seem to exert the best effect when given as close to the time of cerebral insult as possible.

Therapeutic Agents for Cerebral Edema

Urevert.—Lyophilized urea and 10% invert sugar solution is supplied in both 90 Gm. and 40 Gm. bottles. Reduction of intracranial pressure can be accomplished by a dose of 1 Gm. of urea/kg. of body weight. A 90 Gm. bottle of urea is administered over a period of 1–2 hours. Improvement may be seen within 30 minutes. If necessary, urea may be given over a period of 30 minutes, but local irritation as well as vasomotor symptoms may occur. Whenever urea is used, an indwelling urethral catheter should be inserted before the infusion is begun. Care in intravenous infusion is necessary as extravasation will cause tissue sloughing.

Osmitrol.—The mannitol is supplied as a 15% and a 20% solution. The effective dose of 1.5 Gm. mannitol/kg. of body weight can be given over 30–60 minutes. Improvement may be seen within 30 minutes. Up to 200 Gm. mannitol may be given by slow drip over 24 hours.

Decadron.—When used to control postoperative edema secondary to craniotomy for tumor, 10 mg. is given intravenously at the time of anesthesia induction. This is followed by 4 mg. every 8 hours for 3 days. At the end of 3 days the drug may be stopped abruptly. If it is necessary to continue the steroids for more than 3 days, then the dose must be decreased gradually. The same routine may also be used for other types of edema.

Diabetes Insipidus

The antidiuretic hormone is produced under the direct control of the supraoptic and paraventricular nuclei of the hypothalamus. The antidiuretic hormone then passes via the pituitary stalk to be stored in the posterior lobe of the pituitary. It is then released into the bloodstream to be carried to the kidney to regulate reabsorption of urine in the distal tubule.

If there is minimal injury to the neurohypophysis, a temporary diabetes insipidus will appear within 24 hours. Within several days the diabetes insipidus will disappear as the neurohypophysis recovers. With injury to the median eminence (junction of pituitary stalk with hypothalamus), there will be release of the antidiuretic hormone and an immediate diabetes insipidus. After several days the urinary output will apparently return to normal as the posterior pituitary finally discharges the stored antidiuretic hormone. Diabetes insipidus then returns within 3–5 days when the stored hormone is exhausted. If at the time of injury to the median eminence the pituitary gland is also removed, then permanent diabetes insipidus appears within 24 hours.

A urine specific gravity of less than 1.002 is diagnostic of diabetes insipidus. The usual picture is that of a urine volume greater than 6 L., urinary specific gravity less than 1.006, and an increase in the serum sodium level to 160 mEq./L. or more. The serum sodium level is a good indicator of whether the patient is becoming overhydrated (water intoxication) or dehydrated. The best method of knowing the state of the patient's water balance is by obtaining the body weight (each pound is equivalent to 454 ml. of fluid) and a careful recording of intake and output.

Therapeutic Agents for Diabetes Insipidus

Pitressin.—Pitressin is a partially purified fraction of the posterior pituitary. There is 20 units of pressor activity per ml. Since this is short-acting, 0.1–0.5 ml. is given at 3–4 hour intervals.

Pitressin tannate in oil.—A single dose is effective for 24–72 hours and therefore is not used in the early stages of management. The ampule should be warmed to body temperature and thoroughly mixed before injection. Each milliliter contains 5 units of pressor activity. A test dose of 0.3–0.5 ml. should be tried. It is not necessary to use more than 1 ml. per intramuscular injection. It is best to give the injection in the evening and to wait for the polyuria and polydipsia to return before the next injection is given.

Posterior pituitary powder U.S.P.—Dried posterior pituitary powder is supplied in capsules for nasal insufflation. The powder is applied by sniffing a pinch from the back of the hand, blowing it into the nose with an insufflator or rubbing it on the nasal mucosa with the fingertip. The patient uses the powder in accordance with the symptoms—usually every 3–6 hours.

Synthetic lysine vasopressin.—Since the pituitary preparations are of animal origin, some patients will have allergic reactions to the foreign protein. It is then necessary to use the synthetic preparation, which is supplied in both a parenteral and intranasal form.

Chlorothiazide.—Since the thiazide derivatives increase free water reabsorption, they will reduce the urinary volume in diabetes insipidus by approximately 50%. The dosage is: chlorothiazide, 500 mg. twice daily, or hydrochlorothiazide, 50 mg. twice daily. With each dose of thiazide give 1 Gm. KCl by mouth.

POSTSURGICAL MANAGEMENT OF SUSPECT DIABETES INSIPIDUS

1. Accurate fluid and electrolyte assessment must be obtained. This includes recording intake and output, daily weights, daily electrolytes and urine specific gravity.
2. For the first 48 hours keep the patient from becoming overhydrated or underhydrated. In the first 24 hours fluid intake should be 2,000–2,500 ml., and then modified depending on the urinary output. The patient may be allowed ice chips or oral fluids as desired. The tongue should be kept moist and the body weight maintained. If the patient is unconscious, dextrose and water is given intravenously.
3. If at the end of 48 hours the urinary output is greater than 6 L./24 hours, the patient should be given Pitressin. A high urinary volume may represent overhydration and not diabetes insipidus. If the volume is less than 6 L., Pitressin is not given and the body weight is maintained by oral or intravenous fluids. When starting the Pitressin, 0.2 ml. is given subcutaneously and the effect on the urinary volume noted. The dose is repeated every 3 or 4 hours and increased by 0.2 ml. increments at these intervals if necessary. If the patient is overhydrated, the serum sodium concentration will decrease; the patient will then excrete large amounts of urine to combat the overhydration. In Pitressin-resistant diabetes insipidus it may be necessary also to use one of the thiazide derivatives. If there has been

only minimal injury to the neurohypophysis, the temporary diabetes insipidus will disappear within 5–7 days.

Status Epilepticus

Status epilepticus is the state in which a patient goes into a prolonged series of seizures without recovery of consciousness in the interval between seizures. When this process is secondary to an intracranial lesion, it is often difficult to control. If the process is allowed to continue for more than 5 or 6 hours, the patient may suffer a threat both to brain integrity and to life. The patient in status will often have some degree of edema as well as general muscular exhaustion and may become hyperpyrexic. The possibility of low blood sugar as a cause must be considered. During the seizure episode itself the patient must be partially restrained to protect him from injuring himself. It is not always necessary to jam a tongue blade into the mouth; often this knocks out teeth as well as giving the jaw a better surface and leverage for severe biting injuries of the tongue. It is more important to turn the head to one side and pull the lower jaw forward to keep the patient from obstructing his own airway with his tongue. If the status continues for long, it is often advisable to give the patient 50 ml. of 50% glucose intravenously. If a dusky color persists, nasal oxygen should be given. The status must be broken. Any of the following drugs may be helpful.

Sodium phenobarbital, 0.4–0.8 Gm. (6–12 gr.), is given intravenously. If the seizures persist, then after 20 minutes another 0.12 Gm. (2 gr.) is given.

Sodium amytal, although less effective than sodium phenobarbital, is usually more readily available. Dose is 0.5–1.0 Gm. (7.5–15 gr.), slowly given intravenously. Administration must be stopped when the corneal reflex is abolished. If the drug is given too quickly, it may abolish the corneal reflex and result in the cessation of respiration.

Sodium diphenylhydantoin (Dilantin), 150–250 mg., is slowly given intravenously. If necessary, the dose may be repeated and if 30 minutes later the seizures persist, then another 100–150 mg. is given.

Diazepam (Valium), 5–10 mg., is slowly given intravenously at the rate of 5 mg. per minute. If necessary, the same dose may be repeated in 2–4 hours. The drug may be given intramuscularly, but it is less effective than when given intravenously.

Any of the above drugs may stop the seizures. If they do not, then paraldehyde (5 ml. into each buttock) may be tried, and finally general anesthesia may be considered to stop the seizures. A point not to be overlooked when barbiturates are used is that, as the seizure cycle is repeated, it becomes difficult to distinguish between deep barbiturate overdosage and the postseizure stupor.

17

Surgery of the Head and Neck; Infusion Chemotherapy

OSMAR P. STEINWALD, JR., M.D.

Adjunct Surgeon, Rush-Presbyterian-St. Luke's Medical Center; Instructor in Surgery, Rush Medical College

AND

STEVEN G. ECONOMOU, M.D.

Attending Surgeon, Rush-Presbyterian-St. Luke's Medical Center; Professor of Surgery, Rush Medical College

Operations on the head and neck of sufficient magnitude to require intensive postoperative care will usually be operations for cancer of both the head and neck. In addition they include major reconstructive procedures made necessary by destructive cancer surgery. Finally, they are surgical procedures for the immediate care of patients with trauma to the head and neck or for their subsequent reconstruction. The basic care during the immediate postoperative period in all of these patients is similar.

The most common type of cancers for which major head and neck procedures are required are epidermoid cancers of the intraoral region, including tongue, pharynx and larynx and occasionally the salivary glands or malignant melanoma.

Types and Extent of Surgery

The specific type of cancer operation emphasized in this section will be radical neck dissection with in-continuity dissection of intraoral cancer and will usually include hemimandibulectomy. Or the neck dissection may be in-continuity with a laryngectomy. The neck dissection may be bilateral in its extent, either simultaneously or in stages. Both will require special comment and special postoperative care. A knowledge of the basic anatomy as well as the general scheme of the surgery is essential for proper postoperative care of patients. Special attention, however, should be directed toward radical neck dissection, inasmuch as this procedure is included with a contiguous removal of many of the cancers of the area.

RADICAL NECK DISSECTION.—There is general agreement as to what should be removed in a standard radical neck dissection, and these structures are listed in Table 17-1. It is impossible, however, to categorize such a procedure; which structures are removed depends to a great degree on the extent of cancerous involvement of the particular area to be excised.

RADICAL LARYNGECTOMY.—Radical laryngectomy is removal of the larynx and associated lymph nodes with contiguous neck dissection. Removal of the larynx necessitates a permanent tracheostomy as part of the procedure.

RADICAL THYROIDECTOMY.—This is not at present a standardized procedure because there is variation of thought in how best to treat the various types of thyroid cancer. In general, radical thyroidectomy includes the following: an en bloc resection of the lobe involved clinically, thyroid isthmectomy, subtotal removal of the contralateral lobe and of the retrotracheal, retroesophageal and cervical nodes on the involved side. The patients are usually placed on thyroid extract postoperatively. Thyroid extract is begun when oral alimentation is started in a dose of 180 mg. a day, both to prevent hypothyroidism and to suppress the remaining thyroid tissue. Patients must be watched carefully for hypo-

TABLE 17-1.—STRUCTURES THAT ARE, OR MAY BE, SACRIFICED OR MAY BE INJURED AT RADICAL NECK DISSECTION*

	ALWAYS EXCISED	MAY BE SACRIFICED WHEN NECESSARY	MAY BE INJURED AT OPERATION
	Lymph nodes and vessels: fat and fascia		
Nerves	Spinal accessory, ansa hypoglossi, sensory branches of cervical plexus, branches from C_{2-4} to sternomastoid and trapezius, cervical branch of facial	Marginal (mandibular) branch of facial	Lingual, marginal branch of facial, vagus or its superior or recurrent laryngeal branches, phrenic, brachial plexus, cervical sympathetic
Vessels	Internal and external jugular veins and tributaries, variable number of branches of subclavian and external carotid arteries	External, internal or common carotid, thoracic or right jugular lymph duct	External, internal or common carotid arteries, thoracic or right jugular lymph duct
Muscles	Sternomastoid, omohyoid	Platysma, digastric, mylohyoid	
Other structures	Submaxillary salivary gland and lower pole of parotid	Thyroid	Apex of pleura

*From Ewing and Martin: Cancer 5:873, 1952.

parathyroidism (see Chapter 24) and permanent or transitory dysfunction of the recurrent laryngeal nerves with vocal cord paralysis.

SALIVARY GLAND SURGERY.—Removal of parotid salivary gland cancers will frequently necessitate sacrifice of the facial nerve. This leads to a permanent paralysis. When the ophthalmic branch is sacrificed, the lid will droop and not completely cover the eye with blinking, unless a tarsorrhaphy is performed. Special care must be taken to prevent the serious complication of corneal desiccation. This is usually accomplished by instillation of a bland ophthalmic ointment, such as boric acid, into the eye at 4 hour intervals until the patient has regained the ability to close the eye completely with blinking; otherwise a tarsorrhaphy is performed. Facial muscle tone is lost on the side of the facial nerve sacrifice, frequently with drooling of saliva from the side of the mouth. This drooling may contaminate a radical neck dissection wound in the area.

The main needs postoperatively in patients who have surgery of the parotid salivary glands are to know if the facial nerve has been sacrificed and to care for the deleterious effects of the paralysis. A traumatized facial nerve (the main trunk or branches thereof) may function immediately postoperatively, but its function may be absent as soon as several hours later when edema and reaction to the surgery occur. For this reason, it is important to examine patients who have had salivary gland surgery as soon after waking from anesthesia as is conveniently possible to determine whether they have function of the facial nerve. If later it does not function, one can be quite certain (and assure the patient) that function will return. Return of function will usually be apparent within one week following surgery; complete recovery, however, may take several months following trauma to the nerve.

MAXILLECTOMY.—Removal of the maxilla is an uncommon procedure, usually indicated for cancers originating in the antrum or roof of the mouth with extension into the maxilla. The maxilla helps to form boundaries of 3 cavities of the midface, the medial cavity being the lateral wall of the nose, the upper portion of the bone forming the floor of the orbit and the lowermost portion of the bone, the roof of the mouth. Because of the intimate relationship to these cavities, removal causes special problems in that the integrity of these cavities may be destroyed.

A cheek flap is developed to expose the superficial aspects of the maxilla. Following removal of the maxilla a large defect is created, which by necessity communicates directly with the oral cavity. Most often a split-thickness skin graft is placed on the inner surface of this cheek flap to epithelialize the cavity which has been created. This cavity is usually packed rather firmly with petrolatum gauze to aid hemostasis and to prevent regurgitation of liquid into the nose, as well as to maintain the skin graft in its desired position. This packing is usually removed on the third to fifth postoperative day. An obturator made of ordinary commercial sponge material is then placed in the cavity. This is changed daily. Care should be taken in removal of the packing, as it serves as a stent dressing for the skin graft and the graft may be dislodged with the packing change.

A particular problem occurs when the floor of the orbit must be removed. Special reconstructive procedures will have been performed to support the globe of the eye. This should be noted but will not require particular postoperative care except for the usual protection of the cornea.

Postoperative Care

GENERAL CONSIDERATIONS.—Patients undergoing radical neck dissection for whatever reason are usually found in the older age group. Patients with cancers of this area, particularly those with intraoral tumors, are usually heavy smokers and, in addition, frequently have a history of considerable intake of alcohol. One should, therefore, consider possible postoperative problems resulting from these factors. Frequently these patients have had poor dietary habits. This and the discomfort from the tumor often lead to a caloric intake insufficient to maintain the patients' nutrition at a reasonable level. For this reason they may suffer from subclinical malnutrition and be hypoproteinemic, with its attendant difficulties and risks. Malnutrition may cause poor wound healing and increased susceptibility to infection in the postoperative period. Weight loss noted by the patient in the preoperative period may alert the surgeon to the presence of malnutrition. Frequently the patients are hypovolemic and require volume replacement of intravenous fluids and blood in excess of that lost during surgery or that needed for daily requirements. Intrinsic liver disease because of malnutrition and alcoholic intake will frequently be present, as will chronic bronchitis and obstructive lung disease secondary to many years of smoking.

Postoperative orders for care of patients with major head and neck surgery are determined by the extent of resection.

Airway and tracheostomy care.—The primary concern in postoperative care of patients having surgery of the head and neck is maintenance of a clear airway. In virtually all patients in whom the pharynx or oral cavity has been entered, a tracheostomy will have been performed. (Tracheostomy care is described in Chapter 4.) It is essential to humidify the air entering the tracheal stoma. Therefore all patients require a high humidity tracheal collar, the mist being supplied by either aerosol or ultrasonic nebulization. Mucolytic agents have not routinely been used. There must be aseptic, meticulous and repetitive attention to suctioning of the tracheobronchial tree. To re-emphasize, maintenance of an adequately functioning airway is by far the most important aspect in the care of these postoperative patients, and attention to detail in this area is mandatory.

Antibiotic therapy.—All patients undergoing procedures in which the oral cavity will be entered should have antibiotic therapy begun 1 day prior to surgery. Penicillin and streptomycin have been quite satisfactory. Procaine penicillin, 600,000 units intramuscularly every 12 hours, should be given for the first several days. It can be given by the oral route when the patient has begun alimentation. Streptomycin, 0.5 Gm. intramuscularly every 12 hours, should be given with an order for its cessation after 5–7 days of therapy. There is no indication for antibiotic therapy if the oral cavity or pharynx has not been entered.

Suction catheters.—The skin flaps for the radical neck dissection are usually developed deep to the platysma muscle and this will be the only covering of the carotid artery postoperatively. Suction catheters are placed immediately beneath the skin flaps and exteriorized through counterincisions inferior to the lowermost portion of the dissection. These catheters are placed on suction in the operating room and should be resumed immediately on admission to the intensive therapy unit. The suction should be continuous but must not be so strong as to cause the catheters to collapse. In some instances a self-contained suction apparatus will be sufficient but a Gomco unit set on "high" is more dependable.

Dressings.—Light dressings are preferable to heavy compression-type dressings. The adherence of skin flaps is dependent upon suction rather than external compression. An added benefit of light dressings made possible by the use of continuous suction is that any changes which occur beneath the skin flaps will be immediately detected rather than hidden by large, bulky compression dressings.

Intraoral care.—Patients with an intraoral suture line frequently will have an excess of saliva, both because it is secreted in excess and because it is not being swallowed. This saliva should be suctioned as necessary from the side opposite the suture lines. The patient tilts the head toward the uninvolved side and the saliva is suctioned as it pools in the floor of the mouth or buccal-gingival sulcus. This is done with a soft rubber catheter, with a tubing setup distinct from that used for the tracheostomy.

Postoperative positioning.—Following radical neck dissection and recovery from anesthesia, the patient is placed in a position of comfort with the head elevated approximately 30 degrees. This allows for better venous drainage of the head and neck. Inasmuch as the internal jugular vein has been sacrificed on the side of radical neck dissection, no pillows are placed behind the neck region and no compressive dressings are used. These may further compromise drainage in this region. If a bilateral neck dissection has been done, either simultaneously or in stages, the elevated head position is essential. Frequently these patients are most comfortable in an almost sitting position. An attempt is made to keep the head in a straight forward position without undue flexion of the neck or lateral rotation. Placing sandbags on either side of the head for support has not been routinely done but may be useful in some cases.

BILATERAL NECK DISSECTION.—Patients who have undergone bilateral neck dissection with sacrifice of both internal jugular veins should receive steroids before and for 72 hours following the second neck dissection. Dexamethasone has been used in a preoperative dose of 10 mg. intramuscularly followed postoperatively by 4 mg. intramuscularly every 6 hours for 72 hours. Steroids decrease endothelial vascular damage because of their antiinflammatory action and allow for better venous drainage from the head and neck region, thus preventing significant elevations of intracranial pressure. In addition, these patients are allowed to become somewhat hemodiluted to minimize the possibility of venous sludging and consequent venous thrombosis.

Cerebral edema.—If cerebral edema occurs after bilateral neck dissection when steroids have been used, 50 ml. of a 50% dextrose or 25 Gm. of mannitol may be given intravenously. This will cause a transient decrease in intracranial pressure by a shift of fluid to the intravascular space. Some have recommended removal of cerebrospinal fluid by lumbar puncture when there is increased intracranial pressure. This procedure, however, should be reserved for emergency situations or used when all other attempts at reduction of intracranial pressure have failed. It is important to prevent hypoxia and hypercarbia, as these cause a significant increase in intracranial pressure. Recognition of increased intracranial pressure in these patients is important. Most often, if present, these patients will be slow to waken from anesthesia. They will usually complain of severe headache, may be lethargic or combative and will be somewhat confused. On examination the fundi show rather marked venous congestion. Papilledema is not usually a part of this picture. Its absence does not mean that the intracranial pressure is normal. Evaluation of facial edema and cyanosis of the face is not a reliable index of increased intracranial pressure. Almost all patients with bilateral neck dissection will be somewhat cyanotic in the face for the first 48–72 hours.

Tracheostomy.—Patients with bilateral simultaneous neck dissection should routinely have a tracheostomy, regardless of entry into the oral cavity. The larynx is involved in the generalized edema, causing these patients to be susceptible to upper airway obstruction.

PAIN CONTROL.—Patients with radical neck dissection usually do not require large amounts of narcotics for control of pain. The flaps are usually anesthetic since the cutaneous nerve supply has been severed during the operation. It would be a serious error to give patients with major head and neck surgery repetitive doses of narcotics for restlessness, as this may be the sign of increased intracranial pressure or of hypoxia. Arterial blood gases may be drawn if hypoxia or hypercarbia is suspected and appropriate therapy instituted. Oxygen, nasally or by tracheal collar, should be started if indicated, or the patient may be given sodium bicarbonate if acidotic. The amount depends on the degree of acidosis of the patient and is calculated from the base excess value (see Chapter 6). Only rarely will these patients be alkalotic and even more rarely will they require treatment with ammonium chloride for correction.

POSTOPERATIVE ALIMENTATION.—The postoperative feeding of patients should not be a particular problem if the oral cavity, pharynx or esophagus have not been entered in the dissection. These patients can be allowed a clear liquid diet on the morning following surgery. They are advanced to a soft diet and finally to the preoperative diet, the progression depending on the particular patient and his ability to tolerate general feedings. Intravenous fluids may be stopped as soon as oral alimentation is adequate.

Procedures in which the esophagus, pharynx or oral cavity have been entered pose a particular problem in postoperative feeding. A nasogastric feeding tube will have been passed at the time of operation. (A small caliber polyethylene tube has been most satisfactory for this purpose.) Postoperative insertion is difficult and may pose a risk to the suture line. If the patient has not wakened from anesthesia, placement of a tube can best be accomplished with a finger guiding the tube in the posterior pharynx to prevent its entry into the trachea. In the patient who is awake placement of this tube is somewhat more difficult but should be done on the day of surgery before considerable edema has occurred in this area. An attempt is made to pass a small tube down the posterior wall of the pharynx and esophagus into the stomach. Considerable care should be taken that the trachea is not entered. These small tubes may require cooling to facilitate passage and should be well lubricated prior to insertion. Sometimes considerable difficulty occurs in attempting to pass a small caliber tube and in this instance a larger caliber tube such as a Kaslow #9 may be used. If gagging, retching or choking occurs with repeated attempts at passage, the procedure should be abandoned.

Tube feedings of clear liquids may be begun on the day following surgery and increased slowly to prevent gastric dilatation and vomiting. Any of numerous liquid high-protein, high-carbohydrate diets may be used. This can be diluted in equal amounts with water and graduated to full strength. Approximately 2,500 ml. of volume and 1,500–2,000 calories are ideally given. Intravenous therapy can usually be discontinued by the third or fourth postoperative day. Tube feedings usually are continued for 7–10 days postoperatively. Oral alimentation is then begun. If liquids are not tolerated at this time, the patient is encouraged to swallow mushy foods which have some substance. Frequently patients will be able to swallow food with substance but because of tissue distortion or lack of fine tongue movement will not be able to prevent liquids from entering the trachea. In patients with a laryngectomy with a tight esophageal closure it may be wise to leave the feeding tube in place an additional week and have the patient swallow liquids around the tube. This serves to stent the esophagus and prevent early stricture formation.

In operations in which the posterior tongue or tonsillar fossa has been resected, a different type of swallowing problem exists. With loss of substance in this area and fixation of the base of the tongue, elevation of the tongue against the soft palate is not possible. Thus, normal swallowing cannot be initiated. Attempts at swallowing in some of these patients will lead to nasal regurgitation or to aspiration of the swallowed material. If aspiration occurs, it should immediately be suctioned from the tracheostomy tube which should be left in place until the patient can swallow adequately.

VOLUME REPLACEMENT.—Blood loss during head and neck surgery will vary considerably, but between 500 and 2,000 ml. of blood will be lost during a standard radical neck procedure, more if this is combined with a laryngectomy or intraoral tumor excision. Persons concerned with the postoperative care of these patients should regularly monitor the hemoglobin or hematocrit levels as well as blood volume determinations so that appropriate volume replacement can be given. Albumin, 5% solution given intravenously, may be quite helpful in providing volume and at the same time maintaining hemodilution. Hemodilution promotes venous flow and prevents sludging, thereby hopefully diminishing the incidence of venous thrombosis. These patients, however, should not receive anticoagulants or Dextran, since these agents may enhance postoperative bleeding.

Immediate Complications and Their Management

RESPIRATORY COMPLICATIONS

ASPIRATION PNEUMONIA.—The necessity for an adequate airway in patients with head and neck surgery has been stressed. Patients with major surgery of the head and neck involving intraoral entry as well as laryngeal dissection should be closely monitored during their first attempts at oral ingestion. Such patients should be given water first so that aspiration will not be a serious complication. Later jello, pudding, farina and similar foods are offered. Should aspiration occur, the tracheobronchial tree must be immediately aspirated and flushed with small amounts of normal saline solution. Aspiration pneumonia may be a sequel and should be treated with special attention to tracheal toilet as well as intensive antibiotic therapy. Should serious aspiration occur, the patient should be started immediately on a course of steroids. A dose of 200 mg. of hydrocortisone should be given intramuscularly, followed by 50 mg. every 6 hours for 2 days, then 25 mg. every 6 hours for 2 days.

ATELECTASIS.—Atelectasis may occur in the immediate postoperative period. This is best prevented by repetitive aspiration of the tracheobronchial tree. The normal cough reflex is impaired with a tracheostomy tube. This will cause retained secretions and a tendency to atelectasis. Atelectasis is treated by aspiration via the nasotracheal route or with a catheter through the tracheostomy stoma. Occasionally a bronchoscopy for aspiration of retained secretions may be required. Following bronchoscopy the patient may benefit from intermittent positive pressure breathing to maintain expansion of the involved areas. However, there is great risk to the patient if a pressure respirator is used. Excessive pressure may cause injury with possible disruption of the intraoral suture line. It should, therefore, be used only under circumstances in which a lesser alternative is not available. The pressure setting should not exceed 20 cm. water.

PHRENIC NERVE INJURY.—Temporary or permanent injury to the phrenic nerve may occur during a radical neck dissection. This will cause an elevated hemidiaphragm on the affected side, which causes a decrease in pleural volume and may lead to an increased incidence of atelectasis. An elevated hemidiaphragm may be suspected on clinical examination but should be confirmed by a portable chest x-ray. There is no particular treatment for this condition except for continued attention to maintenance of adequate lung volume by deep breathing. Intermittent positive pressure ventilation may be used if there are no oral suture lines. Six 15-minute periods of treatment with the positive pressure respirator each day, with the pressure setting not above 20 cm. water, should be sufficient to maintain lung expansion.

PNEUMOTHORAX.—With dissection in the supraclavicular fossa, the apex of the pleural cavity may be entered. This causes a pneumothorax of varying degree which may or may not be apparent at the time of surgery. Postoperative physical findings of decreased breath sounds and decreased motion of the involved hemithorax may suggest pneumothorax but this should be confirmed by portable chest x-ray in the upright position. If the pneumothorax is more than 20% in volume, the patient should have a thoracic catheter placed in the second intercostal space at the midclavicular line under local anesthesia. If, however, the pneumothorax is less than 20% in volume and the patient exhibits no respiratory distress, it may be safe to temporize while the pneumothorax absorbs. In any case, serial portable chest films will be required to determine whether or not lung expansion is occurring.

Postoperative Hemorrhage

PRIMARY HEMORRHAGE.—Primary postoperative hemorrhage is found in 2–3% of neck dissections and usually occurs within the first

24 hours. Replacement blood transfusions should be given as soon as possible. The hemorrhage may be severe enough to require emergency reoperation.

SECONDARY HEMORRHAGE—CAROTID ARTERY BLOWOUT.—Secondary postoperative wound hemorrhage occurs in approximately 6% of radical neck operations. This hemorrhage usually begins between the third and tenth postoperative days but may be delayed as long as 3 weeks. Secondary wound hemorrhage is arterial in nature and usually from the carotid arterial system. This bleeding is massive but is usually heralded by premonitory bleeding in small amounts. Most patients with spontaneous hemorrhage from the carotid artery have received x-ray therapy within the previous year and usually have residual cancer at the operative site. The other common causes of carotid artery blowout are wound breakdown secondary to tissue necrosis or fistula formation and wound infection.

Management of carotid artery blowout.—Immediate treatment is mandatory if patients with carotid artery blowout are to be saved. Control of hemorrhage is of prime importance and this should be performed by the patient or by the first person seeing the patient with spontaneous hemorrhage. Control is by finger pressure at the site of bleeding; the pressure must be firm enough to prevent continued arterial hemorrhage. The patient must be placed supine and 2 intravenous infusions should be begun. These are usually done by cutdown technique. The patient's vital signs should be carefully monitored and replacement of volume should be given immediately. Preferably this will be blood which has been cross-matched previously and is available in the blood bank. However, if blood is not available, O negative blood should be given.

No attempt should be made to move the patient until the hypotension has been adequately treated and the vital signs are stable. If the bleeding is adequately controlled, no attempt is made to relieve the person applying the pressure to the bleeding site. The patient is taken to the operating room with pressure being applied to the bleeding site. The surgeon, who is gowned, then applies pressure to the critical area himself and the area around his sterile hand is prepared with an appropriate antiseptic. The neck is then draped and the wound opened widely to expose the bleeding vessels. This is usually done under general anesthesia. The bleeding site is located and suture ligatures are placed above and below the area of bleeding. It is necessary to be sufficiently distant from the area of bleeding to ligate the vessel in an area where there is no obvious infection or tumor present. The common or internal carotid arteries are usually the sites from which the hemorrhage occurs. This necessitates ligation of the common carotid artery inferiorly and the internal carotid artery superiorly.

Complications of carotid artery blowout.—The mortality rate of ligation of the common carotid or internal carotid arteries is high. The incidence of cerebral complications and mortality varies directly with the degree of hypotension noted before ligation of the common or internal carotid arteries. Hypotension is associated with a substantial increase in morbidity and mortality. For this reason it is essential to prevent hypotension in these patients or at least to restore the blood pressure to the normal prehemorrhage level prior to attempted direct control of the arterial bleeding. Direct pressure on the bleeding area should provide sufficient time for replacement of blood volume to reestablish the blood pressure to a normal level.

Contributing factors of carotid artery blowout.—The following 3 precautions may be employed to decrease the incidence of spontaneous hemorrhage of the carotid artery: (1) When removal of the adventitia is necessary, it may be helpful to rotate a muscle flap over the carotid artery, which is most easily done with the levator scapulae muscle; (2) skin incisions which lie over the carotid artery are to be avoided to minimize a wound fistula directly over the carotid artery; (3) prophylactic antibiotics must be used if the oral cavity has been entered to prevent wound infection.

If the patient is classified as a high-risk individual (wound necrosis, infection, previous radiation, residual cancer or arterial repair) in whom carotid artery blowout is apt to develop, then a few precautions should be taken. The patient should be tactfully instructed to apply direct pressure himself should a sudden hemorrhage appear and then to call for help. Nursing personnel should be likewise instructed about the necessity for immediate direct pressure over the bleeding site. Finally, orderlies, aides and volunteers should be alerted to the necessary immediate action of direct pressure over the hemorrhage site.

Infection.—Primary severe wound infection in head and neck surgery is not common. Most often the infections are staphylococcal or streptococcal and if they are treated adequately and promptly, there should be no significant delay in wound healing. Infection in this region is most commonly found if the oral cavity has been entered in the dissection. Almost invariably the wound infection is associated with hematoma under the skin flaps. Infection is treated by opening the wound, evacuating the hematoma and providing drainage for the infection. A Penrose drain should be placed in the incision to maintain drainage. Compresses saturated with physiologic saline solution at room temperature should be placed on the infected area for 2 hours and then removed for 2 hours. This sequence should be continued for the first 24 hours and then the wet packs used for 2 hours 4 times each day. The compresses should be continued until there is no apparent infection. This usually occurs by 72 hours after initial drainage. It is important that room-temperature, moist packs be used; hot packs may cause necrosis of the skin flaps. When the wound is initially drained, it should be cultured and sensitivity tests performed. Broad-spectrum parenteral antibiotics should be begun immediately. Oxacillin, 500 mg. intramuscularly every 6 hours, has been favored for hospital acquired infections. If necessary, this antibiotic therapy can be changed when sensitivities have been reported. These should be ready within 24–48 hours following wound culture.

The occurrence of fever postoperatively in patients having surgery of the head and neck is not indicative of an established infection unless the fever exceeds 101 F. rectally. This level has been arbitrarily chosen as a normal response to the tissue trauma and reaction in the head and neck region. The fever may persist for 72 hours but then will spontaneously abate. Should the fever exceed 101 F. rectally, a cause other than the primary surgery itself should be sought. Atelectasis in the postoperative period must first be excluded before immediate postoperative fever is attributed to "tissue reaction."

NECROSIS OF SKIN FLAPS.—During the immediate postoperative period it is imperative that the skin flaps be adherent to the underlying structures. Nourishment of the flap occurs by new vessel growth from underlying tissues as well as by the remaining intact vessels of the flap. Hematoma beneath the flap, with or without infection, as well as previous irradiation, will retard the development of new vessels and thus increase the incidence of skin flap necrosis.

GASTRIC COMPLICATIONS.—Significant gastric complications occur more frequently in patients undergoing surgery for cancer of the head and neck region than for patients requiring surgery for cancer in other parts of the body. The incidence of gastric bleeding in the postoperative period is just under 2% in these patients; this represents a 4-fold increase over the incidence found in patients undergoing surgery for cancer in other areas. Peptic ulcer and hiatal hernia are the 2 commonest sites for postoperative hemorrhage after head and neck surgery.

Treatment of postoperative upper gastrointestinal hemorrhage in these individuals should be no different from its treatment in other patients. This includes blood replacement as required, nasogastric intubation with continuous lavage of the stomach with iced skimmed milk or antacid solution, close monitoring of vital signs and hemoglobin and hematocrit levels, plus anticholinergic medication such as probanthine, 15 mg. intramuscularly every 6 hours. If these methods are not sufficient to control the hemorrhage, surgical intervention will be required. If a particular patient previously had peptic ulcer or is thought to be a high risk for peptic ulceration, this patient should be treated prophylactically in the postoperative period with antacids, anticholinergics and frequent feedings, either orally or through feeding tubes. In the immediate postoperative period blood recovered from the stomach may merely be blood which has been swallowed during or immediately following the procedure. Or the source may be leakage of an intraoral suture line; the latter is rather unusual, and the patient must be suspected of having peptic ulceration or bleeding from hiatal hernia.

LYMPH FISTULA.—A lymph fistula may develop if the lymphatic

duct in the lower neck or supraclavicular region has been injured. Almost invariably this occurs on the left side of the neck with damage to the thoracic duct. Lymph may drain through the wound or, as is usually the case, through the drain site on the third to fifth postoperative day. Confirmation of this diagnosis and its differentiation from serous exudate is performed by giving the patient a small amount of milk orally or through a feeding tube. Milk causes lymph to appear chylous in nature. Frequently a lymph fistula can be controlled by a pressure dressing placed over the lower neck or supraclavicular region with maintenance of suction through the indwelling catheters. The drainage from a lymph fistula may vary greatly in volume. It is usually in the range of 1,500 ml./24 hours but may be up to 6 L./day.

The lymph fistula will usually close within a week with pressure dressings. During the period of lymph loss, it is important to monitor the serum electrolytes. Lymph is approximately isotonic with respect to extracellular fluid. Approximately 20% of ingested fat will be lost with the lymph fistula, as well as a small amount of protein. Volume and electrolyte loss should be replaced by intravenous infusion if the loss is great. Nutritional deficit should be corrected by increasing caloric alimentation. If drainage is considerable and persists for longer than a week, it may be necessary to open the wound and ligate the open duct.

Oral cutaneous fistulae.—Following laryngectomy or intraoral resection, oral cutaneous fistulae may develop. Fistulae following laryngectomy may be present in from one-fourth to one-half the cases. The majority of fistulae will heal spontaneously within a few days but as many as 6% will not, necessitating prolonged hospitalization and often multiple surgical procedures to close the fistula.

Irradiation complications.—*Supervoltage radiation.*—Preoperative irradiation with cobalt-60 or other high-energy sources has been used in head and neck cancer before surgical extirpation. In patients treated with a total of 2,000 rads to the entire neck region in 5 equal treatments on successive days who have been studied extensively, there have been no demonstrable adverse effects of radiation therapy with respect to the operative procedure itself or the incidence of postoperative complications. There seems to be a statistically significant reduction in cervical recurrence of cancer with preoperative irradiation of this nature.

Orthovoltage radiation.—The incidence of postoperative wound complications following orthovoltage radiation therapy is twice that found when no radiation therapy is used. Complications to be expected following orthovoltage irradiation include wound infection, necrosis of skin flaps, separation of wound edges, oral cutaneous fistula and rupture of the carotid artery. The incidence of carotid artery rupture following preoperative orthovoltage therapy has been twice that found when no preoperative radiation therapy was given. In addition, rupture of the carotid artery occurs 3 times more frequently in patients in whom a fistula or skin slough has developed. In this group, oral cutaneous fistulae take longer to close, and massive skin sloughs occur more often. Patients who have had orthovoltage irradiation preoperatively are more susceptible to laryngeal obstruction secondary to laryngeal edema requiring urgent tracheostomy. Preoperative radiation therapy is not associated with an increased incidence of hematoma, infection or fever.

INTRA-ARTERIAL INFUSION CHEMOTHERAPY

Intra-arterial cancer chemotherapy in the head and neck region has been used for several years. The methods are varied and the technique is still considered experimental. Individual responses to different chemotherapeutic agents are not entirely predictable. The applications of the procedure are limited by the toxicity of the drugs and, to some degree, by the technical considerations and mechanical problems of the infusion itself.

Technical Considerations

Catheter placement.—For therapy of head and neck tumors, the intra-arterial infusion catheter must be placed into the origin of the external carotid artery. This is most advantageously accomplished by placing the catheter in a branch which may be ligated or divided without compromising the blood supply to the area of desired infusion. The most successful method is to place the catheter retrograde into the superficial temporal artery under local anesthesia, then to thread the catheter down to the origin of the external carotid artery.

If it is not possible to advance the catheter via the superficial temporal artery into the origin of the external carotid artery, the superior thyroid artery may be used. If this is not possible, the origin of the external carotid artery may be isolated and a catheter placed in this area.

If the area to be infused crosses the midline, bilateral catheters must be placed into the external carotid system. Should the thyroid gland be the desired area of infusion, then the inferior thyroid artery as well as the superior thyroid artery must be infused. An infusion catheter should be placed into the origin of the thyrocervical trunk, from whence the inferior thyroid artery originates, to infuse this area satisfactorily.

Verification of catheter position.—The area of effective infusion via the intra-arterial catheters may be verified by injecting 3–5 ml. of a 5% fluorescein solution into the arterial catheters. The head and neck area are then exposed to ultraviolet light in a darkened room, and the area of infusion will fluoresce. Adjustment of catheter position is then performed in the operating room and a check of the area of infusion can be done any time in the postoperative period, again by injecting the fluorescein solution. Fluorescence of the sclera of the eye indicates that the catheter has been advanced too far and that the internal carotid artery is also being infused with fluorescein distributed to the ophthalmic artery, the first branch of the internal carotid. The catheter should then be withdrawn a short distance and rechecked.

METHODS OF INFUSION.—There are many methods for infusion of the chemotherapeutic agent. The simplest is to dissolve the agent in 5% dextrose and water and place it into a plastic infusion container. Continuous infusion is then provided by a Fenwal Pressure Infusor, which is placed over the bag to maintain sufficient pressure to overcome the arterial flow. This method is particularly desirable because it is simple, air free (no risk of air embolus), inexpensive and allows most patients to be ambulatory.

An entirely portable device is known as the Sage Microflow Syringe. The 20 ml. syringe is battery operated and permits the patient full ambulation. Another portable device is a miniaturized chronometric infusion apparatus devised by Watkins.

For bedridden patients a high volume infusion assembly can be devised. This employs several 1-L. bottles hung in tandem (minimizing the possibility of air embolus) and connected to a peristaltic pump which is electrically driven and can be regulated to infuse the agent at a predicted rate.

CHEMOTHERAPEUTIC AGENTS

ALKYLATING AGENTS.—The alkylating agents most useful in treating cancer of the head and neck are nitrogen mustard, phenylalanine mustard and cyclophosphamide (Cytoxan). They are all toxic to the hemopoietic system, the principal complication being pancytopenia. A complete blood count should be done daily.

ANTIMETABOLITES.—The three antimetabolites currently used are the folic acid antagonists, the purine antagonists and the pyrimidine antagonists. Methotrexate is the folic acid antagonist most commonly used; it is infused intra-arterially in a dose of 50 mg./day. In addition, citrovorum factor is given intramuscularly in doses of 6 mg. every 6 hours. Citrovorum factor is a folic acid analog and must be given simultaneously with Methotrexate to control the systemic toxicity of the Methotrexate. Most patients can tolerate a total dose of approximately 300 mg. of Methotrexate by arterial infusion if citrovorum factor is added. The earliest sign of local toxicity is oral ulceration. In addition, a macular, pustular skin rash may develop over the chest, neck and back. Systemic toxicity is most often manifested by bone marrow depression. Gastrointestinal complications such as nausea, vomiting and diarrhea are common but are not indicative of toxicity.

Routine Care

Routine care of patients undergoing infusion chemotherapy in the head and neck region is not complicated. Care is directed to maintaining the intra-arterial infusion at the desired rate. If the patient is receiving intra-arterial Methotrexate in the range of 40–50 mg./day, that patient *must* receive citrovorum factor, 6 mg. intramuscularly every 6 hours. This is exceedingly important because the patient receives a potentially lethal dose of Methotrexate if the citrovorum factor is omitted. In addition, those patients with impaired renal function who are receiving Methotrexate should be carefully monitored for early signs of toxicity. Most of the Methotrexate is excreted in the urine; any renal impairment therefore increases the possibility of systemic toxicity.

Patients receiving systemic infusion chemotherapy should be monitored daily with respect to hemoglobin and hematocrit values, white cell count and platelet count. All the chemotherapeutic agents affect the hemopoietic system when used in therapeutic doses. The alkylating agents are more likely to affect the erythrocytes, while the folic acid antagonists and the fluoridated pyrimidines usually depress the white cell count and the platelet count. Because of the leukopenia associated with the chemotherapeutic agents, the ability of the body to resist infection is depressed. Should the blood cell count become lower than 2,000 cells/mm.^{3}, the patient should be placed on antibiotic coverage as well as given protective isolation, and the infusion should be stopped.

Complications

Complications in infusion chemotherapy may be divided into two major groups: the technical problems related directly to the infusion technique and the problems arising from the toxicity of the drugs administered.

Technical complications.—*Clotting of blood in the intra-arterial catheter* is the commonest complication. The clots can usually be dislodged by irrigating the catheter with a small amount of heparinized saline solution. This is best done with a small tuberculin syringe. Clotted catheters must not be irrigated, however, if the tip of the catheter is near the internal carotid artery because of the risk of introducing an embolus to the brain.

Dislodgment or kinking of the intra-arterial catheter may necessitate repositioning of the catheter, using fluorescein solution to indicate the area of infusion. Catheters should be secured to the skin, preferably by multiple pieces of tape rather than by direct suture.

Leakage of infusates may occur at the site of entry of the catheter in the skin. A significant volume suggests that the catheter tip is outside the artery. The patient must then undergo another surgical procedure to replace the catheter in its desired position.

Inflammation of the area around the entry of the catheter through the skin is controlled by frequent use of warm compresses. Most often this localized inflammation can be prevented by frequent cleansing of the area and daily applications of antibiotic ointment.

Hemorrhage may occur either from the tumor because of necrosis caused by the chemotherapeutic agent or at the time of removal of the catheter. If the catheter has been tied in place using a rubber band, removal should not be followed by hemorrhage since the elasticity of the rubber band will cause closure of the artery. If the catheter has not been ligated with a rubber band, upon removal of the catheter local pressure must be placed at this area for at least 15 minutes to prevent significant hemorrhage.

Cracking or leakage of a catheter will require placement of a new catheter. Most often this problem can be eliminated by using a resilient polyvinyl catheter of small diameter rather than a larger, stiff catheter.

DRUG TOXICITY.—Use of chemotherapeutic agents in the dosage range required for control of cancers in this area will result in some toxic effects of the drugs. Early toxic effects in fact are helpful and indicate that the patient is receiving adequate dosages of the chemotherapeutic agent. The persons involved in care of patients receiving chemotherapeutic agents in this dosage range must be thoroughly familiar with the particular agent being used and the early signs of toxicity. Specific toxic signs and symptoms have been discussed under the heading Chemotherapeutic Agents.

REFERENCES

1. Clifford, P.: The administration of chemotherapeutic agents in the treatment of advanced head and neck cancer, J. Laryng. & Otol. 78:350, 1964.
2. Duff, J. K., *et al.*: Antimetabolite-metabolite cancer chemotherapy using continuous intra-arterial methotrexate with intermittent intramuscular citrovorum factor: Method of therapy, Cancer 14:744, 1961.
3. Freund, H. R.: Postoperative Care—Complications and Sequelae, in Freund, H. R. (ed.): *Principles of Head and Neck Surgery* (New York: Appleton-Century-Crofts, Inc., 1967).
4. Ketcham, A. S., and Hoye, R. C.: Spontaneous carotid artery hemorrhage after head and neck surgery, Am. J. Surg. 110:649, 1965.
5. Mason, J. H.; Ediger, A. J., and Webb, R. S.: Intra-arterial infusion cancer chemotherapy, S. Clin. North America 48:79, 1968.
6. Royster, H. P.: Complications of Surgery for Cancer of the Head and Neck, in Artz, C. P., and Hardy, J. D. (eds.): *Complications in Surgery and Their Management* (Philadelphia: W. B. Saunders Company, 1967).
7. Vanderberg, H. J., *et al.*: A comparison of wound healing between irradiated and non-irradiated patients after radical neck dissection, Am. J. Surg. 110:557, 1965.

18

Thoracic Surgery

L. PENFIELD FABER, M.D.

Attending Surgeon, Director Section of Thoracic Surgery, Rush-Presbyterian-St. Luke's Medical Center; Associate Professor of Surgery, Rush Medical College

AND

JOHN W. HENGESH, M.D.*

Fellow in Cardiovascular-Thoracic Surgery, Rush-Presbyterian-St. Luke's Medical Center; Instructor in Surgery, Rush Medical College

Preoperative Preparation

SINCE THE ACTIVITY in an intensive care unit can be alarming, patients undergoing thoracic surgery should be involved in an educational and, if indicated, a therapeutic program before operation. Prior information derived from the medical or nursing staff promotes cooperation and eases apprehension.

The physician should instruct the patient in a proper cough effort. When available, physical therapists can reinforce and supplement this instruction. The patient should be made aware of the critical need for vigorous coughing after surgery. It is often necessary to emphasize that coughing will not harm the lungs or chest.

In chronic obstructive and chronic inflammatory processes, preoperative preparation is necessary to render the tracheobronchial tree as free from secretions and organisms as possible. The regimen includes bronchodilators, humidification, intermittent positive pressure breathing and preoperative antibiotics. Patients who smoke should stop as soon as the possibility of a thoracotomy is considered. It is preferable to stop smoking 10–14 days before surgery.

*Supported in part by United States Public Health Service Grant No. 1T12HE05808.

Surgical soap showers are begun several days before surgery. The axilla, chest wall and groin are scrubbed for 30 minutes once or twice daily.

Physiologic Alterations

VENTILATION.—Ventilation is altered by several factors. Anesthesia has a depressant effect on the respiratory center, with a resultant decrease in tidal volume. Incomplete elimination or metabolism of the anesthetic agent further decreases the tidal volume. Large doses of preoperative medication, particularly in surgery of short duration or in debilitated patients, further impair ventilatory efforts. Administration of narcotic analgesics early after surgery potentiates respiratory depression.

Pain and associated muscle spasm make the patient reluctant to maintain adequate respiratory excursion. This causes decreased alveolar ventilation, therefore reducing blood gas exchange.

Hypoventilation results in hypoxia, hypercarbia and respiratory acidosis. There are normal compensatory mechanisms that serve to limit hypoventilation. The initial change is an increase in respiratory rate, which then results in a near-normal minute ventilation. Hypercarbia causes a reflex increase in tidal volume and alveolar ventilation. This mechanism is mediated through the respiratory center and is inhibited by anesthetic agents and narcotics. Hypoxia causes a reflex increase in tidal volume and respiratory rate. This response is mediated through chemoreceptors in the aortic and carotid bodies. Further untoward alterations in ventilation are caused by pre-existing diseases such as kyphoscoliosis, emphysema, restrictive lung disease or a paralyzed diaphragm.

MECHANICS.—Airway resistance may be increased by several mechanisms. Irritating anesthetic gases and manipulation of the lung stimulate secretions which narrow the lumen of the bronchi. Clots which enter the respiratory tract during resection also increase airway resistance by causing turbulent flow. These factors, in addition to pre-existing asthma, predispose to postoperative bronchospasm. A narrow or long endotracheal tube is also a cause of increased airway resistance during spontaneous respiration.

Airway obstruction prevents the lung from returning to its resting expiratory volume, thus increasing the functional residual capacity. Expiration is then active rather than passive. Increase in resistance requires greater inspiratory effort to generate a higher airway pressure to maintain flow. Active expiration and increased inspiratory effort result in increased respiratory work.

Chest wall and pulmonary compliance are both decreased by surgery. Chest wall compliance is impaired by pain and spasm of the muscles of the thorax. Decreased pulmonary compliance is caused by patchy atelectasis with alveolar collapse and surfactant loss, producing a stiff lung which is difficult to expand. Decreased compliance requires greater inspiratory effort and airway pressure to expand the lung. This effort is reflected by increased respiratory work.

Pre-existing pulmonary diseases such as emphysema, bronchial asthma, restrictive lung disease, mitral stenosis and chest wall deformities also cause alterations of pulmonary mechanics.

VENTILATION-PERFUSION DISPROPORTION.—Ventilation-perfusion (V_A/Q) abnormalities occur secondary to a disproportion of the normal ratio of these functions. Atelectasis is a cause of decreased ventilation whereas pulmonary embolus is an example of decreased perfusion.

The normal V_A/Q ratio is 0.8, which means that there is 1.2 times more blood perfusing the lung than there is air ventilating it. The 3 major factors which affect V_A/Q are compliance, resistance and time.[1] Decreased compliance or increased resistance secondary to changes in surfactant or pulmonary congestion result in uneven ventilation. Alteration in the timing of the respiratory cycle often serves to improve the disproportion.

The effect of the most common V_A/Q abnormality in the postoperative period (low ventilation:normal perfusion) is production of a right-to-left shunt. Mixed venous blood traverses the lung without oxygenation and mixes with arterial blood, resulting in hypoxia. This is illustrated by low arterial Po_2 levels despite inhalation of high concentrations of oxygen. This abnormality is due to patchy or lobar atelectasis and pulmonary congestion. The Pa_{CO_2}, however, is not affected since other hyperventilated areas of the lung compensate and blow off the excess CO_2.

The opposite abnormality (normal ventilation:low perfusion) causes minimal changes in the arterial blood gases. Hypoventilation takes place and the remaining portions of the lung compensate adequately. This V_A/Q abnormality would exist if obstruction of the pulmonary artery occurred. This problem is rare, however, in the early postoperative period. Emphysema and fibrosis will also magnify ventilation-perfusion changes in the thoracic surgical patient. Hypoxia and inefficient ventilation cause the patient to tire rapidly. Oxygen must be supplemented and the abnormal V_A/Q ratios corrected.

LUNG VOLUME.—The decrease in lung volume following most pulmonary resections is usually not significant. Segmental resection, lobectomy and bilobectomy ordinarily do not remove enough functional tissue to impair respiration except in the presence of severe pre-existing disease. Candidates for pneumonectomy require careful preoperative evaluation. On occasion, pneumonectomy may be necessary in spite of poor pulmonary function. In this instance, maximum intensive care is required to support the remaining lung.

Diffusion.—Changes in diffusion result only from the loss of capillary bed and lung tissue by resection. The surgical procedure and anesthetic have little effect on diffusion. The remaining portions of the lung readily compensate for any loss in capillary volume.

Blood gases.—Arterial blood gas values are a direct and indirect measurement of changes in pulmonary physiology. Familiarity with principles of acid-base balance (see Chapter 6) and frequent blood gas analyses aid in detecting changes in condition and in evaluating therapy. A single determination provides inadequate information upon which to plan treatment.

Postoperative Management—General Considerations

Pre-existing diseases often complicate the postoperative course or mask the expected improvement following operation. The presence of emphysema, chronic bronchitis, pulmonary fibrosis and chronic infection serve to increase the incidence of complications and may preclude complete recovery.

The intensive care physician must review the chart and all preoperative studies. He must understand the exact nature of the surgical procedure and any complications encountered during surgery. There must be communication between the intensive therapy physician and the surgical team.

Initial Examination

A thorough examination, including vital signs, is performed by the physician upon admission of the patient to the intensive care unit. This provides a baseline for follow-up examination.

Inspection of the patient raises the suspicion of significant alterations in physiology. The lips and nail beds are examined for cyanosis and the chest wall is inspected for adequate and uniform motion. Dyspnea and utilization of the accessory respiratory muscles indicate airway obstruction, nonfunctioning lung tissue or pulmonary insufficiency. Unilateral hypoventilation may indicate atelectasis, hemothorax or pneumothorax. Dressings are examined to ensure that the chest tubes are secure and that there is no air leak or drainage from around them. The boundaries surrounding the areas of saturation of the dressings are marked and any progression noted. Ordinarily there is little or no bleeding from the incision or chest tube stab wound following thoracotomy. When postoperative wound hemorrhage does occur, the chest tube site is the usual cause.

Examination of the entire chest often requires assistance in turning the patient when recovery from anesthesia is incomplete. Both sides of the chest must be percussed. Dullness to percussion, usually occurring on the operated side, indicates hemothorax. Hyperresonance on either side signifies pneumothorax. Hyperresonance due to a residual space on the operated side may be expected following a major resection or may be related to atelectasis or malfunctioning chest tubes. Palpation of the position of the trachea and percussion of the heart and mediastinum are critical in the detection of mediastinal shifts after pneumonectomy.

Following thoracotomy breath sounds over the remaining lung should be almost normal. Decreased breath sounds indicate compression of parenchyma due to hemothorax or pneumothorax. Tubular sounds indicate atelectasis. Coarse rhonchi indicate retained secretions; expiratory wheezing indicates bronchospasm.

Auscultation of the heart determines the quality and intensity of the heart tones. If the pericardium has been opened during the surgical procedure, cardiac tamponade may occur and muffle the heart tones. The rate and rhythm of the heart should be assessed to identify arrhythmias.

Percussion of the upper abdomen will detect gastric dilatation. Air can enter the stomach during ventilation with a face mask or uncuffed tube. The dilated stomach elevates the left diaphragm, impairs ventilation and predisposes to vomiting and aspiration. Short-term nasogastric decompression prevents these complications.

The extremities should be examined for full range of motion and normal muscle power. Unusual positions on the operating table can cause nerve palsies. Preservation of muscular function requires institution of physical therapy immediately upon discovery of such a complication. Differentiation between nerve injuries, cerebrovascular accidents and arterial thrombosis can usually be readily made.

After the initial examination, a portable chest x-ray is taken. Usually there is sufficient recovery from anesthesia for the patient to sit erect in bed. It is important to take the x-ray in the upright position so that air or blood in the pleural space can be seen. (When the patient is supine, air will assume an anterior position and blood will lie posteriorly, making both difficult to detect by x-ray.) Correlation of the physical findings with the x-ray assures a high degree of accuracy.

In thoracotomy for noncardiac disease, the endotracheal tube is usually removed at the end of the surgical procedure. However, if recovery is prolonged or if the need for assisted mechanical ventilation is anticipated, the patient will arrive in the intensive care unit with the endotracheal tube in place. The operating team must inform the intensive care staff of the reason for prolonged intubation. If it is due to prolonged effects of anesthesia, the endotracheal tube can be removed after adequate recovery. However, if the tube provides a route for assisted ventilation, a program must be outlined for its management.

Sterile technique using a new catheter and gloves is essential during aspiration. Auscultation of the chest must be performed frequently when an endotracheal tube is in place. During the patient's transfer to the intensive care unit the endotracheal tube may enter the right main bronchus and cause atelectasis of the left lung. Decreased breath sounds on either side require immediate repositioning of the tube. Breath sounds will occasionally improve after aspiration of thick secretions obstructing a bronchus. A portable chest x-ray should be taken at this time, with the patient supine if necessary, to check the location of the endotracheal tube and aeration of the lungs.

Pressure-controlled ventilation requires inflation of the cuff. Overinflation causes mucosal necrosis and often subsequent stricture of the trachea. Frequent intermittent deflation ordinarily prevents this complication (see Chapter 4).

If assisted ventilation is no longer necessary, the endotracheal tube should be removed. Spontaneous respiration through an endotracheal tube increases airway resistance and respiratory work. Irritation by the indwelling tube stimulates tracheobronchial secretions while long tubes increase the anatomic dead space.

Vigorous coughing and attempts by the patient to remove the tube usually indicate that extubation will be tolerated. However, the physician must be certain that ventilation is adequate. Measurement of tidal volume with a spirometer is the most accurate method. Careful observation of the patient and arterial blood gas determinations aid in evaluation. The rate and depth of respiration are the most helpful clinical parameters, and the Pa_{CO_2} is the best laboratory test. When an endotracheal tube is removed, it is mandatory that trained personnel be available to reinsert the tube if necessary.

Pain

Thoracotomy incisions are quite painful; adequate analgesia is necessary to minimize discomfort and assure cooperation. The sternum-splitting incision is the least painful and the posterolateral thoracotomy incision the most painful. The anterolateral and axillary approaches fall between the above incisions in relation to pain.

Despite the fact that narcotics depress the cough reflex and the respiratory center, these drugs must be used in measured amounts to permit the patient to cough and ventilate adequately. The drug of choice is morphine sulfate, in the dose range of 6–15 mg. every 2–4 hours. Frequent small doses are more effective than occasional large doses. Individual tolerance to morphine varies; the initial dosage should be 6 or 8 mg. every 2 or 3 hours, 10 mg. of morphine will usually be adequate for an average adult patient.

Administration of morphine before recovery from anesthesia causes further depression of the respiratory center. Coughing, hyperventilation and position change should be timed to coincide with maximum analgesia.

If pain is unusually severe and does not respond to analgesics, an intercostal nerve block may be indicated. Although the effect of the block disappears after several hours, it may interrupt the cycle of muscle spasm and thus afford the patient prolonged relief. Intercostal blocks are rarely needed more than once or twice in the early postoperative period.

Oxygen

All patients receive oxygen following thoracotomy. Supplementary oxygen is necessary to prevent hypoxia secondary to alterations in pulmonary mechanics and ventilation-perfusion disproportion common in this situation.

The route of administration is variable. An oxygen tent with a flow of oxygen at 6–7 L./minute provides an oxygen concentration of nearly 40% and adequate humidity. If higher concentrations are desired, nasal oxygen can be added. Personnel must understand that the oxygen tent should not be a barrier to frequent patient examination and evaluation.

In some cases the nasal route may be preferred. An oxygen concentration of approximately 30% can be delivered by a nasal catheter. The flow rate varies from 1 to 6 L. Administration of nasal oxygen is often uncomfortable because of inadequate humidification and desiccation of the mucosa.

High concentrations of oxygen (above 50%) should be used only when absolutely necessary to maintain adequate arterial oxygenation. A high concentration is best used only intermittently, alternating with lower concentrations. High concentrations over prolonged periods have deleterious effects on the pulmonary parenchyma and may cause fatal complications.

In the routine case, oxygen can usually be discontinued 36–48 hours after surgery. It is stopped when the patient is removed from the high humidity oxygen tent. At this point clearing of secretions is improved, ventilation is adequate, respiratory work has approached a more normal level, the lung has expanded and ventilation-perfusion abnormalities are minimal. However, if hypoxia persists and the patient remains dyspneic, an oxygen-enriched atmosphere must be continued. Such patients will require a gradual detachment from oxygen therapy as the pathologic conditions are corrected.

Position of the Patient

After surgery the patient is most comfortable with his head elevated 30 to 45 degrees. In this position the abdominal organs do not impair motion of the diaphragm. The patient is turned frequently to prevent collection of secretions and alveolar collapse of the dependent portions of the lung. It is uncomfortable for a patient to lie on the operated side, but with the aid of the nursing staff and the use of supporting pillows this position can be achieved.

The afternoon or evening following surgery the patient is assisted in sitting upright. Coughing and hyperventilation are most effective in the sitting position. Most patients can sit in a chair on the day after surgery.

The pneumonectomy patient must not lie on the unoperated side. Such positioning may cause compression of the remaining lung by mediastinal shift from fluid in the pneumonectomy space. Also, dehiscence of the bronchial stump would permit fluid from the pneumonectomy space to enter the remaining lung.

Alimentation

Thoracotomy patients can usually tolerate ice chips or small amounts of clear liquids the evening of surgery. Excess fluid intake may cause vomiting. A full liquid diet is begun on the second postoperative day, and gradually the patient is advanced to a regular diet. To minimize postoperative gastroduodenal ulceration, management of patients with a previous ulcer history should include antacids and appropriate diet.

Intermittent Positive Pressure Breathing

There are specific indications for the use of IPPB. The majority of patients do not require it. Treatment is beneficial in patients with chronic obstructive pulmonary disease and obesity. Following decortication, IPPB can also assist in expanding the lung by utilizing increased airway pressure.

IPPB also has disadvantages. Infection can be transmitted if the equipment is not properly sterilized. Incorrect use can actually result in underventilation. Air swallowing during treatment can cause abdominal distention. One must not rely on the IPPB unit as a substitute for an effective cough.

Dressings

The dressings are inspected following admission to the intensive care unit. The dressings support the thorax during coughing and secure the chest tubes. They should be secure to support the operated thorax, but must not place undue stress on the skin. Tension on the skin will result in painful blisters.

X-Rays

Liberal use is made of portable chest x-rays in the intensive care unit. Since physical findings are not totally reliable in the diagnosis of hemothorax, atelectasis, persistent spaces, early pneumonitis and mediastinal shift, portable chest x-ray service must be maintained on an around-the-clock basis. Daily portable chest x-rays are obtained while chest tubes remain in the pleural space. Whenever a significant change occurs in the patient's condition, a portable x-ray is indicated.

Secretions

Maintenance of a clear airway and removal of secretions are vital aspects in the care of the thoracic surgical patient. Removal of secretions decreases airway resistance, alleviates bronchospasm, alters uneven ventilation, prevents atelectasis and decreases respiratory work. A postoperative increase in the volume of tracheobronchial secretions is related to irritation by anesthetic gases and manipulation of the lung. Secretions are more pronounced after decortication and in patients with chronic obstructive pulmonary disease.

As soon as the patient regains consciousness and can cooperate, coughing and hyperventilation are encouraged. Preoperative instruction, adequate analgesia and erect positioning facilitate coughing. Firm support over the incision will alleviate some of the pain experienced during coughing. The hands of the nurse or a towel held firmly around the chest will adequately support the incision. Excess pressure restricts ventilation and increases pain. Supervised coughing and hyperventilation at regular intervals are more productive than unaided patient efforts. Proper hydration and humidification are mandatory. It is important to supplement fluid replacement by intravenous therapy. Inadequate hydration results in thick, tenacious secretions which cannot be raised.

A high humidity atmosphere is best achieved with a high humidity oxygen tent. If this is inadequate, an additional humidifier can be used. Excess moisture within the tent may be mildly uncomfortable but the benefit easily outweighs this temporary discomfort. Further humidification can be given by periodic use of ultrasonic nebulizers.

Excessive or persistent secretions require nasotracheal aspiration (Chapter 4). Following a single nasotracheal aspiration, the quality of voluntary coughing usually exhibits marked improvement.

Aspiration bronchoscopy is carried out when secretions are excessive and cannot be removed by the usual methods. When bronchoscopy is indicated, there should be no delay. The longer a lobe or segment is atelectatic the more difficult expansion becomes. If bronchoscopy is necessary more than twice during a 24 hour period, tracheostomy is generally indicated. Tracheostomy permits frequent aspiration of tracheobronchial secretions and provides a route for assisted ventilation.

In patients with excess secretions it is particularly important to obtain a daily Gram stain and culture of the sputum. The tracheobronchial flora can change rapidly; therefore, antibiotic coverage must be altered accordingly. In following this routine, treatment of an infection may be instituted before the infection becomes clinically apparent.

Management of the Pleural Space

To achieve complete expansion of the remaining lung, it is essential that air and fluid be removed continuously from the pleural space.

bling, since air no longer escapes from the nonaerated parenchyma. Cessation of bubbling may lead the physician to think that the air leaks have sealed, when actually the lung has collapsed. Atelectasis is a prominent consideration when a tube ceases to function soon after a segmental resection.

Occasionally, the air leak may be much larger than expected from the type of surgery performed. The water-seal bottles and tubing must be inspected to ensure that air is not being drawn into the system from a faulty connection. The dressing around the chest tubes should be elevated and the entry sites examined to determine if the tubes have been partially withdrawn or if air is being sucked around the tube into the chest. Leaking stab wounds may be sealed with petrolatum gauze. If the bottles, tubing and chest tube sites appear satisfactory, one can then assume that the air leak is originating from the pleural space.

Failure of the decortication or breaker bottles to bubble indicates either that they are incorrectly connected or that there is a greater volume of air loss from the lung than can be removed by the suction. The latter problem becomes immediately serious, since air will accumulate in the pleural space, causing tension pneumothorax. The amount of suction must be increased to remove a larger volume of air. The decortication bottles should then bubble. A second solution to this problem is to establish suction only on one water-seal bottle, letting the other act as a vent for any buildup of pressure in the pleural space.

Several chest tube clamps are always kept nearby. If there is a breakage in the system, the tubes can be immediately clamped until another bottle is connected. Chest bottles are always secured to the floor to prevent tipping, and a light is placed under the patient's bed to facilitate accurate measurement of blood loss.

A chest tube can be used to control mediastinal shift following a pneumonectomy. In this instance, the tube is permanently clamped and opened only to remove fluid or air. If the tube in a pneumonectomy space is allowed to remain open, coughing will force air out of the pneumonectomy space and the mediastinum will shift to the operated side. Such significant mediastinal shift causes serious physiologic derangement.

Postoperative Care—Specific Procedures

Pneumonectomy

Following pneumonectomy the cardiovascular system must accommodate to the loss of 50% of the pulmonary vascular bed and diffusing capacity. Minimal pulmonary reserve remains, requiring careful scrutiny of the following details.

Pneumonectomy patients are subject to shifts of the mediastinum. These must be prevented. At the end of the operative procedure, the pressure in the pneumonectomy space is adjusted to a mean of −2 cm.

of water. This positions the mediastinum slightly toward the operated side, permitting optimal expansion of the remaining lung. However, rapid accumulation of fluid or air in the pneumonectomy space can shift the mediastinum to the opposite, or unoperated, side. A significant shift will result in obstruction of the superior and inferior venae cavae, decreased cardiac output, hypotension and cardiac arrest. Mediastinal shift can also cause partial obstruction of the trachea; however, obstruction of the great veins occurs first. Compression of the remaining lung also causes dyspnea due to a critical loss of lung volume.

When a pneumonectomy patient exhibits hypotension or respiratory distress, the first condition suspected is mediastinal shift. Examination may reveal shift of the heart and trachea to the nonoperated side. A portable chest x-ray will confirm this diagnosis, but if the patient is in severe distress, immediate aspiration is mandatory.

If a chest tube is in place, unclamping will allow air and fluid to drain and restore the mediastinal position. If a chest tube has not been used, a large bore needle is placed in the second or third anterior intercostal space and air is aspirated to reposition the mediastinum. This adjustment is best performed with one of the commercially available instruments used for manometric adjustment of the pleural pressure. If this type of instrument is not available, a lubricated 50 ml. glass syringe and 3-way stopcock can be used. Air is withdrawn until slight negative pressure is observed by in-and-out motion of the plunger. Higher friction in disposable plastic syringes precludes their use in regulation of intrapleural pressure.

Care must be taken to prevent excess removal of air and resultant shift to the operated side, again causing caval obstruction and possible injury to the heart by the indwelling needle. A portable chest x-ray should be taken as soon as aspiration has been completed to determine the exact position of the mediastinum.

Usually, during slow accumulation of fluid, the air is decompressed through the operative wound into the subcutaneous tissues. This prevents a buildup of pressure. The pneumonectomy space rarely requires aspiration in the postoperative period.

A large gas bubble within the stomach requires nasogastric aspiration. This is especially necessary following right pneumonectomy, as elevation of the diaphragm compresses the remaining lung.

Nasotracheal aspiration of pneumonectomy patients must be done with great caution. Trauma from the tip of the catheter may cause disruption of the bronchial stump. Because of minimal reserve in this group, severe hypoxia can occur during aspiration. Some surgeons do not allow nasotracheal aspiration of pneumonectomy patients for these reasons.

Intravenous fluid therapy is monitored carefully following pneumonectomy. Excessive intravenous replacement produces hypervolemia and resultant right heart overload. No more than 2,000 ml. of fluid should be given in the first 24 hours, and blood replacement should not exceed losses. If there is any question regarding this volume, a catheter should be placed for continuous monitoring of central venous pressure. It is preferable to remain slightly behind in fluid replacement.

IPPB is not contraindicated, but it should be used only if necessary. The sutured bronchial stump will tolerate 15–20 cm. of water pressure.

If the pneumonectomy patient coughs up blood or thin bloody fluid, dehiscence of the bronchial stump must be considered. The patient is immediately positioned with the operated side dependent to prevent further drainage into the remaining lung. If it is ascertained that there is disruption of the bronchial stump, immediate chest tube drainage is instituted. This procedure is lifesaving.

Pulmonary Resection

The general principles of physiologic care, as previously outlined, apply to all pulmonary resections.

Following segmental resection there is usually a moderate air leak from the lung surface. It is not unusual for the water seal to bubble vigorously. Air leak following lobectomy is often small except in those with incomplete fissures.

Following sleeve resection (Fig. 18-3), temporary loss of ciliary function results in collection of secretions just distal to the bronchial anastomosis. For this reason, bronchoscopy is performed on the first or second postoperative day to ensure complete clearing of secretions.

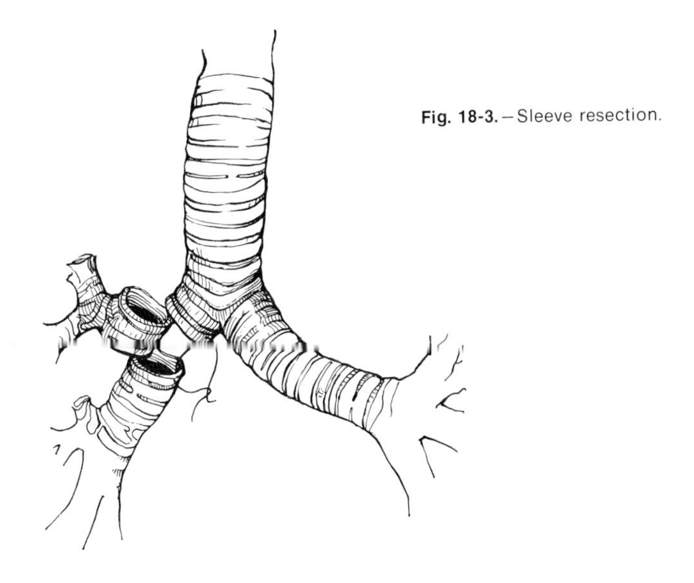

Fig. 18-3.—Sleeve resection.

Bronchoscopy may be repeated if secretions again collect or if expansion is incomplete. Nasotracheal aspiration is avoided, but IPPB can be used at low pressures (10–15 cm. water) if indicated. A sleeve resection is otherwise treated similarly to other types of pulmonary resection.

Pulmonary Decortication

Decortication is the removal of fibrinous material adherent to the visceral pleura to permit expansion of the underlying lung. The fibrinous covering usually results from chronic hemothorax or empyema. Often the underlying lung has been atelectatic and "trapped" for weeks to months. Postoperative expansion may be difficult. The patient must ventilate as vigorously as possible. Expansion may be aided by the use of IPPB at high pressures (20–30 cm.). It is also helpful to have the patient use blow bottles or to blow up a rubber glove. The latter will cause hyperventilation and increase airway pressure.

Particular care must be taken in the management of secretions following decortication. Secretions from the previously atelectatic lung are excessive, and incomplete removal impairs expansion. Daily bronchoscopy may be required for several days.

The raw lung surface following decortication often results in large air leaks. Complete removal of air from the pleural space is essential to promote expansion.

Esophageal Resection and Reconstruction

Surgical diseases of the esophagus are usually accompanied by weight loss and debility. Fluid management in the postoperative period must be precise.

Prolonged exposure of body cavities during thoracoabdominal procedures results in major fluid losses. These losses must be considered in the fluid replacement plan. Significant plasma loss also requires graded replacement. Urine output, specific gravity and osmolarity are measured hourly and influence subsequent intravenous therapy. It is mandatory to maintain accurate intake and output records. Flow sheets are used routinely after this type of surgery. Vitamins should be added to the intravenous fluids, particularly vitamin C to promote wound healing.

These patients should receive absolutely nothing by mouth until an oral contrast x-ray demonstrates a properly functioning anastomosis. In most cases this x-ray examination is not performed until 10 to 14 days following surgery. A clear liquid diet is begun and slowly advanced only after a satisfactory result has been confirmed.

If a nasogastric tube is in place, it must be secured to prevent accidental dislodgment. If the tube is accidentally removed, it may be replaced only after consultation with the operating surgeon, since it is hazardous to pass a tube through a recent esophageal anastomosis. Specific orders for irrigation and aspiration of these tubes are outlined by the individual service (see Chapter 12).

Colon interposition ordinarily includes a neck incision for the esophagocolic anastomosis. The dressings should be changed daily and the wound carefully inspected to detect evidence of anastomotic leak. This is characterized by the collection of saliva in and around the wound. It is important that the drains remain in position should a leak occur. The nasogastric tube is removed upon return of intestinal peristalsis.

The management of secretions and pulmonary therapy are the same for any patient undergoing thoracotomy. Chest tubes are removed when they cease to function.

Thymectomy

Thymectomy is beneficial in the treatment of certain cases of myasthenia gravis, particularly in young women whose disease is of recent onset. The postoperative care of these patients is formidable and requires extremely careful supervision.

The postoperative morbidity and mortality of thymectomy for myasthenia gravis are mainly related to pharmacologic crises, manifest as respiratory and circulatory emergencies. For this reason the patient should be studied before surgery and the reponse to oral anticholinesterase agents evaluated. The minimal dose consistent with normal mastication and swallowing is administered. It is most important to provide a vital capacity of at least 1,800 ml. and a normal Pa_{CO_2}, Pa_{O_2} and pH.

On the day before surgery the anticholinesterase is either reduced or withheld to decrease the likelihood of a cholinergic crisis in the postoperative period. Respiratory depressant drugs such as morphine should be avoided in the preanesthetic medication. Atropine or scopolamine is given to avoid autonomic reflex mechanisms during surgery.

Following surgery strict attention must be afforded to respiratory dynamics. Respiratory insufficiency may occur because of anticholinesterase deficiency, splinting of the chest wall, and atelectasis. If the vital capacity is less than 1,800 ml., tracheostomy is necessary to maintain adequate exchange. Patients with borderline pulmonary function can be assisted with an endotracheal tube and mechanical ventilation for a 24-hour period. If at the end of this time the blood gases, pH and vital capacity are adequate, the endotracheal tube is removed. If these parameters are not satisfactory, a tracheostomy is indicated.

Sudden unexplained deaths have occurred in the immediate postoperative period which may be related to specific lesions of the myocardium. For this reason hematocrit, hemoglobin and serum electrolyte levels must be monitored closely.

Three types of myasthenic emergencies can occur in the postoperative period. All result in respiratory insufficiency; each requires specific drug therapy. For this reason attention is directed to supporting ventilation before institution of drug therapy.

The first type of emergency is the myasthenic crisis from undermedication. Tensilon is given to these patients, 1.0 mg. intravenously, and if muscular strength improves, one of the longer-acting anticholinesterases, such as neostigmine, is then begun. The cholinergic side effects of neostigmine may be counteracted by prior administration of atropine, 0.4–0.6 mg. intramuscularly.

The second, a cholinergic crisis, results from overmedication. This is manifested by muscular weakness and increased bronchial secretions leading to respiratory insufficiency. Atropine, 0.4–1 mg., is given intravenously, with subsequent doses of 0.3–0.4 mg. every 3 to 5 minutes until a therapeutic effect is obtained.

The third type of emergency occurs when antibiotics, which are given either prophylactically or for specific infections, potentiate the already present myasthenic neuromuscular block. These antibiotics include streptomycin, neomycin, kanamycin and polymyxin. When antibiotics are given, careful selection must be used to avoid this hazardous side effect.

Complications

ATELECTASIS.—Atelectasis is defined as collapsed and airless pulmonary parenchyma. It may be patchy, segmental or lobar in nature. It is usually related to ineffective cough and inadequate removal of tracheobronchial secretions. Inspissation of secretions in a segmental or lobar bronchus causes distal collapse of that portion of the lung. The first indication of postoperative atelectasis is a precipitous rise in temperature to 102 or 103 F. The pulse and respiratory rates increase. Although cyanosis may not be manifest, shunting of blood through nonventilated parenchyma does cause hypoxia. Physical examination reveals dullness to percussion and tubular breath sounds in the area of atelectasis. A portable chest x-ray will verify the clinical impression.

Therapy is directed to removal of the obstructing secretions. Coughing, nasotracheal aspiration and bronchoscopy are used as indicated. The longer an atelectatic portion of a lung is allowed to remain deflated, the more difficult it becomes to expand. Bronchoscopy should be repeated as necessary. Total atelectasis of one lung is a definite indication for bronchoscopy. In this instance the airway can be cleared most efficiently by aspiration of secretions through the bronchoscope. Atelectasis should not be treated with IPPB. The increased airway pressure serves only to drive the secretions distally and compound the difficulty.

Atelectasis occurring repeatedly on a surgical service suggests that the staff is rendering insufficient care in stimulating adequate coughing and clearing of secretions.

SUBCUTANEOUS EMPHYSEMA.—Subcutaneous emphysema occurs commonly after pulmonary resections and especially after pneumonectomy if tube drainage is not used. Residual air in the pneumonectomy space is forced out through the incision into the subcutaneous tissues, while fluid accumulates within the space. The residual air often dissects into the tissues of the neck and anterior chest wall. The condition is usually not progressive and generally stabilizes within 48 hours. Subcutaneous air is then absorbed in the next 10 or 12 days.

Following pulmonary resection or decortication, the chest tubes ordinarily evacuate air from the pleural space, thus minimizing subcutaneous emphysema. On occasion, however, subcutaneous emphysema can be massive. Dissection of air along the fascial planes can cause closure of the eyelids and massive enlargement of the scrotum.

The presence of massive subcutaneous emphysema demands immediate investigation. The commonest cause is tube obstruction either by clot or by external compression from the patient's lying on the tubes. Collection of air within the pleural space then forces the air into the subcutaneous tissues.

A second cause of emphysema is malposition of the chest tube, allowing the fenestrations of the tube to lie in the subcutaneous tissues. When necessary, a chest x-ray may be taken for confirmation. The external portion of the tube is cleansed with alcohol and the tube is advanced an appropriate distance. This method carries some danger of introducing infection into the pleural space, but it is generally safer than inserting a new tube.

If the subcutaneous emphysema is progressive and, despite all efforts, the chest tubes fail to function properly, a chest x-ray will usually identify an area of pneumothorax. Under such circumstances it is mandatory that a new chest tube be inserted into this space. This will allow continuous removal of the accumulating intrapleural air and prevent progression of the subcutaneous emphysema.

After initial resolution of subcutaneous emphysema following pulmonary resection, sudden recurrence indicates disruption of a bronchial or parenchymal suture line. Chest tube drainage is necessary to prevent further accumulation of air. The surgeon will then determine whether reoperation is necessary or conservative tube drainage should be continued.

Development of subcutaneous emphysema in a tracheostomy patient who is on assisted or controlled ventilation indicates that the tracheostomy tube may have slipped from the tracheal stoma to a position within the mediastinum. The air from the respirator is then forced into the tissues, resulting in subcutaneous emphysema. This complication can also occur from tight closure of the subcutaneous tissues and skin around a tracheostomy tube. An additional cause is rupture of blebs and pneumothorax during assisted ventilation.

Massive subcutaneous emphysema is distressing to the patient but is not painful. Careful explanation to the patient and his family regarding the cause of emphysema will usually allay apprehension. Airway obstruction from subcutaneous emphysema almost never occurs. Needle aspiration of the eyelids can be performed to permit the patient to see. If the emphysema is uncontrollable, a small incision is made on the upper anterior chest wall under local anesthesia and the subcutaneous air is expressed.

BRONCHOSPASM.—Bronchospasm can be a problem in patients who have chronic obstructive lung disease or a previous history of asthmatic bronchitis. Airway resistance and respiratory work are significantly increased.

As soon as generalized wheezing is detected, appropriate therapy must be instituted. Aminophylline can be given slowly intravenously or by rectal suppository. Arrhythmias can result from rapid injection. Aminophylline is best given over a 30-minute period in a 50 ml. intravenous rider. Isuprel may be given by aerosol inhalation or IPPB, if tolerated. Isuprel, 0.5 ml. of a 1% solution, is added to 1.5 ml. of saline. Sedation should be used cautiously.

If the patient fails to respond, intravenous administration of hydrocortisone may be used. The initial dose is 100 mg. Rapid tapering is begun as soon as the bronchospasm can be controlled by conventional therapy. Persistent severe bronchospasm may necessitate tracheostomy and controlled ventilation with a volume respirator.

BLOOD LOSS.—Drainage from the chest tubes should be measured and recorded hourly. Continued excessive blood loss requires careful scrutiny. A loss of 500 ml./hour for 2 or 3 hours usually requires reoperation.

Following decortication or pleural stripping, patients will sometimes exude large amounts of fluid from the pleural space. This often begins in the second 12 hours after surgery. If there is any question as to the composition of the drainage, determination of the hematocrit is helpful. Excessive plasma loss from the pleural space will often necessitate infusion of albumin.

CARDIAC ARRHYTHMIAS.—Approximately 10–15% of patients undergoing lobectomy and segmental resections will have a cardiac arrhythmia in the early postoperative period. Cardiac arrhythmias have been documented in as many as 30% of pneumonectomy patients. The exact cause for this high incidence of arrhythmia is unknown. Postulated causes include hypoxia, sudden increase in pulmonary vascular resistance and stimulation of receptors within the great vessels. Atrial flutter and fibrillation are the most common arrhythmias encountered. As soon as a postoperative arrhythmia is detected, appropriate therapy is undertaken (Chapters 20 and 21).

In view of the significant incidence of postoperative arrhythmias in patients undergoing thoracic surgery, many surgeons routinely employ preoperative digitalization in patients over age 50. There is some debate regarding the efficacy of preoperative digitalization, but most reports suggest a decreased incidence of postoperative arrhythmias.

LARGE AIR LEAKS.—Large air leaks are seen most commonly after segmental resections, pulmonary decortications and resections in emphysematous patients. The major factor contributing to the persistence of a large air leak is failure of the underlying lung to expand completely. When a raw, leaking surface of the lung is adjacent to the parietal pleura, fibrinous deposits serve to close small parenchymal leaks. However, in the presence of a space, air leaks tend to persist.

Common factors contributing to failure of the remaining lung to expand are atelectasis, hypoventilation, chest tube malfunction and inadequate suction. If any of these factors are detected in conjunction with a persistent air leak or space problem, appropriate steps should be taken. Suction as high as 30 cm. of water pressure may help to decrease the space. On occasion, a third chest tube will be needed to assist in expansion. Less often, reoperation may be necessary for suture closure of a persistent leak.

HYPOVENTILATION.—Despite all efforts, inadequate ventilation may persist. The pathophysiologic alterations result in progressive deterioration. This will be evidenced by a rising Pa_{CO_2}, a falling Pa_{O_2} and respiratory and metabolic acidosis. Under these conditions it will be necessary to institute assisted or controlled mechanical ventilation. Initially the preferred route is via an endotracheal tube. Often 24–36 hours of assisted ventilation is adequate to allow recovery. If the hypoventilation persists beyond this time, tracheostomy is usually indicated. The technique of prolonged respiratory support is discussed in Chapter 5.

PARALYZED VOCAL CORD.—The left recurrent laryngeal nerve may be traumatized during radical left pneumonectomy. It may also be damaged when a mediastinal lymph node dissection is done. The right recurrent laryngeal nerve is rarely injured due to its high anatomic position.

Damage to the recurrent laryngeal nerve results in paralysis of the ipsilateral vocal cord. Approximation of the vocal cords is impossible and the patient cannot generate an effective cough. This is evidenced in the early postoperative period by extreme hoarseness and a grossly inadequate cough. If the patient has an ineffective cough from vocal cord paralysis, and secretions are accumulating, it is beneficial to inject the paralyzed cord with glycerin. The injection will cause the cord to expand and the vocal cords will then approximate. With vocal cord closure, an effective cough is restored. The glycerin is dissipated in 48–72 hours and the injection may have to be repeated.

REFERENCE

1. Peters, R. M.: Coordination of ventilation and perfusion, Ann. Thoracic Surg. 6:570, 1968.

19

Cardiac Surgery: Pediatric

MILTON WEINBERG, JR., M.D.

Attending Surgeon, Rush-Presbyterian-St. Luke's Medical Center; Associate Professor of Surgery, Rush Medical College

IN THIS CHAPTER on the intensive care of children undergoing cardiac surgery, the material to be presented will cover not only the postoperative period but also the preparation of the child for surgery and certain aspects of the operative management. Additionally, certain subjects which are discussed elsewhere in this book—for example, anesthesia, monitoring, tracheostomy and respiratory care—will be dealt with as they apply specifically to children, and as they are seen from the view of the surgeon responsible for the overall care of the patient, as opposed to the rather narrower view of the discussant concerned with a particular phase of care.

Margins for error in children are not great. One would urge the surgeon who operates upon a child not to look here for a set of orders which will cover every contingency likely to arise in the course of a child's care. No area lends itself less well to routine orders. It will be our goal to be as specific as possible in describing concepts, techniques and procedures, but it is our hope that the reader will recognize in these pages a plea for intense observation of the patient, not just the chart, the chemical values and the monitoring devices, and above all, a plea for concern and true affection for the child. The latter attitudes will not only yield the satisfactions inherent in seeing a child recover from an illness and then grow and develop in years of follow-up, but will more immediately make evident the subtle changes in physical signs that characterize the response of children to injury and treatment—signs that will surely not be recognized by the unconcerned surgeon.

The location and assignment of personnel to the pediatric intensive care unit deserves brief attention. There are obvious advantages in having this unit adjacent to the operating room, minimizing transportation distances postoperatively and probably making surgical and anesthesia personnel more closely available to the child in an emergency. These considerations, however, must be weighed against the advantages of placing the unit on the pediatric floor, which in our judgment is the preferable arrangement if adequate personnel and equipment can be made available. Mixing adults and children in the same unit is grossly unsatisfactory from the standpoint of patient care and particularly from the standpoint of the environment for the child. A separate intensive care unit on the pediatric floor ideally surrounds the child with familiar sights and personnel in the critical and rather frightening postoperative period and permits the application of equipment and procedures adapted to the specialized care.

Depending upon the policies of the institution, responsibility for the care of a child admitted for cardiac surgery may fall at one time or another to the pediatric service, the cardiology service or the cardiac surgery service. Without any thought of limiting the involvement or the essential cooperation of the other services, it is our opinion that responsibility for care in the postoperative period should lie with the surgical service. Whatever the assignment of responsibility in a particular hospital, rules regarding orders and procedures should be clearly defined.

Preoperative Preparation

There are no set rules for determining how detailed explanations of forthcoming procedures to a given child should be. In general, it is my opinion that no explanation is helpful in a child under 3 or 4 years of age. Up to age 8 or 10, explicit descriptions are best avoided, and large quantities of relaxed assurances and great affection are called for. The teenagers—restless, sensitive, volatile and anxious while alert, inquisitive and energetic—will require much technical detail coupled with empathy and abundant reassurance. Parents should be allowed to stay with the child the morning of operation until he leaves the floor for the operating room, and they should be allowed to see the child again in the intensive therapy area as soon as it is reasonably possible. This is important in helping to establish for the child that his parents have endured this ordeal with him.

Whenever possible, in a child old enough to establish recognition, it is helpful to have him know before operation the nurses who will care for him postoperatively. A 2-year-old taught to cough before operation will cough most effectively for the instructor with whom he practiced, and this principle will apply to most aspects of cooperation in children. Effective preoperative instruction at age 2 or 3 includes coughing, blowing up balloons and deep breathing exercises. Many children can be taught to use IPPB apparatus at 3 years of age. It should be emphasized that these ventilators should be used only with a mouthpiece that the child learns to hold himself, never with a strapped-on mask. If he cannot use the equipment effectively by his own efforts, the technique is better discarded than forced.

MEDICATIONS

DIGITALIS AND DIURETICS.—Digitalis preparations, usually digoxin, are continued through the day before operation in most children being prepared for open or closed cardiac surgery. Dietary restrictions of water and sodium and intensive diuresis are seldom imposed upon children as they so frequently are in adults, and the consequent arrythmias of digitalis intoxication and potassium depletion following cardiopulmonary by-pass occur only in the exceptional situation. In that rare child requiring unusually vigorous measures to control congestive heart failure and water retention, loss of 5–10% of initial body weight by diuresis may result in electrolyte depletion. As in adults, potassium salts should be administered parenterally or by mouth preoperatively, and digitalis preparations and diuretics should be withdrawn 24–48 hours before a planned open heart procedure with cardiopulmonary by-pass. In the children in whom cardiopulmonary by-pass is not utilized, excessive intraoperative and postoperative losses of fluid and electrolytes by renal excretion do not ordinarily occur, and digitalis and diuretics may be continued to the day of operation despite vigorous preoperative diuresis. Attention to adequate replacement of potassium salts is of course fundamental to proper therapy in all patients undergoing treatment for congestive heart failure.

ANTIBIOTICS.—Prophylactic antibiotics usually are not given to children before operation. This general rule is not meant to exclude the use of appropriate antibiotics in specific circumstances. Nose and throat and perineal cultures are taken in all children admitted to the hospital, and the presence of a beta-hemolytic streptococcus is a specific indication for the administration of penicillin. A single injection of long-acting benzathine penicillin G suspension will effectively eliminate this organism.

The culture of a coagulase-positive staphylococcus from the nasopharynx or anal areas does not ordinarily demand therapy in the absence of evidences of infection. Antibiotic sensitivities should be obtained. Prophylactic antistaphylococcal therapy with intravenous methicillin or cephalothin is begun preoperatively only if implantation of a prosthetic valve is planned.

Staphylococcal skin infections are not uncommon in children, particularly adolescents. Whenever possible, these infections should be controlled prior to the child's admission to the hospital, but adequate control may require administration of appropriate antibiotics before and after operation.

A regimen of prophylactic antibiotic therapy with intravenous methicillin or cephalothin beginning the day before operation and continuing throughout the operative and postoperative periods has been established for adults in whom cardiac valve replacement is planned. We have avoided this preoperative use of the antibiotic in children unless the presence of a staphylococcus has been established, but have administered the drugs in the same manner during and after operation as established in the adult regimen, 16 Gm. of methicillin being added to the priming fluid of the pump-oxygenator in patients weighing 100 lb. or more. Postoperatively the patient is given 2 Gm. of methicillin every 6 hours until he is taking oral feedings freely. Thereafter he is given 2 Gm. sodium oxacillin by mouth every 6 hours for approximately 7 days. In smaller children the dosage of the antibiotic is appropriately reduced. Cephalothin may be substituted for methicillin in the same dosage schedule. In patients sensitive to penicillin consultation should be obtained regarding antibiotic therapy.

SEDATIVES.—Preanesthetic medications for sedation and an anticholinergic action are generally ordered according to commonly available age and weight tables. We have preferred to give no sedative or narcotic drugs to children under 1 year of age. Under 3 months of age we have usually given no premedication, but have frequently administered atropine intravenously in the operating room when the cardiac rate has slowed in response to the altered respiratory mechanics or manipulation of the heart.

MANAGEMENT OF DIET

The usual diet order for "nothing by mouth after midnight" should not be applied to infants and small children. Infants on bottle feedings every 3 or 4 hours should have their regular feedings continue to within 6 or 8 hours of operation, and should be given an additional last feeding of 60–90 ml. water 4 hours before the scheduled time of operation. A child under age 2 who usually has his last feeding before going to sleep at 8:00 or 9:00 P.M. should be given water to drink at midnight and nothing by mouth thereafter for operation at 8:00 A.M.

Dehydration should particularly be avoided in cyanotic children with high hematocrit readings, whatever their ages. These children should be awakened during the night before operation and given water at 10:00 P.M. and again at 2:00 A.M. if operation is scheduled in the early morning. If operation is scheduled later in the day, water should be offered to within 6 hours of operation or intravenous fluids should be started.

Operative Management

It is not our purpose to discuss the many aspects of the operative procedure which obviously affect the postoperative course. Certain features of this period, however, deserve special attention.

Infants who require an incubator on the pediatric floor with controlled heat, humidity and oxygen should be brought to the operating room in the same equipment and should remain in the functioning incubator until all preparations are completed. The temperature in most operating rooms is kept at 70 F. or less, and an exposed infant will quickly lose significant body heat in this atmosphere.

In general, children should not wait in a hallway or a waiting room of the operating suite in unfamiliar surroundings and attended by strangers. The call to surgery should be timed so that the child is moved directly from the floor into the operating room and anesthetized without undue delay. It is our feeling that most children should be anesthetized before any manipulations whatsoever are done, including the placement of blood pressure cuff, electrodes or intravenous cannulas. Suffice it to say that an experienced anesthesiologist will rarely if ever find it necessary to restrain a struggling, terrified child to induce anesthesia.

Secure placement of venous cannulas for the administration of blood if necessary and of fluids and medications is essential to the safe management of the child for at least 48–72 hours during and after operation. Venesections will be necessary in most infants and children under 2 or 3 years of age. Cannulas introduced by percutaneous puncture can usually be placed in older children unless central venous placement is desirable for central venous pressure monitoring. We usually rely upon 1 peripheral venous catheter in infants and children under age 4 or 5 who undergo closed heart procedures. If cardiopulmonary by-pass is planned, we prefer to have 1 peripheral venous catheter and 1 central venous catheter, the latter introduced by venesection into the median basilic vein or occasionally into the saphenous vein. In older children we usually have 2 venous catheters, both peripheral for closed procedures, 1 peripheral and 1 central for open heart procedures. The central venous catheter should be radiopaque or contain a radiopaque line for identification of position by x-ray, and preferably should have a Luer-fitting adapter at one end. A connecting tubing containing injection sites should be interposed between the cannula and the fluid administration set so that changes in sets can be accomplished without disturbing the fixation of the cannula to the limb. All blood administered during and after operation should be passed through a coil placed in a warming unit thermostatically controlled at temperatures approximating 98 F. In infants a scalp vein needle with attached tubing introduced into the injection site nearest the cannula is useful for the administration of medications with a minimum of delay and flushing volume. All fluid administration sets should contain a pediatric volume-measuring set, and the sets used solely for fluids other than blood or its substitutes should contain droppers which deliver a volume of approximately 1/60th of a milliliter per drop. Sets for the measurement of central venous pressure are widely available and commonly used now in all surgical disciplines.

We do not commonly use arterial cannulas for continuous monitoring of systemic blood pressure in children. Monitoring of arterial blood pressure from the cannula utilized for inflow from the pump-oxygenator to the patient provides systemic blood pressure readings in the period just before cardiopulmonary by-pass and in the period immediately after by-pass. If arterial pressure monitoring seems desirable after decannulation, a catheter is easily brought out of the site of repair of the artery and may be left in for a day or two without a significant incidence of complications in children over 3 or 4 years of age. If the aorta has been used for the inflow cannulation and an arterial catheter is felt to be essential in the postoperative period, the ulnar, brachial or femoral artery may be utilized, although we have rarely found it necessary to follow such a course.

ANESTHETIC MANAGEMENT.—The selection of anesthetic drugs, relaxants and materials is properly the province of the anesthesiologist. The surgical team has a critical interest in the effects that carry over into the postoperative period, however, and we consider it important to comment upon certain aspects. The most critical of anesthetic considerations, in our judgment, is the depth of anesthesia, particularly in infants. Concentrations of agents which are totally inadequate for the anesthetization of a normal infant will frequently severely depress a child with hypoxia or a markedly reduced cardiac output because of a congenital cardiac anomaly. The surgeon and the anesthesiologist should be prepared to discontinue all anesthetic agents and permit the child to wake up partially whenever there are evidences of an unexplained decrease in cardiac output during operation. Adequate levels of anesthesia may then be reinstated as necessary. It is our firm belief that a child should never be more than a few breaths away from waking up, except for critical moments such as during the construction of a small shunt when it is essential that the child not move. At the end of operation the child should be awake and vigorous so that assisted or controlled ventilation is unnecessary and the endotracheal tube can be removed. There are, of course, circumstances in which ventilatory support will be essential for hours or days, and it should be instituted without hesitation through an endotracheal tube or a tracheostomy. These circumstances certainly do not include the deliberate suppression of the child's responses so that his respirations may be controlled; rather, they should be limited to brain injury, respiratory inadequacy or an inadequate cardiac output which can be improved by the institution of positive pressure ventilation.

CONTROL OF VENTILATION.—The fact that certain infants must have respiratory support following operation makes the choice of a satisfactory endotracheal tube and adapter a critical one in which the surgeon should take an interest. It has been our observation that the tubes are well chosen by the anesthesiologist to fit the larynx properly. The lumen of the adapter that fits into the tube, however, frequently will be found to reduce the effective airway critically, not so much for the hour or so that the experienced anesthesiology staff controls ventilation in the operating room, but intolerably so for the longer period in the intensive care area where the airway is maintained under less favorable circumstances by less experienced personnel. A surgeon undertaking the care of infants would do well to discuss thoroughly with the anesthesiology staff the selection of endotracheal tubes, adapters and, in fact, all ventilatory equipment including suction catheters appropriate to the sizes of the endotracheal tubes.

Little insight is required to realize that the period on the operating table immediately after application of a dressing to the wound is a time which should be utilized to assess the status of the patient thoroughly. As often as not, however, the youngest man on the surgical team has closed the wound and is the only surgeon left in the room, too little experienced to judge the patient's responses adequately. There is a compulsion felt by all in the room to get the child out and over to intensive care as quickly as possible. The mature judgment of the anesthesiologist and the surgeon should be the deciding factor in whether or not the child should be extubated. If a tracheostomy is going to be necessary, it is most efficiently and safely performed at this point in the operating room with the endotracheal tube in place and the child's ventilation firmly controlled. If the child is not well enough awake to permit removal of the endotracheal tube immediately, an extra 15–30 minutes in the operating room are well spent at this point to avoid sending him to the ward with the tube in place.

TRANSPORTING FROM OPERATING ROOM TO INTENSIVE CARE WARD. —Heat loss and significant depression of body temperature below 98 F. at the close of operation is rarely seen in children over 6 months of age unless growth and development have been severely retarded. These older children are usually transported to the intensive care area in standard beds or cribs. Infants in the newborn period frequently show a drop in body temperature of 2–6 degrees during operation. They should be bundled in warm blankets as soon as dressings are applied and transferred to a previously warmed incubator when cardiac and respiratory stability are assured. If the infant can be extubated, the anesthesiologist should be asked to select an endotracheal tube of the proper size to be attached to the incubator in transit and in the intensive care area so that if an emergency arises, a properly fitting tube will be immediately available. If the infant cannot be extubated, it is likely that ventilatory support will be necessary in transit, since the small tubes that fit in the infant's trachea introduce a factor of high airway resistance to an already compromised cardiorespiratory system. In addition to the endotracheal tube, each bed or incubator should have attached oxygen with tubing for administration by nasal catheter, mask, or ventilator, a hand-operated ventilator with a non-rebreathing valve and adapters for a face mask or endotracheal tube, an oral airway and a laryngoscope with a blade appropriate to the size of the child. Chest drainage tubes are taped at connection sites and usually doubly clamped during transit from the operating room to the ward. If injury to the lungs during operation has resulted in air leaks from pulmonary surfaces, the chest tubes should remain open to the thoracic drainage bottles at all times and should be transported at levels well below that of the patient. If blood loss into the bottles appears to be significant, the tubes should not be clamped, but just as importantly, it is likely that the child should not leave the operating room in this situation. Again, a few additional minutes of observation to evaluate the rate of blood loss are well spent to avoid a frantic return.

The Intensive Care Area

The physical facilities, equipment and drugs necessary in a pediatric surgical intensive care facility do not vary significantly from the basic requirements of the adult unit. These are described in Chapter 20. Personnel requirements include the ability to assign a nurse full time to each patient in the unit if each patient is sufficiently ill. Fortunately, this is seldom necessary when several patients are in the unit but, generally speaking, a cardiac patient returning from the operating room should have the undivided attention of the nurse until he is clearly stable. Space should be allotted in an area of easy access.

Equipment in readiness should include the following: (1) oxygen ready for administration by catheter or mask with a humidifier in the line; (2) suction apparatus with appropriate sterile catheters and connectors and equipment to maintain sterile technique during intratracheal suctioning; (3) an oxygen tent with an adequate humidification system, preferably ultrasonic, for all children except those in incubators; (4) a thermostatically controlled blood-warming unit; (5) ceiling or floor equipment for hanging a minimum of 4 fluid containers; (6) a floor stand for attachment and leveling of a water manometer with a centimeter scale for venous pressure measurements; (7) equipment for exhibiting a continuous electrocardiogram on an oscilloscope, preferably with the ability to record all leads on paper; (8) equipment capable of monitoring arterial blood pressure from an intra-arterial cannula; (9) a mechanical ventilator capable of controlling respiration; (10) a blood pressure cuff of proper size and a stethoscope of reasonable quality. Syringes and needles should be easily within reach of the nurse at the bedside.

Immediately available medications for intravenous injection should include isoproterenol, 0.2 mg./ml.; calcium chloride, 1.0 Gm./10 ml.; lidocaine, 1%; epinephrine, 1:1,000; sodium bicarbonate, 44.5 mEq. in 50 ml. Other drugs such as chlorpromazine, digoxin, deslanoside, quinidine, procainamide, atropine and scopolamine, norepinephrine, heparin and protamine sulfate, and morphine sulfate and meperidine should be available in the unit.

The return to the intensive care unit should initiate specific steps to stabilize the child's position, to allow thorough evaluation of the organ systems and, if necessary, to initiate vigorous and definitive therapy. Definite priorities attend the child's arrival on the intensive care unit. Relegating all other considerations to second place are the immediate placement of a stethoscope over the heart and the location and palpation of a peripheral pulse. It has seemed to me on innumerable occasions that frantic efforts to connect electronic gear have completely excluded the patients from any hope of real evaluation for inordinate periods, during which any catastrophe may occur. A member of the anesthesiology staff invariably accompanies the child to the intensive care ward and usually he can be relied upon to attend to immediate ventilatory needs, whether those needs are merely the observation of an adequate airway and satisfactory chest wall excursion or the maintenance of controlled respirations with a manual ventilator. Attention to the cardiovascular system at this moment is the responsibility of the surgeon accompanying the child from the operating room or the physician assigned to the intensive care unit. While the more sophisticated equipment is being connected, a stethoscope over the heart will permit the physician to judge heart rate and rhythm and palpation of a peripheral pulse will permit judgment regarding blood pressure, cardiac output and peripheral perfusion. With the patient thus under critical observation, other personnel may establish the systems designed to protect, evaluate and treat the child.

Respiratory Management

As indicated earlier, we do not electively impose ventilatory control in children postoperatively, but reserve its use to requisite situations. We are particularly opposed to leaving endotracheal tubes in small children and infants without ventilatory support because of the high airway resistance imposed by the necessarily small tubes. The advantage of access to secretions is more than outweighed by the disadvantages. The child who is returned to the intensive care unit with an endotracheal tube in place has been judged to need respiratory support and that support should be instituted immediately and continued until a later observation indicates that support is no longer necessary.

In general, we do not use assistor ventilators but prefer complete control of ventilation. This control is established by hyperventilation that affords adequate oxygenation and a lowering of the arterial carbon-dioxide partial pressure (Pco_2) to levels which will depress spontaneous respiration. In most instances, adequate oxygenation of the blood – in general, arterial oxygen saturation above 93% – is easily accomplished with inspired oxygen-air concentration of 40% or less. Arterial oxygen partial pressure (Po_2) should not exceed 150 mm. Hg since alveolar oxygen concentrations which produce those higher levels are thought to be injurious to the distal bronchopulmonary units. If the respiratory rate and volume are reduced to the minimum levels that will eliminate all spontaneous respiratory efforts of the patient, then Pco_2 can usually be assumed to have been minimally reduced. Respiratory alkalosis is then at a fixed level since further reduction of minute volume will result in the child's initiating respiratory efforts and probably competing with the machine. Maintaining this minimal level of Pco_2 reduction requires a firm understanding of the mechanics of the ventilator being used and, above all, intense and repeated observations of the patient rather than transient arterial Pco_2 values. When arterial oxygen levels are significantly decreased, the patient's respiratory drive may be maintained by the hypoxemia, requiring increases in inspired oxygen concentrations as well as increases in ventilator rate and volume. The resulting respiratory alkalosis is unavoidable and must be accepted as the least objectionable of the undesirable alterations of blood gases.

Conscious children do not tolerate orotracheal tubes well. If a child capable of biting is to be ventilated for only an hour or so, a bite block may be taped in place to protect the orotracheal tube for this limited period. The tube and the bite block tend to stimulate vomiting, however, and the child must be observed extremely closely. If the child is to be maintained on a ventilator for longer periods, the orotracheal tube should be replaced with a nasotracheal tube or a tube introduced by tracheostomy. The orotracheal tube may be a satisfactory temporary airway in an infant or an unconscious child. It should be noted that most ward personnel will find a nasotracheal tube more difficult to aspirate than an orotracheal tube because of its greater length and generally smaller lumen. This difficulty is usually obviated by lubrication of the aspirating catheter with a water-soluble lubricant.

The overwhelming majority of children undergoing cardiac surgery should return to the intensive care unit without an endotracheal tube and with adequate spontaneous respirations. Infants return in an incubator to which oxygen is flowing and humidification is added. In older children, oxygen is administered by nasal catheter in transit from the operating room and continued by that means during the period of evaluation. They are then placed in a tent with added oxygen and humidification. Most children – and adults for that matter – find continuous oxygen therapy with a mask objectionable. Despite the ability of a mask system to deliver high concentrations of oxygen, therefore, if oxygen is needed beyond the concentrations attainable in a tent, the nasal catheter is better tolerated and is preferred.

The hyperventilation of crying, frequent turning and the occasional stimulation of cough reflex by a catheter introduced through the nose or mouth into the pharynx will adequately evacuate pulmonary secretions in most infants. Holding the infant face down across the knees or over the shoulder and patting the back of the chest will frequently dislodge secretions. Excessive irritation of the pharynx should be avoided and, if secretions accumulate despite the measures described, visualization of the larynx with a laryngoscope and direct aspiration of the tracheobronchial tree should be carried out. If done expertly, this type of aspiration may be repeated at 1–2 hour intervals. When it is done roughly, laryngeal edema can be expected to complicate the child's course further. Direct tracheobronchial aspiration is particularly helpful in the weak, underdeveloped infant incapable of ejecting secretions. Bronchoscopy is occasionally and tracheostomy rarely necessary for the purpose of removing secretions.

Humidification, crying and encouragement to move about and cough will control pulmonary secretions in most children beyond infancy. With persistence and patience, a phenomenal degree of cooperation in coughing and the performance of other activities to stimulate hyperventilation can be obtained. The judicious use of a nasopharyngeal catheter will induce a salutary cough reflex, and the threat of its use will even more often stimulate the child to cough to avoid its application. The trachea cannot often be entered in a small child by blind nasotracheal intubation, however, and persistent fruitless probing of the pharynx will produce little more than a nosebleed and sore throat and a much less cooperative patient. As in the infant, bronchoscopy and tracheostomy will be necessary occasionally for control of secretions.

Temperature Control

Small infants will frequently return to the intensive care area with lowered body temperatures, occasionally as low as 92 or 93 F. The incubator should be kept at 90–94 F. until the infant's temperature reaches 96 F., and then is usually kept in the range of 85 F. Thermometers and thermostats in incubators should be checked periodically, not only by ward maintenance personnel but also by the physicians who are using them.

In the child beyond infancy temperature elevation poses a problem more often than temperature depression. The rectal temperature should be obtained shortly after the child's arrival on the floor and should then be taken at half-hour intervals for the first 2 hours, then hourly for 8–24 hours, depending upon the values obtained. Once the temperature pattern is stable, determination every 4 hours is adequate. The causes of significant temperature elevations immediately after operation are not always apparent. Dehydration during operation, blood and drug reactions and brain injury are among the relatively obscure causes. In children exhibiting peripheral signs of vascular constriction, fever is probably due to poor perfusion of superficial tissues and the consequent inability to lose heat efficiently from skin surfaces. The shivering commonly seen after open-heart procedures can be expected to move temperatures upward. Rectal aspirin given in standard pediatric dosages and a cool oxygen tent will control most temperature elevations in the immediate postoperative period. Cooling blankets and surface sponging with water-alcohol mixtures are used for fever above 104 F. Chlorpromazine given intravenously in increments of 1–2.5 mg. is useful in the treatment of peripheral vascular constriction and the relief of shivering.

Fever persisting or appearing after the first postoperative day is more likely to be associated with recognizable causes, such as atelectasis, obvious dehydration, urinary tract infections when a catheter has been placed in the bladder and, later, wound infections. One would discourage the vigorous pursuit of blood cultures in children with fever within the first 10 days of operation, except perhaps in the child with unexplained fever in the presence of a prosthetic valve replacement. The obtaining of multiple cultures is a thoroughly disagreeable process for the child and in this group bacterial endocarditis is rare during an operative admission. That it may occur in a child with a prosthetic valve, a persistently patent ventricular septal defect or following aortic valvulotomy is undeniable, but it occurs rarely and the cultures should be obtained judiciously with due consideration of its rarity and the disturbance of the child.

Chest Drainage Bottles; Postoperative Blood Loss

Thoracic drainage catheters from the pericardial cavity, mediastinum or pleural cavities are connected to underwater gravity drainage. We have found no advantage in the application of suction to the bottles and have observed a considerable increase in confusion associated with the more complex drainage system. The bottles utilized for small children, certainly those under 50 lb., should have a maximum capacity of 1,000 ml. so that small increments of blood loss can be measured accurately. The bottles should be securely attached to the floor by tape or in a stand designed for the purpose. Blood losses by hour and date should be clearly marked on the bottles and recorded on the ward data sheet. The catheters should not be irrigated, but the tubing profitably may be manipulated by "stripping" or squeezing away from the patient to promote emptying and dislodgment of clots into the drainage bottle.

Chest drainage catheters should be removed as soon as significant drainage has stopped, usually the morning after surgery. In removing the catheters it is well to remember that the thin thoracic wall of small children does not seal the tube tract by overlapping muscle planes as quickly as in adults, and the sponge should be held firmly over the opening and taped securely to avoid ingress of air. We have not used petrolatum gauze over these stab wounds.

It is useful in a small child to relate measured and estimated blood loss to the child's normal blood volume. For practical purposes, normal blood volume may be calculated as 8% of the child's weight, therefore

80 ml./kg. of body weight. Most children should not be allowed to lose more than 10–15% of blood volume acutely without replacement with whole blood or albumin.

It may be noted here that homologous serum hepatitis is seldom apparent clinically in children receiving blood or plasma. It may be assumed, however, that its true incidence is probably the same in children and adults, and the same caution should be exercised in the use of blood products.

Chest X-Rays

Portable chest x-rays are generally taken daily in the intensive care unit in children following cardiac surgery, including particularly the day of operation. In children who are alert and stable, with no physical signs of respiratory problems or evidence of significant blood loss, a chest x-ray is usually obtained 2–4 hours after operation rather than immediately upon arrival on the floor, then repeated the following morning. Areas of unsuspected atelectasis or blood accumulation constitute the major findings in these relatively well children. Children in any distress, with significant blood loss or requiring mechanical ventilation should have a chest x-ray upon arrival on the floor. It seems superfluous to add that the film should be seen, but it is a fact that the x-ray is not infrequently ignored after it is taken. This is particularly true when the staff is busy attending the child in distress, despite the possibility that the cause for the distress may be seen on the film. Obvious abnormalities such as accumulations of blood—in the pleural cavities or manifested by widening of the mediastinum—massive atelectasis and pneumothorax are noted. An endotracheal tube or a tracheostomy tube should always be visualized to be sure that its tip is above the bifurcation of the trachea. The position of the central venous catheter should be noted. When blood loss is persistent, frequent chest x-rays are essential. Clinical signs cannot be relied upon to indicate the gradual accumulation of intrathoracic blood. It is also particularly important to obtain another chest x-ray when previously persistent blood loss ceases, since the cessation may simply be a result of inadequate tube drainage.

Urinary Drainage

There is no need for a urinary bladder drainage catheter in the majority of children undergoing heart surgery. We have not seen a single instance of renal failure after operation, even in several children with known renal disease before operation. Additionally, measurement of urinary output has not been necessary for the evaluation of cardiac output except in the most critically ill child. Our most frequent use of a bladder catheter is in the child undergoing an open-heart procedure when cardiopulmonary by-pass is likely to be prolonged an hour or more. Urinary drainage is not instituted to monitor renal function but to prevent bladder distention, and the catheter is usually removed within a few hours of surgery if the child is stable. Blood-tinged urine following prolonged cardiopulmonary by-pass is common, requires no treatment and invariably will clear in a child. We have also placed indwelling catheters in children with known renal disease, the management of which is, of course, best accomplished with the cooperation of an appropriate consultant in this field. Other indications are for the most part related to central nervous system injury. Specific gravity is measured on all urine obtained by voiding or catheter and is helpful in judging the child's hydration.

Electrocardiographic Monitoring

The electrocardiogram is visualized on an oscilloscope in all children following cardiac surgery. The interpretive signs of cardiac injury and ischemia and the arrhythmias that occur in children are not basically different from those in adults, and they are discussed in Chapters 20 and 21. Certain observations relating to children are pertinent, however. Arrhythmias following cardiac surgery in children are not common and the types of arrhythmias that appear are seldom as chaotic and menacing as those so frequently encountered in adults. The myocardium in a child with congenital heart disease is basically normal and usually capable of competent performance at levels of tachycardia, extrinsic stimuli, electrolyte imbalance and hypoxia that would be intolerable to the adult with rheumatic or arteriosclerotic heart disease. Children with rheumatic and other forms of acquired heart disease are subject to the cardiac dysfunctions characteristic of the specific disorder.

Among the commonest of the abnormal rhythms in children following heart surgery is a nodal rhythm following repair of atrial septal defect of the secundum or primum types. The nodal rhythm is frequently productive of heart rates of 70–80/minute, is without discernible ill effects to the child and usually converts to a normal sinus rhythm within a few days to several weeks. Active treatment is not necessary.

Complete heart block continues to be a serious complication of repair of ventricular septal defect, although an awareness of the usual position of the bundle of His and improved suturing techniques have dramatically reduced its incidence. Particular note of the possibility of its occurrence should be made in the occasional child with a left bundle branch block in the preoperative electrocardiogram, since a right bundle branch block usually accompanies repair of a ventricular septal defect. If a complete heart block is produced and recognized in the operating room, temporary pacing wires should be attached to the right ventricular myocardium and brought out through the skin for control of the heart rate. In most children a rate of approximately 100/minute will produce a satisfactory cardiac output. If the complete heart block persists after 10 days or so of pacing, it will probably be desirable to implant a permanent pacing system, utilizing epicardial electrodes in small children or a transvenous endocardial electrode in larger youngsters. The choice of the route of electrode placement should rest with the cardiac and surgical teams.

A variety of atrial tachycardias are commonly encountered in children operated upon for endocardial cushion defects, Ebstein's anomaly and complete repair of transposition of the great vessels by the Mustard technique. These arrhythmias must be controlled by digitalis preparations, quinidine or procainamide and, if necessary, by direct-current electric cardioversion.

Potassium deficiency or digitalis excess may be manifested by the appearance of premature ventricular contractions, bigeminal rhythms and runs of ventricular tachycardia. Although these rhythms are not often encountered in children, they should be anticipated in the child who has been treated vigorously for congestive heart failure preoperatively, and particularly when commonly used pump dilution techniques result in large urine outputs during and after operation. Such a child should receive 2–4 mEq. of potassium chloride per 100 ml. of urine output to replace potassium as it is being lost. It should be remembered that commonly utilized solutions of potassium chloride containing 40 mEq./100 ml. are highly irritating to peripheral veins and may cause skin sloughs and therefore are most safely delivered into a central venous catheter.

Sudden ventricular arrest or fibrillation is occasionally seen in patients with severe pulmonary hypertension. These episodes may occur without warning and are often refractory to resuscitative efforts. They are best avoided by particular attention to adequate ventilation and acid-base and electrolyte balance in the child with near systemic levels of pulmonary vascular resistance. Suctioning should be performed with great care to avoid a combination of hypoxia and the stimulation of pharyngeal and tracheobronchial reflexes.

The overwhelming majority of the other arrhythmias encountered in children are secondary to hypoxia and will disappear spontaneously with the successful treatment of the hypoxia.

Venous Pressure Monitoring

Techniques and purposes of central venous pressure monitoring are described in Chapter 3 and do not differ appreciably in children. Deserving of re-emphasis, however, is attention to the position of the catheter visualized in the postoperative chest x-ray. Misleading values may be transmitted from a catheter whose tip lies in a jugular or subclavian vein or the right ventricle. In practice, little use is made of central venous pressure monitoring in pediatric cardiac surgery in closed-heart procedures or even in the management of congestive heart failure. However, it is usually employed as a guide to blood volume replacement following cardiopulmonary by-pass with its consequent shifts in blood volume and changes in peripheral vascular resistance.

The levels to which pressures are deliberately elevated to achieve maximum cardiac output should be individualized by the cardiac malformation and by observations made at the operating table relative to the pressure at which cardiac performance appeared to be best. High right atrial pressures are required to fill a right ventricle whose compliance has been diminished by severe right ventricular hypertrophy. The right ventricle in severe pulmonary stenosis or tetralogy of Fallot may require right atrial pressures up to 20–25 cm. of water for maximum filling and achievement of an adequate cardiac output. Conversely, the compliant right ventricle of a heart with atrial septal defect is usually capable of receiving large volumes of blood during diastole without a significant elevation of right atrial pressure. Therefore, following closure of an atrial septal defect, etc., a relatively modest rise in right atrial pressure to 12–15 cm. H_2O may be accompanied by elevations of left atrial pressures to 25–30 cm. H_2O and pulmonary edema because of the inability of the less compliant left ventricle to receive the unaccustomed large volume.

In the operating room immediately following cardiopulmonary by-pass, cardiac performance should be judged in relation to right atrial pressure and a reasonable idea should be formed regarding the central venous pressure at which the heart appears to achieve maximum output. This pressure should be designated as an approximate desirable level in the immediate postoperative course. The consequences of cardiac overload include pulmonary edema, as indicated above, and atrial overdistention with the production of atrial arrhythmias, interference with conduction through the atrium and a fall in cardiac output through inability of the atrium to contract and contribute actively to ventricular filling. Excessively high venous pressure may also contribute to cerebral edema or hemorrhage in a previously injured brain.

Systemic Blood Pressure Monitoring

Intra-arterial blood pressure monitoring in the postoperative period is not utilized often on our pediatric cardiac surgery service. Even though the pediatric intensive care unit should and does have the capability of such electronic monitoring, it is likely that we will continue to use it sparingly, because it is seldom necessary and because standard cuff techniques are satisfactory in most cases for determination of systemic blood pressure. Normal systolic arterial pressure in a small child may range from 80 to 120 mm. Hg. Probably the most common course for variance is in the selection of a blood pressure cuff of proper size. The width of the cuff should be approximately two-thirds the length of the upper arm. A narrower cuff will register blood pressure at higher levels; a wider cuff will register a lower than normal blood pressure.

Mild levels of hypertension – 130/80 to 140/100 – are commonly seen after closure of left-to-right shunts and after pulmonary or aortic valvulotomy. These elevated pressures seldom persist longer than 12–24 hours. Considerably more alarming to nursing and house staff, however, are the higher levels of hypertension encountered after repair of a coarctation of the aorta. Blood pressures of 150/100 are common in children aged 2 to 5, and pressures of 200 mm. Hg systolic and higher are by no means rare, particularly in patients over age 10 or 12. This hypertension does not require therapy. The higher levels usually subside within 24 hours to more moderate levels, which in turn gradually decline to mild at the time of discharge from the hospital. Blood pressure may not fall to normal values until 2 or 3 months following adequate repair of coarctation. The abdominal complications of coarctation repair – abdominal pain, distention, nausea and vomiting and, rarely, bowel necrosis – are in our judgment coincidental to the hypertension and are treated by withholding oral feedings, by nasogastric suction if necessary and, of course, by operative intervention if indicated by the peritoneal signs.

Arterial hypotension in the immediate postoperative period is usually a manifestation of low cardiac output due to hypovolemia or myocardial inadequacy or both, and treatment must be directed to an understanding of the state of reduced cardiac output. A patient who is hypovolemic with normal blood pressures solely due to blood loss is not, and should not be, commonly seen in the intensive care area. As indicated previously, deliberate measurements and estimates of blood loss are essential in children and volume replacement should be instituted for losses approximating 10–15% of the child's estimated normal blood volume. The anemic child should receive blood preoperatively or with the operative incision to assure adequate levels of oxygen-carrying capacity. Despite attention to hemostasis, occasionally a patient will bleed excessively following thoracotomy and require blood replacement or reoperation for control of bleeding.

The tolerated rate of blood loss will vary with the response of the child. A rate of up to 5–7% of estimated blood volume per hour for 3–4 hours might be tolerated in an alert child, warm and dry, who maintains an adequate blood pressure with blood replacement. This rate of loss would probably dictate a return to the operating room for a child who was less responsive or was restless, pale, with cool extremities and a low or marginal blood pressure. Whereas blood loss is relatively easy to quantitate and systemic blood pressure and venous pressure may be measured easily in an older child as guides to blood replacement, infants are considerably more difficult to evaluate. Blood pressure can and should be measured with a cuff and palpation of the radial pulse. The quality of the radial pulse is an excellent guide to blood pressure and cardiac output. Venous pressure can be judged by palpation of the liver, which quickly distends with congestive heart failure, its body firm and tense, its edge blunted. The fontanel also serves as a guide to venous pressure.

Low Cardiac Output State—Treatment

As in the adult, the low cardiac output state associated with myocardial injury and pulmonary vascular obstruction imposes the most difficult management problems in the intensive care unit. These patients typically are those with tetralogy of Fallot subjected to extensive right ventricular outflow reconstruction or repair of ventricular septal defect or of transposition of the great vessels with pulmonary hypertension. In some of these patients, systemic and pulmonary vasoconstriction during cardiopulmonary by-pass persists and is followed by a myocardial effort rendered inadequate by the operative injury. These patients leave the operating room centrally depressed, peripherally cyanotic and cold, and frequently shivering; they have rising rectal temperatures, shallow carotid and femoral pulses and frequently absent radial and pedal pulses. Central arterial pressure may be normal but pressures taken by cuff are low or even unobtainable because of the reduced peripheral blood flow. Venous pressure may be high so that needed blood replacement cannot be sustained. The principles of treatment in this situation include:

1. *Controlled ventilation.*—Not only must adequate air exchange be assured but it is equally important that the calories supplied by the compromised myocardium not be expended in the work of breathing.

2. *Reduction of peripheral resistance.*—The major factor in this resistance is vasoconstriction. We have been most impressed with the response to Thorazine given intravenously in increments of 0.05–0.1 mg./kg. of body weight and repeated at intervals of 30 minutes to 1 hour. The sedation afforded by the Thorazine is an added benefit to the child who is being maintained on a mechanical ventilator. We have been unable to document significant changes in peripheral resistance following administration of massive doses of corticosteroids.

A second significant factor in peripheral resistance is viscosity. Hematocrit levels are ideally maintained at approximately 40%. Volume replacement should be continued with whole blood when hematocrit levels are below 40% and with albumin as the hematocrit goes above 40%. Hematocrits above 50% significantly increase peripheral resistance and cardiac work and occasionally withdrawal of whole blood and replacement with albumin is productive of significant improvement in cardiac output.

3. *Maintenance of maximum myocardial performance.*—We have digitalized all children subjected to a ventriculotomy. Digitalization is begun with digoxin in the operating room immediately after discontinu-

ing cardiopulmonary by-pass. Using standard dosage schedules for parenteral digoxin, half the total digitalizing dose is given intravenously initially, an additional one-fourth is given 4–6 hours later, an additional one-eighth in another 4–6 hours after an electrocardiogram and the last one-eighth in another 4–6 hours. As long as the child shows evidences of a diminished cardiac output, all digoxin—and all other drugs, for that matter—should be given intravenously, since absorption by any other route is unreliable.

Isoproterenol, in our experience, has uniformly produced evidence of an increase in cardiac output by increasing the force of myocardial contraction relative to the accompanying increase in heart rate and by decreasing systemic and pulmonary arteriolar resistance. Dosage is titered to the response, using blood pressure for the most part as a guide to an adequate response. The drugs should be prepared as a solution containing 0.2–1.0 mg./100 ml. of 5% dextrose in water and delivered by minidrop equipment into an intravenous cannula, preferably used for no other medication. The concentration should deliver the planned response with no more than 10–15 minidrops (60 drops/ml.) per minute. In patients with diminished urinary output in the presence of a volume excess, as indicated by persistently high venous pressure and an adequate arterial pressure, diuretics—mannitol, furosemide or ethacrynic acid—should be used cautiously.

Continuing blood loss in these children is poorly tolerated. Chest x-ray should be repeated often to avoid unsuspected intrathoracic accumulation of blood. The possibility of cardiac tamponade, despite an open pericardium, should be kept in mind.

Fluid Requirements

All children are kept on nothing by mouth the day and night of operation. Moist sponges between the lips add to mouth comfort and are eagerly sought by the children.

Routine nasogastric tubes for continuous gastric decompression are unnecessary in children undergoing cardiac surgery. Rarely gastric distention may interfere with ventilation and cardiac output. We have not seen such an instance in a good many years and deplore the routine use of the tube to prevent a most unlikely occurrence.

Intravenous fluids are limited to 5% dextrose in water, administered in amounts of one-half the accepted daily requirements for normal children. The following table may be utilized:

Weight	Amounts/24 Hours
0–10 kg.	50 ml./kg.
11–20 kg.	500 ml. + 25 ml. for each kg. over 10
21 kg. and over	750 ml. + 10 ml. for each kg. over 20

This reduced fluid intake is based upon the concept that fluid is more easily added than withdrawn and that additional fluid may be ordered if the child appears dehydrated during this first postoperative day. Small increments of oral clear liquids are usually begun the morning after operation and the diet is advanced as tolerated with appropriate reduction in the intravenous fluids. In children requiring intravenous support for periods longer than 48 hours careful attention should be given to the administration of properly balanced solutions standard to pediatric care.

Acid-Base Balance

The subject of acid-base balance has been discussed in Chapter 6. It is important, however, to stress the consideration of blood gas determinations at frequent intervals in children who are ill, particularly in infants who are cyanotic or in congestive heart failure. The infant who is acidotic on a metabolic basis expends an enormous caloric output in the work of hyperventilation in the attempt to compensate by blowing off carbon dioxide. Correction of the negative base excess with sodium bicarbonate will dramatically reduce the child's respiratory effort, in addition to achieving the effects described in Chapter 6.

Sedation

Children under 10 years of age require surprisingly little medication for pain postoperatively, and it is our opinion that no standing orders for a sedative or narcotic should be written for this age group. Rather, the restless or uncomfortable child should be seen by a physician and appropriate medication ordered when he is assured that the agitation is not due to hypoxia, intrathoracic bleeding or some other disturbance in the child's clinical course. As indicated before, Thorazine is a useful drug in the restless child, but morphine, Demerol or other medication may be used as preferred in standard pediatric dosage schedules. Again, in the immediate postoperative period all medication should be given intravenously. When the child becomes completely stable, other routes of administration may be used.

Children in their teens do require pain medication and sedation and should have orders for morphine or Demerol in standard dosages for the age and weight.

Allow the parents to spend as much time as possible with the child, consistent with his care and the care of other children in the unit. I would also enter a plea that parents not be asked to help in the child's care by encouraging his coughing or deep breathing or whatever. Their time with the ill and weary child should be spent in dispensing as much tenderness and love as can be packed into the brief visiting period. Children are resilient, generous and forgiving, and hopefully the moments of affection that were displayed by the medical teams and the parents will be remembered more than the pain and the anxieties of the experience.

20

Cardiac Surgery: Adult

WILLIAM E. OSTERMILLER, JR., M.D.*

Former Fellow in Cardiovascular-Thoracic Surgery, Presbyterian-St. Luke's Hospital; Attending Surgeon, St. Joseph Hospital, Santa Ana, California; Assistant Professor of Surgery, University of California College of Medicine (Irvine)

HUSHANG JAVID, M.D., Ph.D.

Attending Surgeon, Rush-Presbyterian-St. Luke's Medical Center; Professor of Surgery, Rush Medical College

AND

ORMAND C. JULIAN, M.D.

Attending Surgeon and Chairman, Department of Cardiovascular-Thoracic Surgery, Rush-Presbyterian-St. Luke's Medical Center; Professor of Surgery, Rush Medical College

INTENSIVE CARE MANAGEMENT

THE DECREASING MORTALITY and morbidity associated with cardiac surgery over the past decade can be attributed to improvements in the training of personnel who care for the cardiac patient, technologic advances in patient monitoring and better understanding of the physiology and pathophysiology of the surgical patient. The intensive care unit has been established to foster this progress.

The team approach is mandatory to the successful management of the patient having cardiac surgery. The more experience the team has,

*Supported in part by United States Public Health Service Grant No. 1T12HE05808.

the smoother its operation will be. Because of periodic turnover of members of the team, these guidelines in management and protocol are presented to help facilitate that period of transition.

Physical Equipment

The physical plant should contain certain basic electronic equipment to measure physiologic parameters necessary in the routine care of these patients. Adquate space is mandatory to permit the placement of electronic equipment and still leave sufficient room for basic nursing care.

MONITORING.—*Electrical activity of the heart.*—The electrocardiograph is connected by paste-on leads and is continuously monitored on an oscilloscope until the patient is stable. Write-out tracings should be available on instant demand.

Arterial blood pressure.—The sphygmomanometer is used in conjunction with a direct arterial pressure, the latter being used mainly during the first 12 hours postoperatively. The arterial catheter is positioned in the operating room. The catheter is kept patent by frequent flushing and proper positioning of the patient's arm. It can be useful for more than 24 hours in most instances. Routes for direct arterial pressure include the ulnar, radial, brachial and internal mammary arteries. It is especially important that all components attached to the arterial and venous monitoring lines be sterile.

Atrial and central venous pressure.—The central venous pressure catheter is placed into a peripheral vein and threaded into a central intrathoracic venous channel. Important factors in technique are: maintain strict sterility; utilize large bore (19 gauge) tubing; be certain that the tip is not against the wall or valve of the vein; use a blunt-tipped catheter and do not force it. Catheters can be placed: by percutaneous puncture of the subclavian or antecubital veins; by cutdown of the external jugular, antecubital or cephalic vein, or by direct right atrial placement at time of surgery.

The *left atrial pressure* is helpful when the right atrial pressure does not reflect the pressure in the left atrium. The left atrial pressure is an index of the function of the left ventricle and its end diastolic pressure in the presence of a normally functioning mitral valve. The oscilloscopic pressure curves from the left atrial catheter are also useful in determining obstruction or incompetence of the mitral valve.

Electrolytes and blood gases.—Apparatus for rapid analysis is situated nearby.

VENTILATION.—Equipment should include an adequate selection of endotracheal tubes, connectors, a hand ventilator bag, a respirator, sterile suction equipment, a laryngoscope and a tracheostomy set.

RESUSCITATION CART.—The success of resuscitation depends upon prompt recognition and treatment of the catastrophe. The resuscitation cart should include a defibrillator, the essential medications outlined here, a hard board on which the patient can be placed for closed chest massage, and instruments required for intubation of the trachea and manual ventilation. The direct-current cardiac defibrillator should be in usable condition and all equipment and medications readily located. The minimum list of drugs to be stocked includes:

	Concentration	How Supplied
1. Autonomic blocking agents		
a) Atropine sulfate	0.4 mg./ml.	20 ml. vial
b) Chlorpromazine hydrochloride (Thorazine)	25 mg./ml.	1 ml. amp.
2. Cardiac drugs		
a) Digoxin	0.25 mg./ml.	2 ml. amp.
Digoxin *pediatric*	0.1 mg./ml.	1 ml. amp.
b) Deslanoside (Cedilanid-D)	0.2 mg./ml.	2 ml. amp.
c) Ouabain	0.25 mg./ml.	2 ml. amp.
d) Quinidine gluconate	80 mg./ml.	10 ml. vial
Quinidine sulfate	100 mg./ml.	2 ml. amp.
e) Procainamide (Pronestyl)	100 mg./ml.	10 ml. oral
f) Procaine hydrochloride	10 mg./ml.	30 ml. vial
g) Diphenylhydantoin sodium	50 mg./ml.	2 ml. (100 mg.) 5 ml. (250 mg.) } Steri-Vial
h) Propranolol hydrochloride (Inderal)	1 mg./ml.	1 ml. amp.
i) Lidocaine hydrochloride (Xylocaine)	10 mg./ml. 20 mg./ml.	50 ml. vial 50 ml. vial
3. Sympathomimetic drugs		
a) Epinephrine (Adrenalin hydrochloride) 1:1,000	1 mg./ml.	1 ml. amp.
Epinephrine suspension (Adrenalin in oil)	2 mg./ml.	1 ml. amp.
b) Norepinephrine (Levophed)	1 mg./ml.	4 ml. amp.
c) Ephedrine sulfate	50 mg./ml.	1 ml. amp.
d) Aramine (Metaraminol bitartrate)	10 mg./ml.	1 ml. amp. 10 ml. vial
e) Mephentermine sulfate (Wyamine sulfate)	15 mg./ml.	1 ml. vial
f) Isoproterenol hydrochloride (Isuprel)	0.2 mg./ml.	1 ml. amp. 5 ml. amp.
g) Phenylephrine hydrochloride (Neo-Synephrine)	10 mg./ml.	1 ml. amp. 5 ml. vial
4. Miscellaneous		
a) Sodium bicarbonate 7.5%	44.6 mEq./50ml.	50 ml. amp.
b) Calcium chloride	100 mg./ml.	10 ml. amp.
Calcium gluconate	100 mg./ml.	10 ml. amp.
c) Magnesium sulfate 10%	100 mg./ml. (16.2 mEq./20 ml.)	20 ml. amp.
50%	1 gm./ml.	2 ml. amp.

d) Vitamin K_1 (AquaMephyton)	10 mg./ml.	1 ml. amp. 5 ml. vial
e) Heparin	1000 units/ml.	1 ml. amp. 10 ml. vial
	5000 units/ml.	1 ml. amp. 10 ml. vial
	10,000 units/ml.	4 ml. vial
f) Aminocaproic acid (Amicar)	250 mg./ml.	20 ml. vial
g) Protamine sulfate	10 mg./ml.	5 ml. amp.
h) Corticosteroids		
Solu-Cortef	50 mg./ml.	2 ml. vial
	125 mg./ml.	2 ml. vial
Solu-Medrol	40 mg./ml.	1 ml. vial
	62.5 mg./ml.	2 ml. vial
i) Aminophylline	25 mg./ml.	10 ml. amp. 20 ml. amp.
	250 mg./ml.	2 ml. amp.
j) Sodium amytal		125 mg. amp. 250 mg. amp. 500 mg. amp.
k) Valium	5 mg./ml.	2 ml. amp.
l) Mannitol	250 mg./ml.	50 ml. amp.
m) Furosemide (Lasix)	10 mg./ml.	2 ml. amp.
n) Sodium ethacrynate (Edecrin)	1 mg./ml.	50 ml. vial

Preoperative Planning

The patient is usually evaluated in the hospital from 2 to 7 days before surgery, depending on the severity of the illness. During this period, baseline physiologic parameters are obtained with the following: (1) a complete blood count (CBC) and urinalysis; (2) serum electrolytes and blood urea nitrogen (BUN); (3) a barium-swallow 4-view chest x-ray; (4) an electrocardiogram; (5) hematologic and clotting survey, including a prothrombin time, clotting time, partial thromboplastin time, platelet count, euglobulin lysis, fibrinolysis and serum fibrinogen levels; (6) major and minor group blood typing; (7) assessment of pulmonary function (a thorough evaluation is performed when impaired function from primary or secondary pulmonary pathology is present); (8) renal function tests (if an abnormality exists in the urinalysis or if the BUN is elevated, the renal function is studied in more detail); (9) liver function tests (liver function is evaluated when there is clinical evidence of hepatic dysfunction; this is generally prehepatic in origin. When primary hepatic disease is present, operation is deferred, if possible, until liver function returns to normal). (10) The psychologic status of the patient is evaluated and special care is taken to alleviate apprehension and correct misinformation.

An important aspect of the preoperative training of the patient is done by a nursing member of the team. This professional complement interviews the patient several days before surgery, explains procedural and environmental aspects of the intensive care unit and establishes rapport (see Chapter 15). The nurse assists in the care of the patient during his stay in the intensive care unit.

The countdown to heart surgery is initiated several days prior to the event. The patient is instructed in breathing with a positive pressure device, is taught to cough effectively and is shown diagrams and pictures of the equipment which will be integral to his care in the postoperative period. Two days before surgery digitalis is discontinued. Potassium supplements are intensified, particularly in the depleted patient. Soap showers are taken several times daily and the night before surgery, a depilatory is applied. Twelve hours prior to surgery, the patient is started on 4 Gm. methicillin by intravenous rider every 6 hours.

Patient Monitoring

Operating Room

The arterial and venous pressure, electroencephalogram and electrocardiogram are continuously monitored during surgery, particularly when cardiopulmonary by-pass is used. Frequent acid-base and electrolyte determinations are made. These, in conjunction with the pulse rate, urine output and rectal temperature, are used to determine the physiologic status of the patient.

A large diuresis of water and electrolytes occurs, particularly when a nonblood hemodilution prime is used. The acid-base level is adjusted as necessary; 40–100 mEq. of potassium replacement is usually required during the operative procedure. Cardiac medications are utilized as required throughout the operative period.

Prior to termination of by-pass most of the blood in the oxygenator is reinfused in an attempt to re-establish adequate central and peripheral perfusion. The degree of vasoconstriction is proportional to the length of cardiopulmonary by-pass. Additional blood and peripheral vasodilators may be needed to improve the peripheral circulation. The patient is kept in the operating room until stable to allow safe transfer to the intensive care unit. This may require additional time, during which appropriate treatment is accomplished. Fatal incidents are more apt to occur if the patient is unstable prior to transfer.

The patient is transferred in the bed which he will occupy for the next several days. The endotracheal tube is in place and the anesthetist ventilates the patient during transfer, utilizing a manual breathing bag.

The surgical team assists in the movement of the patient while attending urinary, chest, intravenous and arterial catheters. Palpation of a major artery during transfer gives valuable information regarding the pulse and blood pressure. Prior to the patient's arrival in the intensive therapy unit, arterial and venous transducers are adjusted and the electrocardiogram is made ready for monitoring.

Intensive Care Unit

Clinical observation.—The most important aspect of the care of the postoperative patient is the moment-to-moment bedside clinical evaluation. A general assessment of condition can be accomplished while the patient is being attached to the monitoring devices.

Ventilation.—This is the first order of priority. During transport to the intensive care unit with an endotracheal tube in place, the patient is usually overventilated. The resultant hypocarbia and apnea allow for easier transition to respirator ventilation. Anoxia can result if ventilation is left unattended. If spontaneous respiration is present prior to placement on the respirator, the ventilator is set at a higher than usual minute volume, thereby accomplishing the same purpose. Occasionally the endotracheal tube may slip into a main bronchus, ventilating only one lung. Comparison of expansion of each side of the chest, auscultation of the lungs and the position of the tube on chest x-ray confirm the location.

Postoperative mechanical ventilation is continued for variable periods. In the good-risk patient without complications, extubation can be accomplished soon after surgery. If the opposite is true, mechanical assistance may be prolonged, on occasion, several weeks. Most patients are assisted for 6 or 8 hours, after which they are weaned away from the respirator and extubated within 12 hours. In general, it is poor practice to remove an endotracheal tube during the night shift.

The ventilator used is optional, but the one preferred by us is a volume respirator. An endotracheal or tracheostomy tube without an inflated cuff is used to produce an open system. Ventilation of the lung can be checked by observing expansion of the chest and by auscultation of breath sounds. Once hypocarbia (manifested by lack of respiratory effort) is induced, the ventilation is decreased to allow unimpaired ventilation without producing severe respiratory alkalosis. The color of the skin and mucous membranes, the cooperation of the patient and the expansion of the chest, in most instances, provide information as to the adequacy of oxygenation.

Oxygen should be discontinued (oxygen administration rarely exceeds 10 L./minute and should average 2–5 L./minute) prior to weaning the patient from the respirator. The patient is allowed to breathe off the respirator for increasing increments of time. During these periods he is observed to see how well he can ventilate on his own and whether he is able to maintain an arterial oxygen saturation greater than 90%. If these criteria are met, the tube is removed. A laryngoscope and a sterile endotracheal tube are kept nearby in case reintubation is needed. The tracheobronchial tree and oropharynx are suctioned before and after removal of the tube. Following extubation the patient is placed in a humidified oxygen environment and encouraged to cough frequently.

Circulatory assessment.—Circulatory distress may be present even when a normal central blood pressure is recorded. The quality of the peripheral pulses, the warmth of the extremities, capillary filling and color of the skin indicate the adequacy of peripheral perfusion. The urine output, body temperature and state of consciousness are further indicators. Early correction of hypovolemia, poor perfusion and acidosis serves to minimize the later sequelae of these conditions.

Central nervous system and renal evaluation.—Following ventilatory and circulatory assessments, other parameters can be quickly and thoroughly evaluated. The state of consciousness, the motor and sensory function, pupillary position and response and the presence of pathologic reflexes will affirm the presence or absence of central nervous system damage.

Kidney function is evaluated by the volume and concentration of the urine. The urine output usually is in excess of 100 ml./hour in the early postoperative period, particularly following hemodilution cardiopulmonary by-pass.

MONITORING OF THE PATIENT.—Although there is no substitute for experienced clinical evaluation, the measurement of physiologic parameters is necessary to follow the postoperative cardiac patient. These measurements include the arterial, central venous and left atrial pressures, the electrocardiogram, urine output, fluid balance, arterial gas studies, acid-base and electrolyte determinations, body temperature and chest drainage. Other measurements occasionally recorded are general laboratory measurements such as bleeding and clotting factors, renal and liver function tests, blood volume measurements and cardiac output. Daily chest x-rays and electrocardiograms are routine.

Arterial pressure.—Continuous monitoring of the arterial pressure is one of the most valuable parameters available during and after surgery. The level of the pressure and the slope of the curve help to detect changes in cardiac output and peripheral resistance.

The arterial cannula is usually placed in the ulnar or radial artery percutaneously or by cutdown prior to surgery. The extremity used for monitoring depends upon the procedure planned and coexistent disease. If severe arteriosclerosis is present without a suitable peripheral vessel available for cannulation, more central arteries may be utilized. When resection of a descending thoracic aortic aneurysm is contemplated, the right arm is used for cannulation, whereas for resection of an ascending aortic aneurysm the left arm is used. This is because the subclavian artery on the side of the aneurysm may require partial or total occlusion, thereby impairing an ipsilateral arterial measurement. Similar conditions occur when performing a subclavian-pulmonary artery shunt. For this reason arch aneurysm operations require lower extremity arterial cannulation. The side opposite the one used for cardiac catheterization is routinely cannulated; if both sides have been used, the better one is utilized or an alternate site is chosen.

The length of time the catheter is patent is directly related to the frequency of irrigation. An irrigation of heparinized solution (5–10 ml.) every 30 minutes is generally enough to keep the cannula patent for 12–24 hours. When direct arterial pressure measurement is no longer needed, the cannula is removed and firm pressure is applied to the entry site for 5–10 minutes. Hemorrhage following removal of the catheter is uncommon.

Central venous pressure.—The central venous pressure measurement is an indicator of cardiac performance and volume load, thereby aiding in the diagnosis and treatment of abnormal circulatory states.[8] It is important to have a continuous reading of the central venous pressure to evaluate the response of the heart to a fluid load and to various medications, and to compare this value with the cardiac output and peripheral perfusion.

A catheter of adequate caliber (14–18 gauge) is placed in a central vein within the thorax. The catheter can be introduced percutaneously or by cutdown into the antecubital or external jugular veins, or by subclavian puncture. The zero point of the central venous pressure measurement is placed at the mid-right atrial level, which corresponds approximately to the anterior axillary line in the fourth intercostal space. An unusually high or low reading in itself can be helpful. The usual normal central venous pressure is from 5 to 12 cm. of water. A very low central venous pressure indicates volume depletion, whereas a high venous pressure may indicate volume overload or cardiac failure. Other causes for high central venous pressure include: (1) placement of the catheter into the right ventricle, or tricuspid insufficiency (fluctuation with the heart beat); (2) impingement of the catheter against a valve or vein wall (little or no fluctuation with respiration); (3) an inaccurate zero level.

Patency is maintained with a very slow infusion of heparinized solution (150–200 ml./24 hours). Antibiotic ointment is applied to the entry site to decrease the incidence of infection. These catheters have remained in place for as long as a week; however, the infection rate is minimal if they are removed within 48 hours. If long-term central venous measurement is required, a percutaneous subclavian venous catheter is the most likely to remain patent and least likely to become infected.

Left atrial pressure.—Although not utilized in every patient, measurement of the left atrial pressure is of great value in the postoperative management of the critically ill cardiac patient. Left atrial pressure is helpful in the assessment of blood volume and the functional capacity of the left ventricle. The left atrial pressure reflects the filling pressure of the left ventricle when the mitral valve is normal.[3] Information obtained from the left atrial catheter includes:

1. Assessment of volume. A low left atrial pressure may be due to hypovolemia or the inability of blood to reach the left atrium. Causes of the latter condition include elevated pulmonary vascular resistance, poor right ventricular compliance and mechanical obstruction of the right side of the heart. Treatment is directed toward increasing the filling pressure, improving the function of the right ventricle or removing the obstruction. An elevated left atrial pressure can be due to hypervolemia, poor left ventricular compliance, or incompetence or stenosis of the mitral valve.

2. Compliance of the left ventricle. Elevated left ventricular end diastolic pressure secondary to heart failure or decreased compliance can cause the low output syndrome. Therefore, higher filling pressures are needed to support adequate cardiac output in such conditions. The elevated left atrial pressure is transmitted to the right side, causing a concomitant elevation of the central venous pressure.

3. Cardiac tamponade. Patients who have cardiac tamponade characteristically demonstrate an elevation of the right atrial pressure to equal the left atrial pressure, which remains static. These pressure curves may be helpful in the differential diagnosis and treatment of low cardiac output.[6]

4. Status of the mitral valve. The postoperative function of the mitral valve can be evaluated by inspection of left atrial pressure tracings. Controlled left atrial hypertension may be helpful in the treatment of low cardiac output, while keeping the pressure below the level of pulmonary edema (35–40 cm. of water).[6] Special care is taken to prevent emboli due to injection of clot or air into the left atrium.

Electrocardiogram.—The electrocardiogram is monitored until the patient is electrically stable. Lead 2 is generally preferred. Oscilloscopic and direct writer tracings aid in the detection of arrhythmias, which occur most commonly in the first 24 hours. Most often serious arrhythmias may be prevented by early treatment of their precursors. A standard electrocardiogram is taken once daily.

Temporary pacing wires are attached to the right ventricle and atrium and either atrial or ventricular pacing is utilized, depending on the need. The pacing wires and a salt bridge to the right or left atrial catheter can also be used to obtain special tracings.

Ventilation.—The patient is ventilated at a fixed rate according to physiologic requirement. Oxygen is administered in a 20–40% mixture in the early postoperative period. The ventilation status is assessed by clinical evaluation, arterial oxygen and carbon dioxide content and the acid-base status.

Urine output.—Although a simple measurement, the hourly urine output is one of the most accurate parameters of perfusion if renal function is normal. Serial monitoring of the specific gravity, osmolarity, blood urea nitrogen, serum and urine creatinine and urine sodium and potassium concentrations help to measure renal function or its rate of improvement following renal damage. Although circulating antidiuretic hormone and aldosterone serum levels are usually elevated following surgical trauma, the hemodynamic improvement ordinarily results in a paradoxical increase in urine output as compared with the preoperative volume.

Fluid balance and chest drainage.—Despite accurate recording of fluid balance, the need for additional volume is predicated more on evaluation of the clinical status and physiologic parameters. An accurate record of fluid intake and output is kept hourly and the adult patient is limited to approximately 1,500 ml. of fluid intake daily. Low left and right atrial pressures, decreased urinary output and cool, cyanotic extremities with poor pulses indicate hypovolemia. If a normovolemic patient with a low cardiac output has a poorly compliant ventricle or increased pulmonary or peripheral vascular resistance, further volume may be needed. As gradual postoperative vasodilation takes place, additional increments may be required.

The drainage of the chest catheter is carefully followed and blood is replaced at the same rate that it is lost. In the routine postoperative patient, periodic stripping of the chest tubes is necessary to decrease clotting of the tubes. If persistent milking of the tubes does not clear the line of liquid blood, continuous significant bleeding is probable. If there is excess drainage, reoperation will be necessary. The chest tubes are usually removed within 36 hours, at which time oral intake usually replaces intravenous fluid.

Chest x-ray.—A portable chest x-ray taken prior to surgery can be used to compare the size of the heart in postoperative chest x-rays if the same distance from the x-ray tube to the patient is maintained. A chest x-ray is taken in a semi-upright position shortly after the patient arrives in the intensive care unit. Factors to be checked on the film are the placement of the chest tubes, expansion of the lung, size of the heart and the location of the endotracheal tube and central venous catheter (Chapter 14). Serial x-rays are taken as needed, usually at least once daily. On occasion metal clips are placed on the heart and adjacent pericardium in such a manner as to be useful in the diagnosis of cardiac tamponade. All chest x-rays on intensive care patients are filed in the intensive care unit so that comparisons can be made when needed.

Acid-base balance and electrolytes.—Acid-base levels and serum electrolytes are monitored during surgery and at intervals thereafter. In the intensive care unit determinations are made shortly after stabilization on the ventilator and 1–2 hours later. In normal perfusion states with assisted ventilation, a mild respiratory alkalosis will persist throughout the early postsurgical period. The resultant hypocarbia abolishes the respiratory drive and permits controlled ventilation. A mild respiratory alkalosis is well tolerated and presents no hazard to acid-base compensation.

Metabolic acidosis requires immediate correction. This is directed at improvement of cardiac output, reduction of peripheral resistance and administration of bicarbonate. One ampule of sodium bicarbonate (44 mEq.) is given slowly intravenously for every 2 mEq./L. base deficit, but no more than 4 ampules (176 mEq.) are given prior to redetermination of the base deficit. If a large amount of bicarbonate is required or if the serum sodium is over 150 mEq./L., an artificial buffer (tromethamine) may be used. The amount administered will depend on the severity of acidosis, but should not exceed a total dose of 500 mg./kg. This buffer is avoided in the presence of renal failure. Serial acid-base determinations will guide total dosage.

Serum electrolytes are also measured at frequent intervals. Potassium depletion is the most common electrolyte abnormality which occurs during and following cardiopulmonary by-pass. Factors influencing this depletion are: (1) the use of diuretics; (2) hemodilution cardiopulmonary by-pass; (3) insufficient potassium supplementation, and (4) increased losses secondary to respiratory alkalosis (Fig. 20-1). Hypokalemia in the digitalized patient predisposes to cardiac arrhythmias and impairs cardiac function.

The following regimen decreases the likelihood of potassium depletion and its complications: (1) routine potassium administration in patients on diuretics; (2) increased oral or intravenous supplements if deficits exist or if further diuresis is required; (3) replacement of losses during and after surgery. The urine volume, along with serial serum and urine potassium measurements, guides the rate of administration. During surgery 60–100 mEq. of potassium are routinely required. After surgery administration should be equal to losses but not exceed 40–60 mEq./hour. Excessive losses may be reduced by spironolactone (Chapter 13).

The potassium balance averaged in 20 patients (Fig. 20-2) reflects the importance of potassium monitoring. Hyperkalemia in excess of 6 mEq./L. in the presence of renal failure requires aggressive therapy (Chapter 9). This includes: (1) exchange resins – sodium polystyrene sulfonate, 30 Gm. rectally once or twice daily (adults); (2) insulin plus a hyperosmolar sugar solution; (3) dialysis – peritoneal lavage or hemodialysis, and (4) sodium bicarbonate.

The serum sodium is often low in the postoperative cardiac patient

Fig. 20-1. – Factors which are responsible for potassium balance.

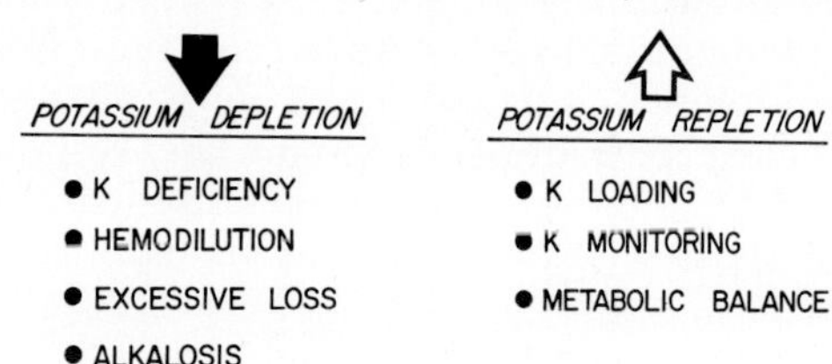

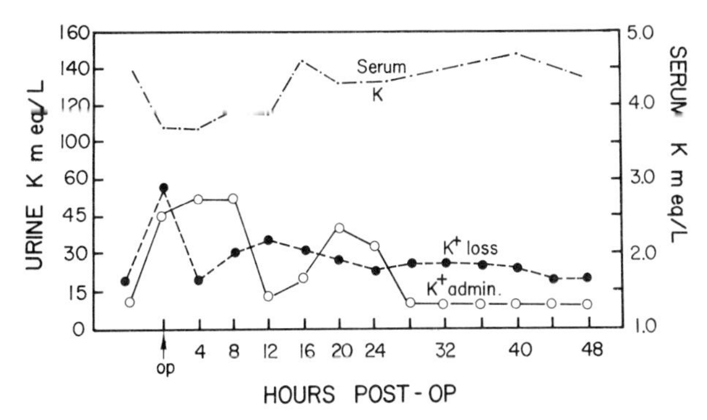

Fig. 20-2.—Potassium loss, administration and serum levels: average in 20 patients during and following open heart surgery.

because of chronic sodium restriction, hemodilution by-pass and postoperative dilutional hyponatremia. Hyponatremia does not require treatment unless the serum sodium drops below 120 mEq./L. Diuresis and fluid restriction usually correct the dilutional hyponatremia. Strict sodium restriction precludes intravenous salt solutions and allows only a 500–1,000 mg. sodium diet in the postsurgical period. Hypernatremia may develop when large amounts of sodium-containing solutions are used for cardiopulmonary by-pass or are administered in the treatment of acidosis.

The serum calcium is determined postoperatively, and hypocalcemia is routinely considered as a cause of poor myocardial function. Hypocalcemia may be dilutional or related to alkalosis or to infusion of citrated blood. Slow intravenous infusion of 500–1,000 mg. of calcium chloride corrects this condition.

Magnesium deficiency may occur in chronically ill patients on prolonged intravenous therapy. The symptoms and signs may simulate those of hypocalcemia. The usual dose is 50 mEq. magnesium sulfate administered intravenously over 4–6 hours.

Blood volume.—Blood volume studies following cardiopulmonary by-pass are not reliable. During this period, however, the chromium-labeled red cell determination gives more accurate results than RISA.

Cardiac output.—Cardiac output studies are not routinely done in the postoperative period. The output of the heart can be fairly well assessed by the measurements previously described.

Coagulation studies.—A preoperative coagulation survey is done on all patients and deficiences are corrected prior to surgery. If bleeding problems occur during or after surgery, the survey is repeated to include a clotting time, platelet count, fibrinolysin and euglobulin lysis levels, plasma fibrinogen concentration, prothrombin consumption, partial thromboplastin time and prothrombin estimation. Often several factors are deficient.

Other tests.—Baseline evaluation of hepatic and renal function and measurement of various serum enzymes are also obtained.

Computerized monitoring.—Many centers are now using computers to record, store and feed back data. This increase in efficiency serves to guide patient care rather than to substitute for clinical examination.

RECOGNITION AND TREATMENT OF COMPLICATIONS

Complications which follow heart surgery may be related to preexisting disease, a complication of surgery or errors in postoperative management. In many cases several factors are implicated.

Postoperative Hemorrhage

Postoperative bleeding is due to inadequate hemostasis or to defects in the coagulation mechanism.

Bleeding from a systemic vessel or cardiac chamber is unlikely to stop without reoperation. Sites usually involved are intercostal vessels, cardiotomy wounds and great vessels. Reoperation for bleeding following cardiopulmonary by-pass is necessary in from 5 to 7% of patients.

The following are indications for re-exploration.

1. If bleeding is exigent, the patient is promptly returned to the operating room.

2. Blood loss of 150–200 ml./hour for 4–6 hours signifies serious bleeding which is often from a specific site(s). Continued blood loss at this rate without operative intervention can result in hemothorax, pericardial tamponade or transfusion coagulopathy.

3. Blood loss of 100 ml./hour for 10–12 hours, particularly if there is no downward trend or if hemothorax occurs, is also an indication for re-exploration. Even after cessation of bleeding, any significant hemothorax should be evacuated if the patient is in satisfactory condition to tolerate another procedure. Removal of blood results in immediate improvement in pulmonary function and minimizes the likelihood of captive lung and empyema.

COAGULOPATHY.—Patients most prone to develop clotting problems are those who have:

1. A previous history of clotting deficiency.
2. An abnormality on clotting survey.
3. Cyanotic congenital heart disease, particularly with evidence that elevated circulating fibrinolysins are present.
4. A prolonged pump time, which often causes sequestration and destruction of platelets, hemodilution of clotting factors and elevation of circulating fibrinolysins.

5. Inadequate heparin neutralization. From 50 to 100% of the total heparin dose is reversed with protamine sulfate. The total dose of heparin used during by-pass depends on the length of by-pass but averages 4–5 mg./kg. Protamine should not be administered in excess of 2 mg./1 mg. of heparin or antithrombin factors can be a cause of bleeding.

6. Liver disease. Prothrombin and fibrinogen are depressed.

7. Renal disease.

8. Multiple transfusions. Acid citrate dextrose (ACD) blood, particularly if 2 or 3 weeks old, is deficient in platelets and most clotting factors.

Recognition and treatment of coagulation defects are outlined in Chapter 8.

Cardiac-Related Complications

Postoperative cardiac problems are categorized into technical complications, the low cardiac output syndrome, congestive heart failure, myocardial ischemia and cardiac arrhythmias.

Technical Complications

Bleeding.—Technical causes of postoperative hemorrhage include bleeding vessels, leaking suture lines and rupture of surgically thinned myocardium. Frequently hemorrhage is not manifest until the blood pressure reaches or exceeds the level present when closing. Common sites of suture line bleeding are: (1) the aortic root, (2) ventricular vent wounds and (3) ventriculotomy and atriotomy sites. Rupture of thinned myocardium may follow debridement of a calcific mitral valve leaflet or excess resection of infundibular stenosis.

Bleeding into the pericardial sac can cause pericardial tamponade. The impaired venous return results in hypotension, decreased pulse pressure and increased venous pressure. A paradoxical pulse of greater than 10 mm. Hg is usually present. The paradoxical pulse is difficult to diagnose while the patient is on the respirator.

Sudden cessation of bleeding after moderate to severe bleeding via the chest tubes suggests accumulation within the pericardium or thorax. Enlargement of the mediastinum on the chest x-ray assists in the diagnosis of tamponade (see Fig. 14-4, *B*). It may be difficult to differentiate acute heart failure from cardiac tamponade. With tamponade the venous pressure tends to rise more rapidly and to higher levels, particularly in the upper extremities. The presence of pulsus paradoxus and the tendency to occur in association with excessive drainage from the chest tubes add further confirmation. Heart failure is more apt to develop slowly and to have an element of pulmonary edema and is accompanied by hypervolemia. Cardiac tamponade requires immediate reoperation.

Heart block.—Surgically induced heart block is usually temporary and can occur up to 48 hours or more after surgery. Temporary conduction defects are caused by suturing or removal of tissue near the bundle or its branches, resulting in edema or hemorrhage with subsequent temporary atrioventricular or bundle branch block. Permanent heart block is caused by: (1) encirclement of the conduction system with a suture; (2) transection of the bundle or its branches and (3) impingement of a rigid prosthesis on the conduction system.

Heart block which occurs during surgery is readily recognized. If it occurs during the placement of a suture in the beating heart, removal of the suture may immediately restore conduction. Often sutures are placed while the heart is fibrillating and conduction dysfunction is not apparent until after defibrillation or for several days. For this reason, temporary pacing wires are routinely employed. When necessary, permanent pacing electrodes are implanted.

PROSTHETIC VALVE DYSFUNCTION.—Dysfunction is caused by: (1) obstruction to opening of the valve; (2) ball valve dislodgment and (3) failure of the ball valve to seat properly. A poorly functioning prosthetic valve is often related to a technical error. Placement of a large prosthesis in a narrow aortic root or small ventricular chamber can impair forward flow. Low cardiac output or arrhythmias may result, often preventing disconnection from extracorporeal support. Failure to remove papillary muscles and chordae tendineae, inadequate resection of valve tissue or foreign bodies in the heart can also impair valve function. Formation of blood clots on the valve leads to hemodynamic abnormalities and distal emboli. Ball valve variance is unlikely to occur in newer valves.

MYOCARDIAL INFARCTION.—Most commonly myocardial infarction following open heart surgery is related to coronary atherosclerosis. However, technical factors can cause coronary artery injury and myocardial damage. Damage can be produced by the following mechanisms: (1) ligature occlusion of an artery; (2) laceration of the coronary artery causing a coronary-cardiac fistula; (3) damage to or obstruction of the coronary ostia, and (4) embolization. The coronary artery can be damaged by a suture during replacement of both the aortic and mitral valves. These injuries are infrequent and are optimally repaired at the same operation. Coronary-cardiac fistulae usually occur following ventriculotomy. Impairment to coronary circulation during or following extracorporeal by-pass can be caused by intimal disruption and emboli of air, fibrin or calcific debris. The prosthetic valve rim may obstruct the coronary ostia.

Subendocardial necrosis.—The etiology of subendocardial infarction following open heart surgery is not known. It differs from myocardial infarction secondary to coronary artery occlusion in that it is subendocardial in location and does not follow the coronary artery distribution. This entity can occasionally be recognized in the postoperative period. It is characterized by cardiac arrhythmias, particularly of ventricular origin, and the low output syndrome. The electrocardiogram may show evidence of subendocardial ischemia or infarction. Postoperative mortality is probably related to the degree of myocardium involved.

CONGESTIVE HEART FAILURE. – Surgically induced congestive heart failure is much less common than that due to inherent cardiac disease. The degree of pre-existing disease in the myocardium determines how readily it can withstand surgical trauma. Congestive heart failure can be due to (1) the production of a new hemodynamic abnormality or (2) failure to correct existing cardiac pathology.

Production of a new hemodynamic abnormality can result from: (1) mitral insufficiency following mitral commissurotomy; (2) left ventricular outflow obstruction from a large mitral prosthesis or aortic outflow obstruction from an aortic prosthesis; (3) breakdown of an annuloplasty; (4) perivalvular leak, and (5) shunting of blood following closure of a septal defect.

Congestive heart failure may develop postoperatively because of the insult of surgical trauma added to an already compromised heart. Some of the more common instances of failure to correct existing cardiac pathology are: (1) failure to open the mitral valve at closed mitral commissurotomy; (2) replacement of only one valve when other significant valvular pathology is present; (3) failure to correct aortic insufficiency during resection of an ascending aortic aneurysm, and (4) inadequate resection of nonfunctional tissue in a ventricular aneurysmorrhaphy.

The onset of congestive heart failure secondary to surgically related causes is variable. If the hemodynamic abnormality is severe and the cardiac reserve limited, the onset may be rapid and unremitting. If failure can be controlled during the early postoperative period, surgical correction can be deferred until a more optimal time. In the presence of severe hemodynamic abnormalities and unremitting failure, early operative repair is mandatory.

Low Cardiac Output Syndrome

Intrinsic myocardial disease is the commonest cause of poor myocardial contractility. This often is the result of long-standing uncorrected cardiac disease from coronary insufficiency, hemodynamic abnormalities, metabolic imbalance, congenital heart disease or myocardiopathy. The addition of surgical trauma to an already diseased myocardium can result in the low output state. Further, uncorrected pathology or production of new lesions also cause low output. The following is a list of conditions which can cause the low output syndrome.

Anatomic Abnormalities

Inadequate repair of cardiac defects (pulmonary or aortic stenosis)
Obstruction of the left ventricular or aortic outflow tract after valve replacement
Ventricular septal obstruction of the outflow tract after repair of tetralogy of Fallot

Inadequate function of a poorly developed ventricle after shunt repair
Clotting of a prosthetic valve

Physiologic Abnormalities

Metabolic aberrations. Acid-base and electrolyte imbalance can impair cardiac function. Acidosis, hypocalcemia and hyperkalemia can decrease the effectiveness of myocardial contraction.

Arrhythmias. Ventricular arrhythmias severely impair cardiac output. A decrease in ventricular filling can result from tachycardia and uncoordinated atrioventricular contractions. Bradycardia (particularly less than 50/minute) can also result in a low cardiac output.

Anoxia. There are many causes of myocardial ischemia. The commonest are coronary insufficiency, inadequate coronary perfusion and inadequate ventilation or pulmonary perfusion.

Decrease in ventricular compliance. Long-standing heart disease, either from congenital or acquired pathology, produces changes in the ventricle to alter its compliance.

Pulmonary hypertension. Elevated pulmonary vascular resistance leads to decreased flow to the left heart.

Clinical manifestations.—The clinical appearance of this syndrome is that of poor perfusion, manifested by generalized vasoconstriction and cold, cyanotic, pulseless extremities. Associated findings include an elevated central venous pressure, a decreased pulse pressure, anuria or oliguria, poor cerebration and decreased cardiac output. The arterial blood pressure is probably one of the least reliable parameters. Hypotension is an indication of advanced deterioration. Arrhythmias and metabolic and electrolyte imbalance are often secondary to low cardiac output and, in turn, precipitate a vicious cycle leading to pulmonary edema, ventricular fibrillation and death.

The longer the delay in treatment of the low output syndrome, the less the chance of reversal. Patients untreated for 4–6 hours often will not respond to treatment. If there is no response to early treatment over the first 6 hours, the low output state is usually irreversible.

Treatment.—Treatment is aimed at improving cardiac output, reducing peripheral vascular resistance and correcting metabolic deficits. Attention should be paid to:

1. Correction of technical abnormalities.
2. Evacuation of pericardial tamponade.
3. Correction of metabolic imbalance. Sodium bicarbonate or other buffering agents can be used for this purpose.
4. Correction of electrolyte imbalance. Potassium and calcium deficiencies impair cardiac output. Potassium chloride can be given in intravenous rider solutions of up to 60 mEq./hour. Calcium chloride is given as an intravenous bolus of 500–1,000 mg. over 5 minutes. Rapid administration of either may result in cardiac arrest.
5. Correction of arrhythmias. Arrhythmias may be caused by hypoxia, electrolyte imbalance, myocardial infarction, mechanical trauma

or metabolic deficits. Treatment of arrhythmias is incomplete without attention to the underlying cause.

6. Decrease in peripheral resistance. Peripheral vasodilators decrease peripheral resistance and increase perfusion while decreasing cardiac work and oxygen consumption. Although peripheral vasodilators are occasionally effective when used singly, most often volume replacement and inotropic agents are necessary. The following peripheral vasodilating medications can be used.

Chlorpromazine is given in an initial intravenous 5 mg. dose. If this does not produce the desired effect, further increments may be given to a maximum intravenous dose of 25 mg. over 2–4 hours. Additional agents are utilized if an adequate response is not obtained. A disadvantage of chlorpromazine is central nervous system depression which can delay the diagnosis of brain injury in the early postoperative period.

Corticosteroids in large doses are useful in the treatment of severe vasoconstriction. High doses (hydrocortisone, 150 mg./kg., methylprednisolone, 30 mg./kg., or dexamethasone, 6 mg./kg.) are administered in a single intravenous bolus and repeated in 4–6 hours if necessary.[5]

Phenoxybenzamine (1 mg./kg. via intravenous rider over 1–2 hours) or *phentolamine* produces vasodilation, but these drugs are not in common use.

7. Inotropic agents used in the low output state include those given below.

Isoproterenol has an inotropic and peripheral vasodilator effect. Isuprel (0.4 mg.) in a 100 ml. rider is titrated to produce the desired response. Usually 1 gamma/minute is administered initially. Increasing amounts may be needed as the patient becomes less responsive. This medication is especially suited for bradycardia or heart block associated with low output. In the presence of ventricular irritability or tachycardia, other medications should be used.

Metaraminol (Aramine), phenylephrine (Neo-Synephrine) can be given as an intravenous bolus or rider. Metaraminol, 1–2 mg./ml., and phenylephrine, 0.2–0.5 mg./ml., are administered at a rate required to maintain a satisfactory blood pressure.

Epinephrine has both a central and peripheral action. However, its use is limited because of its tendency to cause myocardial irritability. It is useful in resuscitation to improve the quality of fibrillation prior to defibrillation.

Levarterenol is a potent vasoconstrictor and when used alone may decrease the chance for reversal of the syndrome. It may be beneficial when used in conjunction with peripheral vasodilators.

8. Volume infusion is generally necessary to improve the circulatory status for the following reasons: *(a)* Peripheral vasodilation: the increased vascular space following the administration of vasodilator agents requires volume infusion to sustain or improve cardiac output.

Therefore, volume replacement with blood or plasma expanders accompanies the use of peripheral vasodilators in most instances. *(b)* Decreased ventricular compliance: poorly compliant ventricles with high end diastolic pressures require elevated filling pressures to propel the blood into the ventricular chambers adequately. Therefore, volume may be needed when "normal" venous pressures are present. *(c)* Pulmonary hypertension: increased pulmonary resistance requires maintenance of higher right-sided pressures to provide an adequate cardiac output. This condition can be differentiated from poor left ventricular compliance by the normal left ventricular end diastolic pressure in the presence of primary pulmonary hypertension.

Congestive Heart Failure

Biventricular congestive heart failure in the postoperative patient is present more often than single chamber failure. The differential diagnosis between congestive heart failure and the low output syndrome can be difficult. The cardiac output may be normal during the early phase of congestive heart failure and later peripheral vacoconstriction and low cardiac output may develop.

Left heart failure is characterized by elevated left ventricular end diastolic pressure and elevated left atrial pressure and occasionally mitral insufficiency. Pulmonary venous pressure of over 35–40 mm. Hg results in pulmonary edema. This is generally transmitted to the right heart, causing right heart failure as well. Postoperative causes of left heart failure are: (1) poorly compliant and poorly contractile left ventricle; (2) inadequate correction of valvular stenosis or insufficiency; (3) an increased volume load following the correction of shunts; (4) ventriculotomy, and (5) myocardial ischemia or infarction.

In *right ventricular failure* there is an elevation of the right ventricular end diastolic pressure, elevation of the right atrial and central venous pressures and occasionally tricuspid insufficiency. The systemic veins are engorged, the liver and spleen enlarged and ascites and edema are usually present. Causes of right heart failure are: (1) inadequate repair of pulmonary valvular or infundibular stenosis; (2) pulmonary hypertension (particularly following closure of a septal defect); (3) a poorly compliant right ventricle; (4) ventriculotomy; (5) inadequate repair of an Ebstein's anomaly; (6) tricuspid insufficiency, and (7) a hypoplastic ventricle.

Pulmonary hypertension and elevated vascular resistance may not significantly improve for several months and even then not completely. When a volume excess is presented to a poorly compensated heart, cardiac failure will result. This margin of tolerance to slight excesses in volume can be extremely narrow.

Treatment.—The objective of treatment in congestive heart failure is to decrease the load on the heart and improve ventricular performance. Hypervolemia is usually treated by diuresis and occasionally by phlebotomy while digitalis improves ventricular function (Chapter 21).

Myocardial Ischemia

Coronary atherosclerosis is a major contributing factor in the morbidity and mortality of surgery for acquired cardiac disease, while myocardial infarction is the most common cause of death following myocardial revascularization. Myocardial ischemia or infarction following cardiac surgery is often difficult to recognize. Myocardial infarction can cause ventricular arrhythmias, congestive failure and the low output syndrome. Electrocardiographic changes and enzyme elevations occur with major infarctions. However, minor infarctions may escape detection due to slight changes in these parameters which also occur secondary to surgery.

Treatment is similar to that outlined in Chapter 21, except that more attention must be directed to ventilation and tracheobronchial toilet because of the postoperative state.

Arrhythmias

Arrhythmias of major or minor significance occur at some time in the pre- or postoperative course of most cardiac surgery patients. Not infrequently, preoperative supraventricular arrhythmias are converted to normal sinus rhythm during surgery, and every attempt must be made to preserve this state. A description of common arrhythmias and their relationship to various conditions and cardiac surgical procedures is included in the following text.

Supraventricular arrhythmias.—*Atrial fibrillation.*—This is characterized by an irregular irregularity as demonstrated by the electrocardiogram (Fig. 20-3). The diagnosis is usually not difficult and is typified by the auscultatory manifestations of irregular rhythm, pulse deficit and variable intensity of the heart sounds. Atrial fibrillation is likely the most common supraventricular arrhythmia present in patients requiring cardiac surgery. It is present preoperatively in many individuals with mitral valve disease and its presence in aortic valve disease indicates either concomitant mitral involvement or increased

Fig. 20-3.—Atrial fibrillation.

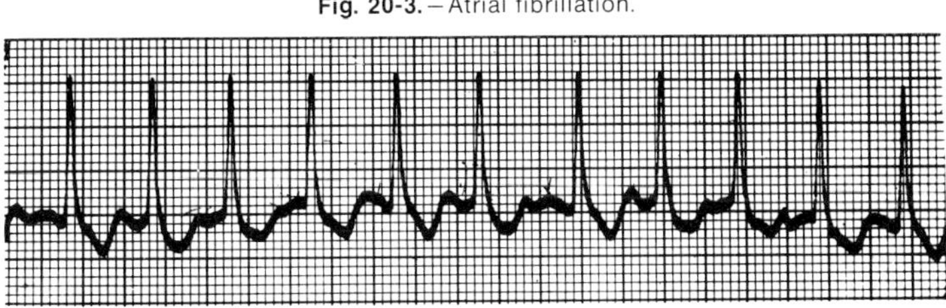

left atrial pressure due to poor left ventricular compliance. In severe aortic valvular disease atrial fibrillation may be present preoperatively or follow elevation of left ventricular end diastolic pressure.

If atrial fibrillation is present at the time of surgery, an attempt is made to convert the heart to normal sinus rhythm following repair. The success of conversion is related to the size of the left atrium, the compliance of the left ventricle and the amount of fibrous replacement of the left atrium.

Atrial fibrillation is treated by control of the ventricular rate with digitalis. Most adult patients who have open heart surgery are digitalized preoperatively, thereby abrogating the need for complete redigitalization in the postoperative period. Later, if the ventricular rate is well controlled, cardioversion to normal sinus rhythm may be attempted.

Atrial flutter.—Atrial flutter is not as common postoperatively as atrial fibrillation. Atrial fibrillation or premature atrial beats may revert to atrial flutter. Atrial flutter with a 2:1 response is suspected in the presence of a regular apical rate of 140–180/minute. The electrocardiogram (Fig. 20-4) demonstrates the "saw-tooth" atrial P waves.

The ventricular rate is dependent upon the degree of atrioventricular block and generally varies from a 4:1 to a 2:1 ratio. Atrial flutter is more difficult to control with digitalis than atrial fibrillation. If digitalis does not improve the ventricular rate, an external direct current shock may be necessary for conversion. This is especially necessary in the acute episode when hypotension or congestive heart failure supervene. Propanolol, 3–5 mg. (in 1 mg. increments) can be given intravenously to assist in the regulation of resistant supraventricular arrhythmias. Its use, particularly in the early postoperative period, must be carefully monitored since hypotension and congestive heart failure can result from depression of myocardial contractility.

Paroxysmal atrial tachycardia.—Paroxysmal atrial tachycardia (PAT) occurs with and without block. Both entities are somewhat uncommon in the early postoperative period but occur one to two weeks after surgery. PAT without block may indicate insufficient digitalis whereas PAT with block is generally indicative of digitalis toxicity.

PAT without block occurs with a ventricular rate of 140–220 beats/minute. The rate is regular and the P waves are usually superimposed on the preceding T waves with normal QRS complexes. This rhythm may be interspersed with a normal sinus rhythm. Carotid sinus pressure may temporarily or permanently terminate the attack. If vagal

Fig. 20–4.—Atrial flutter.

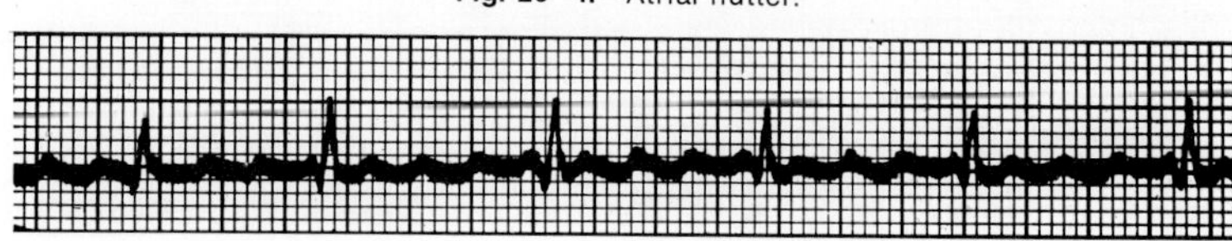

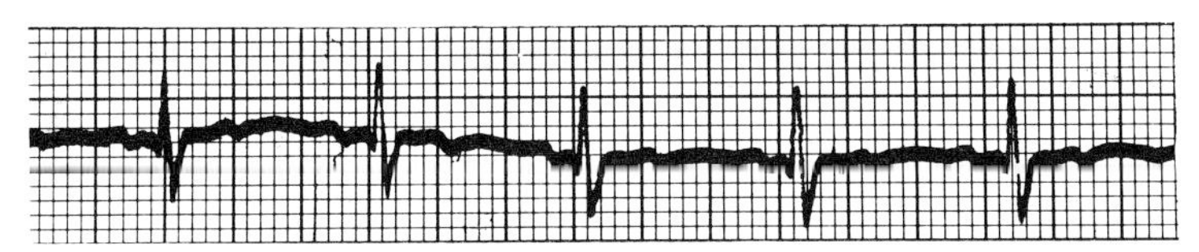

Fig. 20–5.—Atrial tachycardia with 2:1 block.

stimulation does not relieve this arrhythmia, digitalization should be instituted.

PAT with block is seen in potassium depletion and digitalis toxicity. The rate may be regular or irregular, varying from 100 to 180/minute. The electrocardiogram may show a 2:1 block (Fig. 20-5) with occasional periods of 1:1 conduction, or may be of a Wenckebach type. Usually the block can be increased with carotid sinus pressure.

The treatment of this condition is to discontinue digitalis and to administer potassium, if necessary. If cessation of digitalis or supplementation with potassium fail to correct this arrhythmia, 200 mg. of intravenous Dilantin, 200 mg. of intramuscular quinidine or procainamide (100 mg./minute intravenously) can be given.

Premature atrial contractions.—Such premature contractions are common following heart surgery, particularly mitral valve surgery. Atrial premature beats are characterized by an abnormally shaped P wave followed by a normal QRS complex (Fig. 20-6).

An irritable atrial focus causes depolarization of the remainder of the atria if the impulse is initiated after the previous refractory period. If the AV node has repolarized, the impulse will spread into the ventricles. This evidence of atrial irritability often precedes atrial fibrillation or flutter. The treatment is quinidine, 200–300 mg. intramuscularly every six hours.

VENTRICULAR ARRHYTHMIAS.—*Ventricular premature beats.*—Generally, ventricular premature beats precede ventricular arrhythmias. Predisposing causes include hypoxia, digitalis intoxication, acidosis, myocardial infarction, hypopotassemia and trauma. Ventricular premature beats are wide, bizarre and show multifocal QRS complexes which do not follow atrial complexes (Fig. 20-7). This arrhythmia is one of the commonest occurring after open heart surgery and, if more frequent than 3–5 beats/minute, requires therapy to prevent progression

Fig. 20–6.—Premature atrial contraction.

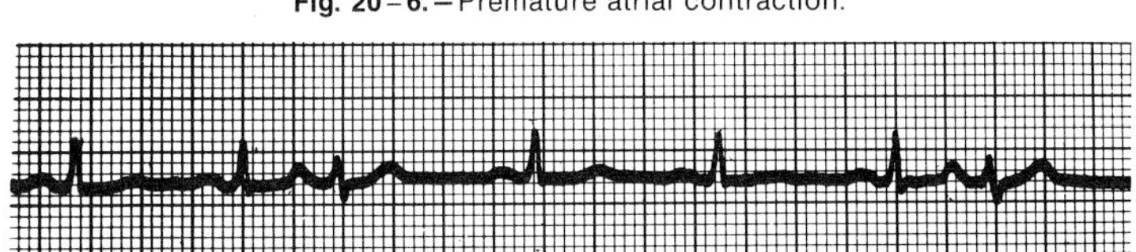

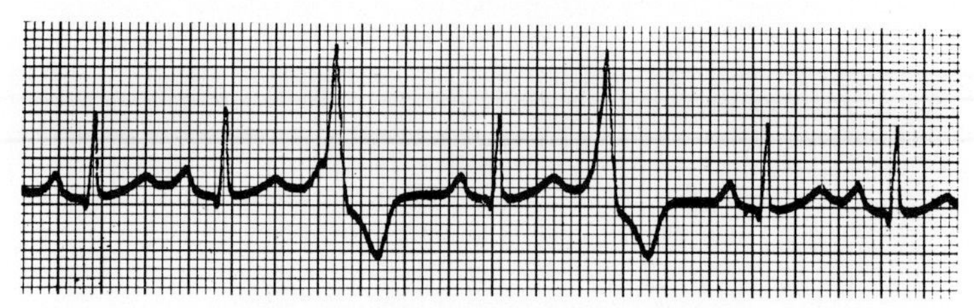

Fig. 20-7.—Premature ventricular contraction.

to more serious arrhythmias. Treatment should be directed at the etiology, although suppression of cardiac irritability is required by one or more of the following agents.

Lidocaine (Xylocaine) is given in an initial intravenous bolus of 25 mg. The onset of action is rapid and the duration of action is short. If sustained suppression is required, a lidocaine drip of 0.5–4 mg./minute may be used. Other medications or cardiac pacing may be required to prevent toxicity from high concentrations or prolonged therapy.

Quinidine in doses of 200–400 mg. every 6 hours is administered intramuscularly. This will often decrease the need for the intravenous lidocaine drip.

Procainamide may be used initially or substituted for quinidine if the former is not well tolerated. The intravenous dose should be 100 mg./minute, not to exceed 1 Gm. Orally 2–4 Gm. a day can be given in divided doses.

Diphenylhydantoin can be given intravenously in a 200 mg. bolus every 6 hours. It is particularly helpful in replacing lidocaine when sensitivity or side effects to that drug are present.

Propanolol can be used in the treatment of ventricular arrhythmias if precautions in its management are recognized (see Chapter 21).

Ventricular tachycardia.—Ventricular tachycardia is characterized by rapid, broad QRS complexes (Fig. 20-8). The associated decrease in the cardiac output frequently leads to ventricular fibrillation. The treatment is the same as that for premature ventricular contractions. Direct-current shock is administered as soon as the tachycardia is

Fig. 20-8.—Ventricular tachycardia.

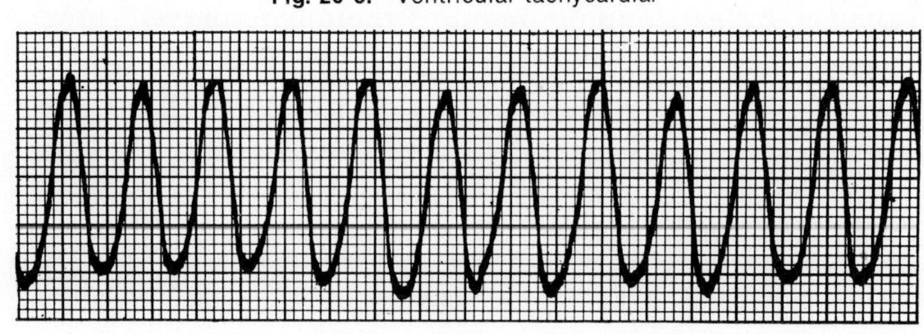

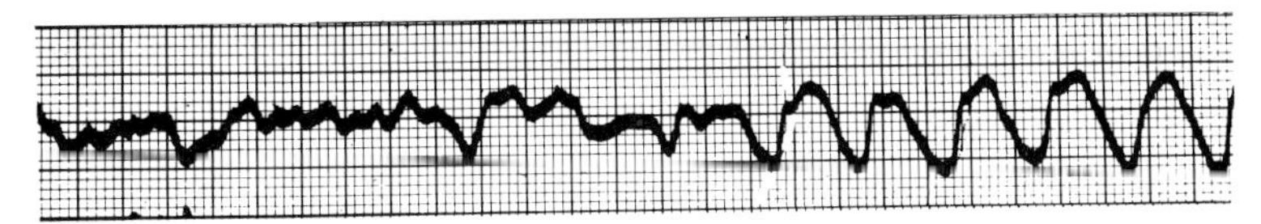

Fig. 20-9. – Ventricular fibrillation and tachycardia.

recognized, and conversion should be completed within 1 or 2 minutes to prevent cerebral damage. If conversion cannot be completed within this interval, external cardiac massage is necessary to maintain cardiac output until conversion can be accomplished. Larger amounts of lidocaine may be given if the 25 mg. bolus is not effective. Most often 50 mg. or more will be required to suppress the irritable focus. Following resuscitation, lidocaine, dilantin, quinidine, and/or cardiac pacing are indicated to prevent recurrence. Correction of acidosis during this period is essential.

Ventricular fibrillation. This fatal arrhythmia demands immediate treatment and is an ominous sign of the patient's general status (Fig. 20-9). The prevention and treatment are the same as those for ventricular tachycardia.

NODAL AND ATRIAL-VENTRICULAR RHYTHMS.–*Nodal tachycardia.* –Nodal rhythms occur not infrequently following cardiac operations. Additional causes include thoracotomy, digitalis toxicity, myocarditis, acute infarction and atropine. The rate is usually 70–130 but may be as high as 180 beats/minute. In the example shown in Figure 20-10 there is an intermediate "high" nodal tachycardia with retrograde atrial depolarization.

The usual cause in the postoperative patient is hypokalemia with digitalis toxicity, and the tachycardia should be treated accordingly. Occasionally in the treatment of a slow nodal rhythm with atropine, a nodal tachycardia will result.

Nodal rhythm.–In a nodal rhythm (45–100 beats/minute) the impulse is initiated at the node (Fig. 20-11). The causes of slow nodal rhythms are: halothane anesthesia, ischemia of the sinus node and trauma to the sinus node. Temporary dysfunction secondary to surgical trauma may not become manifest until hours or days following surgery. Treatment is needed when slow rates decrease cardiac output. Management includes the following: (1) atrial or ventricular pacing to adjust the rate to maximal cardiac output; (2) isoproterenol, utilized in an intravenous drip to maintain the rate between 80 and 110 (0.5–4 gamma/

Fig. 20-10. – Nodal tachycardia.

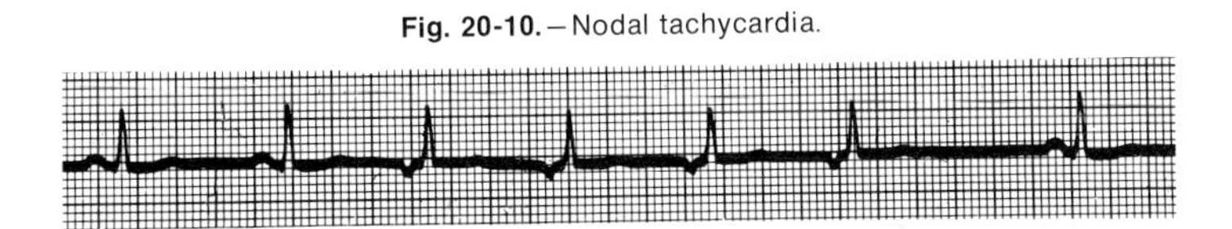

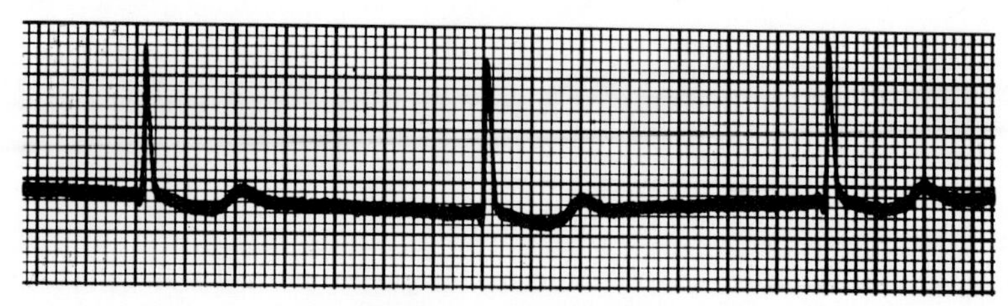

Fig. 20–11.—Nodal rhythm.

minute); (3) intravenous atropine, 0.5–1 mg. intravenously, given in smaller doses (0.2 mg.) and increased as needed to increase the rate.

ATRIOVENTRICULAR DISSOCIATION.—Varying degrees of AV dissociation and block may occur postoperatively, the most common being first degree heart block. Examples of second and third degree heart block are given in Figures 20-12 and 20-13.

The degree to which heart block or dissociation occurs depends on the degree of trauma to the conduction system. Trauma to the conduction system can occur in the following repairs: ventricular septal defect, tetralogy of Fallot, ostium primum and cushion defects, aortic and tricuspid valve replacements and repair of Ebstein's anomaly. If the conduction block occurs during surgery, the chances of a permanent defect are more likely than if it occurs in the postoperative period.[10] When heart block occurs during surgery, a temporary ventricular pacing wire is utilized. Later, if the patient requires permanent pacing, a transvenous pacemaker is inserted. If heart block is present prior to surgery or if tricuspid valve replacement is complicated by heart block, an epicardial pacemaker is implanted.

OTHER ARRHYTHMIAS.—Although not all arrhythmias can be discussed in this chapter, several other categories require mention.

Digitalis-induced arrhythmias.—Although alluded to previously, the more commonly encountered digitalis-induced arrhythmias are: (1) ectopic ventricular contractions, (2) ventricular tachycardia, (3) ventricular fibrillation, (4) nodal rhythms and AV dissociation, (5) PAT with block and (6) AV block.

Fig. 20–12.—Second degree heart block.

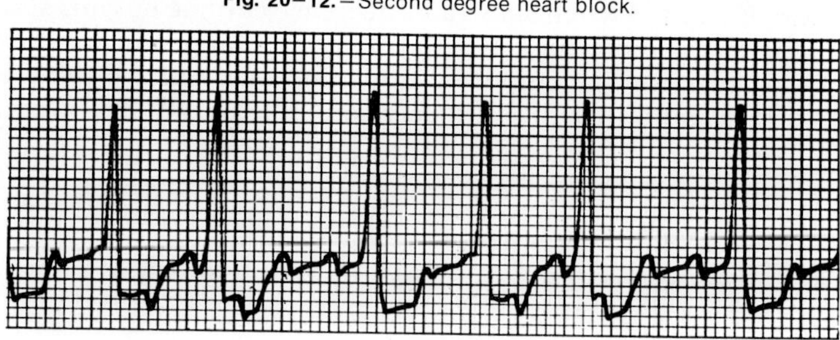

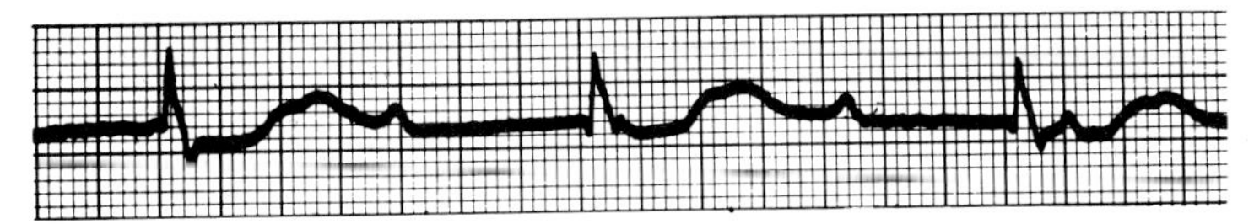

Fig. 20–13.—Third degree heart block.

Surgery causes unique problems regarding digitalis sensitivity in the body tissue. Vagal reflexes and hypoxia potentiate digitalis toxicity.[2] Acetylcholine and succinylcholine can produce serious ventricular arrhythmias in the poorly digitalized patient while changes in acid-base balance (acidosis) and electrolyte balance (hypokalemia) render the myocardium more susceptible to digitalis.

Electrolyte imbalance and digitalis sensitivity.—In *hypokalemia* (serum K^+ below 3.5 mEq./L.), the toxic dose of digitalis may be as little as 40% of the normal digitalizing dose. The potassium loss which occurs with nonblood hemodilution cardiopulmonary by pass often exceeds expectations. Also, postoperative losses may be considerably more than expected. As much as 600 mEq. potassium loss has been recorded in a 24-hour postoperative period (Fig. 20-14).

The following precautions are utilized to avert fatal arrhythmias. (1) Digitalis is discontinued at least two days prior to surgery. (2) Potassium supplementation intentionally exceeds the usual maintenance dose. The amount and route of administration depends on the depletion of body reserves. Twelve to 24 hours before surgery additional potassium is given to keep serum levels at 4.5–5 mEq./L. (3) Careful moni-

Fig. 20–14.—Potassium losses were massive in this patient, who had aortic and mitral valve replacement.

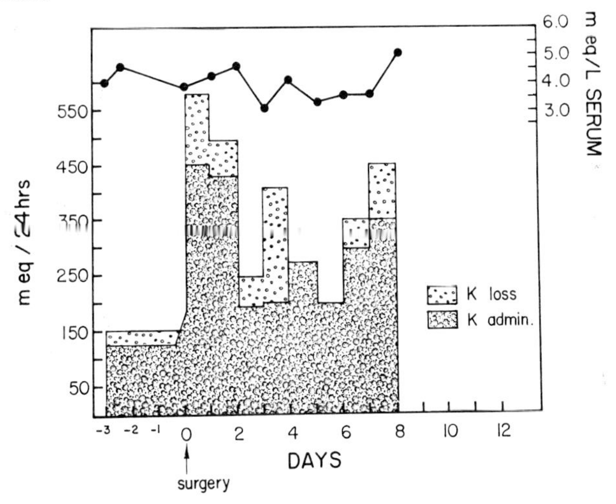

toring of potassium intake, losses and serum levels is done throughout the operative and early postoperative period with losses replaced as they occur.

Calcium given by intravenous infusion may potentiate digitalis toxicity, particularly when given rapidly.

Magnesium deficiency can also potentiate digitalis toxicity. Patients who have chronic debility, large and long-term losses of gastrointestinal secretions or hepatic insufficiency and who have been on prolonged intravenous fluid therapy are prone to develop this deficit. Therapy consists of magnesium sulfate, 500–1,000 mg., given every 2–3 days via intravenous rider.

Wolff-Parkinson-White syndrome.—This syndrome occurs with some degree of frequency in the following anomalies: (1) atrial septal defect; (2) ventricular septal defect; (3) idiopathic hypertrophic subaortic stenosis; (4) tetralogy of Fallot; (5) transposition of the great vessels; (6) tricuspid atresia; (7) endocardial fibroelastosis; (8) Ebstein's anomaly; (9) coarctation of the aorta and (10) coronary artery disease.

It can occur in the postoperative patient with myocardial infarction and digitalis excess. If it was not present preoperatively, these two conditions should be suspected. The electrocardiogram (Fig. 20-15) shows a short PR interval, an abnormal QRS complex, and generally there are paroxysms of recurrent tachycardia. The hemodynamic effects may be detrimental, especially with tachycardia. Treatment should be directed at the etiology. Quinidine is occasionally beneficial in a dosage of 200–300 mg. every 6 hours.

Postoperative cardiac pacing.—The postoperative conditions in which cardiac pacing is utilized are: (1) complete heart block, (2) slow nodal rhythms, (3) incomplete heart block where atrioventricular dysfunction causes decreased cardiac output, (4) abnormal rhythms from ventricular irritability, (5) sinus bradycardia and (6) supraventricular arrhythmias except in PAT with block.

The routine placement of pacing wires has significantly decreased morbidity and mortality. When indicated, atrial or ventricular pacing can enhance cardiac performance and prevent fatal arrhythmias.

It should be stressed that arrhythmias are symptoms of underlying problems which require recognition and treatment. Life-threatening

Fig. 20–15.—Wolff-Parkinson-White syndrome.

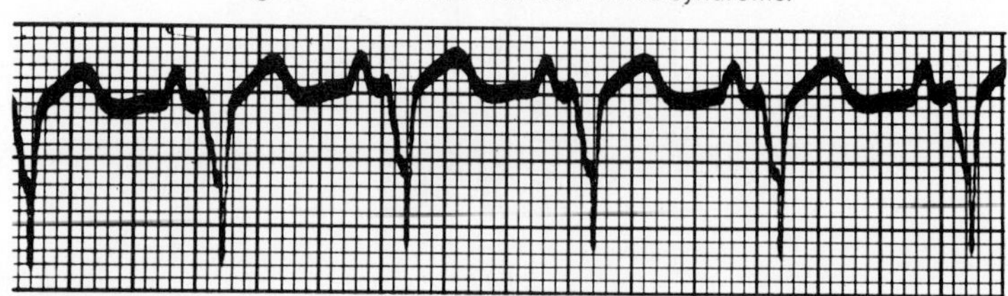

arrhythmias can be managed as outlined; however, if the etiology is overlooked, treatment of the symptom is often ultimately unsuccessful. The most important treatable causes of severe postoperative arrhythmias are: (1) hypoxia, (2) hypokalemia, (3) digitalis intoxication and (4) hypotension with poor myocardial perfusion. The following causes of arrhythmias are inherent in the disease or produced by its surgical treatment: (1) myocardial or subendocardial infarction, (2) myocardial fibrosis, (3) surgical trauma, including cardiopulmonary by-pass, (4) trauma to the conduction system and (5) other intrinsic myocardial disease.

Pulmonary Complications

No other physiologic parameter is so important as the maintenance of pulmonary ventilation with adequate arterial oxygenation. Proper evaluation of the preoperative pulmonary status, careful management of the lungs during surgery and attention to small details in postoperative care decrease morbidity and mortality.

Preoperative evaluation.—The assessment of pulmonary function prior to surgery begins with the history and physical examination. Further investigation is required when there is primary pulmonary pathology, evidence of a pulmonary embolus, chronic pulmonary infection or chronic pulmonary changes due to cardiac disease. In the presence of pulmonary pathology, investigation of pulmonary function and preoperative preparation are carried out as outlined in Chapter 18.

Operative management.—Pulmonary complications are reduced and vital capacity less affected when median sternotomy is used instead of a thoracotomy. Blood gases are monitored throughout the procedure, particularly during cardiopulmonary by-pass. Intermittent inflation of the lungs during extracorporeal circulation decreases postoperative atelectasis.

Postoperative management of ventilation.—The endotracheal tube is left in place from 4 to 36 hours in the adult. Although it should be removed as soon as possible, intubation for as long as 36 to 48 hours rarely causes significant complications. If the patient requires assisted ventilation for longer periods, a tracheostomy is performed. Mechanical ventilation is continued if there is any doubt regarding the adequacy of spontaneous ventilation. This is particularly true in the presence of pulmonary hypertension, increased pulmonary resistance and chronic pulmonary disease.

If the following points are followed in the management of ventilation postoperatively, pulmonary complications can be reduced: (1) adequate ventilation; (2) sighing of the patient (at least every 30 minutes); (3) careful aseptic suctioning of the trachea and bronchi; (4) correct positioning of the endotracheal tube; (5) maintenance of mechanical ventilation until the patient has been observed off the respirator for a satisfactory period (1–2 hours) with adequate spontaneous respiration and arterial saturation.

POSTOPERATIVE COMPLICATIONS.—*Inadequate ventilation.*—Atelectasis is the most common cause of inadequate ventilation. Intrinsic and extrinsic bronchial obstruction and low tidal volume are contributing factors. The peak incidence is in the immediate postoperative period and treatment must be aggressive. (See Chapter 18.)

Additional factors causing inadequate ventilation include the inability of the respirator to ventilate adequately, improper setting of the respirator, and competition with the respirator (Chapter 5). Volume controlled respirators are most efficient in patients with poor compliance of the lung and chest wall. Competition with the respirator is a manifestation of hypoxia and contributes to its progression. Hand ventilation with 100% oxygen initiates hypocarbia and assists in transfer to the mechanical unit. Occasionally sedation is beneficial and in extreme situations muscular paralysis is necessary.

Pulmonary infection.—Inadequate removal of tracheobronchial secretions is the major cause of postoperative pulmonary infections. Early extubation, aseptic technique and aggressive therapy minimize this problem (Chapters 4 and 18).

Pump-lung syndrome.—Patchy pulmonary edema, hemorrhage and atelectasis occasionally follow cardiopulmonary by-pass. Although infrequent, pump-lung syndrome is associated with a high morbidity and mortality. Diffusion defects, pulmonary AV shunting, hypoxemia and decreased pulmonary surfactant comprise this syndrome. Parenchymal pulmonary hypoxia may be the underlying cause.[12] A similar situation can follow prolonged mechanical ventilation. Treatment consists of improving ventilation and administration of corticosteroids to decrease pulmonary interstitial edema.

Renal Complications

Renal dysfunction in the postoperative period is usually a complication of abnormalities which have been existent prior to or occur during or after surgery. Postoperative renal failure is more likely to occur in a previously compromised kidney. The routine preoperative evaluation uncovers the majority of pre-existing pathology. The usual causes of postoperative renal insufficiency are hypovolemia, the low cardiac output syndrome, severe tricuspid insufficiency or right heart failure. Other causes of renal insufficiency include inadequate perfusion during by-pass, renal artery obstruction and red cell destruction with hemoglobinuria. Evidence of renal dysfunction can occur at any time in the postoperative period but its onset is usually within the first 24 hours. Oliguria of less than 20 ml./hour should initiate both diagnostic and therapeutic maneuvers (Chapter 9). Other evidence of dysfunction can include a normal or increased urine output associated with a fixed specific gravity and elevation of the BUN, serum creatinine and serum potassium levels.

Hypovolemia is manifested by low central venous and systemic pressures, vasoconstriction and high specific gravity. Volume is replaced as indicated. The therapy of low cardiac output has been described.

In the presence of acute renal failure (Chapter 9), fluid intake must be limited. Administration of digitalis is modified and nephrotoxic medications are discontinued or restricted. Mild elevation of serum potassium is controlled with ion exchange resins while toxic levels require dialysis.

Central Nervous System Damage

Central nervous system abnormalities following heart surgery are manifestations of cerebral emboli, cerebral edema, cerebral vascular insufficiency or psychotic disturbances. Although the exact etiology may be obscure, the following points may be helpful in differentiation.

Cerebral edema and air embolism often cause a diffuse injury pattern without localization. Emboli of clot, calcific debris, cerebral thrombosis and hemorrhage tend to produce focal signs. Diffuse cerebral signs and unconsciousness in the postoperative patient generally indicate a better prognosis than the presence of focal signs with unconsciousness. However, regardless of localization, persistence of severe neurologic deficits for more than 48 hours is associated with a poor prognosis.

Embolization of thrombi which have formed on prosthetic valves usually occurs later in the postoperative period. To decrease the incidence of this complication, oral anticoagulation is begun after removal of chest tubes (36–48 hours following surgery) unless specific contraindications exist. Contraindications to early anticoagulation are: (1) central nervous system damage, (2) bleeding abnormalities, (3) postoperative hemorrhage and (4) associated pathology in which the hazard of bleeding is significant.

Treatment of cerebral injury is directed at reduction of cerebral metabolism and edema while supporting other physiologic functions (Chapter 16). Cerebral edema is treated with total body hypothermia to 32 C. Osmotic agents extract further fluid from the brain. Corticosteroids are routinely used.

Psychotic aberrations occur in a significant number of patients following open heart surgery. Symptoms can be manifested as disorientation, memory disturbance, bizarre motor restlessness, visual hallucinations, depressed intellectual function or frank psychosis (Chapter 11).

Anatomic neurologic deficits are associated with the majority of psychologic abnormalities.[7] Other factors which seem to be important in the genesis of psychologic disturbances are severe preoperative depression, advanced age and prolonged extracorporeal circulation.

Infection

Postoperative infection is listed in the order of its occurrence following heart surgery: (1) pulmonary infection, (2) urinary tract infection, (3) thrombophlebitis, (4) wound infection and (5) endocarditis.

Prophylactic antibiotics are routinely employed to decrease the incidence of infection. To be effective, antibiotic coverage is required preoperatively, during the operative procedure and in the postoperative period. Adequate blood levels of the antibiotic should be present during exposure to infectious organisms. Intravenous methicillin, 4 Gm. every 6 hours, is begun 12 hours prior to surgery and continued after surgery until the patient is able to take oral medications. At that time oxacillin, 1 Gm. every 6 hours, is substituted.

The diagnosis and treatment of the most common infections are discussed in appropriate sections of this volume.

Endocardial infections occur in a small group of patients following heart surgery.[1,9] Endocarditis can become manifest several days to several years postoperatively, although it usually occurs within the first 6 months. The clinical course can vary from subtle febrile episodes to an acute fulminating course rapidly leading to death. The following are clinical findings often noted in endocarditis: (1) shaking chills and fever; (2) finger clubbing; (3) petechiae; (4) splenomegaly; (5) changing heart sounds and murmurs; (6) systemic emboli and (7) renal, cerebral and peripheral manifestations of embolization. Once the diagnosis is established by blood culture, appropriate antibiotic treatment should be aggressive and massive. If a prosthetic valve is the site of infection, it should be replaced following control of the bacteremia.

Cardiac Arrest and Resuscitation

As with most entities in medicine, the best treatment for cardiac arrest is its prevention. This section will deal specifically with cardiac arrest in its relation to the patient in the intensive care unit.

RECOGNITION OF CARDIAC ARREST.—Cardiac arrest is that condition in which cardiac contractions are absent or ineffectual, resulting in insufficient cardiac output to maintain vital functions of the organs. One of the main objectives of the intensive care unit is the control and prevention of conditions which lead to cardiac arrest. Both clinical and electrophysiologic monitoring help to achieve this goal. Inadequate ventilation, hypoxemia, cyanosis, peripheral vasoconstriction, low output syndromes, cardiac arrhythmias, poor renal function, mental stupor and acidosis are signs which alert the clinician to impending catastrophe.

CARDIOPULMONARY RESUSCITATION.—The success of resuscitation is directly related to the speed of recognition and institution of treatment. Satisfactory resuscitation requires properly trained personnel, continuous monitoring and readily available resuscitation equipment and medications. Resuscitation equipment which should be at the patient's bedside has been outlined earlier. When indicated, it is particularly important to have appropriate medications already drawn into the syringe to expedite their administration. These medications include sodium bicarbonate, 1 amp.; 1% lidocaine; calcium chloride, 1 amp.; 1 ml. of epinephrine 1:1,000, and diphenylhydantoin, 250 mg. Their use is outlined in Chapter 21. The direct-current defibrillator should be ready for immediate use. Endotracheal tubes, laryngoscopes and a hand respirator bag with connectors should also be readily available.

The following are important points in resuscitation.

1. Following recognition of the arrest, additional personnel should be summoned.

2. Ventilatory control must be established. If an endotracheal tube is in place for mechanical ventilation, this can be continued; however, hand ventilation is used for the optimal control of respiration. Ventilation and external cardiac massage are coordinated to provide 1 inspiration between every 4 to 6 sternal compressions.

3. Place a hard board under the patient's back to facilitate cardiac massage. External cardiac compression is performed with the palm of the hand placed over the lower sternum and compression toward the spine at a rate of 60–80 times/minute. The sternum should be depressed 1½ to 2 in. Excess compression can cause rib fracture, contusion and laceration of the heart and great vessels and disruption of cardiac or sternal repair. The effectiveness of massage is best measured with direct arterial monitoring.

4. Direct-current defibrillation. In the postoperative patient it is preferable to defibrillate immediately after the onset of ventricular tachycardia or fibrillation. If the defibrillator is ready for use, its direct administration is preferable to massage and will reduce the complications associated with the latter. The direct-current defibrillator is superior to the alternating-current defibrillator and should be used for external defibrillation in the following manner: After application of electode paste, one electrode is placed over the base of the heart and the other over the apex. Defibrillation is then accomplished, using 100 watt-seconds. Voltage can be increased in increments up to 400 watt-seconds if necessary.

5. Open chest cardiac massage. This mode of resuscitation is not used frequently because of the effectiveness of closed chest massage. When external massage does not adequately compress the heart, as in the presence of severe emphysema, pericardial tamponade or an immobile chest, open cardiac massage should be instituted. In the postopera-

tive patient the chest is best opened through the previous incision if this will lend itself to cardiac massage. The usual incision for open chest cardiac massage is via the left fourth or fifth intercostal space with massage of the heart inside the pericardium. The heart is compressed against the sternum or between the palms of both hands.

Management following cardiac arrest is directed at prevention of recurrence. Acidosis, hypoxia and electrolyte imbalance require correction.[4] Antiarrhythmic agents or cardiac pacing should be used to suppress irritable foci. The therapy of low cardiac output, cerebral and renal insufficiency and complications related to specific procedures have been outlined.

ROUTINE ORDERS following open heart surgery

1. Vital signs every 15 minutes until stable, then every hour.
2. Endotracheal tube to ventilator (adjusted by physician and inhalation therapist). Take patient off respirator every 30–60 minutes and hand ventilate for 5 minutes (if no sighing mechanism on respirator).
3. Suction oropharynx and through the endotracheal tube as often as needed and at least every hour with small sterile catheters. Conclude with irrigation of 10 ml. sterile saline and send 1 aspiration specimen daily for culture and sensitivity.
4. Attach arterial blood pressure line to transducer; irrigate at least every 30 minutes with 5–10 ml. of heparinized saline (250 units/150 ml.).
5. Attach central venous pressure (atrial catheter) line for measurement; record pressure every 30 minutes. Keep open with 500 ml. 5% dextrose/water and 2,000 units heparin.
6. Total intravenous intake to equal 1,500 ml. 5% dextrose/water in 24 hours.
7. Antibiotics: 4 Gm. methicillin every 6 hours to be given in intravenous solution over 30 minutes.
8. Attach electrocardiograph for continuous monitoring. Obtain standard electrocardiogram daily.
9. Urinary catheter to gravity drainage. Measure output and specific gravity every hour.
10. Chest tubes to underwater seal–strip tubes every 30 minutes or as often as needed to keep clear.
11. Nasogastric tube to low Gomco suction; record output every 8 hours; irrigate every 2 hours with 30 ml. sterile water.
12. Adjust bed to elevate head at 30 degrees. Turn patient every 2 hours as tolerated.
13. Check peripheral pulses every 30 minutes and record.
14. Check level of consciousness every 30 minutes and record.
15. Observe for drainage on dressings and notify staff if progressive.

16. Blood gases to be obtained on admission to intensive therapy and as often as needed.
17. Obtain serum K^+, Na^+, CO_2, Ca^{++} on entry to intensive therapy and every 8 hours (or as often as needed).
18. Prothrombin time, clotting time and platelet count on admission to intensive therapy, then daily prothrombin time.
19. Hemoglobin, hematocrit and urinalysis 2 hours after surgery and each A.M.
20. Portable chest x-ray in semi-upright position on admission to intensive therapy and each morning.

REFERENCES

1. Amoury, R. A.: Infection Following Cardiopulmonary Bypass, in Norman, J. C. (ed.): *Cardiac Surgery* (New York: Appleton-Century-Crofts, Inc., 1967).
2. Baum, G. L., *et al.*: Factors involved in digitalis sensitivity in chronic pulmonary insufficiency, Am. Heart J. 57:460, 1959.
3. Braunwald, E., *et al.*: Left atrial and left ventricular pressures in subjects without cardiovascular disease: Observations in eighteen patients studied by transseptal left heart catheterization, Circulation 24:267, 1961.
4. Chazan, J. A.; Stenson, R.; and Kurland, G. S.: The acidosis of cardiac arrest, New England J. Med. 278:360, 1968.
5. Dietzman, R. H., *et al.*: Low output syndrome: Recognition and treatment, J. Thoracic & Cardiovas. Surg. 57:138, 1969.
6. Fishman, N. H.; Hutchinson, J. C.; and Roe, B. B.: Controlled atrial hypertension: A method for supporting cardiac output following open-heart surgery, J. Thoracic & Cardiovas. Surg. 52:777, 1966.
7. Javid, H., *et al.*: Neurological abnormalities following open-heart surgery, J. Thoracic & Cardiovas. Surg. 58:502, 1969.
8. Longerbeam, J. K., *et al.*: Central venous pressure monitoring: A useful guide to fluid therapy during shock and other forms of cardiovascular stress, Am. J. Surg. 110:220, 1965.
9. Lord, J. W., *et al.*: Endocarditis complicating open heart surgery, Circulation 23:489, 1961.
10. McGoon, D. C.; Ongley, P. A.; and Kirklin, J. W.: Surgical heart block, Am. J. Med. 37:749, 1964.
11. Mundth, E. D., and Austen, W. G.: Postoperative intensive care in the cardiac surgical patient, Prog. Cardiovas. Dis. 11:229, 1968.
12. Balis, J. V., *et al.*: The role of pulmonary hypoperfusion and hypoxia in the post-perfusion lung syndrome, Ann. Thoracic Surg. 8:263, 1969.
13. Rosky, L. P., and Rodman, T.: Medical aspects of open-heart surgery, New England J. Med. 274:833, 886–893, 1966.

21

The Cardiac Patient Requiring Major Surgery

A. JERALD ROTHENBERG, M.D.*

Former Fellow in Cardiorespiratory Diseases, Presbyterian-St. Luke's Hospital; Co-director of Coronary Arteriography and The Heart Center, Department of Medicine, Grant Hospital, Chicago, Illinois

AND

RICHARD A. CARLETON, M.D.

Attending Physician and Director, Section of Cardiorespiratory Diseases, Rush-Presbyterian-St. Luke's Medical Center; Professor of Medicine, Rush Medical College

PREOPERATIVE EVALUATION

The patient's status should be evaluated by means of a complete history and physical examination, chest x-ray, electrocardiogram and routine examination of the blood and urine before any surgical procedure is undertaken. Among the questions to be answered are: (1) Is there any evidence of heart disease? If so, what type? (2) Is there any evidence of other organ system disease which may affect the cardiovascular system, such as cerebral vascular disease, orthostatic hypotension, syncope, chronic obstructive lung disease or genitourinary disease? (3) What recent medications has the patient been taking and what toxic reactions and allergies does he have?

HISTORY OF HEART DISEASE.—Patients with stable coronary artery disease tolerate surgery quite well. However, increasing angina is often a herald of infarction and is thus a contraindication to surgery, unless the surgical condition contributes to the angina, for example, anemia

*Supported in part by United States Public Health Service Training Grant No. HE09923-03.

from a bleeding tumor or fever secondary to a tumor or other pathology. Three weeks of bed rest may stabilize the angina, decrease the risks of surgery and not significantly modify the prognosis, even in surgery for cancer. Elective surgery should not be performed less than three months after a myocardial infarction; this is the time required for the infarct to be converted into a firm scar with the development of some collateral blood supply. This is also the time after which the risk of intraoperative and postoperative arrhythmias is lessened. Patients with aortic valvular disease and those with cyanotic congenital heart disease present an increased risk to surgical procedures. An important question is whether the nature of the surgery predisposes to postoperative congestive heart failure; for example, will a ventriculotomy be performed? Has the patient with mitral stenosis previously had pulmonary congestion at times of paroxysmal tachycardia? These patients will require preoperative and continued postoperative digitalization.

Correction and Improvement of Cardiac Status

High Output States

Any disorder which markedly augments the cardiac load such as fever, hyperthyroidism, arteriovenous fistulae or hemoglobin levels below 8.5 Gm./100 ml. should be sought and corrected prior to any surgical procedure.

Overt Congestive Heart Failure

These patients should be treated to decrease the demands on the circulation. Generally, this can be accomplished with bed rest. This must include mental repose as well. The duration of the rest will vary with the severity of heart failure and the response to the total regimen. Bed rest is designed to reduce the demands on the heart so that the venous pressure will be reduced, the blood pressure will be diminished and the renal blood flow will be maintained as near normal as possible. Sodium intake should be restricted. Those with mild congestive heart failure should be restricted to 2 Gm. of sodium per day. This means that these patients can have regular food cooked and served with no salt added. Those with moderate congestive failure should have sodium restricted to 1 Gm. daily and those with severe failure to 0.5 Gm. In severe heart failure in which glomerular filtration is markedly reduced, water intake may have to be restricted to 1,000–1,500 ml./day to prevent hyponatremia. Patients with moderate degrees of failure generally show normal water excretion.

Digitalis is used to increase the force of myocardial contraction and, in patients with rapid ectopic atrial arrhythmias, to decrease atrioventricular conduction and slow the ventricular rate. The speed with which digitalization is undertaken will depend upon the status of the patient. Rapid digitalization should be avoided when slower

TABLE 21-1.—DIGITALIS PREPARATION AND DOSAGE

	Oral Digitalization				Maintenance		Parenteral Digitalization			Excretion	
Preparation	Av.	Range	Absorption	Peak Effect, Hr.	Av.	Range	Av.	Range	Maximum Effect	Action Regression	Action Gone
Digitalis leaf	1.2 Gm.	1–2 Gm.	20%	8–10	0.1 Gm.	0.05–0.25 Gm.				2–3 da.	2–3 wk.
Digitoxin	1.2 mg.	1–2 mg.	100%	8–10	0.1 mg.	0.05–0.25 mg.	1.2 mg.	1–2 mg.	4–12 hr.	2–3 da.	2–3 wk.
Digoxin	3 mg.	2–5 mg.	90%	3–6	0.5 mg.	0.25–0.75 mg.	1.7 mg.	1.5–3 mg.	1–2 hr.	8–10 hr.	2–6 da.
Gitalin	5 mg.	4–8 mg.	75%		0.5 mg.	0.25–1.0 mg.				2–3 da.	8–12 da.
Digilanid	4 mg.	3–8 mg.	20%	6–8	0.40 mg.	0.33–0.66 mg.				1–2 da.	1–2 wk.
Ouabain							0.5 mg.	0.4–0.7 mg.	30 min.	8–12 hr.	1–3 da.
Lanatoside C							1.6 mg.	1.2–2 mg.	1–2 hr.	16–36 hr.	3–6 da.

methods are adequate; oral administration is often better than parenteral administration because lower peak blood levels are attained. Table 21-1 gives the most commonly used digitalis preparations and their digitalizing and maintenance doses. In general, those preparations which act quickly also produce shorter periods of toxicity in the event of overdosage. It is preferable to avoid preparations with long durations of effect in the setting of surgery in cardiac patients. Digoxin often permits rapid action, a stable degree of effect and acceptably short periods of toxicity. If time permits, conversion from a long-acting preparation to digoxin may be advisable preoperatively.

DIGITALIS INTOXICATION.—The signs of digitalis intoxication may be: (1) Gastrointestinal changes—anorexia, nausea, vomiting—often occur first. (2) Visual disturbances—blurred vision, yellow vision, halos around dark objects, diplopia—may be early signs. (3) Neurologic manifestations—headache, fatigue, psychosis, delirium and confusion—may be misleading. (4) Cardiac arrhythmias-premature ventricular contractions, often producing bigeminy, second or third degree AV block or paroxysmal tachycardia—are often the first and most life-threatening signs, especially with rapid parenteral digitalization. For this reason all patients who are digitalized rapidly should be monitored closely. (5) Skin rashes may occur. Gynecomastia is common, but is not really a toxic manifestation.

Treatment.—The first step in therapy is to discontinue the digitalis. Potassium should be administered if the serum level is less than 4.5 mg. and AV block is not present. There is evidence that calcium potentiates the effect of digitalis on cardiac irritability and cardiac conduction. Some observers feel, therefore, that reduction of hypercalcemic states by the use of chelating agents will produce an inhibiting effect on cardiac arrhythmias. Sodium ethylenediaminetetraacetic acid (EDTA), 4 Gm. dissolved in 500 ml. of 5% dextrose and water, given over a period of 2 hours, may control the arrhythmia. Dilantin, 100–200 mg. intravenously, has also been shown to be valuable in ventricular irritability due to digitalis. Propranolol will often control ventricular tachycardia which occurs in digitalis intoxication; up to 4 mg. may be given intravenously over 4 minutes, but an important danger of depressing myocardial contractility exists with this drug. All intravenous medications should be given while the electrocardiogram and blood pressure are monitored.

DIURETICS.—Diuretics are useful adjuncts for the patient in congestive heart failure, especially those with edema, effusions or anasarca. There are various diuretics available, but the most commonly used are the organomercurials, the thiazides and related compounds, the aldosterone antagonists, and ethacrynic acid or furosemide. The dosages of the more common diuretics are given in Table 21-2.

Mercurial diuretics act primarily on the proximal convoluted tubules of the kidney. They inhibit the sulfhydryl enzymes, preventing the

TABLE 21-2.—DOSAGE SCHEDULE OF THE MORE COMMONLY USED DIURETICS

DRUG	ROUTE OF ADMINISTRATION	DAILY MAINTENANCE DOSE	DURATION OF ACTION (HR.)
Mercurials			
Meralluride (Mercuhydrin)	I.V. or I.M.	1–2 ml. every 2–3 days	6–9
Mercaptomerin (Thiomerin)	Sublingual	1–2 ml. every 2–3 days	6–9
Thiazides			
Chlorothiazide (Diuril)	Oral or I.V.	500–2000 mg.	6–10
Hydrochlorothiazide (Hydrodiuril)	Oral or I.V.	50–100 mg.	8–12
Chlorthalidone (Hygroton)	Oral	50–100 mg.	48–72
Methyclothiazide (Enduron)	Oral	2.5–5 mg.	24
Spirolactones			
Spironolactone (Aldactone-A)	Oral	100–200 mg.	
Phenoxyacetic acid derivative			
Ethacrynic acid (Edecrin)	Oral or I.V.	100–300 mg. oral 50–100 mg. I.V.	1–3 oral 1/2–1 I.V.
Anthranilic acid derivative			
Furosemide (Lasix)	Oral or I.V.	40–160 mg. oral 40 mg. I.V.	1–3 oral 1/2–1 I.V.

reabsorption of sodium and chloride, which are then excreted with an osmotically equivalent amount of water. These drugs are given parenterally; generally 1–2 ml. is given intramuscularly at 2 or 3 day intervals. For maximum effect the serum chloride level should be over 80 mg. The important side effects include hypersensitivity reactions, electrolyte disturbances, rarely bone marrow depression and mercurialism.

Benzothiadiazines (thiazides) exert their principal effect on the proximal convoluted tubules. They enhance excretion of sodium, chloride, bicarbonate and potassium ions; ammonia excretion is depressed and the urine is alkaline. Since these agents are kaluretic, supplemental potassium may be needed (especially if the potassium level falls below 4.5 mEq./L.). Patients in congestive heart failure often need about 45–75 mEq. daily in addition to the usual dietary intake of approximately 60 mEq. daily.

Spironolactones are competitive inhibitors of aldosterone at the renal tubular level. Best results are usually obtained with the concomitant administration of another diuretic, especially of the thiazide group, or with a corticosteroid. These drugs are not useful for emergency purposes, because it may take 7 to 10 days for the maximum diuretic action to occur. The usual oral dose is 25 mg. 4 times daily.

Ethacrynic acid reacts with the sulfhydryl groups, impairing absorption of sodium and chloride, probably in the ascending length of the loop of Henle. The oral dose is 50–100 mg. once or twice a day. Diuresis is expected in 2–3 hours. The intravenous dose is 50 mg.; the response, often massive, occurs in 30–60 minutes.

Although it is a different chemical compound, *furosemide* has a similar site and mechanism of action to ethacrynic acid. The usual oral dose is 40 mg. once or twice daily. The intravenous dose is usually 40 mg. with a prompt diuresis resulting within 15–30 minutes. Both agents are capable of producing a "contraction alkalosis" due to large urinary loss of water, sodium, chloride, hydrogen and potassium, without an equivalent bicarbonate loss. This can be corrected by cessation of these compounds and the administration of chloride in the form of potassium chloride, ammonium chloride or lysine monohydrochloride.

Incipient Heart Failure

Recognition of minimal or early congestive heart failure is difficult but important. The presence of a third heart sound, a pulsus alternans, or nocturnal angina or angina decubitus may be the first sign of early heart failure. These patients may require digitalization, a mild diuretic, sodium restriction and bed rest, as described above, before surgery can be performed. Digitalization of patients without heart failure augments the risk of arrhythmias because appropriate guidelines for assessing the completeness of digitalization are absent. Moreover, digitalization can be accomplished promptly when indicated postoperatively. For these reasons, "prophylactic" digitalization is rarely indicated.

Preparation of Patient for Emergency Surgery

If the patient with severe congestive heart failure is in pulmonary edema, the head of the bed should be elevated; 5–10 mg. of morphine sulfate may be given intramuscularly, or 4 mg. intravenously for the severely agitated patient or for the patient in shock with poor perfusion. Fifty mg. of ethacrynic acid or 40 mg. of furosemide given intravenously may effect a prompt decrease in blood volume. A rapid-acting cardiac glycoside should be administered to the patient who is not digitalized; a rapid ventricular response to atrial fibrillation is an indication for additional digitalis in the patient already on digitalis. Aminophylline, in a dosage of 250 mg. given slowly intravenously, may relieve bronchospasm in pulmonary edema; oxygen and rotating tourniquets should be utilized.

Rapid correction of milder congestive heart failure in preparation for emergency surgery is best accomplished by mild diuresis or, in the patient with a rapid ventricular response to atrial fibrillation, by the addition of supplements of 0.125 mg. of digoxin each 4 hours until the ventricular rate is controlled.

Angina Pectoris

Patients with ischemic heart disease can be subdivided into two groups. Patients with a recent myocardial infarction or with recently changed intensity and frequency of angina pectoris have a markedly increased frequency of arrhythmias and infarction with anesthesia and surgery. Patients with an old infarct and no or mild angina pectoris generally undergo surgery uneventfully. Angina pectoris which occurs in patients requiring surgery is commonly abolished by sedatives such as morphine or barbiturates and bed rest.

If the patient is anemic, he may require blood transfusions (best done with packed cells) to relieve angina. The hemoglobin should be maintained above 9 Gm. The nitrates, long or short acting, can be used

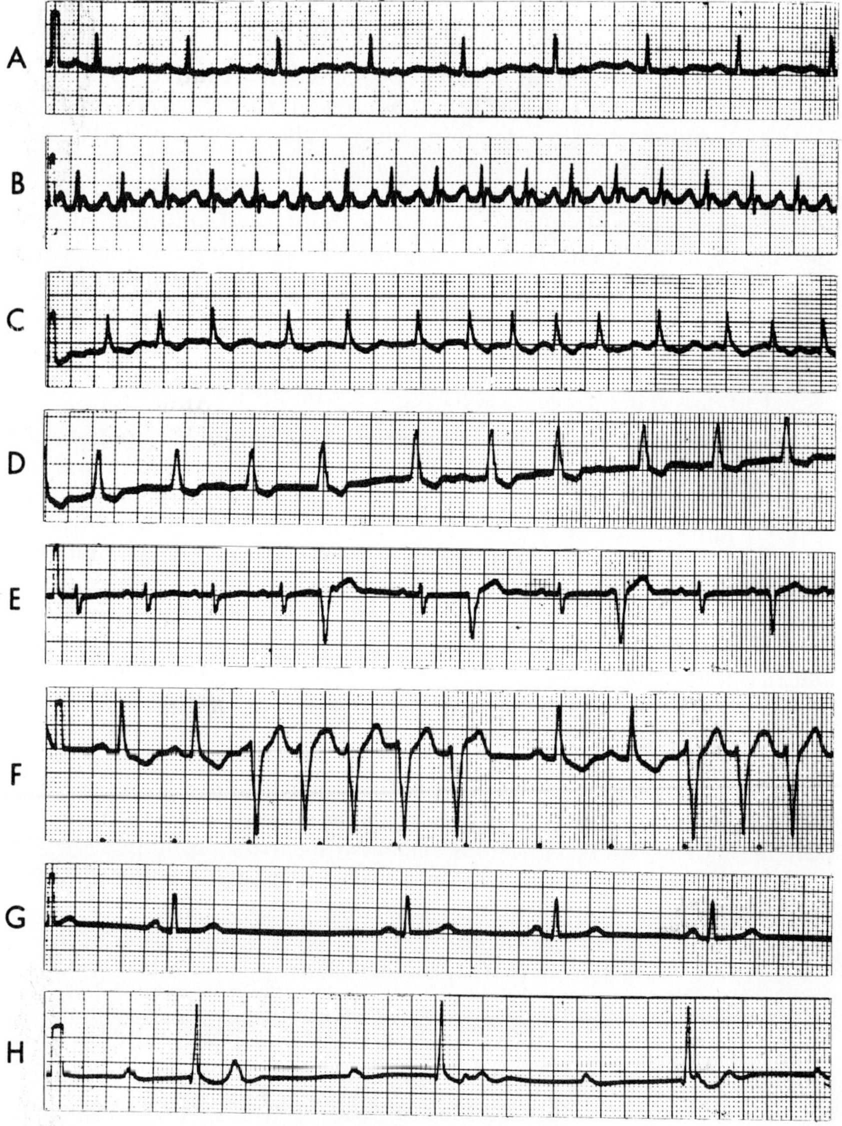

Fig. 21-1.—Legend on facing page.

for symptomatic relief. Oral administration of glyceryl trinitrate, 5–15 mg. 4 times daily sublingually or orally, pentaerythritol tetranitrate, 10–20 mg. 4 times daily, or isosorbide dinitrate, 10 mg. 4 times daily, provide relief. Propranolol in the wide range of oral dosage of 40–240 mg./day can be used in intractable cases but is hazardous when given acutely in preparation for emergency life-saving surgery because it decreases myocardial contractility.

Arrhythmias—Tachycardia

Figure 21-1 displays illustrations of common arrhythmias.

Correction of acid-base imbalance and/or hypokalemia.—Alkalosis and hypokalemia may precipitate ventricular arrhythmias because hypokalemia increases conduction through the AV node and decreases ventricular conduction; a decrease in Pco_2 increases atrial and ventric-

---

Fig. 21-1.—**A,** atrial tachycardia with 2:1 AV block. The P waves occur at a rate of 150/minute. The ventricular rate is 75/minute. This arrhythmia is most commonly seen with digitalis intoxication.

B, atrial flutter with 2:1 AV block. The undulating baseline consists of flutter waves at a rate of 310/minute. The ventricular rate is 155/minute. The degree of AV block can often be increased transiently by vagal stimulation (for example, carotid sinus massage). Digitalis preparations will increase the AV block and slow the ventricular rate.

C, atrial fibrillation with a moderately rapid ventricular response. Often with atrial fibrillation, the ventricular response will be very rapid; for example, the rate between cycles 7 and 11 is 160/minute. Digitalis will slow the average ventricular rate by increasing the degree of AV block. The diagnosis is primarily based upon the positive evidence of atrial fibrillation shown by the rapid, irregular atrial activity seen in the intervals between QRS complexes. This is well seen between the third and fourth QRS complexes. The gross irregularity of the ventricular rate corroborates the diagnosis.

D, atrial fibrillation with a moderate ventricular response. Here, there is also an intraventricular conduction disorder. The underlying atrial fibrillation can be identified from the baseline irregularity, especially between the third and fourth QRS complexes. The wide (0.10 second) QRS complexes in patients with an intraventricular conduction disorder may be erroneously called ventricular complexes of a ventricular tachycardia. This is seen in the ninth through the eleventh complexes.

E, normal sinus rhythm with parasystolic ventricular premature beats. Beats 5, 7, 9 and 11 are ventricular premature beats. Each is dissociated from the atria and is followed by a compensatory pause. The independent P wave immediately precedes beat 9. Beat 11 has an intermediate type of QRS complex reflecting a dual source of ventricular depolarization—the ventricles are partially depolarized by an impulse which originated in the atria (P-R interval = 0.16 second) and by an impulse which initiates the premature ventricular systoles. Fusion beats of this type prove the existence of AV dissociation and, therefore, prove that a ventricular focus is producing the premature systoles. The presence of fusion beats similarly can be used to distinguish ventricular tachycardia from atrial tachycardia with an associated intraventricular conduction delay.

F, normal sinus rhythm with paroxysms of ventricular tachycardia. AV dissociation is present during the ventricular tachycardia as shown by the independent P waves which continue through the tracing. The timing of each P wave is indicated by a dot.

G, sinus bradycardia. A sinus pause of 1.9 seconds is shown. Sinus bradycardia is common in the healthy population and has no import. In the presence of cardiac disease, bradycardia of any type may permit re-entrant ventricular premature beats to appear.

H, normal sinus rhythm, rate 70/minute, with complete AV block and a slow escape rhythm, probably originating in the bundle of His, at a rate of 29/minute. The presence of a slow ventricular rate often permits re-entrant ventricular beats or paroxysms of ventricular tachycardia. The generic therapy is to increase the ventricular rate, usually by cardiac pacing.

ular excitability. These changes appear to be related to the Pco_2 and the relationship of intracellular and extracellular potassium. Acidosis both decreases myocardial contractility and, when severe, predisposes to ventricular tachycardia or fibrillation. Chapter 6 discusses the treatment of acid-base derangements.

Hypokalemia due to potassium losses from diuretic administration or from the gastrointestinal tract merits special attention in any consideration of arrhythmias. Either atrial or ventricular premature beats or paroxysms of atrial or ventricular tachycardia may be produced. Prevention is the best cure; losses of potassium in urine or other body fluids should be measured and replaced. After the fact, potassium should be given to raise and maintain the serum potassium concentration above 4 mEq./L. Oral administration of as much as 40 mEq. every 4 hours can quickly restore body potassium stores. Potassium chloride can also be given intravenously in concentrations not to exceed 80 mEq./L. and with delivery rates not to exceed 40 mEq./hour. This material must be given into a securely cannulated central vein.

PACING.—Intrinsically slow heart rate (for example, sinus bradycardia or second to third degree AV block) provides an opportunity for reentry arrhythmias to appear. Bigeminal atrial or ventricular premature beats are the hallmarks of these arrhythmias. While often benign, they may lead to atrial or ventricular tachycardia, flutter or fibrillation. Atropine, 1 mg. intravenously, will often abolish sinus bradycardia. Particularly if a high degree of AV block is present and is the setting of episodes of ventricular tachycardia, a temporary transvenous right ventricular electrode catheter can be inserted. A battery powered pacemaker can then be used to control ventricular rate. This step will often abolish these arrhythmias.

DRUGS.—Four drugs share similar antiarrhythmic properties. Each slows the rate of diastolic depolarization of many abnormal rhythm-generating foci. Each also slows conduction in myocardial tissue and may thus stop re-entrant arrhythmias. These drugs are quinidine, procainamide, lidocaine and diphenylhydantoin. Each of these drugs is contraindicated in patients with AV block. Cardiac toxicity of these drugs is often preceded by prolongation of the QRS complex and the Q-T interval. An additional drug, propranolol, shares many points of similarity in the suppression of arrhythmias but does so predominantly by blocking β-adrenergic stimuli. Each of these drugs depresses myocardial contractility; quantitative differences exist, with propranolol, quinidine and procainamide most heavily influencing contractility.

Quinidine has its greatest use in slowing the atrial rate in an effort to convert atrial fibrillation and atrial flutter. Quinidine is also of value in abolishing or preventing supraventricular and ventricular tachycardias or premature systoles. The toxic side effects include nausea, vomiting, diarrhea, fever, rash, thrombocytopenia and cinchonism. The average dose is about 300 mg. every 6 hours, given orally or intramuscularly. The range is 200–400 mg. every 4–6 hours.

Procainamide has the same pharmacologic effects as quinidine. The dose is generally 500 mg. to 1 Gm. every 4–6 hours. This drug can be given intravenously at a rate of 100 mg. a minute to convert ventricular tachycardia; severe hypotension can occur.

Lidocaine has the major advantage of rapid onset and short duration of action. It is given intravenously as a bolus of up to 50 mg. or as an intravenous drip. The dose should not exceed 300 mg./hour. Lidocaine is generally used for ventricular arrhythmias, primarily ventricular tachycardia. The side effects, including lethargy, alterations in vision, convulsions and respiratory arrest, quickly disappear with cessation of the drug.

Diphenylhydantoin is effective primarily in ventricular arrhythmias such as unifocal or multifocal premature ventricular beats and in arrhythmias due to digitalis intoxication. For acute arrhythmias the intravenous dose is 250 mg., given over a 5-minute period. The oral or intramuscular maintenance dose is 100–200 mg. every 4–6 hours. The dose should not exceed 1,200 mg. in 24 hours. Disorientation, ataxia and other neurologic disorders occur with toxic levels.

Propranolol is a β-adrenergic blocking agent and exerts its major antiarrhythmic effect by this action. Thus this drug, by blocking the effects of norepinephrine and epinephrine on the heart, may stop or prevent many types of arrhythmias, including ventricular tachycardia.

Propranolol and other β-blocking agents also block the inotropic effects of natural or synthetic adrenergic amines. The resulting decrease in the force of contraction may suffice to precipitate or augment congestive failure. For this reason, β-blocking agents are usually contraindicated for patients who have congestive heart failure. The usual oral dose is 10–30 mg. 3–4 times a day. The intravenous dose is 1–4 mg., given at a rate of 1 mg./minute.

SYNCHRONIZED CARDIOVERSION.—Cardioversion is often of value in the correction of rapid atrial or ventricular arrhythmias. It is rendered more dangerous in the presence of excess digitalis. Ventricular tachycardia or fibrillation may occur. In general, cardioversion, except for ventricular fibrillation, is contraindicated in arrhythmias caused by digitalis toxicity. It is often used electively to convert atrial flutter or fibrillation. In elective use the patient should receive 200 mg. of quinidine sulfate every 6 hours for 24 hours prior to cardioversion. Digitalis is withheld on the morning of the procedure and 200 mg. quinidine sulfate is given intramuscularly 1 or 2 hours before cardioversion. The procedure is performed after the administration of 12–15 mg. of diazepam intravenously for sedation amnesia. Generally conversion will occur with discharges of 100 watt-sec. In case of failure the energy is increased in increments of 100 watt-sec. until 400 watt-sec. is reached.

ARRHYTHMIAS – BRADYCARDIA

Bradycardia may have any of 3 major deleterious effects. Hearts which have restricted stroke volumes may be unable to provide an adequate cardiac output; an idioventricular rhythm in complete AV block may be unstable and unreliable, producing episodic standstill and Stokes-Adams syncope; as noted previously, re-entrant ventricular premature beats or tachycardia may occur.

Atropine, 0.6 – 1.4 mg. intravenously, will often correct sinus bradycardia and, uncommonly, will reduce the degree of AV block.

β-Adrenergic stimulation, for example with 2–4 μg./minute of intravenous isoproterenol, will accelerate pacemaker cells of the sinus node, AV node or idioventricular foci in the Purkinje system. This drug markedly increases both myocardial contractility and oxygen consumption and is thus metabolically a costly antiarrhythmic agent. Isoproterenol will usually accelerate the sinus rate when given for sinus bradycardia, or an idioventricular rate when given to patients with AV block.

Endocardial pacing with a pacing catheter is the primary mode of therapy for sustained bradycardia. Atrial pacing is technically difficult with catheters; therefore, ventricular pacing is used to treat either sinus nodal or AV nodal disorders. Once pacing is established in patients with AV block, the previously contraindicated rhythm-suppressant drugs such as quinidine and lidocaine can be used to suppress ventricular premature beats.

Stabilization of Potential Risk Factors

Diabetes mellitus should be under adequate control before surgery is undertaken. On the day of surgery the patient will not have any food. The dose of insulin should be adjusted to avoid hypoglycemia. Also to be considered is the amount of intravenous glucose the patient will receive during the surgical procedure. There should be frequent tests for glucosuria.

Pulmonary insufficiency from chronic bronchitis or emphysema can be controlled and improved by instituting a program designed to reduce bronchial irritation. Cessation of cigaret smoking is the initial step. Expectorants are helpful to liquefy secretions. The iodides are the most common agents employed. Ten to 15 drops of saturated potassium iodide solution, 1 Gm./ml. in water or juice, can be given 3 or 4 times a day. Other agents, such as terpin hydrate, glyceryl guaiacolate and ammonium chloride, are also available. Mucolytic agents, such as acetylcysteine, reduce the viscosity of mucus and pus and may be administered by aerosol in a dosage of 3–5 ml. of a 20% solution every 4 or 6 hours. The use of mucolytic agents may cause a marked increase in tracheobronchial secretions; patients with an ineffective cough should receive these agents only under close surveillance. Tracheal aspiration may prove necessary to maintain an airway. Bronchodilators such as isoproterenol administered by nebulizer or aminophylline suppositories may provide minimal improvement. Rectal irritation is a common complication of aminophylline suppositories. Antibiotics are indicated if the patient is producing purulent sputum. Usually a broad spectrum drug such as ampicillin, 500 mg. four times daily, or tetracycline, 500 mg. four times daily, can be started after cultures have been obtained. Instruction in postural drainage, pursed-lip breathing and slow, deep respiratory excursions several times a day may help to preserve the bellows function of the thorax. Intermittent use of positive pressure breathing devices may also aid in failure, especially if a mucolytic agent is added.

Antihypertensive therapy with catecholamine-depleting (for example, reserpine, guanethidine) or blocking agents (propranolol) or with monoamine oxidase inhibitors (alpha methyldopa) optimally should be withheld for 2 weeks before surgery. (See Chapter 1.)

Prophylaxis of Endocarditis

Patients with congenital or valvular heart disease or those who have valvular prostheses have an increased risk of contracting bacterial endocarditis and thus should be protected with preoperative antibiotics in any procedures likely to produce bacteremia. Those having dental, nose, throat or other procedures where alpha streptococci abound should be given 600,000 units of penicillin intramuscularly the day before the procedure and for 3 days after the procedure. The patient should receive 600,000 units of aqueous penicillin intramuscularly one-half hour before the procedure. For abdominal or genitourinary procedures, when there is a risk of an enterococcal infection, 0.5–1 Gm. of ampicillin should be given orally or intramuscularly the day before surgery, the day of surgery and for 3 days after the procedure. An alternate regimen combines penicillin and streptomycin or, in patients allergic to penicillin, kanamycin (15 mg./kg. intramuscularly). During or immediately after the surgical procedure 3 blood cultures, one hour apart, should be obtained.

Anticoagulants

Patients receiving anticoagulants for previous pulmonary emboli, ischemic heart disease or implanted prosthetic valves pose little problem in elective surgery. Merely stopping the anticoagulant for 3 or 4 days usually suffices to return the prothrombin time to normal values; this process can be hastened by the intramuscular administration of 5–10 mg. of vitamin K_1. Preparation of the anticoagulated patient for emergency surgery must rely heavily upon vitamin K_1 in doses of up to 20 mg. intramuscularly. Rarely the press of time may require partial exchange transfusion with fresh blood.

POSTOPERATIVE MANAGEMENT

General Measures

The postoperative care will depend on the type of surgery. In general, certain principles prevail. In the previously orthopneic patient elevation of the head of the bed may improve comfort and ventilation. Abdominal distention should be avoided by the use of a nasogastric tube. The patient should be encouraged to cough and begin to exercise and be mobile in bed. Elastic stockings may improve peripheral venous drainage and prevent thrombophlebitis and pulmonary emboli.

Fluid and electrolyte balance should be closely observed and regulated by accurate records of intake and output of fluids and electrolytes, by monitoring the central venous pressure and by careful clinical assessment. If the central venous pressure and urine output remain adequate, 800 ml./$m.^2$ of intravenous fluid daily can be safely administered. If fluids or blood must be given, 5% dextrose in water with enough sodium to balance losses may be given. Packed cells instead of whole blood should be administered to correct normovolemic anemia. The serum potassium should be kept above 4.0 mEq./L. Any acid-base imbalance should be corrected, as outlined in Chapter 6. Oral fluids should be resumed as soon as possible.

Anticoagulants, when indicated, may be started or reinstituted approximately 48 hours after surgery. Initially, use of heparin is preferable because the short duration of action permits prompt cessation if bleeding occurs. The dosage should be adjusted to double the control clotting time one-half hour before the next 4-hourly dose. After cardiopulmonary bypass the prothrombin time is commonly prolonged. Sustained anticoagulation can often be achieved by administering prothrombin depressant agents as the initial anticoagulant.

Major Cardiac Complications

CONGESTIVE HEART FAILURE. – The increased administration of parenteral fluids, increased amounts of blood loss and the development of postoperative infection are the usual causes of postoperative congestive heart failure in the cardiac patient. Treatment is the same as that described under Overt Congestive Heart Failure.

MYOCARDIAL INFARCTION. – Myocardial infarction should be constantly suspected in the surgical cardiac patient, particularly one who has experienced hypotensive episodes, as the usual signs and symptoms may not be present or may have been masked by anesthetics or analgesics. Mild to moderate hypotension with adequate perfusion may be the first manifestation. Arrhythmias, varying from multiple premature ventricular contractions to runs of supraventricular or ventricular tachycardia, may be present. Congestive heart failure and pulmonary edema may be the only indication of a myocardial infarction. Enzyme analyses are of limited value due to the tissue trauma from surgery, but electrocardiograms may show typical ST-T segment changes and the presence of Q waves. Therapy should be the same as for any myocardial infarction. Anticoagulation should be instituted when it is surgically permissible and extended bed rest should be instituted. The usual coronary precautions should be maintained.

ARRHYTHMIAS.—Arrythmias may occur postoperatively and may be relatively benign or life-threatening. Electrocardiographic monitoring and analysis of electrocardiographic recordings which demonstrate both P waves and QRS complexes are the only means of establishing the nature of arrhythmias. Figure 21-1 displays selected examples of common arrhythmias.

Sinus tachycardia is one of the most common arrhythmias seen postoperatively. The rate varies between 100 and 150; it is regular and slows gradually with carotid sinus massage. It is usually secondary to fever, hypovolemia or anoxia. Therapy is usually directed towards the underlying cause. Specifically, digitalization will not correct sinus tachycardia, even at toxic levels, except as a secondary response when congestive heart failure is improved.

Supraventricular tachycardias may represent atrial tachycardias, nodal tachycardias or a group of undetermined origin. The rate is usually 150–200 beats/minute and is very regular. Carotid sinus massage either has no effect or abruptly slows the rate with restoration of sinus rhythm; the tachycardia may abruptly return. This arrhythmia may occur in patients without cardiac disease; such patients may be perfectly comfortable. Generally reassurance and sedation will restore normal sinus rhythm. Vagal stimulation, vasopressors (Neo-Synephrine, 0.5–1 mg. intravenously over 2–3 minutes) or rapid digitalization may be used to restore normal sinus rhythm. The sudden slowing in rate with carotid massage or intravenous Neo-Synephrine can also be used to distinguish an atrial tachycardia from a sinus mechanism.

Premature atrial contractions are usually benign but may be an indication of more serious arrhythmias to follow. When frequent, these can be treated with quinidine, 200–400 mg. every 4–6 hours.

Ventricular premature beats may be benign but may also occur with a myocardial infarction, impending congestive heart failure, with hypokalemia and with digitalis intoxication. The therapy will depend on the underlying cause, as discussed previously.

Atrial fibrillation is characterized as a rapid ventricular rate and an irregular rhythm in the presence of atrial fibrillatory waves. In the undigitalized patient the rate is generally over 100 and may be as fast as 180/minute. Carotid sinus pressure may produce transient slowing. Digitalis is the drug of choice for slowing the rate. It can be given orally to the patient who is not in distress. If more rapid slowing of the rate is desired, a fast-acting preparation should be given parenterally. In instances when the tachycardia is producing hypotension or secondary arrhythmias, direct-current countershock should be used.

Atrial flutter is similar to atrial fibrillation. The atrial rate varies from 250 to 350. The ventricular response in the undigitalized patient is generally in the ratio of 1 ventricular beat for every 2 flutter waves, but variable degrees of block may be present. This arrhythmia is rather unstable and more resistant to slowing with digitalis than atrial fibrillation. Synchronized countershock is the treatment of choice. The degree of AV block can often be increased and the ventricular rate controlled with digitalis if countershock fails.

Paroxysmal atrial tachycardia with block is due to digitalis intoxication 80% of the time. The atrial rate is between 150 and 240; there is usually a 2:1 AV block. The P waves are often small and spiked and demonstrate a ventriculophasic response. (The P-P interval around the QRS complex is shorter than the P-P interval between the QRS complexes.) It is important to differentiate this rhythm from atrial flutter with 2:1 block. In flutter the electrocardiogram demonstrates faster atrial activity with "sawtooth"-appearing P waves, an uneven baseline and no ventriculophasic atrial arrhythmia. If this is due to digitalis, the drug must be discontinued. Potassium chloride, 60 mEq. in 100 ml. 5% dextrose in water, can be given over a 1–3 hour period. Diphenylhydantoin may also revert the rhythm. Direct current cardioversion is contraindicated because countershock may cause ventricular tachycardia in patients with digitalis intoxication.

Ventricular tachycardia is manifested by a rapid, usually regular rate. The rate usually varies between 150 and 220. There is often a slight irregularity with wide bizarre QRS complexes, AV dissociation and an occasional fusion beat or ventricular capture. This arrhythmia is generally life-threatening and must be treated promptly. When perfusion is maintained, lidocaine, 50 mg. given intravenously, will often cause conversion. Subsequent ventricular premature beats can often be suppressed with a slow lidocaine infusion of less than 300 mg./hour. If systemic perfusion is ineffective, direct-current countershock should be employed immediately. Repetitive ventricular tachycardia generally is due to an underlying metabolic cause. Acid-base and electrolyte imbalances should be corrected. Sustained irritability should be treated with quinidine, diphenylhydantoin, procainamide or lidocaine, as described previously.

When these arrhythmias occur because of an intervening bradycardia, the basic heart rate should be increased with atropine, isoproterenol or temporary pacing, all of which have been described under the section Arrhythmias—Bradycardia.

CARDIAC ARREST.—Cardiac arrest is due to ventricular fibrillation or asystole. Ventricular fibrillation which is noted within 30 seconds should never lead to cardiac massage. Immediate direct-current defibrillation should be attempted. The defibrillator electrodes optimally should be placed with 1 under the back and 1 over the precordium; in this way the danger of shock to the nurse or physician is minimized since only 1 electrode is held. Alternatively, 1 electrode can be placed over the cardiac apex and the other, held by a second person, at the upper right sternal margin. Only if this is unsuccessful, or if more than 30 seconds have elapsed, should external cardiac compression be begun.

External massage should be given 80–100 times/minute with the patient on a solid surface. Respiration should be begun immediately, preferably with tracheal intubation and a manually operated valved bag at rate of 12–16 times/minute. Cardiac massage should be suspended momentarily during each exhalation. Acidosis should be corrected with 45 mEq. of sodium bicarbonate given every 5–10 minutes intravenously, with the exact amount to be gauged by the blood pH and Pco_2. The effect of the external cardiac compression can be assessed by noting the femoral or carotid pulsations. Subsequent efforts at defibrillation should be repeated when acidosis has been corrected and oxygenation has been achieved. If no spontaneous cardiac activity occurs after several minutes, 0.2–0.4 mg. of isoproterenol or 0.3–0.5 Gm. calcium gluconate intracardiac may increase the force of contractions.

If cardiac action is restored but there is sinus bradycardia or AV block, ventricular pacing can be instituted. This can either be done by inserting a temporary pacemaker under fluoroscopic control through the jugular vein into the right ventricle or by the percutaneous insertion of a small pacing wire into the ventricle through the anterior chest wall.

SHOCK.—Shock is a state of circulatory failure manifested by mental stupor, weakness, hypotension, peripheral vasoconstriction, acidosis and decreased renal function. The blood volume and heart rate may be high or low depending upon the cause. In the postoperative patient the commonest causes of shock are (1) blood loss, (2) cardiogenic, as from acute myocardial infarction and (3) infectious, as with septicemic shock.

As soon as shock is recognized, therapy should be instituted. The patient should be placed in the horizontal position and kept warm. An airway should be maintained and oxygen administered. If the central venous pressure is less than 8 cm. H_2O, plasma expanders such as salt-poor albumin or graded blood transfusions should be administered. If congestive heart failure is present or if the patient is in atrial fibrillation or atrial flutter, digitalis should be added. β-Adrenergic drugs such as isoproterenol or α-adrenergic stimulating agents such as methoxamine, phenylephrine, metaraminol or angiotensin may be given in a dose sufficient to maintain a blood pressure of 70–80 mm./Hg or the minimum level adequate to provide tissue perfusion. When perfusion is inadequate due to intense peripheral vasoconstriction, peripheral vasodilators such as chlorpromazine, 5–12 mg. intravenously, phenoxybenzamine, 1–2 mg./kg. intravenously, or prednisone, 30 mg./kg. intravenously, will often produce peripheral vasodilation. Simultaneously the venous pressure may fall; usually the use of peripheral vasodilators requires simultaneous expansion of blood volume with blood or albumin to sustain perfusion.

Pulmonary Complications

Pulmonary complications are frequently encountered in the postoperative patient and are generally associated with fever and tachycardia and often with augmented congestive failure. The commonest causes of these complications are discussed below.

The patient with *pulmonary emboli* may have, in addition to fever and tachycardia, pleuritic chest pain, bronchoconstriction, dyspnea and hemoptysis. The chest x-ray may be normal; if pulmonary infarction has occurred, a density may be noted, usually in the lower lobes. The electrocardiogram may show only a sinus tachycardia, a right axis shift, right bundle branch block or an S_I, Q_{III} pattern. The primary therapy for pulmonary embolism is anticoagulation with heparin, the clotting time maintained at about twice the control value at the time of the next dose. An adequate initial dose is usually 10,000 units given intravenously. In addition, symptomatic therapy with oxygen and sedation can be used. Recurrent emboli in the face of adequate anticoagulation may necessitate inferior vena caval ligation or plication. If cardiovascular collapse from a massive embolus has occurred, pulmonary embolectomy must be considered.

Atelectasis is frequently encountered and is generally due to pooled bronchial secretions occluding a bronchus. This is generally manifested by fever, tachycardia, dyspnea and decreased heart sounds with bronchial breath sounds and dullness to percussion over the involved area. Persistent and conscientious nasotracheal toilet and patient cooperation in frequent coughing can prevent this complication. When a major bronchus has been occluded, bronchoscopy may become necessary. Occasionally aspiration of intestinal contents can also occur and rapidly produce inflammation and a chemical pneumonitis. Prompt bronchoscopy and bronchial lavage may minimize the inflammatory reaction. Steroid therapy has been advocated for this.

Management after Cardiac Surgery

The same principles regarding fluid, electrolyte and acid-base balance which have been discussed previously apply to patients after heart surgery. In addition, careful observations must be conducted for incomplete correction or disruption of the correction of the initial cardiac defect, for example, the appearance of regurgitation through a valve prosthesis. The management of arrhythmias is similar to that after noncardiac surgery.

CARDIOGENIC SHOCK.—In addition to the complications already mentioned, one which is quantitatively more common after cardiac surgery is the overwhelming problem of cardiogenic shock, with its components of hypotension, low cardiac output and poor renal, cerebral and peripheral perfusion. The patients suffering from the low cardiac output syndrome can be usefully subdivided into two groups: those in whom the disorder is correctable and those in whom it may only be modifiable.

Correctable disorders.—Many patients return from cardiac surgery with, or subsequently develop, *hypovolemia* due to bleeding or excessive diuresis. The hallmark is a low central venous pressure. Commonly this state can be reversed by volume repletion with blood or albumin given in increments of 100 ml. while the central venous pressure, the arterial pressure, the urine output and the peripheral perfusion are monitored.

Arrhythmias per se may cause very low cardiac outputs by (1) removing effective atrial systole, (2) a rapid ventricular rate or (3) an unphysiologically slow ventricular rate. The therapy for these arrhythmias has been previously discussed.

Disruption of the surgical corrective procedure may, if detected, lead to a second, successful effort to reduce a massive shunt or correct a faulty valvular prosthesis.

In the presence of a low cardiac output and an elevated central venous pressure, *pericardial tamponade* from cardiac bleeding must be considered even in the absence of the classic clinical features. An enlarging cardiac silhouette seen on serial x-rays may permit a tentative diagnosis (see Fig. 14-4). Pericardial aspiration or surgical re-exploration may be lifesaving.

Herniation of the heart through a widely opened pericardium is rare but promptly correctable. This produces overt cardiogenic shock and a unique radiographic appearance (see Fig. 14-8, *B*).

Modifiable disorders.—In general, other causes of the low output syndrome relate to intrinsically poor myocardial function. Intraoperative myocardial infarction, residual myocardial damage from the lesion for which surgery was performed and diverse metabolic derangements may all be causally related. The treatment is the same as that for congestive failure and for shock. Optimal ventilation, prevention or prompt correction of atelectasis and prompt treatment of pulmonary infections will permit high pulmonary vascular resistance beds to open. Correction of acidosis is crucial. Peripheral vasodilation may increase perfusion without adding hypertension to the burden on the heart. Isoproterenol can exert an inotropic effect, at a high metabolic cost, in addition to that produced by full digitalization. The major therapeutic aims of increased perfusion at a decreased cardiac load may, in selected instances in the future, be attained by circulatory assist devices. The passage of time at reduced cardiac work loads may permit even badly damaged ventricles to heal and become smaller and more efficient pumps.

OTHER COMPLICATIONS.—*Central nervous system* complications are common after cardiac surgery, ranging from major cerebral infarction due to emboli through transient periods of disorientation and confusion. The former is generally fatal. The latter are transient and probably reflect transient cerebral hypoxia. Optimal oxygenation is mandatory. Large doses of corticosteroids (30 mg./kg. daily for 2 days) may reduce cerebral edema. Active or passive physiotherapy should be started as soon as the wound permits.

Several complications of cardiac surgery occur or are detected days to weeks after operation and will only be mentioned briefly.

Postpericardiotomy syndrome, of unknown origin, occurs as early as 10 days after surgery. Fever, pleuritis and pericarditis are common. Rarely are pleural or pericardial taps necessary. The major importance lies in distinguishing this disorder from bacterial endocarditis, pneumonia or pulmonary emboli and myocardial infarction. Salicylates or, uncommonly, steroids may prove necessary.

Intravascular hemolysis, especially with valvular prostheses, may lead to the insidious appearance of anemia and reappearance of congestive heart failure. Rarely this complication requires reoperation for correction of a leaking prosthesis.

Bacterial endocarditis should be suspected and sought in any patient with sustained fever after cardiac surgery; antibiotic prophylaxis during surgery does not prevent this complication.

22

Major Abdominal Surgery

ALEXANDER DOOLAS, M.D.

Assistant Attending Surgeon, Rush-Presbyterian-St. Luke's Medical Center; Assistant Professor of Surgery, Rush Medical College

UNDERSTANDING PRE- AND POSTOPERATIVE CARE is essential to the successful completion of major abdominal surgery. Because certain aspects of the care of patients having various types of major abdominal surgery are similar, they will be considered first.

Postoperative Orders in Major Abdominal Surgery

1. *Vital signs.*

The vital signs include pulse, blood pressure and respiration. They should be evaluated at frequent intervals in order to perceive changes in the patient's condition. An example of a schedule is as follows:

q	5 minutes	×	30 minutes
q	15 minutes	×	1 hour
q	1/2 hour	×	2 hours
q	1 hour	×	4 hours
q	2 hours	×	2 hours, then 4 times daily

These orders are routinely begun in the recovery room until the patient's condition is stable, after which he is sent to the intensive care unit. In addition to the vital signs the patient's color, skin turgor, temperature, quality of respirations and general behavior are observed. The nursing staff is of great help in assessing the patient's condition.

2. *Pain medication.*

The most effective pain medication is morphine sulfate. The usual dose is 10–15 mg. intramuscularly every 4–6 hours as required for young, heavier patients. For elderly patients 3–5 mg. intramuscularly every 2–3 hours as required will give analgesia without hypnosis. Other analgesics are Demerol in doses of 50–100 mg. given every 2–6 hours and Talwin in doses of 15–30 mg. given every 2–6 hours. Analgesics should be given cautiously to patients who have carbon dioxide retention associated with emphysema or asthma to avoid respiratory depression and hypotension.

In shock and other conditions in which the peripheral circulation is impaired, analgesics must be given intravenously in one-fourth to one-third the usual dose.

3. *Nothing by mouth (N.P.O.).*

After extensive surgery a paralytic ileus develops which necessitates gastric drainage. Ingestion of liquids will cause gastric dilatation and hypersecretion, emesis and fluid and electrolyte depletion. Patients who have had esophageal anastomoses must be on N.P.O. for at least 10–12 days, due to the high incidence of anastomotic leaks, fistula and abscess formation.

The decision to allow oral intake depends on the type of surgery performed and on evidence that the gastrointestinal tract functions well. Absolute evidence of a properly functioning gastrointestinal tract are the passage of flatus, a flat abdomen and a scanty gastric aspirate. The presence of bowel sounds alone is a poor evidence of adequate gastrointestinal function.

After gastrointestinal function has been established, the gastric drainage is discontinued. The oral intake is begun with small volumes of clear liquids, usually 60 ml., given every hour, then advanced to a clear or full liquid diet on the following day, and then gradually to a solid diet. As a rule, most patients who have had major surgery start on an oral diet the sixth or seventh day. If nausea and abdominal discomfort or abdominal and gastric distention occur after oral intake, the following causes must be sought: paralytic ileus, segmental ileus, a partially obstructed anastomosis, peritonitis, abscess or a mechanical bowel obstruction. Nasogastric drainage should be reinstituted and oral intake discontinued.

4. *Record fluid intake and output (I & O).*

"Intake" includes all intravenous fluids, riders, oral intake and irrigating solutions. "Output" includes urine, fistula, wound and gastrointestinal drainage. In exceptional cases the fecal output is also measured. The fluid and electrolyte balance can only be properly maintained if good intake and output records are tabulated.

5. *Nasogastric tube or gastrostomy to low Gomco suction. Irrigate with 30 ml. normal saline and aspirate every 2–4 hours.*

The major function of gastric drainage is to allow escape of swallowed air. The volume of gastric aspirate in uncomplicated cases is approximately 400–1,000 ml. daily. Foley-type gastrostomies may function better on free drainage than on suction since the latter may draw the gastric mucosa into the perforations, thus blocking the outlet. The distance from the nose to the stomach should be noted on the nasogastric tube to allow the tube to lie uncoiled in the body of the stomach. The tube is taped to the nose with care to prevent pressure necrosis and occlusion of the opposite naris. All gastric drainage tubes should be irrigated with 30–60 ml. normal saline every 2–4 hours to maintain patency. The aspirations must be gentle to avoid mucosal trauma and bleeding.

Gastric aspiration is discontinued when the drainage is minimal, the abdomen is flat and the patient passes flatus. The adequacy of gastric emptying can be tested by instilling 60 ml. of water every hour for 3 hours, keeping the tube clamped between instillations and aspirating the tube the fourth hour. A volume of less than 60–90 ml. indicates adequate gastric emptying.

6. *Jejunostomy tube to free drainage. Irrigate with 30 ml. normal saline every 2–4 hours.*

In the absence of a distal obstruction, a feeding jejunostomy drains little fluid. The jejunostomy is placed on free drainage for 2–3 days, then clamped or used for feeding. To keep the tube patent, it is irrigated with 30 ml. normal saline every 2–4 hours. Aspiration usually yields only a few milliliters and therefore is not necessary. In prolonged periods of gastric retention the patient may be fed through the jejunostomy if there is no distal obstruction. The feedings consist of a blenderized high-calorie, high-protein diet. The gastric aspirate may be saved in a refrigerator and pumped into the jejunostomy as needed. The feedings should be administered slowly throughout the 24 hours to prevent dumping symptoms. A Baron pump serves this purpose well. Occasionally diarrhea may accompany high volumes of feeding. This is corrected with 5–10 ml. of Lomotil or paregoric given every 4 hours.

7. *Sump drains to high Gomco suction. Do not irrigate.*

Sump drains are used in procedures in which it is important that the drainage be brought to the outside with certainty. These drains are placed on high Gomco suction and are sutured to the skin to prevent accidental removal. A safety pin passed through the sump will prevent loss of the drain into the wound after it has been advanced.

Sump suction is discontinued in 3 or 4 days or when the drainage decreases to negligible quantities, thus allowing the patient to ambulate more easily. The schedule of drain advancement depends on the type of surgery and the indications for the employment of drains which will be discussed separately.

8. *Urine volume and specific gravity every 4 hours.*

Many patients having major abdominal surgery have an indwelling Foley catheter inserted prior to surgery. In its absence, the patient must void within 8–10 hours after surgery when permitted. Standing, listening to running water and a moist, warm towel placed on the lower abdomen may help the patient void. The patient is catheterized if he is unable to void or does so only in small amounts. The decision to leave an indwelling catheter will depend on the type of surgery performed, previous symptoms of prostatic hypertrophy and the need to measure the urinary output.

The urinary output is a sensitive indicator of cardiac output and blood volume. The minimum acceptable urinary output is approximately 30 ml. an hour. If the patient's condition is stable, the urinary volume and specific gravity can be measured every 4 hours. If, however, the patient is hypotensive, is bleeding or is hypovolemic, the urinary volume is measured every hour. As the patient's condition improves and the urinary volume increases to acceptable levels, measurement may be done less often. In 3–4 days when the patient is ambulatory, the Foley catheter is removed after a culture and colony count are obtained. The patient should be urged to void 6–8 hours after removal of the catheter. Patients who have had extensive pelvic surgery require a catheter for a longer time.

9. *Intravenous fluids*

During the first postoperative day 2 large intravenous routes are preferred so that whole blood or other colloid solutions may be given rapidly without disturbing the schedule of the routine fluids. One of these catheters may be centrally located for measuring the central venous pressure.

This section will not deal with the calculations of intravenous fluids, which is discussed elsewhere. Fluid orders should be written accurately and completely, for example:

Bottle #1		1,000 ml. 5% D/W	
	with	1 amp. multivitamins	
	with	500 mg. vitamin C	× 8 hours–8 A.M. to 4 P.M.
	with	1,000 units heparin	
Bottle #2		1,000 ml. 5% D/0.45NS	
	with	1,000 units heparin	× 8 hours–4 P.M. to 12 A.M.
Bottle #3		1,000 ml. 5% D/W	
	with	500 mg. vitamin C	
	with	20 mEq. KCl	× 8 hours–12 A.M. to 8 A.M.
	with	1,000 units heparin	

Heparin prevents the clotting of blood which may back up into the intravenous catheter. Potassium is usually withheld the first day or given in very small amounts, since there is a great K^+ release from damaged or lysed cells during surgery and from the transfused blood. Five Gm. or 75 mEq. of Na^+ are given during the first day as a rule. It has been found that small quantities of Na^+ maintain an adequate urinary output.

Fluid orders are written at the same time each day after checking the electrolyte and fluid balance of the preceding 24 hours. A flow sheet is essential in complicated cases.

10. *Turn, cough and hyperventilate (TCH) every 2 hours. Dangle four times a day for 10 minutes. Walk patient four times a day for 5 minutes when tolerated.*

These orders are intended to help the patient raise secretions from the tracheobronchial tree and to maintain venous flow in the legs. In addition, they decrease incisional pain and promote a sense of well-being. Prolonged sitting and dangling cause venous stasis, so that walking is preferred when the patient's condition permits.

Because of incisional pain, discomfort and fear, many patients have difficulty with coughing. These patients should be helped to cough after pain medication is given and while they clutch a pillow against the abdomen. A scultetus binder lends comfort to the patient but slides over the chest if not applied properly and thus embarrasses ventilation. An overhead frame and trapeze will allow the patient to maneuver in bed more easily.

11. *Electrolyte and blood urea nitrogen (BUN) determinations.*

These tests are usually required the day after surgery. The frequency of subsequent determinations will depend on the difficulty of maintaining fluid and electrolyte balance.

12. *Hemoglobin and hematocrit.*

Hemoglobin and hematocrit determinations should be made directly after the operation as a reference point. After 24 hours the fluid compartments have usually equilibrated and further changes in these determinations indicate blood loss, hemoconcentration or hemodilution. A change of 1 Gm. of hemoglobin or 3% of the hematocrit usually indicates a loss or gain of 1 unit of whole blood in the absence of laboratory error.

13. *Sleep medication.*

Sleep medication should not be ordered the first few postoperative days. If the patient takes a hypnotic, he may suffer pain without fully awakening to ask for pain medication, thus spending a restless night. After 2 or 3 days Seconal, 100 mg. at bedtime as required, given intramuscularly or orally, may be ordered. Older patients may require a milder hypnotic.

14. *Antiemetics.*

Antiemetics should be withheld until gastric dilatation and the improper function of drainage tubes have been excluded. Postoperative nausea is usually limited to the first 6–12 hours and may be related to pain medications. Tigan, 200 mg. intramuscularly, or Compazine, 10 mg. intramuscularly, given every 6 hours as required, are useful antiemetics.

15. *Antibiotics.*

Antibiotics may be indicated for a known or probable infection or contamination after cultures have been taken. The intermittent administration of antibiotics as riders in 5% D/W every 6 hours over a 15 minute period is the most effective method. This does not substitute for adequate drainage of contaminated and infected areas.

Parenteral Hyperalimentation

Nutrition is an important aspect of the pre- and postoperative care of the patient in the intensive care unit. Parenteral hyperalimentation is defined as the parenteral administration of necessary nutrients in sufficient quantities to maintain a positive metabolic state.

Bony and soft tissue trauma leads to a generalized breakdown of body proteins in greater quantities than would be expected from the amount of tissue injured. The severity of this catabolic response depends on the extent of the injury, the degree of sepsis, the physical condition of the patient and the duration and degree of starvation and immobilization. As yet the mechanism for the catabolic response to injury has not been clearly understood.

It has been shown that the mortality and morbidity after gastrectomy for pyloric stenosis in poorly nourished patients is much higher than in those patients who are well nourished. Hypoproteinemia may result in dehiscence, wound infection, delayed gastrointestinal motility, decreased tolerance to acute blood loss and decreased antibody production.

The need for maintaining nutrition in surgical patients has been recognized. However, a practical method for supplying large quantities of nutrients to surgical patients parenterally has been slow in development. Three factors prevented this achievement: (1) the ever-present rapid development of phlebitis in peripheral veins, (2) septicemia following long-term use of peripherally placed catheters and (3) the previous belief that a positive nitrogen balance could not be achieved after major trauma. In 1968, however, Dudrick[1,2] was able to achieve consistently, and for prolonged periods of time, a positive nitrogen balance with associated weight gain and healing of wounds and fistulae in pre- and postoperative patients. There were no instances of thrombosis or septicemia. This achievement is attributed to the method of administration, which involves the percutaneous insertion into the subclavian vein of a large polyethylene catheter which is then advanced into the superior vena cava. Infection and phlebitis are not serious problems for the following reasons: (1) the use of sterile surgical technique, (2) the fact that rapid flow in the subclavian vein prevents stasis and bacterial growth around the catheter, (3) the infusion of the hypertonic solution into the superior vena cava where it is rapidly diluted, (4) frequent changes of the intravenous tubing and meticulous care of the puncture site.

SUBCLAVIAN CANNULATION.—The patient is placed in the Trendelenburg position to increase filling of the subclavian vein. A small folded sheet is placed beneath the upper thoracic spine to hyperextend the shoulders. The upper anterior chest on the side selected for puncture is scrubbed with soap and the skin is defatted with ether and prepared with iodine and alcohol.

The physician performing the catheterization wears a surgical

Fig. 22-1.—Subclavian cannulation.

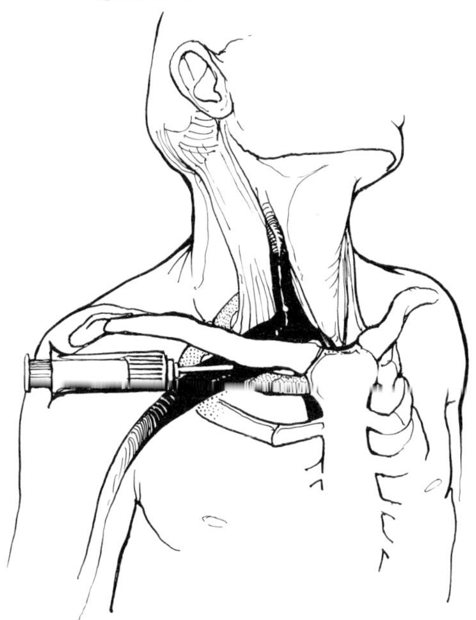

mask, cap and gloves. A skin wheal with 1% Lidocaine is made at approximately the midpoint of the clavicle and just below it. A 2-in. #14 needle is connected to a 3 ml. syringe. The needle is inserted through the wheal into the subcutaneous tissue and is advanced under the clavicle and in front of the first rib, parallel to the frontal plane of the chest toward the suprasternal notch. Care is taken to avoid puncturing the pleura or the subclavian artery by keeping the needle parallel to the frontal plane of the chest. A rush of blood indicates entrance into the subclavian vein, after which the needle is advanced slightly and an 8-in. #16 polyethylene catheter is inserted (Fig. 22-1). If the patient is in the Trendelenburg position, air will not enter the vena cava. The needle is withdrawn, its tip is bent back with a hemostat and the catheter is sutured to the skin. A topical antibiotic is applied to the puncture site and an occlusive dressing is placed over both the puncture site and the junction of the catheter with the intravenous tubing.

Care of the catheter.—Long-term subclavian catheterization is safe. Sepsis and pulmonary embolization are rare. To maintain the sterility of the catheter, the intravenous tubing and the occlusive dressing are changed every 3 days, the skin prepared with iodine and alcohol and the topical antibiotic reapplied. Other intravenous fluids or medications should not be given through this route. The changing of solutions must be accomplished carefully to prevent contamination.

NUTRITIONAL REQUIREMENTS.—Whereas 40 Gm. of protein and 1,500 calories are the daily requirements for a resting individual, 200 Gm. of protein and 3,000–5,000 calories may be required in postoperative patients to maintain a positive nitrogen balance. A positive nitrogen balance in postsurgical patients may be achieved through gastric feedings containing 0.3 Gm. nitrogen/kg. and 30 calories/kg. daily.[4] More recently a positive nitrogen balance has been repeatedly achieved by supplying as much as 0.45 Gm. nitrogen/kg. and 60 calories/kg. daily parenterally.[3] For a 50 kg. individual this is approximately 140 Gm. of protein and 3,000 calories daily. The caloric needs are supplied with a 50% D/W solution and the protein requirements with protein hydrolysates (Amigen or Aminosol). Each 500 ml. of 50% D/W supplies 1,000 calories, and each 1,000 ml. of 5% dextrose with 5% amino acid supplies 6 Gm. nitrogen and 200 nonprotein calories. The ratio of nitrogen to calories should be 1:200 or 1:150.

Potassium plays an important role in the maintenance of nutrition. It is believed that K^+ helps dextrose and nitrogen enter the cell and thus is required in greater amounts than those found in routine fluids. The ratio of potassium to nitrogen in the cell is 3 mEq. K^+ to 1 Gm. nitrogen. In the catabolic state, however, some cells lose as much as 15 mEq. K^+ for each 1 Gm. nitrogen lost and therefore patients on parenteral hyperalimentation frequently require 100–200 mEq. K^+ daily for the reparative process.

Postoperative patients have a transient intolerance for glucose manifested by a diabetic glucose tolerance curve. This, as a rule, persists for no more than a few days because the pancreas is stimulated by dextrose and the various amino acids to produce more endogenous insulin. In some patients, however, extremely high blood sugar levels occur, which could lead to glycosuria, dehydration and electrolyte loss. These patients, as well as diabetics, require exogenous insulin. Regular insulin or Lente insulin may be given. Usually 20 units of regular insulin every 6 hours or 20 units of Lente insulin every morning controls the glycosuria. If high glucose levels persist, the insulin requirement may be increased to 20 units for each 1,000 calories or each 250 Gm. glucose administered.

The requirements for NaCl are approximately 5 Gm. or 75 mEq. daily in addition to that lost from other sources. To avoid the infusion of large fluid volumes, these requirements may be supplied by a 5% NaCl solution.

Other electrolytes such as calcium and phosphorus are added periodically as needed. Patients with high output fistulae or those who have not had an oral diet for a week will require 5–10 mEq. of magnesium daily. Other trace elements are not required until after the first month of total parenteral nutrition. After this time the needs may be supplied with infusions of 1 or 2 units of fresh unpooled plasma weekly.

Vitamins supply the proper enzyme systems for the utilization of nutrients. The minimum daily requirements of vitamins A, B, D and E must be supplied daily. Vitamin C in doses of 1,000 mg. increases the rate of wound healing and therefore should be used in this amount. Vitamin K may be given weekly in doses of 10 mg. Vitamin B_{12} and folic acid may be used as indicated.

Heparin in doses of 1,000 units is placed in each bottle to prevent clotting of blood in the catheter.

Preparation of solutions.—For optimum utilization the protein hydrolysates and caloric requirements must be infused simultaneously. Unfortunately amino acids cannot be preserved for great periods of time when mixed with hypertonic glucose; therefore, these solutions must be mixed daily. A relatively simple method of mixing is as follows: Through intravenous tubing, 1,000 ml. of amino acid solution and 500 ml. of 50% D/W solution are infused into a 2,000 ml. Travenol vacuum plasma collecting unit and the tubing is discarded. The other nutrients are added by needle and syringe. For intravenous infusions a #18 needle is inserted into the air inlet site and the tubing is inserted into the outlet site. One such bottle supplies 1,500 ml. of fluid, 1,200 nonprotein calories and 6 Gm. of nitrogen.

An alternate method of preparation is as follows: 250 ml. of fluid is poured out of a 1,000 ml. amino acid bottle and 350 ml. of 50% D/W added, resulting in a volume of 1,100 ml. with 4.5 Gm. of nitrogen and 850 nonprotein calories. Since the volume of the bottle is 1,200 ml., there is ample room for the addition of various other nutrients. The disadvantage of this method is the waste of solutions and the increased possibility of air-borne contamination.

MAINTENANCE OF ELECTROLYTE AND NUTRITIONAL BALANCE.—Parenteral hyperalimentation should not be instituted until after the first postoperative day or until the patient's blood volume and electrolytes are stable. Most patients may be started on 3,000 ml. fluid, 12 Gm. nitrogen, 2,400 calories, 5–10 Gm. NaCl and 100–120 mEq. KCl.

The patient's weight, electrolytes, blood sugar and BUN should be checked daily and the cardiorespiratory status should be evaluated frequently. The nursing staff should be instructed to infuse the solutions at an even rate throughout the 24 hours and not try to "catch up," in order to avoid glycosuria and waste of nutrients. Persistent glycosuria or an elevated blood sugar level may be controlled with 20 units of regular insulin subcutaneously every 6 hours or 20 units of Lente insulin subcutaneously daily for each 1,000 calories. Care must be taken to avoid hypoglycemic episodes by discontinuing the insulin when the blood sugar falls below 160 mg./100 ml. Most patients will not require insulin.

If the patient tolerates the infusion, more nutrients may be given by increasing the rate of administration. If the plasma vacuum collecting bottle is used, an additional 500 ml. of protein hydrolysate may be added to each container.

Reactions to the amino acid solutions are few. They include flushing, tachycardia, tasting the solutions and transient febrile episodes which may respond to slowing of the rate of administration.

Cirrhotic and uremic patients may be started on 1,500 calories and 25–50 Gm. of protein daily. The quantities may be increased or decreased depending on the patient's tolerance.

INDICATIONS.—Parenteral alimentation is indicated in: (1) preoperative preparation of malnourished patients; (2) postoperative complications in which the gastrointestinal tract does not function properly; (3) gastrointestinal diseases which benefit by rest, such as ulcerative colitis and regional enteritis; (4) anorexia due to carcinomatosis or cancer chemotherapy, and (5) cirrhosis or uremia.

Complications Common to Major Abdominal Surgery

EARLY COMPLICATIONS (24–48 Hours)

HYPOTENSION.—Hypotension is usually a result of hypovolemia. It may lead to myocardial or cerebral infarction and renal damage. Hypovolemia is the end result of preoperative dehydration and weight loss, miscalculated operative blood loss, postoperative hemorrhage and fluid sequestration in the operative area. Other causes of hypotension are myocardial infarction, hypoventilation, overdose of narcotics, adrenal insufficiency and catecholamine depletion due to preoperative antihypertensives. A complete history and examination of the patient and his record usually lead to the correct diagnosis.

Hypotension due to catecholamine depletion responds to intramuscular administration of 10–20 mg. Vasoxyl or 2–10 mg. Aramine and plasma expanders. For more rapid action the drugs can be given intravenously in one third the intramuscular dose. Adrenal insufficiency is treated with 100 mg. Solu-Cortef given rapidly intravenously or in 50 ml. of 5% D/W.

Overdose of narcotics may result in sufficient hypoventilation to require respiratory assistance. The blood pressure is maintained with Aramine or Vasoxyl given intramuscularly or intravenously. Lorfan is antagonistic to the action of Demerol and morphine in the dose of 1 mg. intravenously. If improvement after 1 dose occurs, 1 or 2 more injections of 0.5 mg. may be given intravenously in 3–5 minutes.

Hypovolemia should be prevented. Weight loss due to chronic disease is accompanied by a constricted blood volume, and in spite of normal hemoglobin and hematocrit values a blood volume determination should be performed preoperatively. Deficits are replenished with whole blood over a period of days. The evening before surgery 1,000 ml. 5% D/0.45NS is given to prevent dehydration and to maintain an adequate urinary output. Blood, albumin and saline solutions are given during surgery to keep up with losses.

In the recovery room the central venous pressure, urinary output and the vital signs are carefully observed. A low or decreasing venous pressure and a low urinary output with or without tachycardia or hypotension signify hypovolemia. The anesthesia record and the operative note may reveal inadequate intraoperative blood replacement. A hemoglobin and hematocrit determination at this time will provide a reference point.

The diagnosis and treatment of hypovolemia and impending hypotension must be rapid to avoid the serious consequences. Overtransfusion can be avoided by observing the central venous pressure and frequently examining the lungs for wheezes or rales.

HEMORRHAGE.—Hemorrhage should be suspected in all patients having had extensive surgery and in those who are hypotensive. There are 4 types of hemorrhage: intra-abdominal, gastrointestinal, incisional, and diffuse due to clotting disorders.

Intra-abdominal bleeding.—This type of bleeding may originate from any vessel in the area of dissection. It may manifest itself almost immediately after surgery or many hours later. It may be heralded by an unusual amount of sanguineous drainage from the drains, or it may only be perceived by a falling hemoglobin or hematocrit reading. Rarely the bleeding is so extensive that it results in hypotension and abdominal distention. Rapid transfusion of whole blood is necessary. If more than 3–5 units are administered with no improvement, exploration is usually necessary. The patient can withstand a second operative procedure better than repeated hypotensive episodes and multiple transfusions.

Intraluminal bleeding.—Early gastrointestinal bleeding usually originates from anastomoses. Gastric anastomoses bleed more extensively than small or large bowel anastomoses, due to the abundant gastric blood supply and larger size of the gastric blood vessels. If the gastric aspirate is blood tinged more than 12–24 hours postoperatively, bleeding from the suture line is suspected.

Extensive bleeding will result in a rapid drop in the hemoglobin and hematocrit. Gastric aspiration will be difficult due to clots. Treatment consists of irrigation with large volumes of iced saline solution to decompress the stomach and to constrict the submucosal vessels. Surgery may be indicated after 3–5 units of blood have been administered without signs of improvement. Less extensive bleeding may cease without surgery.

Rarely the bleeding may originate from the gastrostomy site. If the gastrostomy tube has an inflatable balloon, traction may control the bleeding.

Incisional and drain stab wound bleeding.—Dressings which become repeatedly soaked with blood after frequent changes indicate abdominal wound bleeding. The bleeding point is usually located in the subcutaneous tissue and is found after removal of a few skin sutures. With good lighting and retraction a suture ligature can be applied to control the bleeding.

Bleeding from drain stab wounds often originates deep to the anterior sheath. It is best to explore these wounds under local anesthesia in the operating room with sterile technique and with adequate lighting. The incision may require extension for better exposure.

Clotting disorders.—Diffuse intraoperative bleeding in a patient whose clotting was normal preoperatively may be due to (1) increased fibrinolysis, (2) diffuse intravascular thrombosis or (3) depletion or dilution of clotting factors.

Increased fibrinolysis is often associated with liver disease or liver trauma. It is characterized by bleeding from raw surfaces and a normal clotting time but a rapid lysis of the clot. Intravenous administration of 5 Gm. of Amicar as a rider in the first hour and 1 Gm. every hour thereafter for 8–24 hours is the treatment of choice. Amicar is contraindicated in hyperthrombotic states.

Increased intravascular thrombosis also occurs with liver disease, liver trauma or prolonged surgery. There is an increased intravascular clumping of platelets, leading to an increased fibrinolysis. Increased fibrinolysis in turn produces polypeptide chains which may also act as anticoagulants. On occasion intravenous administration of 5,000 units of heparin given every 4 hours has been successful.

Depletion and dilution of all clotting factors occurs after multiple transfusions or after cardiac by-pass. Fresh blood or fresh frozen plasma is frequently helpful.

LOW URINARY OUTPUT.—A urinary output of less than 30 ml. an hour is due to low renal blood flow or renal damage. Low renal blood flow is a result of low blood volume, dehydration or a decreased cardiac output due to myocardial failure. The latter may be diagnosed through physical examination, electrocardiography, determination of appropriate serum enzymes and the presence of an elevated venous pressure.

The Foley catheter should be irrigated to ascertain its patency. The presence of tachycardia, low central venous pressure and high specific gravity indicate hypovolemia. A rapid infusion of 1 unit of albumin and 300-500 ml. of 5% D/0.45NS usually results in an increased urinary output. If there is no response, a 25 Gm. bolus of mannitol is given intravenously. A diuresis indicates severe dehydration or a constricted blood volume and more blood, albumin and intravenous fluids should be administered. If there is no response, the patient has probably suffered lower tubular damage and the volume of fluid thereafter is limited to that of insensible losses, urinary output and gastrointestinal and wound drainage. Potassium is withheld. Renal damage can often be traced to previous hypotensive episodes. Mannitol in a single push given during hypotensive episodes may avert renal damage.

An elevation of the BUN value in postoperative patients often does not indicate renal impairment. An elevated BUN may be due to hemolysis of transfused or sequestered blood, infection, tetracycline, etc. The creatinine in these instances is normal.

Atelectasis.—Atelectasis is the most common early pulmonary complication. It may lead to pneumonia, hypoxia and cardiac arrhythmias. Its frequency is decreased by careful anesthetic and surgical management, early ambulation and coughing. Some patients simply refuse to cough because of incisional pain. A single nasotracheal aspiration of these patients usually clears the secretions and stimulates them to cough more effectively thereafter. In the presence of persistent atelectasis, repeated aspirations will be necessary. Secretions can be made less tenacious and expelled more easily by placing the patient in a high humidity tent and administering intermittent positive pressure breathing for 15 minutes every 4 hours. An alternative method of inducing coughing is by instilling 2 ml. of physiologic saline through a transtracheal catheter every 2–4 hours for 1 or 2 days.

Bronchoscopy is indicated in patients who do not improve with 1 or 2 aspirations and who have x-ray evidence of atelectasis. Repeated bronchoscopy may be necessary in the patients who are too debilitated to clear secretions and in those who are hypoxic.

Late Complications (after 48 Hours)

Prolonged ileus.—Prolonged ileus is usually caused by a low-grade infection or chemical peritonitis secondary to bile, gastrointestinal, pancreatic or serosanguineous fluid accumulation. Electrolyte imbalance must be ruled out. The diagnosis is made by the findings of a high volume of gastric aspirate, a protuberant abdomen, scanty or absent flatus, few or no bowel sounds and abdominal films compatible with adynamic ileus.

Gastric drainage must be maintained until proper function is achieved. Function is evaluated by aspirating the stomach until empty, then clamping the gastric drainage tube, instilling 60 ml. of water every hour for 3 hours and aspirating the stomach on the fourth hour. Aspiration of less than 60–90 ml. at the end of the fourth hour indicates adequate gastric function.

POSTOPERATIVE INFECTION.—Wound infections may be incisional or intra-abdominal.

The *incisional infection* usually manifests itself after the fourth day by fever, increased incisional pain, tenderness and cellulitis. Occasionally a wound infection is manifested earlier by a spiking fever and misdiagnosed as a pulmonary infection. In the early stages there may be no localized signs of infection and only probing of the wound will reveal the purulent accumulation. Incisional infections are treated by opening the involved portion of the wound, obtaining a Gram stain and culture and applying warm saline packs to the wound. Antibiotics are used if there is extensive cellulitis or necrosis or if the fever does not subside, indicating a virulent organism.

Intra-abdominal infections are often associated with colon surgery, anastomotic leaks and extensive dissection. They are manifested by spiking fever, prolonged ileus and, later, abdominal pain and tenderness. If there is evidence of an increasing peritonitis, proper antibiotics and possibly surgical intervention are indicated to drain the source of the contamination adequately. A localized infection or abscess will often resolve with antibiotics.

Locating the position of an abscess is sometimes difficult since in the early stages its only manifestation is fever. Careful examination may reveal a localized tenderness. A rectal examination may elicit tenderness in the pelvis. Frequent mucoid stools indicate rectosigmoid irritation due to an adjacent abscess or phlegmon. Abdominal films may show a haziness or, later, an air fluid level of an abscess. A chest x-ray may show a pleural effusion or elevation of the diaphragm which, on fluoroscopy, may be sluggish or completely immobile.

The treatment of localized intra-abdominal infection consists of appropriate antibiotics after cultures of blood and draining areas are taken, gastrointestinal decompression and use of intravenous fluids if the patient is unable to eat. Surgical drainage is indicated in the presence of increasing pain, tenderness, fever and size of the abscess. On rare occasions an intra-abdominal abscess may dissect into the thoracic cavity, mediastinum or groin.

BOWEL OBSTRUCTION.—Nausea, vomiting, cramping abdominal pain, hyperactive high-pitched bowel sounds, distention and absence of flatus, as a rule, indicate a mechanical bowel obstruction. This differs from adynamic ileus, in which there are sparse or no bowel sounds and the pain is minimal and not cramping. Abdominal x-ray films will show little or no gas in the colon and a dilated small bowel.

The treatment consists of gastrointestinal decompression and careful fluid and electrolyte balance. Passage of a long small-bowel tube under fluoroscopic control must be done early to take advantage of what peristalsis may be present to propel the tube. If this fails, a regular nasogastric tube is inserted and the long tube removed, since small-bowel tubes, due to their great length, are cumbersome and offer great resistance to suction and therefore do not decompress the stomach adequately.

Daily obstructive series are ordered. If after a few days the intestinal obstruction has not been relieved, surgical intervention is usually indicated. With the use of hyperalimentation, patients may be maintained better nutritionally and a longer waiting period may be indicated in selected patients.

Dehiscence.—Distention, obesity, wound infection, malnutrition and severe coughing contribute to the disruption of abdominal incisions. The early manifestation of dehiscence is serosanguineous drainage from a previously dry wound. The patient at times may feel a sudden snap in the wound. Ileus and distention may follow if prompt action is not taken.

If dehiscence is suspected, the abdominal wound is dressed and taped tightly, and the patient taken to the operating room where a more thorough examination is undertaken under sterile conditions. A dehiscence usually requires prompt closure.

"Evisceration" denotes protrusion of viscera out of the wound. Upon discovery the viscera are covered with sterile moist dressings and the patient is taken to the operating room for immediate cleansing and closure.

Delayed gastric hemorrhage.—The stress of surgery, sepsis, major trauma and anxiety are often associated with acute gastroduodenal ulcerations. Other contributing factors are adrenal corticosteroids, salicylates, reserpine, anoxia and intracranial lesions. Salicylates must be used sparingly or not at all postoperatively, since both rectal and oral administration destroy the gastric mucous barrier, thus predisposing to ulceration. Steroids employed in the treatment of septic shock should be discontinued within 24–36 hours, and steroids administered for the support of chronic adrenal suppression should be tapered to maintenance levels in 3–4 days. Anxious patients should be placed on tranquilizers.

The gastric drainage must be observed frequently for bleeding, and gastric drainage tubes should be irrigated every 2 hours with 30 ml. physiologic saline and aspirated gently to assure proper function. Instillation of 30 ml. skimmed milk every 2 hours theoretically helps to buffer gastric acid and does not form thick particles which may occlude the tube. Coffee-ground or red-tinged aspirate after 48 hours must be considered to represent some form of gastric ulceration. The stomach must be irrigated with copious volumes of iced saline solution to reduce the gastric blood flow and to keep it decompressed. In most cases bleeding requiring more than 5–8 units of blood in one day or continuous over several days needs surgical intervention.

The choice of surgical procedure depends on the pathology encountered. Gastric ulcerations are often superficial and multiple, and duodenal ulcerations are, as a rule, deep and discrete and may represent areas of previous chronic peptic ulceration. A discrete, single gastric or duodenal ulceration will often respond to oversewing only. A vagotomy and emptying procedure is preferred, however, if the patient is in satisfactory condition. Generalized superficial gastric bleeding may stop with evacuation of the clots distending the stomach. In this case an emptying procedure only is safest in a very ill patient. A vagotomy on occasion serves to shunt blood away from the mucosa and results in cessation of bleeding. If bleeding is not controlled by these measures, a total gastrectomy is recommended at that time.

Postoperatively these patients often have many complications. Hourly gastric irrigations with ice-cold saline and skimmed milk should be continued. A strict ulcer diet with antacids should be continued for several days after the patient is eating.

OTHER COMPLICATIONS.—The preceding discussion has been limited to complications requiring some special surgical understanding. Other complications which may be found in medical as well as surgical patients are pneumonia, pulmonary embolus, urinary tract infection, phlebitis, fluid and electrolyte imbalance and myocardial infarction. Their treatment is described elsewhere.

Specific Surgical Procedures

PANCREATICODUODENECTOMY (WHIPPLE PROCEDURE)

Pancreaticoduodenectomy is indicated for localized carcinoma of the pancreaticoduodenal area and, rarely, for severe chronic pancreatitis and functional tumors of the head of the pancreas. The care of patients having most types of pancreatic surgery is similar to that following pancreaticoduodenectomy. The mortality and morbidity of this procedure are high, due to the numerous anastomoses, the type of tissue involved, the extensive dissection and the debilitated state of the patient.

SURGICAL PROCEDURE.—The procedure involves the resection of the head of the pancreas, the terminal common duct, the gallbladder, all of the duodenum and 40% of the stomach. Usually the jejunum is anastomosed end-to-end to the remaining transected pancreas and the common duct is anastomosed end-to-side to the jejunum distal to the first anastomosis. Distal to this, the end of the stomach is anastomosed to the side of the jejunum, thus maintaining the continuity of the gastrointestinal tract. Sump drains are placed near the anastomoses to drain serosanguineous fluid and pancreatic or biliary secretions in the event of an anastomotic leak.

PREOPERATIVE CARE.—Patients with pancreaticoduodenal cancer are usually malnourished, hypoproteinemic and hypovolemic. There is a variable degree of liver damage. These patients are placed on a high-calorie, high-protein diet and therapeutic multivitamins, to include 1,000 mg. vitamin C and 5–10 mg. vitamin K daily. The clotting functions are evaluated. The blood volume is determined and if it is low, this is corrected slowly with whole blood. Hyperalimentation should be started a few days preoperatively. Adequate hydration and urinary output are ensured by infusing 1,000 ml. 5% D/0.45NS during the evening prior to surgery. This is not necessary if the patient is receiving hyperalimentation.

POSTOPERATIVE CARE.—The postoperative orders following pancreaticoduodenectomy are similar to those already discussed for other major abdominal surgery. Since oral alimentation may be delayed for from 8 to 10 days, hyperalimentation will be of great help in providing nutrition and promoting rapid convalescence and healing of anastomoses. The drains are not advanced for at least 8 days and until all drainage is minimal and the patient is eating.

POSTOPERATIVE COMPLICATIONS.—The commonest complications following pancreaticoduodenectomy. are (1) fistula, (2) abscess, (3) hemorrhage, (4) hypotension, (5) oliguria and (6) mechanical or adynamic ileus. Other complications, such as atelectasis, myocardial infarction, wound infection, dehiscence and pulmonary emboli, occur with some regularity.

The mortality of jaundiced patients undergoing abdominal surgery is increased. This accounts for the higher mortality in patients having a lesser, palliative procedure for extensive disease causing jaundice. Renal damage occurs more frequently in these instances, but this may be decreased with preoperative hydration.

Hemorrhage, hypotension, oliguria and ileus have been discussed in the previous section. The care of fistulae and abscesses will be discussed.

Biliary fistulae.—Leakage of bile through the suture holes in the common duct may result in 400–600 ml. of bile drainage. This is self-limiting if drained adequately, and ceases over the ensuing 5–8 days. Prolonged biliary drainage or delayed onset of drainage indicates a partial anastomotic disruption for which prolonged suction must be maintained. If there is a distal obstruction, the drainage will continue until the obstruction is relieved. The diagnosis of obstruction may be made on plain abdominal films or on an upper gastrointestinal series with barium or water-soluble contrast material. Total disruption of the anastomosis is rare and is usually caused by an inadequate blood supply to the jejunal limb, or by pressure from an adjacent abscess. Obstructive jaundice and a subhepatic abscess may result. Long-range hyperalimentation and constant sump drainage will help maintain the patient's nutritional status so that he can withstand reconstructive surgery or will hasten closure of the fistula.

Pancreatic fistulae.—Pancreatic fistula drainage is clear and alkaline if not infected. If infected, the enzymes become activated and digestion of the skin occurs. This is prevented by vigorous sump suction and application of protein powders around the fistula. All dressings are kept off the wound. Conservative management usually results in closure of the fistula.

Intra-abdominal abscess.—Despite adequate drainage of anastomotic sites, fluid may accumulate in the subphrenic or subhepatic space and may form an abscess. The diagnosis is made by a spiking fever, ileus, pain and tenderness. Chest and abdominal films may show a pleural effusion, an elevated diaphragm and a distended bowel. The bilirubin and alkaline phosphatase may be elevated. The treatment consists of specific antibiotics, hyperalimentation, hydration and gastric suction if there is an ileus. Most suspected subphrenic or subhepatic infections resolve with this early treatment and do not require surgical drainage.

Biliary Surgery

The results of biliary surgery vary with the indications. Elective cholecystectomy for cholelithiasis bears the best results with a minimal morbidity and mortality. Emergency or urgent surgery for empyema or septic cholangitis is associated with a higher morbidity and mortality. Sphincterotomy, which is occasionally performed for multiple small common duct stones or stenosis of the sphincter of Oddi, is complicated occasionally by hemorrhagic pancreatitis and duodenal fistula. The most difficult biliary surgery and the one with the most variable results is that for common duct reconstruction. The operations of choice are resection of the stenotic segment and reanastomosis or a Roux-en-Y jejunal limb to the proximal common duct.

Surgical procedure.—The surgical technique of cholecystectomy is well known. It is important to ligate all aberrant small biliary radicles and lymph and blood vessels to diminish fluid accumulation. Drains are usually inserted. In common duct exploration the choledochotomy must be securely closed around the T-tube to avoid bile leakage, and the T-tube must drain freely. In performing a sphincterotomy the posterior duodenal wall must not be perforated and the pancreatic duct should be avoided when suturing the duodenal mucosa to the common duct wall by placing the suture only laterally and at the apex. In primary common duct reconstruction there must be no anastomotic tension, and a T-tube should be inserted above and through the anastomosis for decompression and splinting for a period of 6–12 weeks or more. The limb of the

Roux-en-Y is made at least 12 in. long to avoid reflux and tension on the anastomosis. Sump drainage is imperative to drain bile originating from the anastomosis.

PREOPERATIVE CARE.—Patients with obstructive jaundice are usually malnourished and prone to clotting disorders and have a variable degree of hepatocellular damage. Hepatitis must be excluded by history and appropriate laboratory studies. Malnutrition and vitamin deficiencies should be reversed with a high-carbohydrate, high-protein diet and therapeutic multivitamins.

Pyridoxine in high doses is hepatotoxic. Similarly vitamin K must not be given in doses greater than 5–10 mg./day. Medications detoxified by the liver should be given cautiously. A diet high in protein may induce hepatic failure, but most patients tolerate it well.

There is a frequent association of gastroduodenal ulceration in patients with cirrhosis and for this reason they should be on an ulcer diet. Hydration is maintained by infusing 1,000 ml. of 5% D/0.45NS the evening before surgery, thus ensuring an adequate urinary output.

POSTOPERATIVE CARE.—After routine cholecystectomy, gastric drainage is discontinued in 12–24 hours since there has been minimal manipulation of the abdominal viscera. Parenteral fluids are maintained for 48–72 hours, during which time clear liquids may be started. If in 3–5 days there has been no drainage, the drains can be advanced daily and removed on the seventh day. Biliary drainage occurring immediately postoperatively is indicative of transected small biliary radicles or, less commonly, a lacerated major duct. Bile drainage beginning after the third day is rare and, if it is short-lived, may be due to a local accumulation of bile which has broken into the drain site. If bile drainage persists, it may be due to a dislodged tie around the cystic duct stump or damaged major ducts. The drains must be left in place until all drainage ceases and there is no evidence of a local infection.

Patients with more extensive biliary surgery should be kept on gastric drainage and parenteral fluids until there is evidence of gastrointestinal function. This is characterized by the presence of normal bowel sounds, a soft, flat abdomen, passage of flatus and minimal gastric drainage. The presence of bowel sounds alone is not indicative of a functioning gastrointestinal tract.

The advancement of drains is delayed until the fifth day after choledochotomy and they are removed by the tenth day. In common duct reconstruction, anastomotic disruption occurs most commonly around the tenth day, at which time there is maximum anastomotic inflammation and edema. The drains therefore are not advanced until after this time.

T-tubes are allowed to drain by gravity for 5–6 days. On the sixth day, if gastrointestinal function is established, the T-tube may be clamped periodically for increasing lengths of time. If there is no discomfort, it can be clamped continuously after the eighth or ninth day, allowing free drainage for a half-hour period daily to prevent sludging within the tube. An alternative method of determining the proper time to clamp the T-tube is to measure the hydrostatic pressure of the common duct. The normal common duct pressure is 10–15 cm. of water, which is equivalent to the distance from the anterior abdominal wall to the common duct. When the meniscus of bile falls to the level of the anterior abdominal wall as seen through the T-tube, it may be clamped as outlined above.

POSTOPERATIVE COMPLICATIONS.—Subphrenic or subhepatic fluid accumulation, fistula, jaundice and pancreatitis are specific complications associated with biliary surgery. Hemorrhage, hypotension, oliguria, atelectasis and myocardial infarction may occur and have been discussed.

Subhepatic or subphrenic fluid accumulation.—The most frequent complication of biliary surgery is subhepatic fluid accumulation. Lymphatic channels, blood vessels and aberrant biliary canaliculi are transected during biliary surgery. The flow of fluid may not be appreciated during dissection and therefore these structures may not be ligated. In most instances this fluid escapes around and through the drains. In some cases the fluid becomes loculated away from the drain sites, or the drains are inadvertently displaced or advanced too early, thus thwarting escape of fluid. The findings in fluid accumulation are epigastric fullness, abdominal pain and tenderness and ileus. If the diaphragm is involved, there may be pleuritic or referred shoulder pain. There may be a pleural effusion, and the diaphragm may be elevated or immobile. Fever, chills and marked tenderness occur when the fluid becomes infected and forms an abscess. The frequency of this complication may be reduced by ligation of all transected tissue and adequate drainage.

Treatment consists of administration of appropriate antibiotics, prevention of abdominal distention and bed rest. As a rule, conservative therapy results in resolution of the fluid. Surgical drainage is indicated in the presence of an enlarging abscess and a prolonged period of debilitating fever.

Fistulae.—Biliary drainage in the early postoperative period originates from transected aberrant biliary canaliculi or major ducts, inadequate closure of a choledochotomy around the T-tube or a displaced T-tube. As a rule, this is a self-limiting complication if the drainage is adequate. The drains must not be advanced and gastric drainage should be maintained somewhat longer until evidence of chemical peritonitis is excluded and proper gastrointestinal function is present.

Later in the postoperative period the onset of bile drainage indicates a leaking cystic duct stump, a displaced T-tube, a leak in the duodenotomy or sphincterotomy or a delayed drainage of a bile loculation into the drain site. The presence of an elevated amylase level or the finding of food particles in the drainage indicates a duodenal fistula. Fluoroscopy with contrast material will indicate the size and location of a duodenal fistula. T-tube cholangiography verifies the presence of a displaced T-tube or other major biliary duct fistula. When one limb of the T-tube is in the common duct and the other out, the T-tube may be pulled slightly so that both limbs are out to allow closure of the choledochotomy. The T-tube may be left in the abdomen to serve as a drain until the fistula closes. In the absence of peritonitis or an enlarging abscess conservative management is usually successful.

If complete disruption of the duodenotomy occurs, the fistulous drainage may reach a volume of 4,000–5,000 ml. daily. Careful maintenance of a flow sheet is imperative. Hyperalimentation may be lifesaving. The electrolyte content of the duodenal aspirate may be determined for more accurate replacement. If a jejunostomy is present, this fluid can be saved in the refrigerator and pumped into the jejunostomy.

Sump drainage must be re-established if the sump has been removed. This is accomplished by extending the incision of the previous stab wound under local anesthesia and reinserting a sump, with care not to puncture the bowel through forceful manipulation. Digestion of the skin by duodenal fluid escaping around the drains is prevented by frequent bathing and application of protein powders or other protective material on the skin. Dressings keep the wound wet and cause wound digestion.

Pancreatitis.—The serum amylase level as a rule rises significantly after sphincterotomy and, on occasion, after simple instrumentation of the sphincter of Oddi. This rise is usually not associated with abdominal signs or symptoms of pancreatitis and falls to normal within 2 or 3 days. A persistently elevated amylase may signify chronic pancreatitis, pancreatic duct obstruction or a traumatic pseudocyst. Gastrointestinal decompression should be maintained for a longer period. Antacids, anticholinergics and sedation will keep the pancreatic secretions to a minimum. Surgical intervention is not indicated in the absence of compelling signs. An enlarging pseudocyst will require surgical internal drainage. Macroamylasemia must be ruled out in asymptomatic patients.

Rarely, hemorrhagic pancreatitis may develop. In addition to the therapy outlined, blood, calcium, carbonic anhydrase inhibitors and antibiotics in the presence of sepsis are indicated. Surgical intervention is occasionally indicated in the patient with hemorrhagic pancreatitis who is deteriorating on conservative management. The purpose is to drain the pancreas, decompress the abdomen of pancreatic fluid, drain pseudocysts or remove a mechanical obstruction of the biliary tree.

Postoperative jaundice.—Jaundice after major biliary surgery is not uncommon. The more serious causes are retained common duct stone, trauma to the common duct, septic cholangitis or septic shock and hepatitis. Retained stones and trauma to the common duct will often require re-exploration.

Septic cholangitis in the absence of common duct obstruction is treated with systemic antibiotics after wound and blood cultures are obtained. Exploration is indicated if cholangitis persists while the patient is on antibiotics. The patient is explored, preferably directly after a drop in fever. Septic shock is treated in the usual manner with large volumes of fluid, antibiotics and steroids.

Hepatitis after Fluothane anesthesia may be diagnosed by a rise in the serum enzymes and eosinophil count. Serum hepatitis may occur as early as 2–3 weeks after transfusion.

Rarely, the insult of surgery, anesthesia, sepsis, etc., may induce hepatic failure in patients with chronic liver disease. Intravenous glucose supplying 1,000 calories daily will help reduce protein breakdown and ammonia intoxication. Medications toxic to the liver, such as narcotics, barbiturates and large doses of vitamin K and pyridoxine, must be avoided.

Partial Hepatectomy

In the past 15 years the mortality of hepatectomy has decreased as a result of a better understanding of the surgical anatomy of the liver, improved surgical techniques and better pre- and postoperative care. Patient survival and regeneration of liver tissue is possible if as little as 20% of healthy liver has been spared. The operative mortality of a left hepatectomy is 10% and of a right hepatectomy is 35%.

The indications for hepatectomy are primary or metastatic neoplasms, as well as severe hepatic contusions and lacerations which are limited to 1 or 2 anatomic units of the liver. Resection for localized, primary and secondary carcinoma of the liver has resulted in occasional 5 and 10 year survivals.

Surgical anatomy.—In the surgical approach to the liver the lobes are divided according to their vascular supply. There are no cross-communications of the vascular supply and venous drainage among the various lobes and segments. The right lobe of the liver lies to the right of a plane between the gallbladder and the vena cava, is supplied by the right hepatic artery and portal vein and is drained by the right hepatic veins. The left lobe lies to the left of this plane and is divided at the round ligament into a medial and lateral segment, each having its own blood supply and drainage.

Preoperative care.—It is important to have a determination of the blood volume so that deficits can be corrected slowly preoperatively. The entire clotting mechanism is evaluated. The patient's nutrition is improved through hyperalimentation or oral diet while his condition is being evaluated. If the albumin is lower than 3.5 Gm./100 ml., albumin should be administered in large quantities preoperatively. The colon is cleansed with cathartics. Preoperatively Sulfasuxidine 2 Gm. 4 times a day for 5 days, given orally, or kanamycin, 500 mg. 3 times a day for 3 days, given parenterally, reduce the number of ammonia-producing organisms. The patient's hydration is maintained with intravenous administration of fluids started the evening before surgery.

In the operating room, in addition to the hyperalimentation catheter, a central venous pressure and a peripherally placed large catheter are also inserted for rapid blood administration. The hyperalimentation catheter is used for that purpose only to avoid contamination. The central venous pressure catheter may be used for blood replacement.

Operative procedure. – The liver is examined to determine resectability. The porta hepatis is exposed and the vessels isolated. The liver is resected at the interlobar or intersegmental planes, either after first clamping its blood supply at the porta hepatis or by simply transecting the liver with the handle of the scalpel and tying off major vessels as they are encountered. Clamping the blood supply produces a line of demarcation but is not as advantageous as theoretically expected, because the bleeding is still profuse since it is difficult to locate an exact avascular plane. In addition, damage to the remaining liver may result even though the period of arterial occlusion is shorter than the safe 30 minutes.

The transected vessels and bile ducts are ligated with nonabsorbable material. Use of large mattress sutures is avoided because they cause necrosis, which in turn encourages sepsis and rebleeding. A great volume of blood is lost and must be replaced promptly. Hypertonic glucose is administered through the hyperalimentation catheter to prevent hypoglycemia. Large Penrose and sump drains are placed over the raw liver surface to drain blood, serum and bile. A T-tube in the common duct may decrease choledochal pressure, thus reducing bile drainage from the raw liver edge, and may also prevent obstruction of the common duct due to clots, but these effects are controversial.

Postoperative care. – It is extremely important to follow the vital signs and venous pressure closely. Blood is given unhesitatingly if there are signs of hypovolemia. Through the hyperalimentation catheter 500 – 1,000 ml. 50% D/W are given daily to supply calories and prevent hypoglycemia. For the ensuing five to ten days 150 – 500 Gm. of salt-poor albumin are infused daily to prevent ascites and edema, since the liver will not produce proteins during this period. No more than 2–5 Gm. salt are given unless there are extensive gastrointestinal losses, since there is a great salt retention.

Broad-spectrum antibiotics have been found to reduce the incidence of septicemia and liver failure.

The sump drains are left on high Gomco suction for days or weeks as indicated by the amount of aspirate.

Complications of hepatectomy. – Hemorrhage, hypovolemia and hypoglycemia are common early complications (24 – 48 hours). Biliary fistula, subphrenic abscess, septicemia, jaundice and liver failure are frequent late complications of hepatectomy.

Hemorrhage.—Probably in no other general surgical operation is the survival of the patient more dependent on adequate blood replacement before, during and after the operation. Bleeding almost always continues slowly after surgery, but diminishes over a 24–48 hour period. If it persists after 5–7 units of blood have been administered, surgical exploration may be required. The clotting mechanism must be studied and, if abnormal, must be treated as outlined earlier. Necrotic liver tissue may cause hyperfibrinolysis. If the bleeding is unresponsive to Amicar, resection of the necrotic tissue may be necessary to reverse this process.

Bleeding manifested after 48 hours usually signifies necrosis and sepsis of devitalized liver and may require re-exploration.

Hypovolemia.—Splanchnic bed pooling may occur because of a diminished hepatic sinusoidal mass when more than 25% of the hepatic mass has been resected.[5] This results in systemic hypovolemia despite seemingly adequate replacement of calculated blood losses. Equilibration of the blood volume is attained over a period of a few days. Blood is given in spite of seemingly adequate calculated replacement and in the absence of obvious blood losses if the patient presents with a picture of hypovolemia. Other causes of hypovolemia have been discussed.

Hypoglycemia.—In extensive hepatic resection the glycogen stores are diminished, as is the ability of the liver to break down glycogen. Hypoglycemia and death can result. The blood glucose levels, therefore, are checked and through the hyperalimentation catheter 500–1,000 ml. of 50% D/W are given daily for the first 3–4 postoperative days. Then 40 Gm. of amino acids may be added and the amount increased in 10–20 Gm. increments as the tolerance of the patient is evaluated until a maximum of 100–200 Gm. is given daily in 7–10 days.

Biliary fistula.—A large volume of bile mixed with serosanguineous fluid may be aspirated postoperatively through the sump drains. Usually it decreases to insignificant amounts within 7–10 days. When large biliary radicles have been missed and not oversewn, the drainage is prolonged. Suction on the sump drains is imperative to prevent accumulation of bile and the development of bile peritonitis.

Subphrenic abscess.—In the presence of necrotic liver and inadequate drainage of bile and serous fluid, a subphrenic or subhepatic abscess may develop. The manifestations have been discussed. Surgical drainage is indicated if the patient fails to respond to, or deteriorates on, nonoperative management.

Septicemia.—Septicemia contributes significantly to the mortality of hepatectomy. Prevention depends on meticulous surgical technique, adequate drainage of the raw liver surface and drainage of unresolving abscesses. The treatment of septicemia has been discussed elsewhere.

Jaundice.—Jaundice after hepatectomy often is a result of hemolysis of transfused blood and absorption of blood and bile. Two serious causes of jaundice commonly seen in hepatic surgery are hepatic failure and obstruction of the common duct due to clots (hemobilia). Hepatic failure is treated with systemic and intestinal antibiotics, cleansing enemas, adequate caloric intake and avoidance of protein. Common duct obstruction due to hemobilia might be prevented by T-tube insertion during surgery. If a T-tube has not been inserted, administration of antibiotics may prevent a septic cholangitis. Repeated episodes of cholangitis require common duct drainage.

Gastric Resection

Among the various types of gastric resection, there are 2 factors that influence the operative care and complications: the extent of resection and the type of anastomosis. In a partial gastric resection the continuity of the gastrointestinal tract is achieved by anastomosing the end of the stomach to the proximal duodenum, as in the Billroth I method, or to the side of the proximal jejunum, as in the Billroth II method. The anastomosis after total gastrectomy is accomplished by a Roux-en-Y anastomosis between the esophagus and proximal jejunum. In the Roux-en-Y and Billroth II anastomoses the area about the duodenal stump is drained with Penrose or sump drains.

Preoperative care.—Many patients requiring gastric surgery are so malnourished that it is necessary to promote a positive nitrogen balance using the oral route, jejunostomy feedings or parenteral hyperalimentation. Blood volume is restored if depleted. In the presence of achlorhydria the stomach is irrigated to diminish the bacterial count. Prophylactic systemic antibiotic therapy is also necessary in those with achlorhydria. Other preparations are hydration, determination and correction of any clotting disorders and the establishment of adequate infusion sites.

Postoperative care.—Gastric decompressing tubes must be irrigated with 30–60 ml. normal saline and aspirated every 2 hours to prevent plugging with mucus and clots. Plugging of the tubes may result in gastric dilatation, vomiting and suture line bleeding or disruption. Gastric drainage as a rule is maintained for 3–5 days, after which gastric emptying can be tested. The patient may start on clear liquids on the fifth or sixth day. After total gastrectomy a nasogastric tube is usually employed for only 2 or 3 days, but the patient is placed on strict N.P.O. orders for at least 10 days since for this period there is still danger of an anastomotic leak.

The sump and Penrose drains to the duodenal stump and esophagojejunal anastomoses are not advanced until the eighth to tenth day in order to provide an adequate tract should a suture line disruption occur.

The chest tubes used in thoracoabdominal operations are removed on the second or third day or when the lung is expanded and the chest tubes are not functioning. When the esophagojejunal anastomosis is a precarious one, the lower chest tube may be left in for a longer period.

POSTOPERATIVE COMPLICATIONS.—The complications encountered during the first 48 hours are hemorrhage, pancreatitis, jaundice and atelectasis. Those occurring after 48 hours are delayed emptying, duodenal fistula, subhepatic abscess, esophagojejunal anastomotic leak and electrolyte imbalance. Other complications are myocardial infarction, pneumonia, wound infection, dehiscence and thromboembolic phenomena.

Hemorrhage.—There are 2 common sources of postoperative bleeding: intraluminal and intra-abdominal.

The diagnosis of *intraluminal bleeding* is suspected if the gastric aspirate contains fresh blood longer than 24 hours after resection. It may or may not be associated with signs of hypovolemia, depending on the rate of bleeding. Most often the source is a submucosal gastric vessel at the anastomotic site. Other sources may be overlooked pathology, such as ulcers, malignancy or telangiectasia in areas difficult to examine.

The treatment consists of gastric irrigation with large quantities of iced saline to keep the stomach decompressed and to reduce gastric blood flow. Surgical intervention is indicated if the bleeding does not stop after 4–5 units of blood are given in 1 day; if the bleeding continues slowly, requiring 1–2 units daily for several days; or if there is a suspicion that the pathology was missed.

Occasionally the gastrostomy site bleeds, but this can be controlled by traction on the gastrostomy tube if the tube is a Foley type with an inflatable balloon.

The diagnosis of *intra-abdominal bleeding* is suspected when the hematocrit level falls or there is hypovolemia with no evidence of intraluminal bleeding.

Any vessel near the area of dissection may bleed. Occasionally the spleen is ruptured even though it has not been manipulated, since traction of the stomach or colon may avulse the splenic capsule or hilum. Exploration may be required if 3–4 units of blood are needed to maintain the vital signs.

Pancreatitis.—Pancreatitis may result from manipulation of the pancreas, unroofing of a posterior penetrating ulcer or suture ligation of a posterior bleeding point. In such cases a postoperative amylase determination is indicated. As a rule an elevated amylase level does not warrant specific treatment, but when it is associated with abdominal pain and hypovolemic shock, it indicates severe pancreatitis. Treatment consists of gastric drainage, maintenance of fluid and electrolyte balance, and use of carbonic anhydrase inhibitors and of antibiotics in the presence of sepsis. Kanamycin, Keflin and Ampicillin are the antibiotics of choice.

Jaundice.—Postoperative jaundice is often secondary to hemolysis or sepsis. Rarely it may be caused by common duct obstruction and cholangitis as a result of surgical trauma. In these cases surgical correction is usually indicated.

Atelectasis.—Atelectasis is common after gastrectomy and even more common after thoracoabdominal incisions. Its incidence can be reduced by vigorous coughing, ambulation and high-humidity inhalation. Treatment may require nasotracheal aspiration or bronchoscopy.

Delayed emptying.—Adequate gastric emptying is usually evident by the fifth postoperative day, but emptying may be delayed for days to weeks. Usually this is due to anastomotic edema or a bulky, narrow anastomosis. Gastric suction must be continued until the aspirate diminishes. Tube testing of gastric emptying may be performed every 3–4 days. It is important to maintain the patient's nutrition through jejunostomy feedings or parenteral hyperalimentation and albumin infusions. Good nutrition reduces anastomotic edema and improves gastrointestinal motility.

Occasionally the opening of the anastomosis may be delayed for as long as 3 weeks. Up to this time, if the patient is maintained well nutritionally and the surgeon believes the anastomosis was performed well, nonsurgical treatment is the wisest choice.

A delay in emptying beyond 3 weeks usually indicates a mechanical obstruction and may be caused by a variety of conditions. These are: (1) afferent or efferent loop obstruction, (2) a poorly constructed anastomosis, (3) narrowing of the jejunum by the mesocolon if the mesocolon has not been sewn to the stomach and (4) a narrowing of the bowel due to a jejunostomy.

The location of the obstruction may at times be determined on fluoroscopy, using barium or a water-soluble contrast medium. If the obstruction is at the jejunostomy site, removal of the tube may effect relief. An obstruction of the stoma not responsive to conservative therapy requires surgical correction.

Duodenal fistula.—There are 2 factors contributing to duodenal fistula. The first is an edematous and friable duodenal stump due to an active ulcer of the duodenum which makes the gastroduodenal anastomosis or closure of the duodenal stump difficult. The second is obstruction of the afferent or efferent loop resulting in an increased proximal intraluminal pressure and stress on the duodenal stump closure.

The disruption may present with pain and tenderness in the right upper quadrant and bile-stained drainage. Often there is drainage with no pain. In the absence of peritonitis or abscess formation the treatment consists of suction, protection of the skin and careful attention to fluid, electrolyte and nutritional balance.

As a rule, duodenal stump leaks occur 7–10 days postoperatively at the time of maximal edema and inflammation of the anastomosis. A fistula in the early postoperative period may lead to peritonitis and abscess formation more readily since a firm tract has not yet formed. The volume of the fistula may be 1,000–5,000 ml. daily. Hyperalimentation can supply adequate calories and protein to maintain weight and promote healing if the patient is unable to eat due to obstruction of the gastric outlet.

A duodenal fistula associated with a gastric outlet obstruction cannot close. The obstruction should be corrected if it persists longer than 3–4 weeks postoperatively.

Subphrenic or subhepatic abscess.—Abscess formation may result from contamination of walled-off collections of fluid. Such an abscess is often associated with duodenal fistula. Treatment includes antibiotics, parenteral fluids and gastric drainage if obstruction or ileus is present. In the presence of an enlarging mass or unrelenting fever, surgical drainage is required.

Abscess formation as a result of an esophagojejunal leak is associated with a high morbidity and mortality. This type of abscess usually presents with a scanty mucoid drainage on the eighth or ninth day. Food particles and saliva appear at the drain site following ingestion. The patient may have a septic debilitating course and eventually die of the infection. More often the fistula closes with few complications other than a stricture which can later be dilated. The treatment consists of suction drainage, no oral intake and jejunostomy feedings or hyperalimentation. An esophagogram will disclose the extent and location of the fistula and abscess cavity. Antibiotics are usually required. Surgical drainage is indicated if drainage is inadequate.

Electrolyte imbalance.—High output duodenal fistulae lead to dehydration and electrolyte imbalance. Accurate flow sheets are essential and the electrolyte content of the aspirate may be determined for accurate electrolyte replacement. Fluids are given both parenterally and via a jejunostomy, if one is present. In its absence, a catheter for hyperalimentation is inserted in the subclavian vein and 3,000 calories, including 150–200 Gm. protein and all vitamins are infused daily. No patient should die from inanition, dehydration or electrolyte imbalance if the subclavian route for hyperalimentation is employed.

Pelvic Exenteration

The most frequent indication for pelvic exenteration is advanced carcinoma of the cervix limited to the pelvis. Other indications are locally invasive carcinomas of the bladder, rectum and prostate.

A total pelvic exenteration involves removal of the rectosigmoid, uterus, bladder and pelvic nodes. The patient must have a colostomy and some form of urinary diversion. In an anterior exenteration the rectum is spared and in a posterior exenteration the bladder is spared.

There are various methods of accomplishing urinary diversion. The Bricker bladder or ileal conduit is the method employed most frequently. A segment of ileum is isolated, the ureters are inserted into the segment, one end is oversewn and the other is brought out to the skin. The advantages of this type of artificial bladder include constant drainage and limited electrolyte absorption, thus avoiding pyelonephritis and hyperchloremic acidosis, respectively.

An ileocecal bladder is constructed from the isolated cecum and terminal ileum. The advantage is the absence of constant drainage. The disadvantages are the increased incidence of pyelonephritis and the need for periodic catheterization of the segment. A wet colostomy involves implantation of the ureters into the sigmoid colon, thus mixing urine with the fecal stream. The disadvantages are constant drainage, frequent pyelonephritis and hyperchloremic acidosis due to the absorption of electrolytes.

Because the pelvic floor has been partially removed, a pack is placed through the perineal opening into the true pelvis. This supports the viscera, promotes hemostasis through pressure and prevents loculation of purulent material within the pelvis.

PREOPERATIVE CARE.—Preparation includes careful evaluation of renal function, adequate nutrition either orally or through parenteral hyperalimentation, mechanical cleansing and sterilization of the colon, vaginal sterilization with Betadine douches or antibacterial suppositories, correction of blood volume and preoperative hydration. Ureteral catheters inserted prior to surgery are of great help in identifying the ureters if previous irradiation and surgery have distorted the anatomy or if the tumor mass is extensive.

POSTOPERATIVE CARE.—In an uncomplicated postoperative course the care is simple. As a rule the gastric drainage is minimal, making correction of the fluid and electrolyte balance routine. In the first 48 hours, 2 or 3 units of blood may be required if there is extensive pelvic drainage.

The gastric drainage is usually discontinued on the fourth or fifth day. The colostomy begins to function on the fifth or sixth day, and irrigation is not necessary. Oral feedings may be started at this time.

Inadequate urinary output may be due to poor emptying of the ileal conduit. Distal obstruction due to stomal edema is overcome by inserting a straight catheter. When a Foley catheter is used care is taken to prevent pressure necrosis of the stoma by only partially filling the bag. Ureteral catheters, when employed, may be left in the ureters for 4 or 5 days to prevent kinking and obstruction from clots and edema.

The perineal pack is not disturbed for 4–5 days. It is then advanced daily after moistening with saline. This may be a painful procedure and it is advisable to premedicate the patient with a narcotic. After the pack is removed, the pelvic cavity is irrigated with 200 ml. physiologic saline twice daily to remove the accumulated seropurulent fluid. Sitz baths twice daily may be started after a week. Daily inspection and lysis of adhesions and loculations manually will prevent abscess formation.

Ambulation begins on the third or fourth day, allowing time for formation of adhesions which help prevent herniation of the viscera into the pelvis.

COMPLICATIONS.—Pelvic exenteration is frequently associated with complications. Previous irradiation adds to the morbidity by causing inflammation, adhesions and loss of vascularity. The most frequent early complications are hemorrhage, hypovolemia, hypotension and oliguria. Late complications include delayed bleeding, urinary fistula, bowel obstruction, enteric fistula, hyperchloremic acidosis and colostomy complications.

Hemorrhage.—Persistent hemorrhage from the pelvis may be evaluated by removing the perineal pack in the operating room and ligating individual bleeding points. Reapplying the perineal pack more tightly may result in cessation of bleeding. If the bleeding area is not found in the pelvis, a transabdominal approach may be necessary.

Oliguria.—A low urinary output may be due to obstruction of the ileal conduit or ureter. This is verified by inserting a small catheter into the ileal conduit to evaluate the residual. The wet dressings must be weighed since urine leaks around the stoma.

Delayed bleeding.—Delayed bleeding is a result of necrosis of blood vessels due to inflammation and previous irradiation. Bleeding may be massive so that rapid transfusion is required. The source of bleeding may usually be found in the pelvis, and it may be necessary to carry out exploration in the operating room. Individual vessels are oversewn or, if the bleeding is diffuse, the pelvis is packed tightly. If the bleeding source is not found through this approach, a transabdominal exploration may be necessary. Internal iliac artery ligation may be required to control the hemorrhage.

Urinary fistula.—Urinary fistulae originate from a necrotic or traumatized ureter, a disrupted anastomosis or a necrotic ileal conduit.

A fistula occurring early postoperatively is related to surgical trauma. Those occurring later are secondary to necrosis of a devitalized terminal ureter or a disrupted anastomosis. A ligature partially involving a ureter may devitalize its wall at that point, or extensive mobilization of a ureter may devitalize a whole segment. An ileal conduit with poor blood supply or too much tension or one exteriorized through a thick abdominal wall may likewise become necrotic.

A ureteral fistula may be located by performing an IVP, and an ileal fistula is located by endoscopy or by injecting contrast material into the artificial bladder. Small ileal bladder fistulae respond favorably to drainage with an indwelling catheter over 2–3 weeks. Healing may take a month in the presence of previous irradiation. Larger fistulae or necrosis of a segment of ileum require surgical revision.

Ureteral fistulae may close if on a rare occasion a catheter can be inserted past the perforation. Usually this is not possible and a nephrostomy is required. The resulting ureteral stricture may be repaired at a later time.

Bowel obstruction.—Bowel obstruction occurs frequently after pelvic exenteration. Treatment must be prompt. An attempt at passing a long tube must be made early while bowel function is still present. Fluoroscopic control is of help in placing the balloon at the pylorus. If after 24 hours the long tube is not in the duodenum, it should be removed and a nasogastric tube substituted. Hydration and nutrition are best maintained by hyperalimentation. The course of the disease is followed by physical examination and abdominal films. Relief of the obstruction is heralded by passage of flatus, a flat abdomen, a decrease in the volume of gastric aspirate and resolution of dilated small bowel on the abdominal films. Decompression is maintained for 1–2 days after gastrointestinal function is achieved, after which the patient is allowed liquids with the tube in place. Only after an adequate oral intake is tolerated is the tube removed. Surgical relief of the obstruction is generally required when no improvement is seen after 2–3 days.

Small bowel fistula.—A small bowel fistula may occur with or without bowel obstruction. The fistulous tract may exit into the pelvis or through the abdominal wall. Treatment consists of hyperalimentation, hydration, suction on drains inserted in the region of the fistulous tract to prevent digestion of the skin and gastrointestinal decompression if a bowel obstruction is present. In the absence of a bowel obstruction, the patient may be allowed a liquid diet high in calories and protein. Fistulae in irradiated bowel heal slowly and a bypass may be necessary. An obstruction distal to a fistula likewise will require surgical correction.

Hyperchloremic acidosis.—Hyperchloremic acidosis is common with urinary diversion into the sigmoid colon. Occasionally it is seen with an ileal conduit which is too long or which has an obstructed stoma. The typical findings are Kussmaul breathing and an electrolyte picture of high Cl^- and low CO_2. The length of the ileal segment is evaluated with injection of a water-soluble contrast medium. Continuous drainage is maintained with a catheter. Sodium bicarbonate helps correct the metabolic acidosis and large volumes of fluids promote diuresis. After electrolyte balance is achieved, the ileal conduit is revised.

Colostomy complications.—Colostomies present a few serious problems. The 2 most common ones are necrosis of the distal end in a fat patient and subcutaneous infection. If the necrosis is thought to extend below the anterior sheath, a revision or proximal colostomy is required to prevent peritoneal contamination. If the necrosis does not extend below the anterior sheath, a revision is not immediately necessary. The subcutaneous tissue is drained in the event of a localized infection.

Other complications of pelvic exenteration are sepsis, pyelonephritis, inanition, delayed healing of wounds and thromboembolic phenomena.

Splenectomy

Splenectomy is indicated for hypersplenism, traumatic rupture, improvement of surgical exposure and as part of a cancer operation when the splenic nodes are in the drainage route of the malignancy.

This section deals with splenectomy for hypersplenism. Primary conditions in which splenectomy may be indicated are idiopathic thrombocytopenic purpura, congenital spherocytic anemia and, less commonly, idiopathic pancytopenia and neutropenia. Secondary hypersplenism, similarly, may involve all elements or individual elements such as platelets, erythrocytes and neutrophils. It is seen in leukemia, lymphoma, sarcoid, Banti's syndrome, Gaucher's disease, and other conditions. Splenectomy is usually recommended after the bone marrow is shown to be normal or hyperactive and the survival or the peripheral count of the various elements is diminished.

PREOPERATIVE CARE.—Careful preparation of the patient is important. The blood volume is evaluated and replaced slowly with whole blood or packed cells, depending on the red cell mass and the patient's cardiac status.

Many of these patients are on high doses of corticosteroids and thus are unable to respond to stress due to chronic adrenal suppression. Steroid management is outlined in Chapter 24.

The entire clotting mechanism is evaluated. If the platelet count is below 35,000 or there are petechiae or ecchymoses, platelet packs are helpful.

A nasogastric tube is not used in the presence of a low platelet count to avoid nasopharyngeal bleeding. A gastrostomy may be inserted following splenectomy.

Perineal, throat and nose cultures are taken. Reverse isolation is instituted in those patients having white counts below 600–1,000. Antibiotics are not indicated unless a specific infection is present.

POSTOPERATIVE CARE.—As the incision is made, a platelet pack is administered in those patients having a low platelet count, cutaneous hemorrhage and other signs of bleeding due to insufficient platelets. Another platelet pack is given following removal of the specimen. As a result of platelet administration, the platelet count reaches its peak in 2–3 hours. Depending on the platelet count and the condition of the patient, additional platelets may be given in the early postoperative period. As a rule, the platelet count increases within 12 hours of splenectomy. Determinations of hemoglobin, hematocrit and platelets are ordered directly postoperatively and daily thereafter.

Steroid doses are reduced to preoperative levels in 3–4 days and, unless needed for treatment of the primary disease, should be tapered and discontinued prior to discharge. The gastrostomy tube is placed on intermittent suction for 2 or 3 days, after which gastrointestinal function returns and the tube is clamped. The splenic bed drain is removed in 2–3 days unless there is evidence of an infection or drainage.

COMPLICATIONS.—The early complications (first 48 hours) of splenectomy are intra-abdominal hemorrhage, pancreatitis, gastric injury and atelectasis. Late complications (after 48 hours) are subphrenic abscess, septicemia, postsplenectomy fever and mesenteric vein thrombosis.

Hemorrhage.—Even though the splenic bed and splenic pedicle are dry on inspection, hemorrhage occasionally complicates splenectomy, especially if the spleen is extremely large. Bleeding may become apparent by the rapid onset of hypovolemia or by a gradual decline of the hemoglobin and hematocrit values. The clotting mechanism is studied and deficiencies corrected. If the platelet count is below 35,000, 1–2 platelet packs and fresh whole blood are given. Persistent bleeding at a rapid rate requiring 3–5 units of blood should be investigated surgically.

Pancreatitis.—Clinical pancreatitis after splenectomy is not a common occurrence. An elevated amylase level, however, may be found in the fluid aspirated from the splenic bed drain of many asymptomatic patients. Pancreatitis should be considered in the presence of abdominal pain, ileus and elevated amylase 1 or 2 days postoperatively. Supportive treatment is indicated.

Gastric wall damage.—The splenic pedicle is adjacent to the greater curvature of the stomach and the tail of the pancreas. Injury to the pancreas may cause pancreatitis. Injury to the gastric wall may result in a small fistula or in an expanding abscess and peritonitis. The former is treated with gastric and abdominal drainage and the latter with surgical closure and drainage.

Atelectasis.—Irritation of the diaphragm and subphrenic fluid accumulation splint the diaphragm and cause atelectasis of the left lower lobe. This is treated with early ambulation, high-humidity tent and intermittent positive pressure. Bronchoscopy is preferred to nasotracheal aspiration if the platelet count is low.

Subphrenic abscess and septicemia.—Chemotherapy and a depressed white count impair the ability of the patient to combat infection. A subphrenic abscess and septicemia may easily develop. The mortality is high. Initial treatment consists of correcting fluid and electrolyte balance and massive antibiotic administration after proper cultures are obtained.

Postsplenectomy fever.—This is an ambiguous entity. It is a diagnosis of exclusion in patients who have fever but no clinical evidence of infection. In fact, it may represent a variety of conditions such as pancreatitis, a small abscess, atelectasis or phlebitis.

Mesenteric vein thrombosis .—On rare occasions mesenteric vein thrombosis may develop. Its manifestations are fever, ascites, hypovolemia, ileus, jaundice and often rapid progression to death. It is associated with an extremely high platelet count of more than 1,000,000. Normally during the first week after splenectomy the platelet count rises to 500,000 or 1,000,000, after which it falls to a lower level. The method of treatment of a patient with a platelet count above 1,000,000 is controversial. It ranges from the administration of 5,000 units of heparin every 4 hours in patients having a platelet count over 1,000,000 or 2,000,000 to no therapy at all.

REFERENCES

1. Dudrick, S. J.; Vars, H. M., and Rhoads, J. E.: Long term intravenous hyperalimentation, Fed. Proc. 27:486, 1968.
2. Dudrick, S. J., *et al.*: Long term parenteral nutrition with growth development and positive nitrogen balance, Surgery 64:134, 1968.
3. Dudrick, S. J., *et al.*: Can intravenous feedings as the sole means of nutrition support growth in the child and restore weight loss in the adult? Ann. Surg. 169:974, 1969.
4. Riegel, C., *et al.*: The nutritional requirements for nitrogen balance in surgical patients during the early postoperative period, J. Clin. Invest. 26:18, 1947.
5. Stone, H. H., *et al.*: Physiologic considerations in major hepatic resections, Am. J. Surg. 117:78, 1969.

23

Renal Transplantation

WILLIAM G. MANAX, M.D., Ph.D.

Associate Attending Surgeon and Director, Section of Organ Transplantation, Rush-Presbyterian-St. Luke's Medical Center; Associate Professor of Surgery, Rush Medical College

EFFECTIVE MANAGEMENT of patients receiving renal allografts crosses several specialty barriers, involving the interdigitation of efforts of surgeons, internists, hematologists, urologists, immunologists, psychiatrists, pediatricians and neurologists. This interdisciplinary approach has refined our knowledge to the point where we can now state without quarrel that the grafting of kidneys will be practiced with increased frequency and success in the future. Since 1962 the number of patients who have returned to a useful place in society following renal allotransplantation has risen steadily.[11] Transplantations of the heart,[5] liver,[12] lung[4], pancreas[13] and spleen[14] have also been undertaken during this interval and show great future promise.

Achievements made in several areas of transplantation research have been summarized in numerous journals and monographs and will not be recapitulated here. Rather, attention will be focused on specific details of management pertaining to transplantation of the kidney during the early postoperative period.

The Transplant Unit

The possibility that many, or perhaps even most, renal allografts will gradually fail is not a valid argument against further clinical transplantation, for the measure of social, economic and vocational rehabilitation during the period of satisfactory renal function is relatively complete. Moreover, Hume[7] has clearly shown that retransplantation for the indication of a failing first (or even second or third) renal allograft can be carried out with reasonable expectation of success. Because of the rapid progress in this field, it is possible that within 10 years renal allografting may be done routinely in many centers. At the present time, however, such is not the case and for the moment a transplant unit should be in, or a part of, a university teaching hospital.

Before giving a detailed account of postoperative management of patients with renal allografts, a brief description of the basic prerequisites of a clinical transplant unit is in order. The number of beds required for a program averaging 2 transplants per month is approximately 10. Some patients obviously require longer hospitalization than others, and some patients who have been discharged may require readmission for treatment of complications. There should be a facility to accommodate at least 2 patients with recent kidney grafts, and this facility should provide protective measures against infection. The unit should have in its immediate vicinity a small conference room with a blackboard. Equipment to perform a urinalysis should be available, particularly for examination of the urinary sediment. Examinations of a fresh urine specimen should be carried out frequently by the responsible physicians. Ideally, this unit should incorporate a small laboratory for critical hematologic and biochemical determinations. Ultraviolet screening of the doorways, as used by a few groups, is not critical. Because infections in these patients are more frequently caused by endogenous flora than by the extrinsic environment, rigid precautions as provided by the "life island" isolation technique are not indicated. Our own approach in the prevention of sepsis consists of close attention to cleanliness and minimal traffic within the unit.

General Considerations in Management of the Patient

SELECTION AND PREPARATION OF RECIPIENT.—One of the most important aspects in managing a patient with a kidney allograft is the selection of that individual for the procedure. Obviously, the recipient should have irreversible renal disease and should be sufficiently ill to require a transplant, although by no means does this imply that the procedure is a last-hope, desperate therapeutic endeavor. Potential candidates therefore must not develop infections at all costs, nor should they be malnourished or critically ill before definitive operative therapy is planned.

When a patient with chronic renal failure becomes unresponsive to conservative medical measures, then a more definitive form of management must be instituted for maintenance of life. At this juncture, intermittent hemodialysis is usually indicated. The patients are maintained in as optimal a condition as possible by periodic hemodialysis until they receive a renal allograft from a living related or cadaver donor.

Vigorous preparation of recipients is mandatory for satisfactory postoperative results. In addition to eradication of infection, malnutrition and iron and vitamin deficiencies, so common in patients maintained on long-term dialysis, should be corrected before transplantation. Also, elective bilateral pretransplant nephrectomy has several advantages.[15] It eliminates the need for an additional surgical procedure at the precarious time the patient is receiving immunosuppressive drugs, it removes actual and potential foci of infection and it greatly facilitates control of hypertension.

QUALITY OF THE ALLOGRAFT.—The attainment of immediate and satisfactory renal graft function is one of the most important factors in obtaining long-term success. The best indication of initial graft function is the achievement of early postoperative diuresis along with a striking general improvement in the patient's over-all condition.

Several factors influence the quality and function of a renal allograft immediately after transplantation.

Ischemic insult to the renal graft.—Minimization of ischemic insult to the allograft during the period between its devascularization in the donor and its revascularization in the recipient is crucial for attainment of early function. Improvement in the technique of organ transfer and allograft perfusion to flush out the vascular tree (using heparinized 5% low molecular weight dextran in a physiologic solution at 5 C.) is one of the most important steps in attaining prompt graft function. Starzl and associates[24] have clearly shown from study of large series of patients that ischemic periods near to or exceeding 1 hour are unsatisfactory. Without doubt, the shorter the ischemic period imposed on a kidney, the more superior is its immediate function. One must not exceed 40 minutes of ischemia for consistent attainment of good renal function. Facility in the performance of vascular anastomoses stemming from laboratory experience is therefore most significant before embarking on renal allotransplantation.

Incidence of oliguria and anuria.—Immediate anuria or oliguria after renal transplantation indicates absent or sluggish renal function. Most of these failures are technical, immunologic or consequent to prolonged ischemia. When kidneys from living related donors are used, immediate poor function is uncommon; when it is encountered, excessive ischemia and/or tissue incompatibility are the chief causes.

Measures to prevent injurious ischemic effects in the donor kidney during its in vitro environment are indicated. Heparinization by local infusion or by systemic administration to the donor is of value in preventing intrarenal clotting. Goodwin, Mims and Kaufman[2] have demonstrated that arterial flushing with a perfusate containing heparin is more rapid and complete than with perfusates not containing heparin. Hypotensive episodes in donor patients must be religiously avoided to protect the kidney being removed; this is also true for living donors, to ensure maximum security for the remaining single kidney. Finally, when poor function occurs after transplantation, the failure must be ascribed to technical imperfection rather than to more exotic causes such as "acute rejection," unless the latter can be proved with absolute certainty and the former objectively excluded after thorough searching for operative error.

Intensive Care of Patients with Allografts

Postoperative care of a patient with an allograft is unique in that it is concerned so intensively with the prevention of rejection. Most engrafted kidneys behave initially as if they were recovering from acute tubular necrosis; they excrete a dilute urine with a sodium content in the vicinity of 70–100 mEq./L. and potassium ranging from 10 to 17 mEq./L.[18]

A most significant item to bear in mind constantly is that, with successful transplantation, many of the preoperative (and catastrophic) physical and laboratory findings present in these patients are so abruptly reversed that the resulting homeostatic alteration may be sufficiently extensive and rapid to pose a real threat to life. Virtually all patients undergoing renal transplantation are in a terminal phase of disease and at times some hardly can be classified as borderline operative risks. Most are very anemic and preoperative correction of this anemia by blood transfusions risks acute heart failure. At least 95% of recipients have marked muscle wasting and 60–70% have some neurologic disturbance (psychoses, neuropathies, convulsions). Gastrointestinal disorders such as peptic ulceration, ileus, diarrhea or bleeding are common. These features are so often reversed with such rapidity posttransplantation that the change may pass unrecognized and therefore no steps are implemented to manage the adjustment.

A massive diuresis very often begins in the operating room. In patients with kidneys from living related donors, if the ischemia time is minimal, the surgeon may expect hourly urine outputs above 400 ml. for the first 12 hours or more.[25] Starzl reported massive diuresis in one patient to the extent of 2,000 ml. of urine an hour. This individual died 12 hours after transplantation from an acute electrolyte disturbance. Of utmost importance, then, during this initial diuretic phase is appropriate replacement of fluid and electrolytes. Urinary electrolytes (sodium, potassium and chloride) must be measured at least 3 times daily early in the postoperative period, for the urine composition is one of the most informative guidelines in the proper plan of therapy on a day-to-day basis.

Adequate preparation of patients prior to transplantation by hemodialysis has reduced the tendency for massive diuresis to the extent the diuresis may be life-threatening. A good practical rule to remember is that these patients must be given replacement fluids at the same time the diuresis is occurring, but not in such large volumes as to perpetuate the polyuria. Intravenous replacement can be estimated by using a simple empirical regimen after the general range of electrolyte loss has been determined. Generally the patients are given 5% glucose in 0.45N saline in a volume equal to approximately two thirds of the urinary output of each preceding hour. Some clinicians prefer to administer lactated Ringer's solution, utilizing an identical fractional replacement approach. In most cases it is not necessary to replace potassium losses. However, if the diuresis is unusually excessive, the addition of 20 mEq./L. of potassium to the intravenous fluid is in order. This electrolyte pattern ordinarily is the picture seen in successful renal transplant patients; consequently it would seem that electrolyte concentrations are predictable with a great degree of accuracy. Such is generally true, but in the immediate postoperative period it is still necessary to carry out laboratory determinations of serum and urinary electrolytes at least 3 times daily to make sure the electrolyte composition expected is indeed present.

The high urine volumes usually begin to diminish after 24 hours. Even after this period, and even in the face of oral fluids, it is advisable to continue intravenous therapy for another 2 or 3 days, during which time urinary output, although diminishing, is still relatively excessive. The nasogastric tube is removed as soon as possible after operation, according to the usual criteria, and then oral liquids are administered. These patients usually proceed to a bland diet 24 hours after tube removal, depending on the tolerance of the gastrointestinal tract. Weight loss during the first week after operation is invariably present, the extent depending on the degree of preoperative hydration, graft function, fluid and electrolyte replacement and the age of the patient. Indeed, weight loss is striking in some patients.

There are several additional changes in patients after transplantation. The mental improvement is often heightened to euphoria, in contrast to the preoperative state of hopelessness and apathy. Patients are ambulated no later than the second postoperative day unless an unusual circumstance exists. As early as possible a high-calorie vitamin-rich diet is initiated. There is no necessity to impose rigid fluid or salt restrictions until such time as rejection occurs with diminishing renal function.

Attention is paid to sterile precautions during the entire hospital course to the extent that is compatible with reasonable effectiveness. In short, the measures employed by doctors, nurses and other personnel are comparable to the sterile conditions practiced during standard burn treatment.

When practically feasible, the patient is encouraged to engage in whatever reasonable activities he desires outside his hospital room. Hopefully, this environmental change can be accomplished within 5 or 6 days in the company of an encouraging friend or family member, educated to assist in any care necessary during the period of absence from hospital. Such activity is of great benefit and can be done with ease in successful candidates.

An indwelling urethral catheter is inserted in recipients at the time of surgery and removed as quickly as possible afterwards. An effort should be made to remove the catheter by 24–36 hours postoperatively, for the development of bladder or ascending infection is always a threatening possibility. Catheter removal should include culture of the tip. Wound drains are unnecessary insofar as this author's surgical approach is concerned and consequently none of the problems attending wound drainage are encountered.

Most patients are ready for discharge from the hospital 9–14 days after surgery, and physical activity is encouraged. Thereafter patients are seen at frequent intervals on an outpatient basis. An effort is made not to rehospitalize individuals unless mandatory. Some authorities even manage (in some instances) the inevitable rejection crises on an outpatient basis.

Immunosuppressive Drugs and Rejection

Immunosuppressive drug therapy is the key to retention of the foreign graft by the host. While the effectiveness of splenectomy or thymectomy in mitigating the rejection process has not been proved, that of various immunosuppressive drugs has irrefutable documentation.[17] Immunosuppressive drugs are crucial in the prevention of destruction of the foreign renal allograft.

At present azathioprine and prednisone are the immunosuppressive agents in common use. In addition, some groups use sequential radiation to the kidney, giving 150 R on the first, third, fifth and seventh days. During periods of threatened rejection the dose of prednisone is increased as high as 300–500 mg. daily. Intravenous actinomycin C may be administered, or additional local radiation employed during a rejection crisis. Antilymphocytic globulin (ALG) may be used routinely as an adjunctive measure to azathioprine and steroids or given only at the time of rejection.

The most important single drug used in the prevention of rejection is azathioprine (Imuran). Its precise efficacy in preventing or modifying rejection remains enigmatic, although a major action is known to be interference with nucleic acid synthesis in cells. Azathioprine, for its desired purpose, must be administered continuously rather than in response to specific indications of rejection. It is given before, during and after rejection and may be classified as a prophylactic drug. Recipients receiving kidneys from living donors are usually pretreated with azathioprine, the dosage varying from 1.5 to 5 mg./kg./day, starting 1 to 8 days before operation.

From the very beginning of azathioprine therapy the clinician must closely scrutinize the recipient's hematologic profile. The white blood count (WBC) provides the best index of toxicity of azathioprine and is a direct warning of drug overdosage. A reasonable approach in attaining the desirable maintenance dose of this drug is to reach that level possible without causing leukopenia. Thereafter the white blood cell count determines doses beyond which further increases are dangerous. Experience has clearly shown that the best policy is *never* to induce leukopenia with azathioprine deliberately.

Varying degrees of acute tubular necrosis may occur postoperatively, especially if a cadaver kidney is used in a situation in which the donor's death was preceded by a prolonged agonal period of hypotension or where there is a prolonged period between death and removal of the kidneys. Usually the allograft recovers from the ischemic damage, although in some instances recovery takes as long as one month. During a period of acute tubular necrosis the most important therapeutic measure is the reduction of the dose of azathioprine to very low levels. The kidney is the normal route of excretion for azathioprine and excessively high blood levels occur in the absence of renal function.[23] This may in turn lead to bone marrow hypoplasia, aplasia and other complications. During the period of renal shutdown the patient is continued on regular prednisone doses as the principal means of immunosuppression.

The continuity of azathioprine therapy is of major importance and ideally this drug should not be omitted for even a day. An order for azathioprine is written at the same time daily, preferably at 6:00 P.M. The entire daily dose is ingested at one time; divided doses are rigidly avoided to prevent error. Despite the great value of azathioprine for immunosuppression, in most cases it cannot prevent rejection if used as the sole agent.

The value of prednisone as an adjunctive measure to azathioprine for immunosuppression was first appreciated by Goodwin.[3] Most groups now employ the prophylactic use of steroids, usually prednisone, in a pretreatment regimen in a fashion comparable to the use of azathioprine. Prednisone is usually started 1–3 days before transplantation in large doses and continued thereafter in diminishing amounts, until a maintenance dose of 7–10 mg. daily is reached 1 to 1½ months after operation. In our unit 3 mg./kg./day of prednisone (or prednisolone intramuscularly) is administered 24–72 hours preoperatively, in divided doses 4 times daily. At the time of surgery an additional 50–100 mg. of prednisolone is infused intravenously 30 minutes prior to revascularization. After surgery prednisone is coninued, but reduced every 5 days until the desired maintenance dose is reached.

The administration of prednisone is not without continuous danger, necessary as it is for success. Acute gastrointestinal bleeding is always a threat and consequently all patients treated with steroids are placed on a strict ulcer management program.

REJECTION.—Acute or chronic rejection of a renal transplant, either threatened or complete, may present in many different ways and may occur at any time from a few hours posttransplantation to years later. The classic signs of rejection are fever, edema and tenderness of the graft in association with malaise, anorexia and decreased urinary output. Bear in mind, however, that rejection may be present in the absence of these findings, and most often the diagnosis of rejection is made by inference. Some additional findings which may aid in arriving at a diagnosis are lymphocyturia, proteinuria, increased urinary lysozyme activity and elevated urinary alkaline phosphatase level. Renal function tests (in addition to the usual blood urea nitrogen levels, serum creatinine and creatinine clearance determinations) may include: renograms, radioscintigrams, renal blood flow studies, depression of the C^2 fraction of complement clearances (creatinine, inulin, I^{131} hippuran), renal biopsies and immunoglobulin determinations.

For practical purposes the most useful daily indicators of threatened rejection are the sudden appearance of oliguria associated with a rise in BUN, with or without fever. The rise in BUN may not necessarily occur with an accompanying elevation in serum creatinine value, but the more severe rejections are usually associated with an increase in the serum creatinine and a fall in the creatinine clearance. Recently Starzl[20] described the syndrome of early acute rejection incited on an immunologic basis and similar to the Shwartzman reaction. Starzl's thesis is that a chain reaction is caused by renal endothelium inciting an antigen-antibody reaction characterized by local intravascular thrombosis and platelet aggregation. The recommended therapy is treatment with heparin, which carries some degree of success.

Postoperative Complications

Some of the complications have been alluded to in the foregoing discussion. Without question the most serious risks in organ transplantation are specific consequences of immunosuppressive drug therapy. All the possible complications of the administration of steroids have been encountered in patients with engrafted kidneys. Specific toxicity of azathioprine, as mentioned previously, runs the gamut from bone marrow aplasia or hypoplasia to well-documented hepatotoxicity. Infection is by far the most serious complication in these patients and persists as the leading cause of mortality.

INFECTION.—A reservoir of infection resides in the endogenous bacteria present in the recipient. Early in the posttransplant period infections with pyogenic bacteria are the commonest. After long-term immunosuppression, relatively normal antibody responses to a variety of bacterial and viral antigens can be demonstrated. Some suggestions exist, however, of deficits in cellular immunity. Perhaps this is the reason for the prevalence of late bizarre, complicating infections such as those caused by fungi (especially Candida albicans), viruses (herpes zoster, cytomegalic inclusion disease) or protozoa.[16] It is encouraging that there are reports of dramatic recoveries from a variety of these bizarre yet serious infections if specific treatment is implemented without delay, even in patients on immunosuppressive therapy.

When infections occur, the lung is a commonly involved organ.

In addition to the usual pulmonary complications such as pneumonitis or atelectasis, there is a peculiar affliction called "transplant lung syndrome."[6] The characteristic findings in this clinical syndrome are an alveolar-capillary block demonstrated by a fall in arterial Po_2 and oxygen saturation with maintenance of a normal Pco_2. The physical findings are variable, and x-ray changes are consistent with localized, patchy or diffuse pneumonitis. These changes are most often coincident with the onset of threatened rejection and normally disappear with the administration of increased doses of immunosuppressive drugs. If this syndrome is severe, clinical cyanosis and leukopenia are present and an impressively diminished Po_2 and O_2 saturation are present even when the patient is on 100% oxygen.

The precise pathophysiology of transplant pneumonia is obscure. Characteristically it shows direct pulmonary capillary damage with edema and round cell infiltration of the alveolar walls and eventually loss of pulmonary surfactant.[9] A popular theory regarding the etiology of this syndrome is that antibodies directed against the transplanted organ may also cross-react against other host tissues.[10] This explanation could account for the amelioration of the above pulmonary changes with increased immunosuppression.

In all patients, both before and after operation, cultures are taken twice weekly of the nose, throat, skin and urine. These steps provide current information regarding the endogenous bacterial flora of the patients. When an infection arises, it is frequently possible from these data to predict not only the type but also the antibiotic sensitivity of the organism involved.

The choice of antibiotic depends on a number of considerations, including the etiology and site of the infection, the general condition of the patient, the adequacy of renal function and the severity of immunosuppressive drug effect manifested by the patient. Staphylococcal infections are usually best treated with penicillin- G or one of the penicillinase-resistant preparations. For serious gram-negative bacillary infections, chloramphenicol is commonly the antibiotic of choice because it is potent, possesses a broad antimicrobial spectrum and has no increased toxicity in the presence of failing renal function. Tetracycline is less frequently employed than chloramphenicol because of its antianabolic effect with a resulting elevation of the BUN. Bactericidal agents such as kanamycin and streptomycin are also frequently used. Care must be taken to regulate the dosage of these drugs in the presence of renal insufficiency because of the distinct danger of jeopardizing the function of the transplanted kidney. In general, when renal function is impaired, one half the usual daily dose is given every third day.

GASTROINTESTINAL HEMORRHAGE.—Gastrointestinal hemorrhage secondary to duodenal ulceration is common in patients on high doses of steroid therapy. Hemorrhage has a higher incidence during periods of rejection when immunosuppressive agents are administered in high doses. Massive gastrointestinal hemorrhage in this particular patient population is such a lethal complication postoperatively and presents such a problem in management that it is now recommended that any patient with a known gastroduodenal ulcer or a classic history of peptic ulceration undergo appropriate operative therapy for this condition prior to the transplant procedure before he is placed on immunosuppressive drugs.[21]

At the time of rejection crises when high doses of steroids are given, it is mandatory that patients be examined routinely for occult blood in the stools. Starzl reported guaiac-positive stools in 35 of his first 42 patients who received renal allografts.[22]

THROMBOEMBOLIC PHENOMENA.—Thrombosis can be a very specific complication of a renal transplant procedure. First of all, thrombophlebitis may develop in the legs or pelvic veins after vascular operative manipulation, with the distinct possibility of the development of fatal pulmonary emboli. Thromboembolic phenomena are common in those individuals in whom the spleen has been removed, and it is significant that these complications have decreased with the elimination of splenectomy as a routine part of the procedure. Some authorities have gone so far as to recommend ligation and division of the hypogastric veins at the time of transplantation as a precautionary measure against the development of pulmonary emboli.[19] Apart from manipulation of vessels and anastomosis of the external iliac vein, specific dangers are added, rendering patients more susceptible to the development of thrombosis. These patients are emaciated, have muscle wasting and are debilitated and generally inactive prior to surgery. Moreover, there is commonly a marked weight loss in the early postoperative period, further predisposing these individuals to the development of emboli and thromboses.

PANCREATITIS.—Pancreatitis has been reported in kidney transplant recipients as a complication of steroid therapy, but it may also occur as a consequence of viral hepatitis or cytomegalic viral infection.[1] Some investigators have suggested that pancreatitis accompanying renal transplantation may be secondary to an autoantibody type reaction similar to the etiologic mechanism postulated for transplant lung syndrome.[8]

ILEUS.—Following any major operation in a uremic patient there is slow return of peristalsis. It is especially desirable in these patients to remove the nasogastric tube as soon as possible for ease of regulation of fluids and electrolytes. Ileus consequent to retroperitoneal dissection from bilateral nephrectomy is a common occurrence, often prolonged, and can often create a confusing picture postoperatively. Careful hemostasis, compulsive attention to tidy dissection and the avoidance of unnecessary operative maneuvers are important factors in circumventing ileus.

ADDITIONAL COMPLICATIONS.—Steroid-induced diabetes mellitus commonly occurs in transplant patients on high doses of steroids. During periods of treatment for rejection especially, there may be progressive hyperglycemia or glycosuria which may develop over several weeks. In most patients parenteral insulin is not indicated and the alterations in carbohydrate metabolism are rapidly reversed as the doses of prednisone are subsequently reduced.

In virtually all patients on chronic steroid therapy moon facies and abnormal distribution of the body fat occur. It is important, therefore, that patients be informed prior to therapy of the side effects of steroids.

REFERENCES

1. Bourne, M. S., and Dawson, H.: Acute pancreatitis complicating prednisone therapy, Lancet 2:1209, 1958.
2. Goodwin, W. E.; Mims, M. M.; and Kaufman, J. J.: Human renal transplantation: III. Technical problems encountered in six cases of renal transplantation, J. Urol. 89:349, 1963.
3. Goodwin, W. E., *et al.*: Human renal transplantation: I. Clinical experiences with 6 cases of renal homotransplantation, J. Urol. 89:13, 1963.
4. Hardy, J. D.: The transplantation of organs, Surgery 56:685, 1964.
5. Hardy, J. D., *et al.*: Heart transplantation in man: Developmental studies and report of a case, J.A.M.A. 188:1132, 1964.
6. Hill, R. B., Jr.; Rowlands, D. T., Jr., and Rifkind, D.: Infectious pulmonary disease in patients receiving immunosuppressive therapy for organ transplantation, New England J. Med. 271:1021, 1964.
7. Hume, D. M.: Progress in Clinical Renal Homotransplantation, in Welch, C. E. (ed.): *Advances in Surgery* (Chicago: Year Book Medical Publishers, Inc., 1966), vol. 2.
8. Hume, D. M., *et al.*: Renal homotransplantation in man in modified recipients, Ann. Surg. 158:608, 1963.
9. Hume, D. M., *et al.*: Comparative results of cadaver and related donor renal homografts in man, and immunologic implications of the outcome of second and paired transplants, Ann. Surg. 164:352, 1966.
10. Kanich, R. E., and Craighead, J. E.: Cytomegalovirus infection and cytomegalic inclusion disease in renal homotransplant recipients, Am. J. Med. 40:874, 1966.
11. Kidney Transplant Registry: Published report, Peter Bent Brigham Hospital, Boston, Mass., 1969.
12. Lillehei, R. C., and Manax, W. G.: Organ transplantation: A review of past accomplishments, present problems and future hopes, Anesth. & Analg. 45:707, 1966.
13. Lillehei, R. C., *et al.*: Transplantation of the stomach, intestine and pancreas: Experimental and clinical observations, Surgery 62:721, 1967.
14. Marchioro, T. L.; Starzl, T. E., and Waddell, W. R.: Splenic homotransplantation, Ann. New York Acad. Sc. 120:626, 1964.
15. Merrill, J. P.: Medical Management of the Transplant Patient, in Rapaport, F. T. and Dausset, J. (eds.): *Human Transplantation* (New York: Grune & Stratton, Inc., 1968).
16. Merrill, J. P.: *The Treatment of Renal Failure* (2d ed.; New York: Grune & Stratton, Inc., 1965).
17. Murray, J. E.; Wilson, R. E., and O'Connor, N. E.: Evaluation of long-functioning human kidney transplants, Surg. Gynec. & Obstet. 124:509, 1967.
18. Najarian, J. S., *et al.*: Protection of the donor kidney during homotransplantation, Ann. Surg. 164:398, 1966.
19. Starzl, T. E.: *Experience in Renal Transplantation* (Philadelphia: W. B. Saunders Company, 1964).
20. Starzl, T. E.: Personal communication.
21. Starzl, T. E.: Personal communication.
22. Starzl, T. E., *et al.*: Clinical experience with organ transplantation, South. M. J. 58:131, 1965.
23. Starzl, T. E., *et al.*: Clinical problems in renal homotransplantation, J.A.M.A. 187:734, 1964.
24. Starzl, T. E., *et al.*: Factors in successful renal transplantation, Surgery 56:296, 1964.
25. Starzl, T. E., *et al.*: Technique of renal homotransplantation: Experiences with 42 cases, Arch. Surg. 89:87, 1964.

24

Endocrinologic Problems in Surgery

WILL G. RYAN, M.D.

Associate Attending Physician, Rush-Presbyterian-St. Luke's Medical Center; Associate Professor of Medicine, Rush Medical College

HARRY W. SOUTHWICK, M.D.

Attending Surgeon and Acting Chairman, Department of General Surgery, Rush-Presbyterian-St. Luke's Medical Center; Professor of Surgery, Rush Medical College

THEODORE B. SCHWARTZ, M.D.

Attending Physician, Director, Section of Endocrinology and Metabolism and Chairman, Department of Medicine, Rush-Presbyterian-St. Luke's Medical Center; Professor of Medicine, Rush Medical College

FREDERIC A. dePEYSTER, M.D.

Attending Surgeon, Rush-Presbyterian-St. Luke's Medical Center; Professor of Surgery, Rush Medical College

AND

JANET WOLTER, M.D.

Associate Attending Physician, Rush-Presbyterian-St. Luke's Medical Center; Associate Professor of Medicine, Rush Medical College

In the modern hospital, surgery of the endocrine glands is performed with a negligible to small mortality rate, depending on the gland involved and the extent of the operative procedure. Similarly, under most circumstances, significant postoperative complications should be minimal. Careful preoperative evaluation and preparation of the patient is most important in bringing even a seriously ill patient into optimum systemic condition for operation. Careful monitoring of the patient during surgery is essential not only to rectify problems common to any operation but also to anticipate and stabilize the various abnormalities that may be associated with hyper- or hypofunction of the specific endocrine gland under treatment.

The Thyroid Gland

A thyroidectomy is most commonly undertaken for the removal of an enlargement of the thyroid gland. Such a patient may demonstrate varying conditions of thyroid function.

The majority of patients are euthyroid. The enlargement of the gland may be a benign process, such as a colloid goiter or a benign neoplasm, and this may be unilateral or bilateral. If the disease is confined to one lobe, a lobectomy is the treatment of choice. If both lobes are involved, generally a bilateral subtotal thyroidectomy is indicated.

For malignant thyroid disease the operative procedure is generally more extensive and may even require a total thyroidectomy. When there is gross evidence of disease in the cervical lymph nodes at operation, a node dissection is performed and extended to include the paratracheal nodes as well as the retroesophageal nodes. Occasionally elective neck dissections on patients without clinical evidence of metastatic disease are undertaken, but this is less frequently performed now than a few years ago.

Patients with hyperthyroidism that has not responded to medical management or has recurred on such management, as well as patients who have a hyperactive solitary nodule, are also candidates for surgical treatment. If possible, the patient should be euthyroid before surgery. This can be accomplished in most cases by the administration of methimazole or propylthiouracil for 6 weeks to 3 months prior to surgery. (The usual methimazole dose is 10–20 mg. every 6 hours.) Leukopenia is a frequent side effect of the administration of these drugs and should not cause undue alarm. Agranulocytosis, usually heralded by sore throat, is a much more serious, but fortunately rare, complication. Drug-induced skin eruptions are seen more frequently and may usually be controlled by switching from methimazole to propylthiouracil, or vice versa. Potassium iodide (SSKI) 10 gtt. daily for a week to 10 days preoperatively, may provide additional benefit by preventing release of thyroxin as well as apparently diminishing the vascularity of the gland.

Chronic thyroiditis is occasionally an indication for thyroidectomy, as it is sometimes difficult to distinguish from a malignant neoplasm. Acute thyroiditis is rarely an indication for surgical treatment except when an acute suppurative process exists.

Postoperative Complications

Hemorrhage.—Postoperative hemorrhage is the most frequent and potentially life-threatening condition for which the patient must be observed following thyroidectomy. The bleeding may produce a primary problem from blood loss alone or, more commonly, a secondary problem associated with airway obstruction.

The bleeding following thyroidectomy may be either venous or arterial. Venous bleeding usually occurs from small blood vessels and is not commonly a cause of a major complication. It generally results when a small blood vessel which has been clamped is not ligated because the hemostat has fallen off. With coughing or straining during the postanesthesia recovery period, these venous channels may open and produce a puffiness beneath the skin flaps. Occasionally a deeper, larger vein which seemed to be adequately secured may also open up under similar circumstances. Here the complication may resemble arterial bleeding, although the sequential development of the problem is usually a much slower one. The usual venous bleeding rarely requires much in the way of active treatment. The patient should be observed carefully for signs of progression of the hematoma and particularly for signs of airway obstruction, but gentle pressure usually will stabilize the problem and prevent its progression.

Arterial or deep venous bleeding, on the other hand, can rapidly precipitate an emergency situation. In such a case, a patient who has been initially doing quite satisfactorily may suddenly begin to complain of tightness in the neck and difficulty in swallowing and breathing. Examination reveals the neck tissues to be tense and the patient apprehensive. If possible, the patient should be returned to the operating room, but this is not often feasible. Often the wound must be reopened in the intensive care unit or postanesthesia recovery area. Again, if time permits, aseptic technique should be employed. If the patient is becoming cyanotic, however, and there are signs of cardiac arrhythmias, the wound should be opened immediately. The compression is generally associated with blood that has collected beneath the strap muscles. These muscles should be separated and the clot evacuated. The first and foremost consideration is the re-establishment of an airway, and this should be done before any attempt is made to control the source of bleeding. If relief of the pressure from the hematoma is insufficient, a tracheostomy should be performed. Occasionally orotracheal intubation can be accomplished, but the personnel capable of performing this on a struggling, acutely ill patient are rarely available. With the airway re-established and the bleeding temporarily controlled by pressure, the patient should be returned to the operating room for specific control of the origin of the bleeding. If the arterial bleeding has come from the superior thyroid artery, its control may require re-induction of anesthesia since the artery frequently retracts high into the neck and is, therefore, impossible to secure in the conscious patient.

AIRWAY OBSTRUCTION.—Airway obstruction may occur following thyroidectomy from causes other than postoperative bleeding. When a bilateral subtotal or total thyroidectomy has been performed, the possibility of damage to one or both recurrent laryngeal nerves exists in at least 1% of the patients. When the paralysis is unilateral, airway obstruction is usually not a problem unless there is some superimposed complication. Postoperative hemorrhage, as mentioned earlier, may be one of the contributory factors. Edema associated with the dissection, particularly if a neck dissection has been performed with interruption of paraesophageal venous plexus, may develop in the false cords and in the area of the arytenoids, producing respiratory obstruction. Depending on the state of consciousness of the patient, an attempt should be made at direct or indirect laryngoscopy to determine accurately the status of the vocal cords with respect to position and mobility. If an inadequate airway is present, whatever the reason, a tracheostomy should be performed immediately.

THYROID STORM.—Postoperative thyroid storm is the most dreaded complication of thyroid surgery for hyperthyroidism. As mentioned earlier, adequate preoperative preparation will almost invariably prevent this occurrence. Should thyroid storm (marked signs of hypermetabolism and fever) develop, hydrocortisone (Solu-Cortef, 100 mg.) should be administered intravenously every 8 hours during the period of severe stress, and adrenergic blockage should be instituted. Cardiac arrhythmias and dehydration are common. Pre- and postoperative supplements with intravenous glucose further minimize epinephrine release by preventing hypoglycemia. Additional measures include constant surveillance in a quiet, cool, darkened room, sedation (usually with barbiturates or phenothiazines), intravenous fluids, multivitamins and cooling by means of a hypothermia blanket if necessary. Appropriate attention to the eyes will prevent corneal ulceration.

HYPOPARATHYROIDISM.—Hypoparathyroidism is an additional potential complication of thyroid surgery. It is more apt to occur when an extensive dissection has been necessary either for the treatment of hyperthyroidism of a diffuse nature or for the treatment of a malignant neoplasm, particularly when a paratracheal node dissection and radical neck dissection have been undertaken as part of the operative treatment. The hypocalcemia may be transient, associated with an interference to the blood supply of the parathyroid glands, or it may be permanent, secondary to their extirpation. The management of hypocalcemia will be discussed in the section on the parathyroid glands.

PREOPERATIVE EVALUATION AND PREPARATION

On occasion there are compelling reasons, such as unrelated emergency surgery, for the euthyroid state not being attained in a hyperthyroid patient. This requires an accelerated form of treatment aimed at rapid relief of the hypermetabolic state. Adrenergic receptor blockage may accomplish this within 24–48 hours. Guanethidine is administered in doses of 20–60 mg. every 12 hours to provide alpha-receptor blockade. Beta-receptor blockade is accomplished by the concurrent administration of propranolol, 10–20 mg. every 6 hours. Guanethidine-induced postural hypotension and propranolol-induced congestive heart failure must be watched for carefully, particularly in patients with underlying heart disease. The anesthesiologist should be alerted to the use of these drugs. Hyperthyroid patients are inordinately sensitive to adrenergic stimuli. For this reason, adrenergic drugs (epinephrine, norepinephrine) and cholinergic blocking agents (atropine) are either contraindicated or used with extreme caution in this group. Cyclopropane induces endogenous catecholamine release, thus predisposing to cardiac arrhythmias.

The hypothyroid patient should be made euthyroid before any surgery unless there are overriding considerations, such as severe angina pectoris. A hypothyroid patient about to undergo any surgical procedure is extremely fragile and may be unduly sensitive to the effect of anesthetic agents and medications, particularly thyroid. The elderly hypothyroid patient or the patient with heart disease should be given thyroid hormones very cautiously, as arrhythmias and congestive heart failure are prone to develop from therapeutic doses. Ordinary amounts of morphine may cause prolonged sedation or respiratory arrest; an appropriate starting dose is in the range of 0.5–1 mg. Tri-iodothyronine is given in doses of 5–10 μg./day and increased in similar increments every third day until the euthyroid state is obtained or side effects such as angina pectoris or cardiac arrhythmias appear. The therapeutic effect of T_3 may be monitored by improvement in serial electrocardiograms. Preoperative and intraoperative administration of intravenous fluids must be carefully regulated. The myxedematous patient has depressed kidney function and a compromised circulatory system which cannot compensate for minimal volume excess. Acute pulmonary edema is the end result.

Ambulation must proceed slowly in the postoperative period. Supplemental medication increases the metabolic demand and the effect of the medication, alone or in combination with activity, may precipitate angina pectoris or congestive heart failure.

The Parathyroid Glands

Surgery of the parathyroid glands may be undertaken for either primary or secondary hyperparathyroidism as well as for neoplasms of one or more of the parathyroid glands. Usually only a single gland is involved in a neoplastic problem, but all glands must be inspected for evidence of multiplicity of tumor. For hyperplasia, either primary or secondary, particularly associated with chronic renal disease, multiple gland removal is the treatment of choice. Usually there is at least a transient hypoparathyroidism following removal of a parathyroid adenoma or the removal of multiple glands. The treatment varies with the degree of hypocalcemia and with the rapidity of its onset. When the hypocalcemia becomes apparent within 12–18 hours postoperatively, it is liable ultimately to be severe and requires aggressive management.

POSTOPERATIVE HYPOCALCEMIA.—An indication of a developing hypocalcemia can be elicited early by tapping the trunk of the facial nerve to elicit a twitch of the ipsilateral lip (Chvostek's sign); this should be performed during each examination of the patient. The pulse should be monitored for evidence of cardiac arrhythmias. As the status progresses and becomes more profound, severe tetany, laryngeal spasm and acute anxiety states may supervene. The serum calcium should be checked the evening following surgery and at least daily thereafter for several days. However, the clinical evaluation of the patient generally gives indication of an impending problem before the laboratory results are returned.

Asymptomatic mild hypocalcemia may require no treatment except careful observation. Tingling of the lips, fingers and toes or mild tetany should be treated with oral calcium preparations (calcium lactate or gluconate). A convenient and well-tolerated liquid preparation is Neo-Calglucon, which contains calcium equivalent to that in 20 gr. of calcium gluconate in each 5 ml. The usual dose is 15 ml. 3 times daily. Moderate to severe tetany should be treated with intravenous injections or infusions of calcium gluconate or lactate. A syringe, a needle and an ampule of calcium gluconate are kept at the bedside for emergency use. Ten ml. of 10% calcium gluconate may be injected intravenously over several minutes while monitoring the pulse for arrhythmias. Particular caution should be used in patients receiving digitalis since they are more susceptible to the development of arrhythmias. Patients requiring more intensive calcium therapy may be given daily infusions of up to 100 ml. of 10% calcium gluconate in 1,000 ml. 5% dextrose in water.

Prior to correction of the hypercalcemia, obligatory water loss ordinarily results in some degree of dehydration. Hypercalcemia may reduce the effect of antidiuretic hormone on the renal tubules; these patients, therefore, have a hypotonic urine. An initial postoperative oliguria may be present until the volume deficit is gradually corrected. Calcium replacement is not begun unless clinical symptoms and laboratory values require such therapy. Vitamin D is usually withheld for 4–6 weeks except when hypocalcemia is particularly difficult to control. The parathyroid glands usually recover within this period. Calcium is restricted to document a fall in the serum level and thus verify that the appropriate operation has been performed.

Postoperative hypocalcemia may be due to decreased absorption secondary to hypofunction of the remaining glands or to increased deposition into the decalcified skeleton. Urinary calculi, if present, may dissolve or pass, but until they do, the hazard of postoperative renal colic persists.

OTHER COMPLICATIONS. – Both postoperative bleeding and the potential of an obstructed airway secondary to it or damage to the recurrent laryngeal nerves can occur following parathyroidectomy in the same manner as following thyroidectomy. The treatment is the same as outlined earlier in the section on the thyroid.

TREATMENT OF HYPERCALCEMIA. – Rarely emergency surgery may be required in a patient with hypercalcemia for disease unrelated to the parathyroid glands. Mild degrees of hypercalcemia may respond to institution of a low-calcium diet and fluid replacement adequate to produce a diuresis if time permits. More severe symptomatic hypercalcemia requires corticosteroids, usually prednisone, 60–80 mg. daily in divided doses. Usually 3–4 or more days are required before an effect is seen. Intravenous phosphate (Inphos; Kendall Co., Needham, Mass.) has been used as an effective and rapid treatment for hypercalcemia. This mixture of sodium and potassium phosphates (1.5 Gm. phosphorus) is infused slowly over a period of 6–8 hours. Mithramycin, an antibiotic used in the treatment of testicular cancer and more recently in Paget's disease, has been observed to lower serum calcium effectively. It may be given in a dose of 25 μg./kg. body weight daily for several days in acute hypercalcemic states with good results. Both phosphate and mithramycin are limited to investigational use at this time.

The Adrenal Glands

The removal of both adrenal glands is most often undertaken for the treatment of disseminated breast cancer. The removal of the glands for hypertension has, for all practical purposes, been abandoned as the medical management of hypertensive cardiovascular disease has become more effective. Hyperplastic states are the usual cause of Cushing's syndrome and these may or may not be associated with pituitary tumors. Both benign and malignant neoplasms can arise in either the cortex or the medulla, and the symptomatology and potential postoperative complications are, of course, considerably different.

POSTOPERATIVE COMPLICATIONS

Acute bleeding following adrenalectomy is fortunately a rare complication of the operative procedure. The only major vessels of any size associated with the adrenal glands are the central veins, whose size and position are well known. The vein on the right is much shorter than that on the left, and also the right adrenal vein empties directly into the vena cava. It is for this reason that when bilateral adrenalectomy is being performed, the right side is usually done first. If complications arise and the operative procedure is prolonged, it is better to defer operating on the left side than to proceed.

Almost invariably there is a drop of 1–3 Gm. in the patient's hemoglobin level during the first 3 or 4 postoperative days. This is generally not through the drain sites and probably remains in the retroperitoneal tissue. The extent of blood loss may be more apparent than real, however, as part of the drop in hemoglobin may be associated with increased blood volume, which in turn is associated with fluid retention secondary to corticosteroid replacement.

Pneumothorax may occur following adrenalectomy, particularly if the twelfth rib has been resected. This should be kept in mind if the patient becomes dyspneic postoperatively. Closed drainage should be established if the diagnosis is confirmed. Some degree of postoperative ileus is an invariable accompaniment of any retroperitoneal dissection. This is usually not a major problem following surgery of the adrenal glands and these patients generally do not require nasogastric intubation. One should not hesitate, however, to insert such a tube if the abdominal distention becomes significant.

ADRENOCORTICAL INSUFFICIENCY.—Adrenocortical insufficiency can be tolerated for only a short period and is the major complication to be avoided following adrenal surgery. It is advisable to be overcautious rather than undercautious in replacement therapy. Replacement dosage should be instituted at or before surgery in any patient in whom it is suspected that endogenous adrenal steroid production is inadequate. This includes patients who have received corticosteroids for more than a few weeks within the past year, patients with adrenal cortical malfunction from any cause, patients with pituitary disease and patients undergoing either partial or total adrenalectomy or hypophysectomy. Patients with Cushing's syndrome and those who require large doses of corticosteroids for other reasons are likely to be in a protein-catabolic and a potassium-depleted state. This should be corrected by administration of supplemental potassium chloride (4–12 Gm./day) and a high-protein diet for several days prior to surgery. If there is a significant diminution, blood volume should be restored preoperatively by the administration of human serum albumin or blood.

Steroid replacement therapy should begin prior to or upon starting the operation. It is important to administer steroids to cover the period of stress but not to continue for prolonged periods and cause the catabolic effect to interfere with wound healing. Synthetic steroids devoid of mineral-regulating activity should not be used for replacement therapy.

The preoperative preparation consists of cortisone acetate, 100 mg. intramuscularly, and cortisone acetate, 100 mg. orally, at 9 P.M. the evening before operation. This is repeated one hour prior to surgery in the morning. Hydrocortisone is available in the operating room to be given intravenously should it be required during the course of the operation. It is not routinely employed as it is rarely required. Should it be necessary to use hydrocortisone to support the patient during surgery, the steroid is given intravenously in 1,000 ml. of 5% glucose in water through a vein separate from the one being used for the anesthetic and/or routine fluid administration.

The postoperative regimen includes 50 mg. of cortisone acetate (I.M.) every 4 hours for 4 doses, every 6 hours for 4 doses, and then every 8 hours. Fluids are restricted to 2,500 ml. during the first 24 hours; 500 ml. of this is physiologic saline. In addition to the intramuscular cortisone, each 1,000 ml. of intravenous fluid during the first 24 hours contains 100 mg. of hydrocortisone. This intravenous administration is discontinued after the first 24 hours, although hydrocortisone is kept at the bedside for use should it become necessary. On the third postoperative day the administration of cortisone is shifted to the oral route provided the patient is able to tolerate oral feedings. The cortisone is reduced to 25 mg. every 6 hours on the fifth postoperative day, then to 25 mg. every 8 hours on about the seventh or eighth postoperative day. By the tenth postoperative day the patient is usually at the maintenance level of 25 mg. every 8 hours for the first 2 periods of the day and 12.5 mg. for the third period. As an alternative, cortisone acetate, 12.5 mg. every 8 hours, may be combined with fluorohydrocortisone, 0.1 – 0.2 mg. daily. Frequent serum electrolyte determinations and careful check for edema or weight gain are advisable. The possibility of precipitating diabetes from excessive doses of corticosteroids must be considered. When unilateral adrenalectomy has been performed for primary aldosteronism, corticosteroid replacement is unnecessary. In such cases, careful attention to potassium balance is essential to prevent postoperative hyperkalemia. Bilateral adrenalectomy for this disease requires replacement therapy as outlined above.

PHEOCHROMOCYTOMA

The adrenal medulla receives no consideration in adrenal surgery except in patients who have a pheochromocytoma. These patients should be prepared for surgery with an alpha-adrenergic receptor blocking agent as soon as the diagnosis is made. Adrenergic drugs, cholinergic blockers and other agents which cause a relative or absolute increase in sympathetic activity are contraindicated preoperatively. Cyclopropane anesthesia cannot be used for this reason. Phenoxybenzamine (Dibenzyline) in oral doses of 40 – 100 mg. every 12 hours for at least 3 days prior to surgery is commonly used and has made the management of blood pressure during and after surgery less complicated. Despite initial fears, experience has indicated that this drug can be given until the time of operation without causing hypotension unresponsive to pressor agents during surgery. Phentolamine (Regitine) intravenously in doses of 1–5 mg. is used for immediate effect should the blood pressure rise to dangerous levels during surgery. Intravenous norepinephrine (Levophed) and plasma volume expanders should be readily available should hypotension occur following removal of the tumor. Blood replacement should be started during the early phases of anesthesia and continued at a rate sufficient to maintain the central venous pressure, since these patients have a relative hypovolemia due to chronic vasoconstriction. Graded replacement is necessary to sustain the intravascular volume.

Inhibitors of catecholamine synthesis (methyltyrosine) have also been used for preoperative preparation of the patient, but experience with this approach is not as great as the use of alpha-receptor blocking agents. This approach remains experimental.

Propranolol (Inderal), a beta-receptor blocking agent, is useful in the prevention and treatment of the cardiac arrhythmias which may occur in these patients. The oral dose is 60 mg./day in divided doses for 3 days before surgery. Intravenous propranolol may be administered in doses of 1–3 mg. (not exceeding 1 mg./minute) under electrocardiographic monitoring for life-threatening arrhythmias.

Several days after surgery urinary vanilmandelic acid and catecholamine determinations are obtained to verify complete removal of the tumor. Postoperatively the administration of corticosteroids is unnecessary unless bilateral adrenalectomy has been performed.

The Endocrine Pancreas

Total pancreatectomy is a rarely indicated surgical procedure. More commonly a portion of the pancreas is removed, either for the control of hyperplastic islet cell function or the removal of a neoplasm. Pseudocysts of the pancreas are generally treated by internal drainage and complications of this procedure are few. There are multiple types of operations employed in the treatment of chronic pancreatitis and here the potential complications when dealing with chronically inflamed scar tissue are many.

Postoperative hemorrhage is the universal potential complication of any major abdominal surgical procedure and the chance of hemorrhage following subtotal pancreatectomy may be aggravated by splenectomy in conjunction with the pancreatic resection. Because of the frequency of leakage from the anastomotic sites, any operative procedure on the pancreas should be well drained. Early signs of intra-abdominal bleeding may be the appearance of bright red blood on the dressings even before signs of shock become apparent. If initial supportive measures are unsuccessful in maintaining the patient in a satisfactory condition with spontaneous cessation of bleeding, the patient must be returned to the operating room for the control of hemorrhage.

Peritonitis following pancreatic resection is generally associated with a leak at one or more of the various anastomoses. The peritonitis may be associated with a gastrointestinal or biliary leak. Each requires appropriate measures to establish external drainage initially and subsequent corrective management if the leakage does not stop spontaneously.

SURGERY IN THE DIABETIC PATIENT

The diabetic patient presents a major potential challenge in management, whether the diabetes is spontaneous or the result of a surgical procedure. Such management, both during and after surgery, can be complex but it has been our practice to keep it as simple as possible. Patients not insulin-dependent preoperatively have oral medications stopped the night before surgery and are supplemented with regular insulin as necessary postoperatively. It is our practice to discontinue phenformin during any period of stress or illness because of its possible relationship to the precipitation of lactic acidosis.

Insulin-dependent patients are given half their usual long-acting dose on the morning of surgery. It is supplemented with regular insulin as needed on the basis of fractional urine or blood sugar determinations in the acute postoperative phase. The patient is then returned to the former regimen as rapidly as feasible, usually with resumption of food intake.

Regular insulin may be given subcutaneously in doses of 10 (2+ glycosuria) to 20 (4+ glycosuria or acetonuria) units as needed. It is good practice to have a physician order each dose of insulin rather than to have a nurse give it on a scale according to the amount of urine sugar present. The latter approach allows too many errors in management, resulting in hypoglycemia or acidosis. The addition of insulin to intravenous solutions is not recommended.

During anesthesia intravenous glucose should be given continuously to avoid hypoglycemia, which may result in brain damage. Intravenous glucose (50 ml. of 50% solution) should be given rapidly to any unconscious patient in whom there is a possibility of hypoglycemia.

Diabetic acidosis is treated in the usual manner with insulin, sodium bicarbonate, fluids and electrolytes. Bicarbonate is ordinarily necessary for correction of acidosis only if the serum bicarbonate concentration is less than 10 mEq./L. Sodium lactate should not be used for correction of acidosis for reasons to be discussed below.

OTHER METABOLIC PROBLEMS

NONKETOTIC HYPEROSMOLAR COMA.—A special problem which may arise during treatment of a burn patient is that of nonketotic hyperosmolar coma. This syndrome is probably secondary to marked dehydration and usually is associated with hyperglycemia and hypernatremia, but normal or slightly low serum bicarbonate levels. Many patients who develop this syndrome have been receiving corticosteroids and most of them are not diabetic. The treatment consists primarily of the administration of large amounts of fluids and electrolytes to correct the dehydration and insulin to lower the blood sugar. Frequently these patients are insulin-sensitive and hypoglycemia can develop easily.

LACTIC ACIDOSIS.—Lactic acidosis is encountered infrequently but carries a high mortality rate. It may occur spontaneously, due to a defect in the metabolism of lactate. Usually it occurs in association with circulatory collapse, renal or hepatic failure, alcoholism or other causes of tissue hypoxia. The diagnosis of lactic acidosis should be suspected in any patient in stupor or coma who has metabolic acidosis with or without hyperventilation. The diagnosis can be verified by demonstration of plasma lactate in excess of 7 mM/L. Therapy consists of removal of the impediment to tissue oxygenation, withdrawal of all but indispensable medications and correction of acidosis by the administration of sodium bicarbonate. It is reasonable to consider dialysis if lactate excess persists. Hyperbaric treatments to improve tissue oxygenation and injection of methylene blue to convert lactate to pyruvate remain experimental.

HYPOGLYCEMIA.—The surgical management of hypoglycemia is usually associated with the removal of beta cell adenomas of the pancreas which produce excess amounts of insulin. Rarely hypoglycemia is caused by non-insulin-producing retroperitoneal or thoracic sarcomas. After the establishment of a tentative diagnosis, management consists in protecting the patient from episodes of severe hypoglycemia. A trial of diazoxide (for investigational use only) preoperatively to determine its effectiveness in control of the blood sugar is warranted. The response may influence the extent of the procedure undertaken in the event that difficulty is encountered in removal of the tumor.

On an empirical basis, corticosteroids (100 mg. hydrocortisone) should be given on the morning of the operation to prevent hyperpyrexia and death of obscure etiology which has been observed in some of these patients. Glucose should be administered intravenously in amounts to prevent severe hypoglycemia during anesthesia. The blood sugar may be readily monitored during anesthesia with Dextrostix. Blood sugar determinations are necessary during recovery from anesthesia and 3–4 times daily for several days. Often transient hyperglycemia occurs after complete excision because the normal islet cells may be temporarily unresponsive due to the previous long-standing hypoglycemia. Ordinarily treatment with insulin is not required and the islets recover their functional capacity within a few days.

If a surgical cure is not achieved, medical control of hypoglycemia must be instituted. This is most practically accomplished with the use of diazoxide. Effective control has been obtained in some patients for several years. The dose ranges from 200 – 1,200 mg./day. If a small dose is effective, it is best given at bedtime with a bedtime feeding, since nocturnal hypoglycemia is most difficult to control. Larger doses are usually given 3 times daily. The limiting factor in the dosage is the frequency of side effects of the medication. The most troublesome of these is the development of edema, which may lead to congestive heart failure. Diazoxide is an antidiuretic even though it is chemically related to the thiazide diuretics. Cardiac arrhythmias, nausea and vomiting may also be troublesome, usually occurring with doses of 600 mg./day or more. Other side effects include overgrowth of facial hair and eyebrows, postural hypotension, hematologic and dermatologic abnormalities, hyperuricemia, lymphadenitis, gingival hyperplasia and muscle wasting. These are less common and are usually minor in severity. Occasionally a patient may not respond to diazoxide unless it is given as a suspension instead of in capsules. In such instances, in which a near total pancreatic resection has been performed, it may be postulated that the capsules are not adequately digested for release of the medication.

Other hyperglycemic agents such as corticosteroids, ACTH, glucagon and growth hormone may be effective for short-term treatment, particularly when oral medication is precluded. However, they are impractical for long-term use because of adverse side effects.

Metastatic beta cell carcinoma is particularly difficult to manage and responds poorly to medication with diazoxide. Alloxan, which is diabetogenic in animals, has not been of value in those patients in whom it has been used. A newer diabetogenic agent, streptozotocin (for investigational use only), appears to have more promise, having produced tumor regression and normoglycemia in some patients.

The Pituitary Gland

Operations on the pituitary gland are performed not only for primary neoplasms but as a part of the management of disseminated malignant disease, particularly cancer of the breast.

The management of the postoperative intracranial surgical patient has been outlined in Chapter 16. The pituitary gland is occasionally exposed trans-sphenoidally; the postoperative care and potential complications are identical essentially to those for a patient who has undergone a resection of the maxilla (Chapter 17). The most innocuous means of destroying the pituitary, from the surgical point of view at least, is the use of a radioactive implant of yttrium introduced transnasally. The only significant postoperative surgical complication here is a leak of cerebrospinal fluid, and with the present silastic plugs that are used to close the defect in the sella, this has become extremely rare.

Postoperative Complications

The major postoperative considerations peculiar to surgery of the pituitary gland are associated with its multiple endocrine functions. Although surgical procedures on the pituitary gland may affect many or all of the trophic hormones, the only trophic hormone deficiency of any immediate concern is that of ACTH. Any surgically produced or preexisting deficiency of ACTH requires substitution both during and after the surgical procedure with physiologic doses of adrenocortical steroids. Management is similar to that outlined for the pre- and postoperative care of the patient undergoing surgery of the adrenal glands. It must be remembered that, with pharmacologic doses of steroids, underlying diabetes may be unmasked and lead to complications of diabetic acidosis or coma.

Antidiuretic hormone deficiency.—The other immediate problem likely to be encountered in pituitary surgery is that of deficiency of antidiuretic hormone. If adequate amounts of the pituitary stalk are left intact, there may be no deficiency, but if the stalk is removed to a variable extent, an inconstant deficiency of the hormone may result in considerable difficulty in the control of fluid balance. Characteristically there is a triphasic response to surgical damage of the posterior pituitary and stalk. Immediately following the surgery polyuria and polydipsia are present, which usually last from 4 to 5 days. There is then a period of intense antidiuresis which persists for approximately 6 days. This is followed by the permanent polyuria and polydipsia of established diabetes insipidus. It is generally agreed that the initial diuretic phase results from acute damage to the hypothalamus so that stored hormone is not released. The antidiuretic stage results from degeneration of hormone-laden tissue and its release into the circulation. Administration of a water load during the antidiuretic phase will not induce the usual diuretic response. Removal of the posterior pituitary at the time of stalk section will usually prevent the antidiuretic phase.

After diabetes insipidus occurs, there may be variable degrees of recovery, making water balance only a minor problem. The most effective way of showing a deficiency of antidiuretic hormone is to demonstrate a hyposthenuric urine (specific gravity 1.010, 300 mOsm./L.) in the presence of a serum which is slightly more concentrated than normal (290–300 mOsm./L.). This is best done by determination of serum and urine osmolality. In the absence of means to determine osmolality, it may be more simply demonstrated by exhibiting a decrease in urine output and an increase in urine specific gravity to more than 1.015 during a period of dehydration. The usual procedure is to withhold water until the patient has lost 3–5% of his body weight. This ordinarily produces enough dehydration to raise the osmolality of the serum sufficiently to stimulate the osmolar receptors of the hypothalamus.

This will release antidiuretic hormone if the system is functional. The patient must be observed during this period because excessive dehydration may cause hypotension. The normal serum osmolality is in the range of 290 mOsm./L. With adequate dehydration it should rise to approximately 310 mOsm./L. and the normal urine osmolality will ordinarily rise to the range of 500–900 mOsm./L. Depending on the degree of diabetes insipidus, the urine osmolality may only slightly exceed that of the serum or be as high as 300–400 mOsm./L. As an alternative to dehydration for raising serum osmolality, hypertonic saline may be infused (3% NaCl, 0.25 ml./kg./minute for 45 minutes) which results in a prompt decrease in urine volume if antidiuretic hormone can be released.

An error in management occasionally encountered is overhydration. This produces polyuria with a low specific gravity, resulting in an erroneous diagnosis of diabetes insipidus. If the degree of overhydration is severe enough, it can produce water intoxication and cause coma and convulsions.

During the management of polyuria, frequent electrolyte determinations are necessary to guide electrolyte and fluid therapy. It is important to make a correct distinction between diabetes insipidus and overhydration, for treatment with antidiuretic hormone during overhydration may produce acute water intoxication. Diabetes mellitus with glucosuria producing an osmotic diuresis with high specific gravity and osmolality must be considered in the differential diagnosis, but this is easily determined by assessment of urine and blood glucose.

The management of diabetes insipidus consists of the administration of adequate antidiuretic hormone to decrease the urine volume to normal levels with a coincident increase in specific gravity. Initially aqueous Pitressin, which has a duration of action of 4–6 hours, may be given subcutaneously or intramuscularly but should not be given intravenously. For the average postoperative patient 5 units (0.25 ml.) should be given initially and the dose increased to 10 units (0.5 ml.) with subsequent injections, as necessary. It is recommended that aqueous Pitressin injections be repeated at 3–4 hour intervals as required. Aqueous Pitressin may also be administered intranasally by spray or dropper in similar dosage, but this route is not as dependable as parenteral injection. If more prolonged therapy is required, the longer lasting Pitressin tannate in oil may be given after initial control with aqueous Pitressin. The usual dosage is 2.5–5 units (0.5–1 ml.) intramuscularly, at required intervals. The intervals are variable and may be 36–48 hours or more. Pitressin snuff preparations are available for long-term use but are less predictable and therefore not recommended in acute postoperative management. Chlorpropamide (250–500 mg. daily) has recently been found to be useful in management of partial diabetes insipidus. It may produce effective antidiuresis only if there are small amounts of residual antidiuretic hormone present, but should be tried in all patients, since it is much more convenient for long-term therapy.

25

The Patient with Liver Disease

A. WILLIAM HOLMES, M.D.

Attending Physician and Director, Section of Hepatology, Rush-Presbyterian-St. Luke's Medical Center; Professor of Medicine, Rush Medical College

WILLIAM S. DYE, M.D.

Attending Surgeon, Rush-Presbyterian-St. Luke's Medical Center; Professor of Surgery, Rush Medical College

AND

ROBERT J. OVERSTREET, M.D.

Assistant Attending Surgeon, Rush-Presbyterian-St. Luke's Medical Center; Assistant Professor of Surgery, Rush Medical College

ALTHOUGH THE INTENTION of this chapter is to provide information regarding the postoperative care of patients with known liver disease or with evidence of hepatic insufficiency appearing postoperatively, it is essential to consider also preoperative factors bearing on the subsequent course of either kind of patient. For this reason we shall go first into some general considerations regarding the liver and surgery, and then discuss those problems raised by specific operative procedures.

Preoperative Considerations

NORMAL LIVER.—Patients who have normal liver structure and function can ordinarily be expected to withstand surgery well. Although it is often stated that intraoperative hypoxia can injure a normal liver, animal studies would suggest that hypoxia must be severe or protracted to cause hepatic damage.

ACUTE HEPATITIS.—Extensive experience in and since World War II indicates that surgery during the course of acute hepatitis carries a high mortality rate due to postoperative worsening of the hepatitis and subsequent liver failure. Careful study of such patients shows, however, that the major hazard exists in the patient who has not yet reached his peak bilirubin level and is therefore in the worsening phase of the disease. The patient who has passed the point of maximum biochemical abnormalities and whose symptoms have also subsided is in the convalescent phase of hepatitis. If emergency surgery is necessary at this time, the clinical and biochemical manifestations of hepatitis will probably worsen, but there is little risk of hepatic encephalopathy or a fatal outcome.

CHRONIC PARENCHYMAL LIVER DISEASE.—The anticipated response of the patient with chronic liver disease to anesthesia and surgery depends entirely on the kind and the severity of his disease. It is not possible to make all-inclusive statements about "cirrhosis" which will have any value. Two facets of chronic liver disease which bear more or less independently on the outcome of such a patient are cell injury and fibrosis.

Cell injury.—Patients with acute *and* chronic alcoholic liver disease or those with extensive hepatocellular necrosis due to a flare-up of chronic hepatitis will have severe derangements of hepatic conjugating and synthesizing capacities. These can best be detected by finding moderately or markedly elevated serum transaminase activities and such indicators of impaired hepatic synthetic capacity as a prolonged prothrombin time in spite of vitamin K administration or diminished serum pseudocholinesterase activity. The inadequate drug metabolism of these patients applies to anesthetic agents as well, and surgery in such individuals is apt to be fraught with as much hazard as in patients in the early phase of acute viral hepatitis. If there is question about the presence of hepatocellular injury, preoperative needle biopsy of the liver or postponement of the surgery for the purpose of medical treatment should be strongly considered.

Hepatic fibrosis.—The fibrous septa in the cirrhotic liver are rich in vascular channels and contain many arteriovenous anastomoses. These, in addition to the deformed architecture characteristic of cirrhosis, lead to the development of portal hypertension and may well also be a factor in ascites production. Because the development of these fibrous septa is largely independent of hepatocellular function, it is possible for a patient to have marked cirrhosis yet have good hepatocellular function. In considering the cirrhotic patient for surgery, therefore, one must look at these facets independently. The cirrhotic with portal hypertension, and even ascites, can be a perfectly good surgical candidate if the hepatocellular function is good. Two important points should be kept in mind with regard to such patients, however. First, it is obvious that portal hypertension will lead to considerably more blood loss than is usual in abdominal procedures. An elective cholecystectomy for asymptomatic stones should be approached with caution in the patient with portal hypertension. Secondly, if a patient has marked ascites, the sudden loss of abdominal fluid when the abdomen is entered can lead to all the well-recognized complications of massive paracentesis, such as shock or hepatic coma. It is wise, therefore, to try to get such a patient as dry as possible before surgery.

CHRONIC EXTRAHEPATIC BILIARY OBSTRUCTION.—These patients usually have good hepatocellular function and rarely have significant septum formation. Surgery to relieve the biliary tract block is therefore not likely to lead to serious hemorrhagic or metabolic difficulties in the postoperative period as long as adequate parenteral vitamin K (5–10 mg.) is given preoperatively. The one exception is the patient with marked hyperbilirubinemia and this situation will be dealt with in detail on page 424. The presence of suppurative cholangitis, which is quite common in this group of patients, does require special attention. If the patient is to be in optimal condition for surgery and if peritoneal sepsis is to be avoided, cholangitis should be treated preoperatively and for 5–7 days after surgery. The drugs of choice are usually ampicillin, 8 Gm./day, or tetracycline, 2 Gm./day.

CHOICE OF ANESTHETIC AGENT.—The specific agent used during the operative procedure is probably far less important than careful preoperative preparation and evaluation of the patient. The greatest controversy in this area revolves around halothane and Penthrane. It has been suggested, though not proved, that occasionally acute hepatic necrosis develops because of exposure to one or the other of these agents. In the case of Penthrane, nephrotoxicity may rarely occur as well. It is very likely that in the occasional patient acute hepatic necrosis develops after 2 or more exposures to halothane. This is thought to be on the basis of hypersensitivity, and it may be possible to identify individuals who will have this often fatal reaction by the occurrence of unexplained fever and eosinophilia in the early postoperative period. If such signs appear, the patient should be checked clinically and biochemically for evidence of hepatocellular injury (transaminase, bilirubin, prothrombin time), but even if overt liver injury has not occurred, halothane should not be used again in that patient. Despite these rare reactions, there is no evidence for any inherent hepatotoxicity of halothane and it can be used with confidence in patients with pre-existing liver disease if the anesthesiologist feels he can handle the patient best with it.

General Postoperative Problems

Occasionally there are patients in whom abnormalities of hepatic function tests are detected in the postoperative period when results of these tests have been normal before surgery. These may be isolated or combined abnormalities and can best be considered individually.

ISOLATED TRANSAMINASE ELEVATIONS.—The term "transaminase" is used here to represent the whole family of intracellular enzymes, elevated serum activity of which has been used as a reliable indicator of hepatocellular injury: serum glutamic oxaloacetic transaminase (SGOT), serum glutamic pyruvic transaminase (SGPT), lactic dehydrogenase (LDH) isoenzymes, sorbitol dehydrogenase (SDH), etc. Minimal elevations (up to twice the upper normal for a given laboratory) are not unusual after many kinds of surgery and cannot be regarded as indicators of liver injury. An isolated SGOT level in this range may indicate myocardial infarction or pulmonary embolism, and signs of these complications should be sought. Isolated elevation of LDH usually reflects hemolysis and is not surprising if the patient has had multiple transfusions or has an underlying hemolytic disorder. Erythrocyte LDH consists largely of isoenzymes 1 and 2 and is heat stable; hepatic LDH includes isoenzymes 4 and 5 and is heat labile. If appropriate biochemical facilities are available, the distinction can be made readily.

Moderate elevations.—Elevations of 2 to 10 times normal are extremely unusual after uncomplicated surgery and bear investigation. Possible causes are:

1. Postanesthetic liver injury. In this situation serum enzyme activities may well go up before any other hepatic tests show abnormal results. These patients often have nausea and weakness out of proportion to what one might expect from the operation performed and, if the right upper quadrant can be examined adequately, a large, tender liver is often found. There is no specific treatment save for bed rest and observation.

2. Passive congestion of the liver due to venous hypertension. Hepatic congestion produces centrilobular damage causing elevation of serum activity of the enzymes usually associated with the liver. This is best detected by assessment of the patient for signs of congestive heart failure and measurement of the venous pressure. Treatment is obviously that of the underlying cause.

3. Necrosis of organs other than the liver. SGPT and SDH are enzymes which are almost entirely restricted to liver tissue, whereas most others can also be found in other organs. If elevated serum activities of other enzymes (such as SGOT or LDH) are detected and there is no clinical evidence of liver involvement, SGPT and/or SDH should be measured to see if the problem does, in fact, reside in the liver.

Marked elevations.—Elevations more than 10 times normal are extremely rare. They may indicate massive hepatic necrosis, in which case there are almost always concomitant abnormalities of bilirubin and prothrombin activity in addition to clinical evidence of an obviously sick patient with nausea, often mental obtundation and some right upper quadrant pain. The cause may be the coincidental and unfortunate performance of surgery in a patient with unrecognized acute hepatitis, postanesthetic hepatic necrosis or ligation of the hepatic artery. The first 2 are treatable only by supportive measures; if the third is considered a reasonable possibility, a celiac axis arteriogram should be done immediately to visualize hepatic arterial supply.

Marked but transient elevations of serum enzyme activity have also been seen occasionally after severe hypotensive episodes. The enzyme values reported are astronomical (for example, SGOT 6,000, ICD 75,000), but there are no associated abnormalities of other hepatic tests and the enzymes promptly return to normal over the next 3–5 days. This sequence of events may also occur in the patient who has not had any surgery but who has hypotension for some other reason. There is, to our knowledge, no explanation for these findings.

Isolated elevations of alkaline phosphatase.—There are relatively few situations in which alkaline phosphatase alone is elevated. These include:

1. Healing bone. After any procedure in which bone is cut (for example, the sternum-splitting incision for cardiac surgery), the serum alkaline phosphatase activity will rise as healing and osteoblastic activity proceed. This cause of alkaline phosphatase elevation can be identified if serum activity of leucine aminopeptidase or 5′ nucleotidase are measured. All three of these enzymes are excreted by the liver and, if the high alkaline phosphatase is on the basis of a liver lesion, either or both of the others will also be elevated.

2. Recovery from passive congestion or from acute alcoholic liver injury. It is rather common for patients recovering from the acute liver injury of centrilobular congestion or from an alcoholic hepatitis to have a rising alkaline phosphatase. The mechanism of this is not clear but seems likely to be due to focal cholestasis in areas of regeneration.

3. Obstruction of a major hepatic duct. If either the right or left hepatic bile duct has been ligated or if a retained gallstone obstructs either duct, the patient will have a rising alkaline phosphatase on the basis of obstruction of a single lobe. Jaundice often does not develop because the other lobe, with normal drainage, will be able to excrete the excess bilirubin. This syndrome is usually associated with pruritus and there may also be chills, fever, and tenderness due to cholangitis proximal to the obstruction.

4. Drugs. The number of therapeutic agents which can cause cholestasis has grown far beyond chlorpromazine, norethandrolone and methyltestosterone, which were originally thought to be the prime offenders in producing drug cholestasis. For this reason, the list of drugs administered to a patient with an unexplained postoperative elevation of alkaline phosphatase must be looked at carefully and the drugs reduced to the minimum necessary for optimal care. Most tranquilizers and some antibiotics, in addition to some anabolic steroids, have at one time or another been implicated in or proved to cause cholestasis. It is not practical to list each one of these, as any compilation will be out of date 6 months after it is made. This is not to say that

drugs should not be used, but rather that the effects of administered medications should be monitored. If drug-induced cholestasis does occur postoperatively, withdrawal of the drug constitutes adequate treatment. Chronic liver disease has been an extremely rare sequel of this syndrome.

ISOLATED ELEVATION OF BILIRUBIN.—The single cause of postoperative hyperbilirubinemia without elevation of other hepatic function indices is hemolysis. (Surprisingly, direct as well as indirect bilirubin levels may be elevated.) This may be hemolysis of transfused senescent red cells (each unit of whole blood equals about 250 mg. of bilirubin, which is also about the normal daily hepatic excretion of bilirubin), hemolysis of the patient's own red cells in the vascular space due to an underlying hemolytic process, hypersplenism, trauma to cells crossing a vascular or valvular prosthesis or hemolysis of the patient's own cells in a hematoma. Elevation of lactic dehydrogenase activity commonly accompanies this.

Posttransfusion hyperbilirubinemia requires no treatment and will clear over a period of days. Jaundice due to a hematoma does not of itself demand drainage of the hematoma. Immediate treatment of intravascular hemolysis is not always possible or necessary and must be considered on the merits of the individual case. If postoperative hyperbilirubinemia develops for any of these reasons in a patient with underlying chronic liver disease, the jaundice will be much more marked and alarming because of the patient's relative inability to handle a bilirubin load, but care of the patient in this situation should be no different.

ABNORMAL RESULTS OF MULTIPLE HEPATIC TESTS.—In a number of situations results of more than one hepatic test are abnormal in the early postoperative period. These should be analyzed in the same way that one looks at liver chemistries in the nonsurgical patient. It should be emphasized that blood biochemical studies can indicate the pathophysiology present, but the etiology must be derived from clinical considerations. Hepatic tests can be classified conveniently as follows:

1. Tests of excretory capacity (alkaline phosphatase, leucine aminopeptidase, 5′ nucleotidase). Abnormalities of these tests indicate a block in thc biliary tree at some level; they will not differentiate an extrahepatic block such as may occur with a retained common duct stone from intrahepatic block such as may occur with a cholestatic drug reaction.

2. Tests of conjugation and excretion (serum bilirubin, bromsulfalein excretion). These tests measure the capacity of the liver both to carry out a rather simple chemical reaction, namely, the conjugation of 2 substances, and to excrete the conjugated product. Thus they are not terribly valuable in distinguishing hepatic parenchymal disease from an obstructive process. Bromsulfalein excretion is of particularly little value in the patient with obvious evidence of liver impairment because

of its extreme sensitivity and its nonspecificity, which no doubt contributes to the high incidence of false positivity.

3. Tests of synthetic capacity (prothrombin time after 5–10 mg. of parenteral vitamin K, serum pseudocholinesterase level). The substances are synthesized *de novo* by the liver and their activity in the blood indicates reliably the functional capacity of the hepatocytes. Values are not abnormal in a purely obstructive process.

4. Tests of cell membrane integrity (SGOT, SGPT, ICD, LDH IV and V). The transaminases and many other enzymes are normally present in the hepatocytes and leak from the liver cell which has been injured. Elevation of their activity in the serum is, therefore, an indicator of hepatocellular injury. Modest injury may occur in patients with extrahepatic obstruction and cholangitis but major elevations of serum enzyme activities are reliable indicators of hepatocellular damage.

5. Tests which detect abnormal proteins (thymol turbidity, cephalin flocculation, gamma globulin by serum electrophoresis). Though these tests are often looked upon as liver tests, they are, in fact, only indicators of the abnormal kinds or amounts of serum globulin seen in patients with chronic liver disease. They usually give abnormal findings in patients with the myriad of other diseases in which globulin abnormalities exist. Because abnormal proteins are most commonly seen in *chronic* liver disease, these tests are not often of much value in the early postoperative period.

DIFFERENTIAL DIAGNOSIS OF POSTOPERATIVE JAUNDICE.—With this background, one can look at the differential diagnosis in early postoperative jaundice as follows:

Elevated bilirubin and alkaline phosphatase with normal or nearly normal SGOT and prothrombin time.—This combination of abnormalities ordinarily indicates a block in biliary excretion and should raise consideration of drug or postoperative cholestasis or extrahepatic obstruction.

In drug cholestasis the patient will usually complain only of pruritus. Examination is usually unrevealing except for icterus and the occasional presence of a slightly enlarged nontender liver. Review and reduce the list of medications. No other specific therapy is indicated. It is well to remember that jaundice may worsen or remain constant for as long as 3 weeks after the offending drug is discontinued.

Benign postoperative cholestasis is a relatively rare condition of unknown etiology occurring most commonly but not exclusively after abdominal surgery. Such patients are indistinguishable from patients with drug cholestasis. No treatment is indicated; the condition will subside spontaneously without residual.

Extrahepatic common bile duct obstruction is most often seen after biliary surgery, but occasionally patients with other kinds of operations will have common duct obstruction due to stone. Patients with acute extrahepatic duct obstruction often have right upper quadrant and right subscapular pain and such evidences of cholangitis as fever and chills. If cholangitis is present, the liver is quite tender and with or without cholangitis it is often enlarged. If this syndrome develops, possible causes should be reviewed, such as coincidental common duct stone, retained stone missed at surgery, accidental ligation of the common duct or transection of the common duct. Cicatricial stricture will rarely develop soon enough to cause obstructive icterus in the *early* postoperative period. Obstruction alone does *not* require emergency treatment, and indeed it is often wise to allow the patient to recover adequately from operation before considering re-exploration. If cholangitis coexists, however, this must be treated with antibiotics (ampicillin, cephalosporin or tetracycline) because of the very real risk of gram-negative sepsis. Incidentally, a modest amount of periportal hepatocellular necrosis occurs in cholangitis and moderate elevations of SGOT, SGPT, etc., are not surprising.

Elevated bilirubin and transaminase, with normal or nearly normal alkaline phosphatase.—This biochemical picture indicates acute hepatocellular necrosis. The prothrombin time may or may not be prolonged; if it is, the degree of prolongation is a good indicator of the severity of the process. Almost all of these patients complain of nausea and lassitude and only occasionally will they complain of right upper quadrant distress. Possible causes of acute postoperative hepatocellular necrosis are the anesthetic agent, transfusion, an unrecognized viral hepatitis and infarction.

Postanesthetic hepatic necrosis is most commonly associated with halothane but may occur after other anesthetic agents as well. Fever is common, as are eosinophilia and tender hepatomegaly. Often elevated serum enzyme activities will antedate hyperbilirubinemia and this preicteric phase may last as long as 2–3 weeks. The diagnosis is made only by exclusion; there is no specific diagnostic test.

Posttransfusion hepatitis will not occur in the early postoperative period but should be kept in mind. The shortest reported incubation period from transfusion to documented disease is 12 days. One should make a careful search of the record for preoperative transfusions, which may have been given as long as 3–6 weeks before surgery.

Rarely a patient with clinically inapparent hepatitis will be taken to surgery. If this happens, the clinical and biochemical signs of disease will worsen dramatically in the early postoperative period. Except for the eosinophilia, which is much less common in viral hepatitis, these patients cannot be distinguished from those with postanesthetic liver necrosis. There is no specific treatment save for the use of hydrocortisone, 500–1,000 mg. daily intravenously, in patients who develop confusion and asterixis, indicating the onset of hepatic encephalopathy. Though there is no uniform agreement on the use of adrenal steroids in this situation, some authors have found them to be of value.

Hepatic infarction is a rare complication resulting from the inadvertent ligation of the hepatic artery or one of its major branches. Patients in whom this occurs have rapidly increasing jaundice and fever without striking hepatomegaly. Hepatic coma develops within a few days. As indicated earlier, if this complication is suspected, emergency hepatic arteriography is indicated, with a plan to attempt repair should obstruction to arterial supply be found.

Elevated bilirubin, alkaline phosphatase and transaminase. —Marked elevation of all 3 kinds of tests is unusual but has been seen in the early postoperative period in patients who have had extensive surgery, usually vascular, with many transfusions, known or likely hematoma and concomitant renal failure. The degree of alkaline phosphatase elevation has in some patients led to a consideration of exploration for extrahepatic obstruction. It is not clear what causes this picture, which is delineated in detail by Kantrowitz and associates (New England J. Med. 276:591, 1967), but it seems likely to be a result of renal insufficiency, reduced hepatic blood flow and perhaps hepatic hypoxia, all occurring together. Biopsy or autopsy study of the livers of such patients shows only a little congestion and no other striking abnormalities.

Complications of Specific Operative Procedures

There are certain kinds of hepatobiliary surgery associated with specific complications and these are described here.

Portosystemic Shunt

There are 4 major problems which may arise after shunt surgery. The kind of shunt is relatively less important than the fact that one has been done.

Early postoperative oliguria.—This is quite common and such patients may excrete only 15–30 ml. of urine an hour following surgery. On examination the patient usually has a rapid pulse and a narrow pulse pressure. The specific gravity of the small volume of urine which is passed is normal to high. These patients are dehydrated, probably because of the exposure of a large peritoneal surface for long periods during shunt surgery, in addition to loss of ascites and the preoperative fluid restriction and diuretic therapy. If a blood volume measurement is done and if there is no preoperative value for comparison, one can be badly misled, since the usual cirrhotic patient has a large preoperative plasma volume (55–70 ml./kg.), and a postoperative plasma volume of 45–55 ml./kg. (compared to a normal value of 45±6 ml./kg.), while large by the usual standards, represents in fact dehydration for that specific patient. Failure to recognize this often leads to injudicious use of potent parenteral diuretics which only worsen the situation.

If fluid intake in these patients is simply increased, they will respond promptly with a more satisfactory urine flow. The kind of fluid given is important only in terms of sodium restriction. Most cirrhotics, and especially those with ascites, have secondary hyperaldosteronism and will retain sodium tenaciously. This is especially true in the immediately postoperative patient who cannot be given aldosterone antagonists because of the unavailability of the parenteral form of the medication. A maximal sodium intake of 50 mEq./day should be adequate but urine sodium excretion should be monitored to confirm this.

HEPATIC ENCEPHALOPATHY.—In the postshunt patient confusion, asterixis and hyperammonemia may be present either because of excessive ammonia influx (exogenous coma) or because of primary liver cell failure (endogenous coma). Exogenous coma is usually due to 1 of 2 causes: Either the patient went to surgery with blood in the gastrointestinal tract due to recent preoperative hemorrhage, or he was fed postoperatively with more protein than he could tolerate. The former cause is bothersome because the postoperative ileus prevents rapid mobilization and evacuation of the blood, but almost all such patients will respond to the infusion of arginine glutamate. The prime effect of this substance is to stimulate the Krebs urea cycle and tie up more ammonia. The usual dose is 25 Gm. dissolved in 300–500 ml. of 5% dextrose in water and given within a 90-minute time period. If it is effective, the patient's mental state should show evidence of clearing over the ensuing hour. Repeat doses can be given if necessary every 8 hours. If the exogenous coma is due to dietary protein influx, restriction of dietary protein is all that is necessary.

It is mentioned parenthetically that although many kinds of diets have been recommended for the shunt patient in the early postoperative period, it has been our experience that such patients tolerate the usual progression from liquid to soft to general diet very well. If the patient had ascites preoperatively or if ascites has developed following surgery, daily sodium intake should be restricted to 800–1,200 mg. There seems to be no advantage in pushing carbohydrates or arbitrarily restricting protein.

Characteristically exogenous coma is *not* associated with significant changes in blood values which pertain to the liver except for blood ammonia. Endogenous coma, on the other hand, because it is due to primary liver cell failure, is accompanied by significant deterioration evidenced by other hepatic tests such as prothrombin time, bilirubin and transaminases. This early postoperative deterioration can be a grave prognostic sign and probably results from diminution of liver blood flow following surgical revision of the portal circulation. It is, therefore, primarily seen after end-to-side portacaval rather than splenorenal shunt, whereas recurrent varix hemorrhage is more common after splenorenal than portacaval shunts. There is no specific treatment. Many patients will have a transient period of endogenous coma which will clear, but some of these patients will deteriorate steadily and die with liver failure. Arginine glutamate is seldom of help. There seems to be no relationship between early postoperative encephalopathy and the later development of chronic encephalopathy due to protein intolerance which may become apparent 2 months or more after shunt in 10–20% of patients.

RECURRENT GASTROINTESTINAL BLEEDING.—This distressing early postoperative complication may be a sign of shunt thrombosis and recurrent variceal bleeding, but it is more often due to acid peptic disease. It should be recognized that thrombosis of a technically satisfactory shunt is a very rare occurrence. If it occurs, it usually takes place within a few days after surgery and is accompanied by the rapid accumulation of ascites, often with wound dehiscence. We have gained some confidence in the use of the rectal ether circulation time in testing for shunt patency. This test was introduced many years ago as a means of detecting slowed portal flow, and hence portal hypertension. It is worthless for that purpose, but it will demonstrate rapid transport of ether from rectum to lung in the presence of a patent portosystemic shunt. A rectal tube is inserted at least 6 in. and 2 ml. of diethyl ether is instilled into the rectum. The time from instillation of ether to detection of ether in the expired air should be less than 45 seconds and is usually closer to 25 seconds in the presence of a patent shunt. If a shunt is thrombosed, this time is much longer, approaching 2–3 minutes.

Upper gastrointestinal bleeding due to peptic ulcer or gastritis is not rare immediately after shunt and has been said to occur in up to 10% of shunt patients. This can be related to the stress of bleeding varices and subsequent major surgery, but it has also been shown that cirrhotic patients have gastric hypoacidity which, after shunting, is replaced by normal or elevated gastic acid values. The mechanism of this rise in gastric acidity is not clear but may relate to the diversion of gastrin and/or histamine around the liver and consequent decrease in hepatic metabolism of either or both of these substances.

The patient with hematemesis and/or melena after a portosystemic shunt must be handled like any other individual with upper gastrointestinal hemorrhage from an unknown source. Although emergency fluoroscopy of the esophagus, stomach and duodenum may yield valuable information, it is clear that the margin of error of this radiographic study is large. This is particularly true in the patient who has had a shunt, since esophageal varices do not disappear immediately after a shunt and are likely to be seen whether they are the source of bleeding or not. Esophagoscopy, and gastroscopy if necessary, should be done as soon as practical after the onset of bleeding to identify with certainty the source of the bleeding. As more experience is gained with celiac axis arteriography, this may become an acceptable alternative procedure. Subsequent treatment of the patient then depends on the findings at endoscopy. If the patient has recurrent varix bleeding, 20 units of Pitressin given *slowly* intravenously may stop the hemorrhage, but this drug should not be given more often than every 6–8 hours and for no greater period than 48–72 hours because of the reduced hepatic blood flow following Pitressin administration. If bleeding is not controlled by Pitressin, then a Sengstaken-Blakemore tube should be inserted. In either event further surgery will have to be considered, either another kind of shunt (mesenteric-caval, splenorenal) or a direct attack on the esophagus (transection and reanastomosis, varix ligation or esophageal resection with jejunal interposition).

Bleeding ulcer or gastritis should be handled in the usual way and it is difficult to say whether continuous gastric suction is better than continuous or intermittent milk and antacid administration. The hazard in the administration of large amounts of milk relates to its protein content and the consequent danger of hepatic encephalopathy, but the response to this protein load will vary with the individual. Obviously it is desirable to avoid reoperating in such a patient, but if bleeding is brisk and persistent, gastric surgery may have to be considered.

ASCITES FORMATION.—In some shunt patients there may be considerable ascites in the first few postoperative days. As mentioned, this may be a consequence of shunt thrombosis, but it is much more likely to be due to an inordinate sodium load in the intravenous fluid given in the operating room. We have seen a number of shunt patients who have been given 3–6 L. of lactated Ringer's solution during surgery; in almost every one of these individuals ascites began to develop immediately postoperatively. Prevention of this complication is obvious and simple. Specifically avoid the administration of large amounts of sodium to such patients. Once the ascites has developed, however, treatment should be guided by the volume of the fluid accumulation. If the volume of ascites is small or even moderate, if continued accumulation is not occurring and if the patient has no signs of distention or dyspnea, it may be entirely adequate to restrict further sodium intake and wait. If, on the other hand, distention is extreme or accumulation is rapid, it becomes necessary to administer diuretics. Mercurials have been tried in this situation but are seldom of benefit. Mannitol, 25 Gm. by intravenous push, or furosemide, 40 mg. intramuscularly 3 times daily if necessary, are much more likely to be of help. Ethacrynic acid given intravenously should be avoided if possible, since it can occasionally produce a massive diuresis and dangerous hypovolemia and hypochloremia. Paracentesis is also to be avoided, but if the patient does not respond to diuretics and wound disruption threatens, it may be the only alternative. Intravenous infusion of the ascitic fluid removed has been advocated by some to avoid protein depletion; but because of the frequent pyrogenic reactions and the lack of solid evidence of the efficacy of this procedure, we do not favor it. As soon as the patient can tolerate oral medication he should be started on spironolactone, 25 mg. 4 times daily.

Another cause of early postoperative ascites is intrahepatic portal hypertension after end-to-side portacaval shunt. If at the time of surgery the portal vein is clamped and if the pressure measured on the *hepatic* side of the clamp rises briskly, this means that there is extensive communication between the hepatic arterial and portal venous systems. The frequent development of extensive ascites in such patients after end-to-side portacaval shunt has led some authors to suggest that in such a situation a shunt which retains continuity of the portal vein and thereby decompresses the liver, such as a side-to-side portacaval or splenorenal shunt, should be the procedure of choice. If, however, an end-to-side shunt has already been performed, the problem becomes one of stringent treatment of the ascites, which will usually require at least 100 mg./day of spironolactone and 80–120 mg./day of furosemide plus a daily sodium intake not in excess of 1,000 mg. for control.

Because of this propensity for ascites to develop in the postshunt patient, it is wise to avoid the use of drains whenever possible in portosystemic shunt surgery. If it is necessary to drain the peritoneal space, these drains should be removed as soon as possible. A patient who has had abdominal drains inserted and who then forms substantial amounts of ascites will, of course, freely lose the ascitic fluid through the drain sites. Surgical closure of such ascitic fistulae is difficult unless production of ascites is stopped by the use of diuretics.

OTHER PROBLEMS.—There are no other problems peculiar to shunt surgery which need mention here except perhaps for hypersplenism. Many cirrhotics have hypersplenism preoperatively and on occasion (about 20% of patients in our experience) if a shunt is constructed and the spleen left in, exaggerated thrombocytopenia, hemolysis and leukopenia will occur postoperatively. This reaction is almost always transient, subsiding in 7–14 days, and requires no treatment. It is probably the result of increased splenic blood flow following lowering of portal pressure.

PARTIAL HEPATECTOMY

Occasionally in patients with a nonmetastasizing hepatoma or with a single hepatic metastasis from some other resectable primary lesion, it is necessary to remove a portion of the liver. Though this is a formidable surgical procedure, the complications peculiar to the operation are surprisingly few. The most important consideration is that during and immediately after the operation the patient must get substantial amounts of intravenous dextrose, at least 10–15 Gm./hour. In addition, it is wise to monitor the blood sugar every 12 hours for at least the first 3–5 postoperative days. Hypoglycemia (due to the removal of a major glycogen store) is by far the most dangerous early postoperative complication of partial hepatectomy and is almost always preventable. If the right lobe of the liver is resected, hyperbilirubinemia and hypoprothrombinemia may develop as a consequence of the reduced functioning hepatic mass but these will resolve spontaneously. Patients should be watched closely for evidence of blood loss from the large raw surface of liver remaining and for evidence of infection developing in the dead space left by the resected lobe. Therefore, in partial hepatectomy, as well as in trauma to the liver or extrahepatic biliary surgery, it is of utmost importance that *adequate drainage* be established. The large doses of wide spectrum antibiotics given will not be effective unless this therapy is instituted and maintained together with thorough and complete evacuation of blood and bile from about the liver. When the clotting mechanism is normal, bleeding in excess of the expected amount must be recognized promptly and immediate reoperation performed if blood replacement alone is insufficient. Decompression of the extrahepatic biliary tract either by T-tube or by cholecystostomy allows for diagnosis of hemobilia, should it occur. It also serves to vent the biliary system and provide a lower intraductal pressure, thus minimizing the risk of bile peritonitis should there be failure of ligation of all biliary ducts. The T-tube drainage should be maintained for a minimum of 3 weeks and certainly until all sump drains about the liver have ceased to function.

Complications of Surgery for Extrahepatic Obstruction

Oliguria or anuria.—It is important to recognize that, for reasons which are not entirely clear but which may relate to formation of bile casts, oliguria and anuria may occur in surgical patients who have direct serum bilirubin values in excess of 15 mg./100 ml. This was one of the earliest described forms of so-called "hepatorenal" syndrome. It can be prevented by the use of intravenous fluids and mannitol in amounts sufficient to maintain the urine volume in excess of 3,000 ml./day. This fluid push should be started just before surgery and maintained for at least 48 hours after the operation. If this has not been done and the patient has become oliguric, an immediate attempt to induce a water and mannitol diuresis must be made. If the patient is allowed to become anuric, the likelihood of re-establishing urine flow is small and the outcome is usually fatal.

Recurrent obstructive jaundice.—If recurrent obstruction develops after surgery of the common bile duct, the patient will usually complain of right upper quadrant pain and pruritus. Fever and chills will also occur if associated cholangitis is present. The causes of this picture are usually retained stones or ligation or other trauma to the common duct or both hepatic ducts. If the patient has a T-tube in place, the tube should be irrigated to ensure its patency. If this does not relieve the obstruction, a T-tube cholangiogram should be done and will usually indicate the source of the problem. If the T-tube has already been removed or if none was left in at the time of surgery, it will not be possible to localize the obstruction readily and re-exploration must be considered.

As indicated earlier, recurring obstruction is *not* in itself an indication for immediate surgery. Only if the patient has cholangitis which does not respond to antibiotic therapy should one feel forced to reoperate. It is often far better to allow the patient to recover from the effects of the first procedure. Although percutaneous transhepatic cholangiography may be helpful in localizing the obstruction, it should not be done unless one is ready to reoperate because of the particular hazard of a bile leak after puncture of the liver in patients with extrahepatic biliary obstruction.

It should be mentioned that the elevated bilirubin and alkaline phosphatase values characteristic of biliary obstruction will return to normal more slowly in patients who have been obstructed for longer periods. One such patient, who had obstruction and cholangitis for at least 9 months after accidental ligation of her common bile duct, then had the obstruction relieved. The bilirubin and alkaline phosphatase did not reach normal levels until 14 months after corrective surgery. Recurrent obstruction must then be differentiated from slow improvement of hepatic function. The latter situation should not be of concern.

SPIKING FEVER WITH OR WITHOUT CHILLS (ABSCESS FORMATION). – Biliary surgery may be septic because of cholangitis, and patients may have spiking postoperative fever because an abscess develops above, within or below the liver. All 3 kinds of abscess are marked by tenderness in the right upper quadrant. If the abscess is between the liver and the diaphragm, there is often infiltration of the overlying lung, and the right diaphragm may be seen to move poorly or not at all at fluoroscopy. A simultaneous radioisotope scan of liver and lung may show an increased space between these organs and this is the most specific diagnostic procedure in this situation. Intrahepatic abscess may be marked only by fever and a tender liver. The liver is usually enlarged, but in patients with recent biliary surgery liver size is often difficult to assess because of the incision, etc., in the right upper quadrant. Most, but not necessarily all, patients with intrahepatic abscess or abscesses will have a rising or inordinately high alkaline phosphatase activity. If the lesion is larger than 2 cm. in diameter, a radioisotope liver scan may delineate it but a smaller abscess will not produce a defect in a scan. In subhepatic abscess the diaphragm often moves normally, hepatic function tests are not significantly altered and tenderness often extends down into the right midabdomen.

When abscess is suspected, the results of culture and sensitivity studies done on gallbladder or common duct bile at the time of surgery or of subsequent cultures of drainage fluid should be studied and appropriate antibiotic treatment instituted. If no cultures are available or no growth was obtained, then no matter which of the 3 kinds of abscess is present, the infecting organism is likely to be enteric and the treatment of choice is ampicillin or cephalosporin. If the situation is not controlled by antibiotics, re-exploration and drainage may have to be considered.

JAUNDICE, COMA, FEVER AND ELEVATED SGOT.—Patients with this combination of signs have acute hepatic necrosis. As mentioned on page 418, this may be a consequence of surgery and anesthesia unrelated to the specific procedure. The other important cause is hepatic infarction due to accidental hepatic artery ligation. It must be stressed that, if this complication is suspected, early arteriography must be done if a fatal outcome is to be avoided.

26

Peripheral Vascular Surgery*

MARSHALL D. GOLDIN, M.D., M.S.

Fellow in Cardiovascular-Thoracic Surgery, Rush-Presbyterian-St. Luke's Medical Center; Instructor in Surgery, Rush Medical College

AND

JAMES A. HUNTER, M.D.

Attending Surgeon, Rush-Presbyterian-St. Luke's Medical Center; Associate Professor of Surgery, Rush Medical College

Carotid Endarterectomy

INITIAL POSTOPERATIVE EXAMINATION.—Initial postoperative examination includes evaluation of: (1) level of consciousness and motion of the extremities and (2) adequacy of ventilation. Hypotension is occasionally a problem and the usual causes following anesthesia should be considered. An occasional cause peculiar to carotid surgery is described below.

Inspection of the neck and the amount of wound drainage provide a baseline upon which to evaluate postoperative bleeding. The quality of the voice is compared to its preoperative state. Several nerves are vulnerable to injury, and evaluation of these structures is outlined.

The examinations described are performed at regular intervals during the first 24–48 hours.

NEUROLOGIC EXAMINATION.—As the patient awakens, gradual return of consciousness and purposeful motion of the extremities are manifest. Lethargy, coma, deviation of the eyes and tongue toward the operated side, contralateral paralysis or paresis are indications of cerebral damage. Causes include operative ischemia, embolus of air or particulate matter and thrombosis of the operated vessel. The use of a temporary internal shunt ordinarily precludes the likelihood of ischemia. If thrombosis or a large particulate embolus is a consideration,

*Supported in part by United States Public Health Service Grant No. 1T12HE05808.

immediate reoperation and removal of the obstruction may reverse the process. If only a focal deficit is present, reoperation will not be effective; however, gradual improvement of localized lesions is common. Cerebral hemorrhage may occur in a recent area of infarction if revascularization is performed too soon following a stroke. It may be difficult to define the cause of neurologic deficit in a given postoperative patient. Exceptionally, re-exploration of the artery may be necessary to prove vessel patency when the complication is severe.

RESPIRATORY DISTRESS.—Respiratory difficulty following any surgical procedure in the neck area demands immediate attention.

Laryngeal edema.—Laryngeal edema is rare following atraumatic short-term endotracheal intubation.

Pharyngeal obstruction.—Premature extubation is the most common cause of postoperative pharyngeal obstruction. Stroke is a further possibility following carotid artery surgery. Pharyngeal obstruction may be due to injury to the hypoglossal nerves. Denervation of the tongue allows this structure to fall posteriorly and thus obliterate the airway. This problem usually becomes manifest shortly after extubation.

Immediate therapy requires placement of an airway and reintubation. When the patient is fully awake, if removal of the tube is again followed by airway obstruction, tracheostomy is indicated.

Intrinsic laryngeal obstruction.—Laryngeal stridor and obstruction can occur following bilateral abductor vocal cord paralysis. Injury to the innervation of the vocal cords may occur during arteriography, but is more likely to occur as a result of operative trauma to the vagus nerve. Direct laryngoscopy is diagnostic. The treatment is tracheostomy. When the injury is due to edema or hemorrhage, gradual return of function will occur.

Extrinsic laryngeal or tracheal compression.—Extrinsic laryngeal or tracheal compression may be secondary to wound hematoma. Tracheal compression and/or deviation from this cause require reintubation and reoperation. Bleeding from pharyngeal veins occurs under low pressure and rarely results in tracheal compression. Large hematomas are usually caused by arterial bleeding.

HYPOTENSION.—Myocardial infarction should always be considered as a cause of postoperative hypotension.

Hypotension after carotid endarterectomy usually is not secondary to blood loss, since such loss is usually minimal. Treatment includes bed rest in the supine position for 1 to 3 days. Gradual elevation without hypotension can usually be begun on the second or third day. In severe cases, vasopressor support may be required for 1 or 2 days.

HYPERTENSION.—Hypertension occasionally occurs during or immediately following carotid endarterectomy. A significant elevation above the preoperative level requires therapy with hypotensive agents. Rapid control may be achieved by intravenous administration of trimethaphan (Chapter 13).

Examination of the wound.—The size of the neck, tightness of the sutures and respiratory state are all useful parameters to indicate postoperative hemorrhage. Usually drains are employed, but the amount of drainage is neither a constant nor an accurate indication of hemorrhage. Increased tension and swelling most commonly signify this problem and prompt reoperation is mandatory to prevent respiratory obstruction. Careful reintubation should be performed prior to return to the operating suite if the patient is imminently in danger of respiratory obstruction.

Usually the site of hemorrhage is a leaking arterial suture line, but occasionally the pharyngeal venous plexus is implicated. As in all vascular surgery, the incision should never be closed until the anastomosis has been inspected with the patient stable at his or her normal blood pressure.

Nerve injuries.—Several nerves are vulnerable to injury in this area.

Hypoglossal nerve.—This structure innervates the tongue. Injury results in the inability to protrude the tongue. Unilateral injury may cause slurring of speech and difficulty in swallowing. Bilateral injury results in retraction and may cause respiratory obstruction secondary to falling backward and obstruction of the pharynx.

Treatment consists of reintubation in the event of airway obstruction. Once the patient is well awake and careful extubation confirms the diagnosis, tracheostomy should be performed after temporary reinsertion of the endotracheal tube. Gradual return of some function may later allow removal of the tracheostomy.

The cause of injury may be division of the nerve at the upper extent of exposure of the internal carotid artery. Much more commonly, temporary paralysis is secondary to retraction and stretching of the nerve.

Vagus nerve.—This nerve supplies the ipsilateral vocal cord. The voice may be normal if only one cord is out (abductor paralysis). Respiratory obstruction occurs with bilateral paralysis.

If there is unilateral cord paralysis without hoarseness, one can usually wait 6–12 months for function to return. If not, Teflon injection is helpful. Bilateral cord paralysis requires tracheostomy.

This nerve is contained in the carotid sheath. Trauma to the main trunk above the origin of the recurrent laryngeal nerve is probably the most common cause of vocal cord paralysis following carotid surgery. Percutaneous carotid arteriography is a further remote possibility. Direct recurrent nerve trauma is unlikely.

Marginal mandibular nerve.—The marginal mandibular branch of the facial nerve innervates the superficial facial muscles at the angle of the mouth. Drooping of the angle of the mouth occurs with injury to this structure. Gradual return of function usually occurs during the postoperative period but may take weeks to months.

The cause of injury may be retraction at the upper extent of the incision which results in stretching and temporary loss of function. Less commonly the nerve may be severed just before it crosses the angle of the mandible. For this reason, it is wise to make a slight posterior curve at the uppermost aspect of the incision.

Phrenic nerve.—This structure innervates the diaphragm. Injury will result in elevation and paradoxical motion of the diaphragm.

Assisted ventilation and elevation of the head and trunk may be required. This injury may be asymptomatic until discovered on chest x-ray.

The phrenic nerve is located medial to the carotid sheath. It is not exposed during the routine approach. With more extensive procedures, such as carotid subclavian by-pass and radical neck dissection, injury can result in temporary or permanent paralysis of the diaphragm. Injury is suspected clinically upon discovery of compromised ventilation, and diagnosis is confirmed by fluoroscopy.

POSTOPERATIVE ORDERS following carotid endarterectomy

1. Bed rest 24 hours; the patient may sit at bedside the evening of surgery with assistance.
2. Frequent assessment of vital signs, including level of consciousness.
3. Observe neck for change in size or excess drainage.
4. Notify physician immediately of any change in respiratory status.

First postoperative day

1. Drain is removed on the morning following surgery. Ambulation is permitted as tolerated with limited neck motion.
2. Neurologic status is again re-evaluated.
3. Hoarseness, if not present initially, may be now attributed to a reversible process. The usual late causes include laryngeal edema and transient vocal cord paresis.
4. Drooping of the angle of the mouth, when present, is usually manifest immediately after surgery and can be expected to improve if the nerve has not been severed.

Surgery of the Thoracic Aorta

Patients undergoing resection of the thoracic aorta for aneurysm are usually middle-aged or older and have a high incidence of associated diseases. Among the most prevalent are arteriosclerotic involvement of the major vessels, diabetes mellitus, emphysema and cardiac or renal disease. Operative and postoperative complications are largely associated with these diseases and a discussion of each category will be included.

INITIAL EXAMINATION.—Following major resection of the thoracic aorta, a comprehensive examination is essential to uncover early complications which require immediate treatment. Once this examination is complete, attention is directed toward repeated surveillance to expedite discovery of adverse changes in the patient's condition.

Vital signs are measured immediately upon arrival at the intensive care unit. Appropriate treatment is guided by evaluation of adequacy of ventilation and blood volume replacement by the usual parameters. Myocardial infarction may occur in this group and postoperative electrocardiographic changes and arrhythmias may indicate the presence of such a process.

Neurologic examination is divided into 2 categories; the first consists of evaluation of the brain, while the second includes evaluation of the spinal cord. Early examination consists of ascertaining the level of awareness and motion of the extremities.

The pattern of urine flow is usually established during surgery. Oliguria cannot be tolerated by these patients and great emphasis must be placed on maintenance of adequate urinary output and immediate treatment should the volume fall below a minimum of 30–50 ml./hour.

Peripheral pulses are examined and the presence and the quality recorded as in other vascular procedures. Vessels may be occluded by debris, thrombosis or technical defects. Particular attention must be accorded the carotid vessels in this group.

Postoperative hemorrhage almost always occurs during the first 24 hours and is usually manifest during or shortly after surgery. Rapid accumulation of blood in the chest drainage apparatus or pleural cavities is indicative of postoperative hemorrhage. Most commonly the cause is inadequate hemostasis in the operative site. Coagulation defects, however, do occur with a significant degree of frequency following reconstruction of the thoracic aorta.

Most patients require continued ventilatory assistance for hours to days. For this reason the endotracheal tube is left in place and serves as a route for ventilation and tracheal toilet. A common factor causing difficulty in the immediate postoperative period is decreased compliance secondary to emphysema. Much less common is endobronchial hemorrhage originating from the lung parenchyma as a consequence of pulmonary trauma occurring incidental to aortic resection in an anticoagulated patient.

Postoperative Complications—Recognition and Management

Cardiac complications.—Cardiac complications are frequent during and after aortic resection. There is a high incidence of coronary artery disease in this patient group. Manipulation of the heart, cross-clamping of the aorta, disturbed acid-base balance and cardiopulmonary by-pass all have adverse effects on the heart.

Manipulation impairs venous return and can stimulate arrhythmias. Cross-clamping and cardiopulmonary by-pass both impair cardiac output and coronary filling; ventricular dilatation and myocardial ischemia may result. Further impairment to venous return may occur from tension hemothorax.

Congestive heart failure may have an insidious onset and progress to pulmonary edema in the early postoperative period. Increased venous pressure, tachypnea, blood-tinged frothy tracheal aspirate and decreased compliance are indicators of this complication. Early recognition and treatment with fluid restriction, diuretic therapy and digitalization are essential. Massive failure requires phlebotomy. Positive pressure ventilation is a helpful adjunct.

NEUROLOGIC COMPLICATIONS.—Neurologic complications may be divided into central (cerebral) and peripheral (spinal) categories.

Central defects.—Central neurologic defects include coma, hemiparesis, hemiplegia, focal disturbances and psychosis. The mechanism of injury and the degree of neurologic deficit are helpful in predicting the likelihood of recovery.

In general coma denotes a diffuse process, but if the patient responds to stimuli, the prognosis is good. Deep coma persisting for longer than 24–48 hours is usually associated with a poor prognosis. Focal deficits usually exhibit gradual improvement and may remit entirely. Deep coma with a focal deficit signifies severe cerebral damage.

Focal lesions are caused by particulate emboli, thrombosis or hemorrhage. It is never possible to define the prognosis of patients with neurologic complications totally and, because of this, intensive supportive care and optimism must be maintained. Emboli consist of air, debris or clots. Air may enter the vascular system at one of several points. Thrombosis occurs secondary to stenotic vessels or inadequate cerebral perfusion. Fragile vessels and/or excessive perfusion pressure predispose to focal hemorrhage. Diffuse deficits are caused by cerebral ischemia or emboli. Arteriosclerotic narrowing or involvement of cerebral vessels by the dissecting aneurysm, poor oxygenation and temporary cross-clamping are causes of cerebral ischemia.

A comprehensive neurologic examination is performed after surgery and at regular intervals thereafter. Sudden appearance of a focal deficit (hemiplegia, hemiparesis) in a formerly neurologically sound patient should give rise to the suspicion of occlusion of the extracranial carotid system. Preoperative evaluation usually uncovers stenotic lesions in this area. Other causes include emboli and extension of the aortic dissection. If discovered early, all of these processes may be amenable to local surgical treatment.

In those patients exhibiting a generalized neurologic deficit, the administration of steroids (dexamethasone, 8 mg. intramuscularly every 8 hours) is useful to decrease the effects of cerebral edema. When a volume overload is present, rapid diuresis with osmotic or metabolic agents is indicated. Fluid and salt restriction are carried out as in the usual postoperative by-pass patient, but in a more stringent fashion when steroids are used. Mild total body hypothermia (32–34 C.) serves to diminish the metabolic demand of the central nervous system and is a helpful adjunct in such cases.

Peripheral defects.—Acute interruption of the blood supply to the spinal cord results in an immediate deficit which is manifest following anesthesia. Motion and sensation of the lower extremities are imparied and progressive deterioration is often the case. In those patients with severe ischemic damage, spinal shock occurs and is best treated with the patient in the supine position. Vasopressors and volume replacement may be indicated to reverse the sequelae of peripheral vasodilatation and expanded vascular bed. In contrast to central lesions, peripheral lesions may not be manifest until the second or third postoperative day. In gradual thrombosis of segmental or collateral vessels, hours to days are required for the deficit to become apparent. Spinal cord injury may be reversible with amelioration of the lower extremity neurologic deficit.

Patients with spinal cord lesions require local attention to several areas. Loss of visceral innervation requires prolonged gastrointestinal and genitourinary intubation. Loss of somatic sensory and motor innervation requires meticulous skin care and muscle re-education. Decubitus ulcers are more prone to develop in those with impaired innervation.

Renal complications.—Adequate urinary output is an important parameter in following the renal status of the patient. There is a high incidence of pre-existing renovascular disease in this group of patients. Consequently, insults which may be tolerated by the normal kidney assume major importance under such conditions.

Osmotic diuretics are routinely used during surgery and also in the postoperative period as an indicator of renal integrity. In case of oliguria unresponsive to a trial of mannitol (25 Gm.) and ethacrynic acid (200 mg.), the diagnosis of acute renal failure is made.

The etiology of the failure assumes major significance in regard to treatment and the prospect of survival. Hypovolemia should be first considered, since it is readily diagnosed and easily treated. Low urinary volume, low venous pressure and high specific gravity bespeak hypovolemia. Similarly, a response to ethacrynic acid and mannitol indicates either hypovolemia or a successful therapeutic result from this diagnostic regimen in the marginal kidney. In the latter instance, all efforts should be directed toward maintenance of flow. (See Chapter 0.)

Renal arterial obstruction may be due to aortic dissection, thrombosis or emboli. Early detection (intravenous pyelography, angiography, isotope renogram) and repair will permit salvage of some of this group. Parenchymal causes include tubular necrosis secondary to ischemia or hemolytic transfusion reaction.

Once the diagnosis has been established, regulation of fluid and electrolyte balance requires meticulous attention. Often urinary output gradually improves over 2 or 3 days, during which a progressive elevation of the BUN necessarily occurs. After this rise the level remains stable for several days, later gradually returning to the preoperative level.

Hemodialysis is the preferred method for the treatment of acute renal failure or the complications thereof. In almost all situations a temporary dialysis shunt can be inserted under local anesthesia and hemodialysis begun within several hours. Regional heparinization is extremely useful in the early postoperative period or in those with bleeding diatheses. (See Chapter 9.)

PERIPHERAL VASCULAR OCCLUSION.—Thrombotic and embolic occlusions rarely occur following surgery of the thoracic aorta. In cases of dissecting aneurysm, extension of the process to cause a peripheral visceral obstruction is an additional hazard. The presence of pre-existent arteriosclerotic narrowing predisposes to thrombosis or embolic occlusion at these points.

Fragments of intima and thrombi adherent to the inner wall of a vessel or the endocardium are prone to embolize and obstruct at a distal site. Large emboli inevitably lodge at points of major divisions or bifurcations.

Carotid occlusion is manifest by appropriate neurologic deficits and is usually confirmed by clinical examination. An enlarged vessel with a transmitted pulsation is suggestive of dissection while a normal-sized vessel with an exaggerated pulse usually signifies an obstruction distal to that site. Similar clinical findings apply to the extremities and are most easily discerned in the femoral and axillary locations. An occlusion proximal to the site being examined ordinarily causes obliteration of all pulses distal to that level. Visceral occlusions present with prolonged ileus, pain and abdominal distention. The manifestations of renal arterial occlusions are described in the appropriate section.

The site, extent and often the mechanisms of occlusion of visceral vessels are suspected by clinical examination and confirmed by arteriography (renal, celiac, superior and inferior mesenteric arteries). Intravenous pyelography is helpful in indirectly evaluating the renal vessels. Local surgical treatment is performed to revascularize the compromised organ or extremity. Regional or local anesthesia is preferred in most instances. In those cases in which the blood supply to an extremity is marginal but the limb is viable, a temporary delay is reasonable to allow the patient's condition to improve prior to another operative procedure.

POSTOPERATIVE HEMORRHAGE.—Hemorrhage following surgical repair of the thoracic aorta can be divided into 2 categories. Mechanical defects of hemostasis comprise the majority, while the remainder consist of hematologic defects.

In general, a high index of suspicion may be derived during the intraoperative period. Hematologic defects are usually manifest during surgery and may be related to a deficiency of normal clotting factors or to derangement of these factors resulting from operative trauma. Following surgery, inadequate neutralization of heparin or excessive protaminization are additional causes to consider (Chapter 8). Mechanical causes may be suspected when there is a widely exposed mediastinal surface with many potential sites of hemorrhage. Bleeding from the wall of the aneurysm or back-bleeding from intercostal vessels following resection of the descending aorta is not uncommon. Other sites include leaking needle holes in the graft or adjacent aorta and suture line defects.

In the presence of significant postoperative hemorrhage, when mechanical factors are suspect, early reoperation is indicated. If hematologic defects are discovered, appropriate treatment is instituted.

There remains a group of patients in whom neither cause is obvious. Should replacement transfusion and appropriate therapy of likely coagulation defects prove ineffective, we believe that this group should also be re-explored. It is felt that continued nonoperative therapy will most probably have a fatal outcome, whereas exploration and discovery of a significant bleeding site will result in the salvage of some patients in this group. The presence of hemothorax with mediastinal shift is another indication for repeat thoractomy.

RESPIRATORY COMPLICATIONS.—Among the most prominent postoperative pulmonary complications are hemothorax and atelectasis. The former is due in large part to the mediastinal dissection. Incision into pulmonary parenchyma and liberation of pulmonary fibrinolysins further contribute potential sites of hemorrhage. Atelectasis is usually secondary to incisional pain, splinting and failure to cough, but may be related to extrinsic tracheobronchial compression and resultant loss of normal contour.

Significant hemothorax and atelectasis impair ventilation and predispose to infection. When chest tubes do not provide adequate drainage, thoracentesis, additional tubes or reoperation must be considered. Nasotracheal aspiration is frequently required. Refractory lobar atelectasis or total atelectasis of an entire lung are absolute indications for bronchoscopy in such patients. Persistent inability to clear secretions, persistent atelectasis and brain damage constitute indications for tracheostomy. In most cases in this category the volume respirator is the only means whereby adequate ventilation and oxygenation of boggy, traumatized lungs can be achieved. It is not unusual for such patients to require assistance for prolonged periods.

Stretching or distortion of the left recurrent nerve by the pathologic lesion can cause left vocal cord paralysis prior to surgery. Operative dissection may also result in injury to this structure. Injury to the thoracic duct is also related to the procedure and is a further cause of pleural fluid accumulation. Therapy is discussed elsewhere in this chapter.

Division of Patent Ductus Arteriosus

The course following operation for patent ductus arteriosus is in most cases predictable. Possible complications will be discussed.

HEMORRHAGE.—Hemorrhage may occur in the immediate postoperative period and is manifest as hemothorax or mediastinal hematoma. Hemothorax is due to bleeding from the chest wall in the majority of cases. Rarely a slow leak from the aortic or pulmonary artery suture line will result in a mediastinal hematoma at the upper left heart border.

The presence of an accumulation of blood within the thoracic cavity increases the risk of infection, impairs ventilation and may be an indication of continued bleeding. If a significant amount of blood is present and does not drain through the chest tube, reoperation is indicated.

NERVE INJURY.—Operative trauma to the recurrent branch of the *vagus nerve* is manifest as temporary or permanent paralysis of the left vocal cord. Unilateral injury to the main trunk of the vagus nerve below the origin of the recurrent branch is rarely evident unless the contralateral nerve is injured at a later time.

If the vocal cord paralysis interferes with the cough mechanism, a glycerin injection will provide temporary relief and permit further assessment of cord function at a later time.

Operative injury to the *phrenic nerve* results in ipsilateral paralysis and elevation of the diaphragm. On fluoroscopic examination the diaphragm does not move with respiration.

INFECTION.—Infection of the pleural space is rare following elective division of a patent ductus. In those cases in which ligation without division has been performed, there is an increased risk of infection and recanalization.

CONGESTIVE HEART FAILURE.—Congestive heart failure is an uncommon occurrence following the routine patent ductus repair. However, as the pulmonary vascular resistance and pressure increase, reversal of the shunt takes place. Surgical interruption of the ductus in this situation may result in an excessive load on the right ventricle and cause right-sided failure.

Repair of Coarctation

INITIAL EXAMINATION.—The initial examination, in addition to the usual parameters, includes particular attention to the peripheral pulses, chest drainage and the neurologic examination.

Distal pulses. In most cases the distal pulses will have been diminished or entirely absent prior to surgery. Restoration of the pulses to normal is the immediate objective of surgery. However, the rapid increase in perfusion pressure may result in visceral vasoconstriction, a complication which becomes manifest later in the postoperative period (see below).

Hemorrhage.—Bleeding may occur from one of several sites. Some degree of hypertension frequently persists for hours to days and increases the likelihood of bleeding from the aortic suture line or recently divided chest wall collaterals and intercostal vessels. Extrapleural hematoma occurs with somewhat greater frequency in this group due to the chest wall collaterals. Hemothorax from intercostal artery bleeding due to injury by the pericostal closure sutures can occur. Particular care needs to be exercised in thoracotomy closure and the stitches should be inspected after placement.

Cerebral examination.—Hypertension with or without the common association of congenital berry aneurysm is a common cause of stroke in this group. Acute elevations of pressure in the brachiocephalic system during aortic cross-clamping may result in cerebral hemorrhage. Postoperative elevations in significant excess of preoperative levels require temporary lowering to safer levels. Gradual stabilization of the blood pressure will occur over 2–10 days' time.

Spinal cord examination.—In general, cross-clamping of the aorta just above and below the coarctation does not significantly affect the collateral circulation. For this reason, in contradistinction to aneurysms of the thoracic aorta, constrictive lesions are associated with a more ample distal collateral circulation, the congenital types having the most fully developed supply. Only in those cases in which significant collateral vessels are temporarily cross-clamped is spinal cord ischemia a possibility. Exceptionally a mild coarctation may be seen with negligible collateral development.

Later Complications

Thoracic duct fistula.—The presence of milky white drainage from the chest is indicative of injury to the thoracic duct. In most cases this complication may be suspected within the first 24 hours and is confirmed as the character becomes definitely milky white, separates into 2 layers upon standing and increases in volume after meals.

Treatment is conservative; the fistula usually closes during the first week. If the drainage persists without evidence of slowing, the patient's nutritional state is certain to deteriorate. Maintenance of nutrition and surgical ligation of the thoracic duct are indicated at this time.

Postcoarctation syndrome.—Abdominal pain, ileus and distention occur between the second and fourth postoperative days in 5–10% of patients following coarctation repair. This syndrome is secondary to exposure of the visceral arterial system to an increased pulse pressure and arterial flow, which causes vasospasm and intimal damage. Severe forms of the syndrome may result in intestinal ischemia and infarction. Milder forms may simply cause abdominal pain. Symptomatic therapy is adequate in the majority of patients, but in some abdominal exploration is required. Prevention of excessive postoperative hypertension may decrease the incidence of this complication in the small group of patients with paradoxical blood pressure elevation.

Surgery of the Abdominal Aorta

Examination of the patient following major abdominal vascular surgery (bifurcation graft, renal artery, mesenteric revascularization) requires a comprehensive approach. It is most efficient to examine the patient by organ system, once the initial examination has covered the vital functions and the area of surgical therapy.

INITIAL EXAMINATION.—*Ventilation.*—Estimate adequacy of rate and depth of respiration. If ventilation is inadequate due to lethargy, pain or obesity, treat the primary cause if possible, but do not hesitate to institute mechanical ventilation (assisted or controlled, as indicated) to prevent acute respiratory insufficiency.

Blood pressure.—Hypotension is particularly dangerous in the patient with narrowed coronary, cerebral and renal vessels who has a new vascular prosthesis.

Large and rapid volume shifts occur during the operative period. Hypovolemia is the most common early cause of hypotension following major vascular surgery. When the venous pressure is elevated or perhaps even normal, the next most common cause, myocardial infarction, should be considered. Myocardial infarction is the commonest cause of postoperative death after abdominal aortic resection.

Long-term antihypertensive and diuretic therapy deplete catecholamines and electrolytes, respectively. Hypertensive patients, particularly those having renal artery reconstruction, may develop hypotension on the above basis. Prior knowledge of antihypertensive medications facilitates treatment with catecholamines and appropriate electrolytes when the cause of hypotension becomes evident. It is best to discontinue the antihypertensive medications at least 2 weeks prior to elective surgery.

Heart rate.—Hypovolemia and myocardial infarction may affect the heart rate in a similar fashion, thus serving to indicate a state which requires diagnosis and attention.

Peripheral vascular examination.—Note color, temperature and sensation of extremities. Note presence and quality of peripheral pulses and compare with preoperative findings and immediate postoperative results. Pedal pulses are marked with a ballpoint pen by the house staff for later comparison.

Urine volume.—Obtain the anesthesia record to determine the volume during surgery. Refer to the patient's preoperative record to determine presence of pre-existing renal impairment. A minimum of 30–60 ml./hour is necessary to ensure reasonable confidence that RBF is adequate. Specific gravity is an excellent parameter of accuracy of volume replacement if osmotic diuretics have not been used.

Nasogastric tube.—Check position and patency of the nasogastric tube and the function of suction apparatus. If nasal O_2 is used, mark the 2 catheters respectively to avoid the rare but disastrous complication of gastric inflation.

Diagnosis of arterial occlusion.—The color and temperature of the extremities and quality of the pulses should be noted and recorded at regular intervals.

The diagnosis of arterial occlusion is made upon discovering the absence of a previously present pulse. The patient will complain of ischemic pain. The first objective signs include impairment or loss of cutaneous sensation. The extremity becomes pale. Later a faint cyanosis ensues. Muscular weakness is first manifest as decreased force on motion of the first toe against resistance. Gradually muscular swelling occurs. This is an ominous sign, indicating that irreversible muscle damage is soon to occur. The temperature gradually decreases as blood flow is impaired. Comparison of the extremities during postoperative examinations is essential to detect the early changes of vascular occlusion and to facilitate therapy.

Obliteration of previously present pulses following surgery signifies thrombosis of a distal artery or graft and may be related to several factors, some of which are reversible. Occlusion of the iliac vessels results in loss of sensation and pale color above the knee. Occlusion at the level of the superficial femoral artery results in similar findings at the midcalf, while popliteal occlusion causes a change just above the ankle. The results of occlusion are variable and depend on the extent of clot propagation and the presence of collaterals.

Inadequate distal run-off can be suspected on the preoperative arteriogram. In some cases this decision is difficult and can only be made at surgery or even in retrospect after other causes of occlusion have been excluded.

Technical failure may take several forms. Kinking of a long graft, discrepancy of size, distal emboli and improper suturing are all technical factors which contribute to thrombosis, intimal dissection and subsequent occlusion. Immediate arterial occlusion usually results during surgery; however, gradual thrombosis may occur following partial occlusion. Transient hypotension can result in stasis and thrombosis of vessels and occurs more readily in recently operated areas.

Postoperative Complications

Gastrointestinal tract.—Adynamic ileus always occurs following operation on the abdominal aorta. Nasogastric decompression to prevent abdominal distention is desirable for a minimum of 3 days and may be required for longer periods. Occasional bowel sounds detected prior to the third postoperative day should not prompt alimentation, since these are almost always ineffective; further ileus and distention are usually inevitable. For these reasons, nasogastric decompression is maintained for 3 or usually 4 days. Tube testing is performed at the end of this period and the patient is then allowed to begin an oral diet.

The degree of postoperative ileus is directly related to the extent of dissection, the primary disease and additional procedures. Those patients with severe disease requiring prolonged and difficult dissection will usually have a longer ileus. Ruptured abdominal aneurysm characteristically causes ileus for 4–7 days because of the large retroperitoneal hematoma. Lumbar sympathectomy may prolong the ileus 1–2 days.

Prolonged ileus, particularly when associated with abdominal tenderness and distention, raises the suspicion of surgical complications. Often the distention occurs with few additional objective findings, since the pain medications are probably still being given.

On occasion, other causes of prolonged ileus and abdominal pain must be considered. Those to review include the following: (1) hemorrhage and retroperitoneal hematoma, (2) bowel obstruction, (3) rectosigmoid necrosis, (4) intestinal ischemia, (5) pancreatitis, (6) cholecystitis and (7) diverticulitis.

Hemorrhage and retroperitoneal hematoma.—Retroperitoneal hematoma is the most common cause of ileus following aortoiliac surgery. Postoperative hemorrhage should be suspected when continued transfusions are required to maintain the systemic and central venous pressures. Abdominal distention and tenderness are further signs, but a considerable volume of blood can be sequestered in the abdomen before significant changes occur. Intra-abdominal hemorrhage is usually limited to the immediate postoperative period (24 hours), while gastrointestinal hemorrhage usually does not begin until 3–4 days following major abdominal surgery. Gastroduodenal ulcers of this type characteristically bleed or perforate near the end of the first week.

Bowel obstruction.—Adhesive bowel obstruction most commonly occurs 7–12 days postoperatively. Gastrointestinal decompression, preferably with a long tube, is effective in relieving the majority of these obstructions. Wound dehiscence must also be considered at this time. In those obstructions which do not remit within 48–72 hours or which show signs of worsening, or when there is evidence of developing peritonitis, re-exploration is indicated.

Colon necrosis.—Rectosigmoid ischemia is an uncommon complication of abdominal aortic surgery. Blood supply to this area may be compromised following aortoiliac resection, particularly if the internal iliac arteries are occluded and a patent inferior mesenteric artery has been ligated. If there is superior mesenteric artery insufficiency, the complication is even more likely. Abdominal pain and tenderness (out of proportion to that expected in the usual postoperative abdomen) may become manifest shortly after surgery but can be delayed for several days if marginal collaterals retard ischemic necrosis. Abdominal rigidity should never be present following elective abdominal surgery and is a cause for immediate investigation. The diagnosis of rectosigmoid ischemia is made by proctoscopy. Early the mucosa is pale or white; later bluish black discoloration occurs. Sigmoid necrosis requires colostomy or, in rare cases, abdominoperineal resection.

Intestinal ischemia.—Stenosis of visceral vessels may be asymptomatic and therefore unsuspected until bowel ischemia becomes manifest in the postoperative period. Hypotension may result in thrombosis of a previously stenotic lesion. Intestinal ischemia may occur at any time following operation.

Pancreatitis.—Traumatic pancreatitis secondary to upward retraction of the viscera is an uncommon cause of ileus following surgery of the aorta. This usually causes diffuse abdominal tenderness, prolonged ileus and signs of hypovolemia. Most commonly the diagnosis is made by those having a high index of suspicion and is confirmed by serum and urinary amylase determinations. Pancreatitis presents from 24 to 96 hours after surgery.

Cholecystitis.—Biliary tract disease is common after age sixty. Cholelithiasis may lead to acute biliary obstruction during the postoperative period. As in all postoperative patients, the indication for pain medication should be reviewed frequently and care taken to avoid the administration of medication which might mask symptoms of an intraperitoneal complication. Biliary obstruction can occur at any time during or after hospitalization.

Diverticulitis.—Diverticulosis is also very common after sixty. Diverticulitis may have an insidious onset and progress to localized or generalized peritonitis within a short time. Fever associated with left lower quadrant abdominal pain and tenderness are the usual presenting signs and symptoms.

Postoperative hemorrhage.—In the great majority of cases postoperative hemorrhage following surgery of the abdominal aorta is secondary to inadequate hemostasis. There are many sites from which intra-abdominal bleeding may occur following abdominal aortic surgery. Bleeding from the suture line occurs when the sutures are too far apart or fail to include all layers, and from needle holes in thin-walled vessels (particularly after endarterectomy). Bleeding may also occur through the wall of the graft (more commonly with the knitted than with the woven types). Injury to the iliac veins may occur during the dissection and cause considerable difficulty postoperatively with slow but persistent oozing. The bed of the graft, in addition to the adjacent lumbar arteries and veins, serves as another potential site. Through-and-through retention sutures, commonly used in ruptured aneurysms, may lacerate the deep epigastric vessels and cause abdominal wall hematoma or intra-abdominal bleeding. Administration of excessive doses of heparin during aortic repair is uncommon. Neutralization with protamine is usually not required. In the face of postoperative bleeding, if reversal of heparin has not been performed, one-half the usual dose of protamine is given slowly by the intravenous route. The equivalent is 10 mg. protamine/1,000 units of heparin.

Postoperative gastrointestinal hemorrhage is due to stress or peptic ulcer until proved otherwise. On occasion, after age sixty, diverticulitis may present as lower gastrointestinal bleeding. Aortoenteric fistula does not occur in the immediate postoperative period. Rarely is this condition manifest under 6–12 months following surgery.

RESPIRATORY COMPLICATIONS.—Respiratory complications are common following major abdominal vascular surgery. Contributing factors include emphysema, obesity and bronchitis, particularly prominent in smokers. The length of the incision and resultant pain further hinder ventilation.

There are several methods by which postoperative ventilation may be improved. Deep-breathing exercises and intermittent positive pressure ventilation serve to combat hypoventilation and associated dependent congestion and atelectasis. Gastrointestinal decompression prevents elevation of the diaphragm; however, the indwelling tube may in itself impair breathing, coughing and expectoration of secretions.

In patients with marginal pulmonary function, tube gastrostomy serves to circumvent some of the above complications. Inadequate humidification of inhalation therapy treatments dehydrates the tracheobronchial mucosa. Proper attention to respiratory care will prevent the majority of complications associated with this operation. (See Chapter 4.)

GENITOURINARY SYSTEM COMPLICATIONS.—Urine volume is the best parameter of renal blood flow and the state of hydration of the postoperative patient. Several causes of oliguria following aortoiliac surgery must be considered. Appropriate therapy must be instituted prior to progression to an irreversible state. The diagnosis and treatment of hypovolemia has been outlined. The remaining causes of oliguria are related primarily to local problems.

Direct injuries to the ureter include ligation and division, which result in peritonitis, diffuse pain and abdominal distention, usually manifest during the first 24–48 hours. Prolonged cross-clamping of the renal arteries, particularly in those with impaired renal function, may produce enough ischemia to cause renal failure. Cross-clamping below the renal arteries can also result in reflex arteriolar spasm and similar complications. Obstruction to the renal arteries can be caused by thrombosis (usually in already narrow vessels), intimal dissection and emboli, all related to cross-clamping and manipulation of the aorta and renal arteries.

Adequate preoperative and intraoperative hydration helps to maintain renal blood flow. This is especially important in those with some degree of renal impairment and those undergoing vascular reconstruction. Minimal operative ischemia and osmotic diuresis further aid in preservation of kidney function.

All patients require an indwelling catheter. On occasion, the orifices may become obstructed, the tube kinked or a defect in manufacture become apparent. In appropriate cases, replacement of the catheter will remedy the situation.

Urine volume and specific gravity are measured every 2 hours for the first 24 hours, every 4 hours for 48 hours, and then at less frequent intervals. Removal of the catheter should be performed just after return of gastrointestinal function (3–5 days). In general, however, older male patients usually require slightly longer periods of catheterization, undoubtedly related to the size of the prostate in this age group.

A routine urinalysis should be obtained just prior to catheter removal and appropriate treatment instituted as indicated. Careful attention should be accorded this area; urinary tract infection is relatively common following prolonged catheterization and may be a major source of morbidity.

POSTOPERATIVE ORDERS following surgery of abdominal aorta

1. Vital signs every 15 minutes until stable, then hourly.
2. Examine and record quality of foot pulses; also record color, temperature and sensation of extremities with vital signs.
3. Pain medication.
4. Intake and output.
5. Foley catheter to free drainage.
6. Urine volume and specific gravity every 2 hours for 24 hours, then every 4 hours.
7. Nasogastric tube to low Gomco suction.
8. Irrigate nasogastric tube with 30 ml. water or saline every 2 hours and aspirate gently.
9. Turn, cough and hyperventilate every 2 hours.
10. Assist patient to dangle at bedside with feet on chair 4 times a day as tolerated if graft does not cross groin.
11. Intravenous fluids: total of 2,500 to 3,000 ml. in 24 hours in average-sized patient. Total volume and electrolyte concentration modified by urine volume and specific gravity and volume of nasogastric aspirate.
12. Complete blood count and urinalysis evening of and morning following surgery.
13. Electrocardiogram as indicated.
14. Electrolytes second and fourth postoperative days and as indicated.

15. High humidity tent, IPPB as indicated.
16. Chest x-ray as indicated.
17. Continue preoperative antibiotics for 7 days (when used).

HYPOTENSION.—As considered above, hypotension occurring early in the postoperative period is usually secondary to hypovolemia from inadequate volume replacement or persistent hemorrhage. Myocardial infarction may occur during surgery or any time in the postoperative period and is the major cause of mortality in this group. The central venous pressure and electrocardiogram aid in diagnosis of these complications. The presence of chest pain is an important positive finding, but its absence is of no diagnostic significance.

Several abdominal complications which produce hypotension within the first 1–3 days include rectosigmoid or small intestinal ischemia, pancreatitis and urinary extravasation. Each is discussed in appropriate sections. Emphasis must be placed on early and appropriate treatment of hypotension; patients with narrowed cerebral, coronary and visceral vessels cannot tolerate even short periods of reduced flow.

GENERAL CONSIDERATIONS IN POSTOPERATIVE CARE

Numerous aspects of care in the patient who has had aortoiliac surgery require particular consideration. All are related to local factors.

In cases in which the prosthesis crosses a joint, the patient must not acutely flex this area for 3–5 days. At the end of this time gradual flexion is allowed, but the patient is cautioned to refrain from prolonged acute angulation of the joint and to assume a slouching position when seated. These restrictions should not retard the usual postoperative position changes and ambulation. Indeed, sitting at the bedside with assistance should be instituted as soon as tolerated.

Positions which favor venous stasis should be avoided. Venous stasis is especially hazardous in those with pre-existing venous insufficiency. As in all hospitalized patients, the patient's legs should not be permitted to hang over the bed rail or lie flat on the floor. A chair or footstool under the feet affords support and promotes drainage. As the patient progresses from bed rest, he should be encouraged to ambulate and then return to bed, avoiding more than brief chair sitting. Deep thrombophlebitis often follows prolonged periods in a position not conducive to venous return. Diagnosis and therapy of this problem is outlined elsewhere in this chapter.

Prophylactic elastic stockings or bandages may decrease venous stasis and its associated complications. Elastic stockings must fit precisely, while bandages require frequent rewrapping to be effective. Ill-fitting stockings or wrappings may be too tight and cause distal edema or ischemic pain. A further problem is skin necrosis, particularly in patients with vascular insufficiency. The necrosis characteristically occurs beneath the wrinkles of the fabric.

In general, elastic support is not recommended on a prophylactic basis. Prevention of venous stasis is best accomplished by mild elevation of the foot of the bed and minimizing the amount of time the patient sits in a chair.

Of further importance is prevention of decubitus ulcers and skin burns of the heels and elbows. These lesions are particularly prone to occur in thin patients and those with vascular insufficiency. Frequent changes of position and elevation of the heels with a soft bath blanket placed under the calves and moleskin patches are helpful measures.

On occasion following revascularization, reflex arteriolar dilatation results in erythematous engorgement of the leg. This characteristically occurs directly after surgery and remits within 24 hours. It may be differentiated from acute arterial occlusion by persistence of pulses, warmth, hyperesthesia (but no ischemic pain) and lack of sensory deficit. Acute venous occlusion (ileofemoral thrombosis) results in a mottled, bluish white leg; ordinarily it involves the entire extremity. Initially, and unless it progresses to a severe degree, the pulses are not affected.

On the other hand, sympathectomy may produce paradoxical transient arteriolar spasm, resulting in a temporarily pale, cool extremity without other signs of ischemia. This is an uncommon event.

A broad-spectrum antibiotic is begun on the day prior to surgery and is continued for 7 days postoperatively. In this way adequate levels are present during that period when the patient is exposed to the maximum risk of contamination.

Femoral Popliteal Reconstruction

In general, examination of the extremity should parallel that outlined for aortoiliac reconstruction. Properly performed reconstruction in addition to adequate inflow and distal run-off are prerequisites for success. In those with marginal run-off, lumbar sympathectomy may be performed to provide additional cutaneous flow.

Early local complications include thrombosis of the operated segments and hemorrhage in the wound. Thrombosis is related to inadequate flow (inflow or outflow) or technical difficulties (intimal dissection, distal emboli or disparity in size of the graft and artery). Hemorrhage is caused by a leaking suture line, inadequate hemostasis or premature anticoagulation.

A later complication is lymphatic obstruction. This lesion usually occurs 2–7 days after surgery and is manifest as a diffuse swelling from the toes to the knee. The pulse is not affected, the leg remains warm and improvement usually follows bed rest and elevation. Obstruction of the popliteal vein causes erythema, heat and swelling. Treatment includes bed rest, elevation and heparin.

There is some tendency to distal extremity swelling in all patients with femoral popliteal reconstruction. This usually lasts 4–6 weeks and is treated by avoidance of prolonged dependency (for example, sitting) and, in the occasional more severe case, by elastic support.

Thrombophlebitis

Thrombophlebitis varies in severity from a benign superficial process (superficial phlebitis) requiring only supportive treatment to a deep process (deep phlebitis) which may cause pain, tenderness or mild or marked edema and serves as a source of pulmonary emboli. More profound involvement (phlegmasia alba dolens) begins with sudden onset of diffuse swelling and tenderness of the extremity. Initial pallor may be followed by bluish mottling, extensive edema and arterial spasm (phlegmasia cerulea dolens). Division into 2 categories is helpful.

SUPERFICIAL THROMBOPHLEBITIS.—This is characterized by throbbing pain, localized superficial swelling, erythema and increased local warmth. A tender cordlike structure may be palpated beneath the skin. Differential diagnosis includes: (1) lymphangitis, which is associated with regional adenopathy and linear inflammation, and (2) localized cellulitis, in which a break in the skin is usually evident. Furthermore, cellulitis causes diffuse edema while the edema of superficial thrombophlebitis assumes a localized distribution.

Usual sites include those of prior involvement, local trauma and varicosities; most commonly it follows intravenous cannulation for infusion. Distal edema does not occur in relation to superficial thrombophlebitis.

Treatment includes local heat, analgesics and elastic support, in addition to mobilization as soon as pain permits. Heat is most easily applied in the form of a heating pad (low heat). Warm, moist packs tend to cool rapidly and macerate the skin. In those in whom pain is severe or impairs mobilization, Butazolidin, 100 mg. 3 times a day, is useful.

DEEP THROMBOPHLEBITIS.—Deep thrombophlebitis involving the calf veins is characterized by a sensation of fullness of the calf and pain during motion of the extremity. There is tenderness of the calf, pain on dorsiflexion of the ankle (Homan's sign), increased warmth and bogginess to palpation. Mild edema of the foot and ankle and superficial venous distention of the leg may be associated with this type of deep thrombophlebitis. The lack of significant edema serves to emphasize that minimal impairment of deep venous outflow is present.

Differential diagnosis includes severe cellulitis, but well-localized swelling, prominent superficial tenderness and systemic manifestations serve to differentiate cellulitis from the more deep-seated process.

Deep calf phlebitis is a major cause of pulmonary embolism. The inflammation at the initial site of thrombosis serves to provide a secure attachment to the intima of the vein. Embolization rarely occurs from this site. Instead, fragmentation of the distally propagated clot within the lumen serves as a source of emboli.

Treatment is directed toward preventing propagation of the clot by anticoagulation, preferably with heparin. Elastic support and elevation serve to increase venous flow through the deep veins and to prevent stasis. Elevation is achieved best by avoiding bends in the mattress and placing blocks under the foot of the bed. Bed rest should be continued until all pain and swelling have disappeared. Then ambulation is begun and gradually increased.

Deep thrombophlebitis involving the ileofemoral system is characterized by diffuse edema from the toes to the groin with tenderness over the femoral canal. The onset of swelling is usually sudden and follows an acute episode of throbbing pain in the extremity. The swelling often progresses to a massive state within several hours. The involved extremity is warmer than the contralateral side and the initial pallor with fine bluish mottling changes to dusky cyanosis during the ensuing hours.

To cause such extensive swelling of an extremity, it is necessary that major impairment to venous outflow be present. Obstruction of the common femoral vein above the level of the profunda femoris is the lowest level at which this may begin, and indeed the process often extends proximally to the level of the internal or common iliac veins. As venous obstruction progresses, secondary arterial spasm and diminished pulses may compound the problem by further impairing blood supply to the extremity. If obstruction is severe, ischemia and gangrene may follow. At this point the marked edema serves to distinguish between primary venous and primary arterial occlusion, since acute arterial occlusion *does not* cause early massive swelling as seen in acute iliofemoral thrombosis.

Pulmonary Embolism

Pulmonary emboli usually originate from thrombosis of the deep veins of the pelvis or lower extremities. Pulmonary embolus is a frequent, unsuspected autopsy finding in middle-aged and elderly patients. A high index of suspicion must be afforded these individuals. Any unexplained change in course, such as dyspnea, chest pain, confusion, fever or pneumonitis, must be carefully scrutinized to uncover occult emboli.

DIAGNOSIS.—Methodical examination of the lower extremities should be performed at least 1–2 times daily in every hospitalized patient. Inspection of the lower extremities may reveal superficial venous distention on the involved side. Tenderness to palpation is an important finding. Its absence must not rule out the diagnosis. Examination should further include: (1) comparison of size, (2) temperature and (3) consistency of the lower extremities.

Measurement should be made daily at the same level above and below the tibial tubercle. Increased warmth is one of the earliest physical findings and the most common finding in the difficult to diagnose patient. The boggy consistency is secondary to edema of the involved area; however, an intraluminal thrombus with an attachment only at its origin may cause minimal change in the circumference of the extremity. The above signs and symptoms, often absent, may in fact be preceded by cough, fever, chest pain or hemoptysis.

In those cases in which a very high clinical index of suspicion and patient deterioration prevail, heparin in amounts to keep the clotting time at 20–30 minutes is given intravenously as initial therapy and diagnostic efforts are then instituted. Treatment is properly delayed if the diagnosis is uncertain and the patient's condition does not require emergency therapy.

Chest x-ray may be negative in those with a small embolus but without infarction. Larger emboli result in infarction and a wedge-shaped opacity near the periphery. The right lower lobe is the most common site of pulmonary emboli. Still larger emboli can block a main pulmonary artery and cause increased radiolucency of the lung field on the involved side.

Radioisotope lung scan can be performed on short notice and the result is available almost immediately. Isotope scans serve to outline the perfused areas of the lung but do not necessarily indicate the etiology of obstruction of the nonperfused areas. Causes such as pneumonia and atelectasis may mimic the findings seen in embolism.

Pulmonary arteriography is the most accurate tool for the diagnosis of pulmonary embolus. Simultaneous determination of right ventricular and pulmonary arterial pressures add valuable confirmation and some prognostic information.

ANTICOAGULATION.—In the absence of a contraindication to anticoagulation, confirmation of a pulmonary embolus requires immediate anticoagulation with heparin. Contraindications include hematologic disorders with a bleeding tendency and active peptic ulcer. These may be changed to relative contraindications as the clinical situation indicates.

Anticoagulation is maintained with heparin in doses sufficient to prolong the clotting time to 2–3 times the normal control value of 10–15 minutes. The usual dose is 4,000–6,000 units, given by the intravenous route every four hours. The clotting time is determined one-half hour before the next dose. Once regulation has been achieved, clotting times should be checked once daily. Careful observation to detect gastrointestinal or urinary tract bleeding is mandatory. Antacids may be helpful in those who are prone to peptic ulcer disease.

Anticoagulation is successful in the prevention of recurrent emboli in the majority of patients (90%). In the remainder of patients who develop additional emboli despite adequate anticoagulation, ligation or plication of the inferior vena cava is essential.

Following caval interruption, anticoagulation is reinstituted 24 hours later and early ambulation with elastic support is instituted.

EMBOLECTOMY.—Significant elevation of mean pulmonary artery pressure (greater than 30% of mean systemic pressure) and radiographic evidence of 75% occlusion of the main pulmonary artery fulfill the criteria for pulmonary embolectomy in most patients in whom the clinical diagnosis of embolus has been made. Surgery is indicated in any patient in whom the diagnosis is confirmed by arteriography and who is deteriorating despite supportive therapy. The presence of continuing shock is probably the best single indication for embolectomy.

Partial cardiopulmonary by-pass may be lifesaving in the moribund patient. This resuscitative effort may be begun in the ward, followed by transfer to the operating suite for pulmonary embolectomy. Plication or ligation of the inferior vena cava is performed after by-pass has been discontinued.

The recovery period is usually prolonged and the postoperative mortality rate is high. The total mortality in patients undergoing embolectomy is approximately 50%.

Decreased pulmonary compliance is a major factor complicating postoperative ventilation. Volume-controlled respirators are most efficient in the management of this problem. The sequelae of shock and multiple transfusions further add to the morbidity and mortality. Postoperative management following cardiopulmonary by-pass is outlined in Chapter 20.

The general condition of the patient is the most important determinant of ambulation. As pain and edema decrease, ambulation is increased. Elastic support is indicated for one purpose only, to control edema when present. Intermittent elevation is also helpful.

Early anticoagulation is with heparin. Long-term oral agents are continued for 3 months following discharge.

27

Major Urologic Surgery

MALACHI J. FLANAGAN, M.D.

Associate Attending Surgeon, Rush-Presbyterian-St. Luke's Medical Center; Associate Professor of Surgery, Rush Medical College

AND

LOWELL R. KING, M.D.

Chief, Division of Urology, Children's Memorial Hospital, Chicago; Professor of Surgery, Northwestern University

UROLOGY DISPLAYS a high degree of precision and predictability in the diagnosis and treatment of genitourinary tract abnormalities. The urologist frequently is concerned with such divergent problems as those related to the pediatric and to the geriatric age groups. Patient care, therefore, must be grounded in the fundamental understanding and application of basic surgical considerations. Furthermore, the urologist's participation in the care of the patient with endocrinologic and metabolic problems requires understanding of medical as well as surgical principles of patient care. Conversely, a working knowledge of urologic problems is useful and necessary to all physicians, regardless of specialty, who render patient care.

General Considerations

THE CATHETER

The urethral catheter has achieved wide usage beyond the simple purpose of urinary drainage. By varying the size and end of the catheter (Fig. 27-1), multiple objectives can be achieved in the care of patients undergoing urologic surgery. However, in recent years the potential harm from abuse of the catheter has received emphasis. Certainly, the insertion of the catheter for nursing convenience in the patient with urinary incontinence and indiscriminate use of the catheter to determine urinary output is to be considered only in very selected instances. If

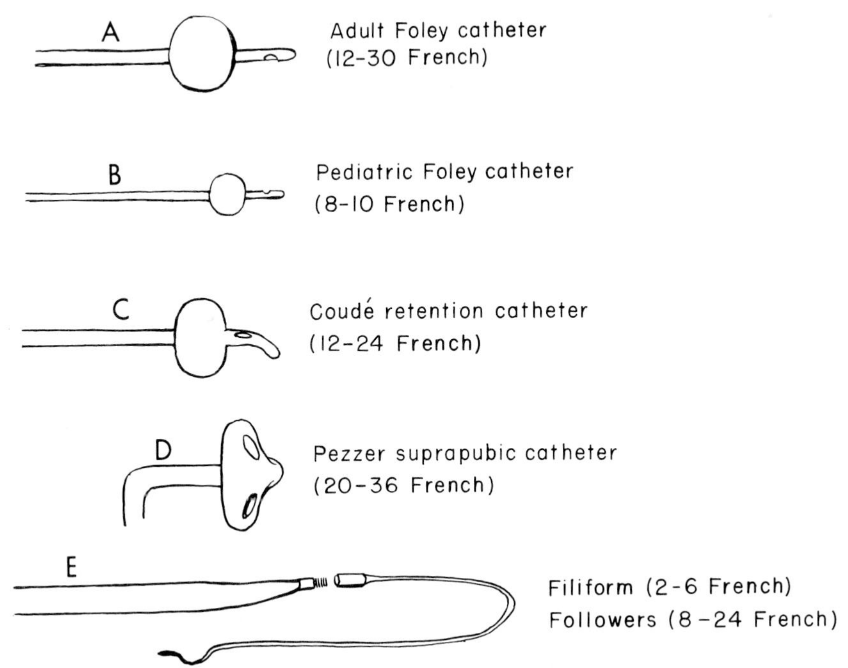

Fig. 27-1.—Commonly used types of catheters. **A,** adult self-retaining catheter (5, 30 and 75 ml. balloon, 12–30 F.); **B,** pediatric self-retaining catheter (3 ml. balloon, 8–10 F.); **C,** coudé olive-tipped retention catheter (5–30 ml. balloon, (12–24 F.); **D,** Pezzer self-retaining suprapubic drain (20–36 F.); **E,** urethral filiform tip (2–6 F.) and threaded Philips catheter (8–24 F.).

an inlying catheter remains in place for more than 48 hours, change from a previously sterile to an infected state must be anticipated, detected and properly treated.

In the current "catheter controversy" it must be emphasized that it is not only the use of the catheter itself that is under question, but the selection of catheter type and size, the technique of insertion and the pre-existing status of the urinary tract, all of which have considerable bearing on the possible harm following its use. The judgment as to the need for catheter use is often left to the least experienced member of the surgical team. In catheterizing the elderly male, selection of a coudé olive-tipped retention catheter (Fig. 27-1, C) will greatly reduce the trauma to the prostate and minimize bleeding and possible sepsis. The simple practice of using liberal amounts of lubricant is often overlooked. Forceful passage of a catheter through a mildly constricted area of the urethra will invariably produce urethral trauma and open vascular channels for contamination and infection. Finally, in the presence of significant residual urine, failure to employ catheter drainage is a far greater danger.

The definitive indications for the use of the urethral catheter are:

(1) drainage of the obstructed or paralyzed bladder; (2) bladder drainage following injury or surgery of the urinary tract or contiguous structures; (3) occasionally for purposes of obtaining an accurate urine sample or carrying out specific urologic studies such as cystography or cystometrography; (4) major surgical procedures during which information regarding renovascular integrity is essential.

The choice of catheter size will vary with the situation for which the catheter is employed. Catheters are measured by diameter in French units, 1 French unit (1F.) being equivalent to 0.33 mm. A normal adult male urethra will accommodate a 20–22 F. size; a normal adult female urethra, 22–24. It is desirable to employ the smallest catheter whenever possible to minimize local urethral and periurethral irritation. The only disadvantage of choosing a small size, such as a 14 or 16 F. catheter, is the tendency toward occlusion with urinary crystals, mucus and blood clots. The chief indication for larger catheters is to ensure good drainage when blood clots which will require irrigation can be anticipated. A large catheter may also be advantageous in long-term catheter use, since replacement and change are apt to be less frequently required.

Adult retention Foley-type catheters (Fig. 27-1, *A*) are available in 3 balloon sizes–5, 30 and 75 ml. For most purposes, a 5 ml. bag is satisfactory. The chief use of a larger size is to provide hemostasis in the region of the prostate and bladder neck in the immediate postprostatectomy period. The use of a large balloon may also be advantageous in the elderly disoriented patient who may inadvertently extract an intact catheter.

Catheter irrigation is ordinarily unnecessary except in instances of hemorrhage from the prostate or bladder. If a catheter fails to drain, irrigation with a small amount of sterile water or saline is permissible to clear any minor accumulation of urinary crystals or mucus. If more frequent irrigations are required to maintain catheter patency, it is better to replace the catheter, since frequent irrigations only enhance the possibility of introducing infection. Often, acidification of the urine with agents such as mandelic acid, methionine or cranberry juice will prolong catheter patency. When prolonged catheter drainage is anticipated, continuous or intermittent closed irrigation systems (Fig. 27-2) using dilute bacteriostatic solutions, such as 0.25% acetic acid, have been shown to delay the appearance and intensity of the bacilluria associated with catheter use.

The non-balloon type of retention catheter (mushroom, Pezzer [Fig. 27-1, *D*], or malecot type) is employed when large-caliber bladder drainage is required, as in the immediate postprostatectomy period or in the paraplegic. Such catheters are usually inserted suprapubically and afford superior bladder drainage. The disadvantage of such catheters is the difficulty associated with replacement because of the inability to maintain a straight suprapubic sinus tract.

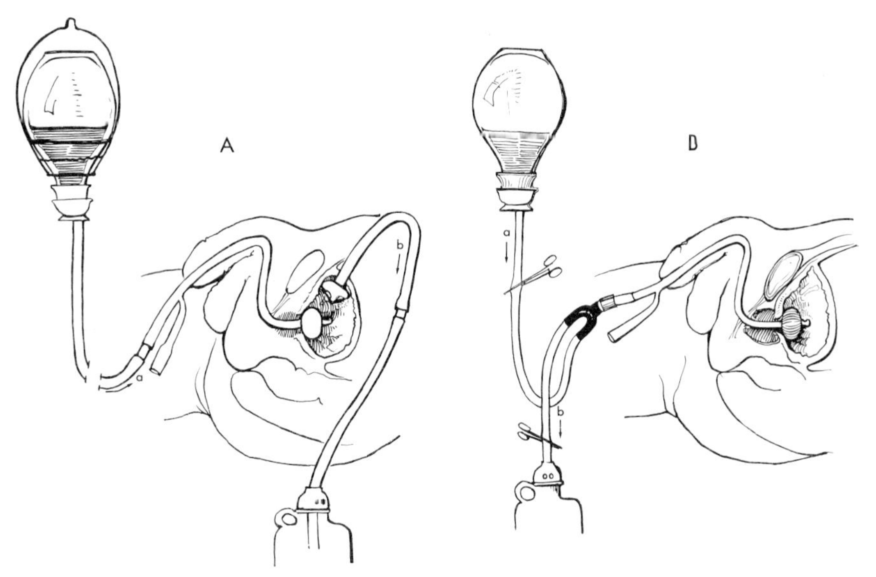

Fig. 27-2. – **A,** 2-way continuous postprostatectomy bladder irrigation. Continuous irrigation is performed by gravity inflow through the urethral catheter (*a*) during simultaneous outflow via the suprapubic catheter (*b*). Frequent observation is necessary to prevent bladder distention if clots obstruct the drainage catheter. **B,** 2-way intermittent bladder irrigation. Intermittent inflow (100–200 ml.) by gravity drainage (*a*) is performed during temporary outflow occlusion (*b*). The outflow tube is kept unclamped at all other times. Isotonic saline is used for bladder irrigation to minimize fluid and electrolyte disturbances.

Urinary infection may result from the use of the catheter. If the catheter is allowed to remain in place for more than 4 or 5 days, bacilluria and pyuria can be expected. The effect of an inlying catheter can be seen on cystoscopic examination if edema and hemorrhage of the posterior bladder wall result from the suction or siphonage effect of gravity drainage. A foreign body reaction in the urethra always occurs with catheter drainage and may lead to severe urethritis, periurethritis and stricture formation. If drainage is anticipated for more than 96 hours, prophylactic use of urinary antiseptics and/or antibiotics is indicated. Urinalysis and urine culture should be obtained at least weekly on all patients with long-term catheter drainage, and specific antibiotic therapy should be employed with or without local bladder irrigations. Such therapy should be continued with adequate hydration and urinary acidification. Once a catheter is removed, follow-up urine cultures must be obtained and, if results are positive, treatment must be continued until subsequent determinations show reversion to negative.

THE URETERAL CATHETER. – Ureteral catheters inserted cystoscopically are of small size – 3–10 F. The tiny catheter lumen is apt to occlude easily and thus should be irrigated with *small* (2–5 ml.) volumes of sterile saline if drainage stops. If drainage cannot be reinstituted, the use of the ureteral catheter may still be advantageous by virtue of its action as a splint for urine drainage around the catheter as well as through its lumen. Further irrigations serve no useful purpose and may introduce contamination and infection into an already compromised ureter or kidney. Occasionally, slight change in the position of the ureteral catheter may yield the sudden return of urinary drainage through the lumen. Ureteral catheters should remain in place no longer than absolutely necessary. In most instances, no harm is done if these catheters are left indwelling for 4 or 5 days. If ureteral catheter drainage is required for more than 9–10 days, more aggressive supravesical drainage measures such as ureterostomy or nephrostomy probably should have been considered initially. The use of a ureteral catheter for more than 4 days in pregnancy is absolutely contraindicated due to the close proximity of the friable ureter and iliac vessels.

Determination of Urinary Output

The normal 24 hour urinary output varies greatly. An output in the range of 400 ml. (20 ml./hour) may be associated with normal renal function. Nevertheless, in instances of oliguria there must be immediate determination of the cause and prompt treatment. Before considering the diagnosis of acute tubular necrosis, the drainage status of the urinary tract must be assessed. Urethral catheterization may yield previously undetected chronic urinary retention. Oliguria or anuria occurring after pelvic surgery may indicate unilateral or bilateral ureteral occlusion which may respond to ureteral catheterization. Urine may drain from other areas such as the wound or the vagina or via abdominal drains. Other factors to consider include the state of hydration and the adequacy of the circulation. Examination of the urine is necessary to determine its color, the presence of clots and the specific gravity.

An often overlooked method to measure renal function is determination of the urea content of the urine. If high, good renal function can be assumed; if low, acute tubular necrosis may be present. These considerations are mentioned because of the many instances of postoperative oliguria or anuria which are not due to parenchymal renal damage. The presence of oliguria per se is not an indication for the use of diuretics such as mannitol or ethacrynic acid. Until the above-mentioned local factors are ruled out, diuretics should not be given. Urinary output of more than 100 ml./hour may be comforting to observe but not always required to indicate adequate renal function.

Egress of fluid suspicious of urinary character may be noted from areas outside the urinary tract. Proof of urinary character may be surprisingly difficult. Measures such as injection of intravenous indigo carmine or methylene blue and determination of the urea content of the drainage fluid may aid in clarifying the problem.

Pre- and Postoperative Problems

EXTRAVASATION.—The presence of urine in any area outside the urinary tract is highly irritating initially and with continued insult produces frank inflammation, sepsis and abscess formation. Whenever the urinary tract is operated upon, extravasation must be anticipated and a source of external drainage, such as Penrose drains, diverting catheters, or both, must be provided. Leakproof closure of an incision in the kidney, ureter, bladder or urethra is the exception rather than the rule. Failure to recognize the need for external drainage will invariably lead to disastrous consequences. Continued extravasation of urine into the peritoneal cavity will result in severe peritonitis, sepsis and uremia. Continued extravasation of urine into the retroperitoneum will produce infection, abscess formation and ureteral obstruction. Continued extravasation in the deep pelvis will lead to severe pelvic cellulitis, peritonitis, abscess formation and renal shutdown. Whenever any doubt exists about the integrity of the urinary tract, external drainage is always desirable.

CONTRAST MEDIUMS.—The high degree of diagnostic accuracy is largely dependent upon the employment of various x-ray contrast studies of the kidney, ureter, bladder and urethra. Contrast mediums are well tolerated by the urinary tract. In instances of allergy to intravenous use of contrast mediums, retrograde injection of dye to outline the kidney and ureter is usually tolerated without incident. However, the instillation of a dye such as Hypaque or Renografin through a ureteral catheter to outline a kidney and ureter is not without hazards. Injection of media under pressure or excess volume (more than 5–6 ml.) may lead to distortion of the pyelographic shadow by blunting of the calices, pyelovenous backflow, pyelolymphatic backflow and severe and prolonged flank pain and pyelonephritis. Another consequence, particularly in the patient with pre-existing renal or ureteral disease, is ureteral edema, oliguria, anuria and possible renal shutdown. Particularly in the latter instance, any indication of induced renal trauma by a contrast medium should alert the surgeon to the possibility of anuria. This situation requires prompt therapy with diuretics, antibiotics and analgesics and possible reinsertion of the ureteral catheter.

URINARY RETENTION AND CATHETERIZATION.—Urinary retention is usually due to either prostatic obstruction from prostatic hypertrophy or urethral obstruction from stricture formation. The patient may or may not have experienced prior symptoms suggestive of outlet obstruction. This is particularly common in the postoperative period after surgery on contiguous pelvic structures. The presence of suprapubic dullness and pain establishes the diagnosis but may not be obvious on examination. Whenever doubt exists, urethral catheterization must be employed.

Urethral catheterization is a precise surgical procedure. Properly performed, it is of inestimable value to the patient. If improperly performed, grave local and systemic complications may occur, particularly in the male. The urethral meatus should be thoroughly cleansed with antiseptic solution such as aqueous Zephiran and, with the physician employing sterile gloves, a generous amount of lubricant is applied to the tip of the catheter. The anterior urethra is placed on slight tension and slowly and carefully negotiated with a 16 or 18 F. catheter. If obstruction is encountered, relubrication of the catheter may be helpful. The catheter should never be forced through an area of obstruction. If such approach is unsuccessful, an assessment of the cause of obstruction is necessary. If prostatic obstruction is the cause, a coudé or curved tip catheter (Fig. 27-1, *C*) may pass the elongated and angulated posterior urethra. Prostatic obstruction may also be bypassed by insertion of a flexible stylet (Fig. 27-3) into the lumen of a standard retention catheter. If obstruction is due to urethral stricture, use of filiform dilators (Fig. 27-1, *E*) should be considered. A filiform 2–6 F. catheter is initially passed beyond the stricture and then into the bladder. The end of the filiform is then attached to a larger dilator (Philips) and the stricture gradually dilated. The dilator may then be taped in place (Fig. 27-4) or removed and replaced with a retention catheter.

The advisability of using a retention-type catheter or a straight catheter will depend on the anticipated duration of the need for the catheter. Urinary retention in the young patient after a herniorrhaphy, for instance, certainly can be expected to be short-lived. On the other hand, retention in the elderly male may not be. In general, repeated catheterizations are potentially more harmful to the patient than the use of one retention catheter for several days.

Urinary infections.—Efforts in the diagnosis and treatment of urinary infections are directed primarily to detection of the offending organism, proper antibiotic therapy and general measures toward the prevention and management of bacteremic shock. It must be remembered, however, that the anatomic source of infection must be identified and properly eradicated. Failure of response to the medical

Fig. 27-3.—Flexible stylet (mandrin) to facilitate insertion of retention catheter. **A,** incorrect insertion, **B,** correct insertion.

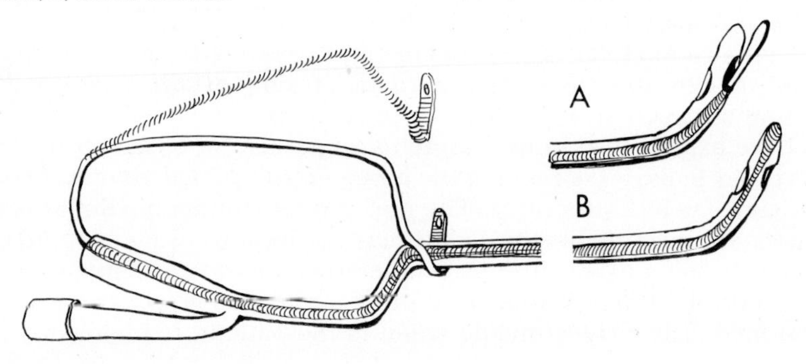

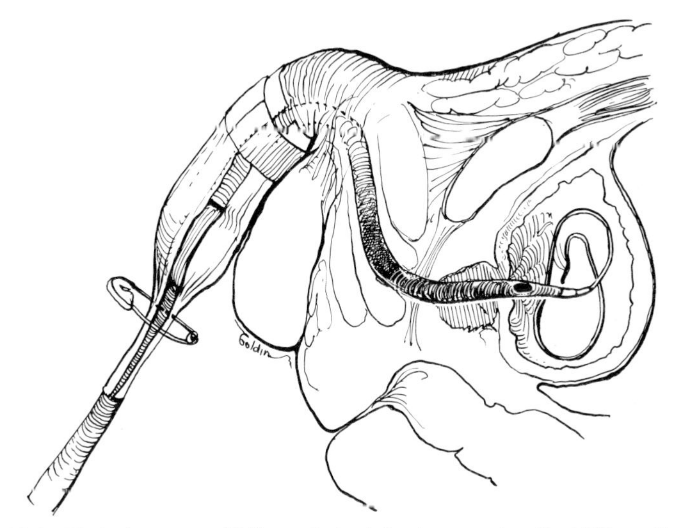

Fig. 27-4. – Method to secure Philips catheter following use of urethral filiform. Note hole of catheter inside the bladder and coiling of the filiform.

treatment of pyelonephritis indicates an undrained source of infection; this could be a perinephric abscess, infected hydronephrosis, renal carbuncle, renal calculus or polycystic kidneys. Recurrent cystitis may indicate bladder calculi, diverticula or lower urinary tract obstruction from prostatic or urethral obstruction. An underlying prostatic or urethral stricture may be the cause of poorly controlled and recurrent epididymitis.

Urologic Surgery

Surgery of the Kidney and Ureter

The kidney and ureter are ordinarily exposed retroperitoneally by reflecting the peritoneum medially. Whenever the kidney or ureter is operated upon, external drainage must be employed postoperatively. Utilization of the flank position, so common in renal surgery, may render ventilation more difficult, since the kidney rest tends to splint the contralateral side. Poor expansion of the operated side tends to occur due to pain. For this reason it is important to encourage deep breathing and coughing postoperatively despite such discomfort.

The pleural reflection may descend inferiorly or even be adherent to Gerota's fascia, rendering entrance to the pleural space likely. Pleural repair without postoperative pleural drainage can usually be accomplished. However, external closed drainage must be employed if closure is inadequate. Failure to do so is associated with pneumothorax and pleural effusion.

Postoperative hemorrhage from the renal fossa is rarely encountered when operative hemostasis is satisfactory. The presence of large amounts of bloody drainage from the incision may initially appear alarming but the fluid usually consists primarily of urine. After partial nephrectomy delayed hemorrhage may be anticipated and, if it occurs to any serious degree, will require immediate reoperation. Extrinsic pressure to control renal hemorrhage is usually ineffective.

Nephrostomy is undertaken for a variety of indications, the major one being adequate drainage of the urine from an operated kidney (Fig. 27-5). The nephrostomy tube is ordinarily of the Pezzer type and is inserted through the lower pole of the kidney. Failure of drainage of urine from the nephrostomy tube requires immediate investigation. Occlusion with clots should be corrected by irrigation with small amounts of saline (30–60 ml.). Overdistention of the renal pelvis by irrigation may produce bleeding and sepsis and should be avoided. Repositioning of a nephrostomy tube should only be undertaken after consultation with the operating surgeon, since only slight positional changes may lead to complete tube malfunction. Inadvertent removal of a nephrostomy tube from an incision is a urologic emergency. The sinus tract of the tube, often oblique and tortuous, may close in a matter of minutes. The tract must, therefore, be kept open with any available straight tube.

Plastic revision for ureteropelvic junction obstruction with hydronephrosis (pyeloplasty) commonly includes nephrostomy tube drainage and an additional splinting catheter traversing the repaired area (Fig.

Fig. 27-5.—**A,** urinary drainage via nephrostomy. **B,** nephrostomy tube drainage with ureteral splint following pyeloplasty.

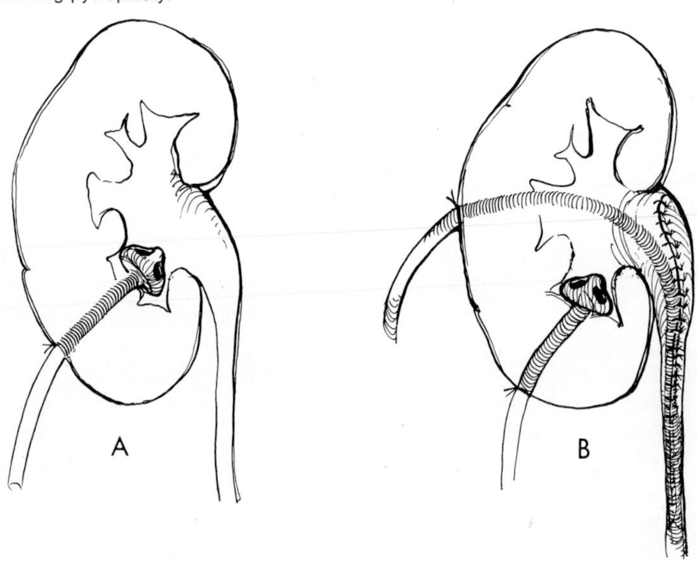

27-5, *B*). Since both tubes emerge from the wound, it is important to recognize the difference between the two. Inadvertent position change or removal of either tube may lead to serious complications.

Surgery of the Prostate

The term "prostatectomy" as applied to routine prostate surgery is incorrect. The entire prostate gland is not removed in surgery of benign prostatic hypertrophy; only the central adenomatous portion involved with hypertrophy is excised. The peripheral cortex of the prostate, which is composed of compressed normal prostatic tissue, remains intact. Total prostatectomy includes complete removal of the prostate gland and seminal vesicles and is employed only in instances of cancer of the prostate in which the disease is confined to that structure. Nevertheless, for purposes of identification, the term "prostatectomy" will be retained in the discussion as denoting operative removal for benign prostatic hypertrophy.

Operative excision is carried out by two routes, the endoscopic (transurethral) method (Fig. 27-6, *A*) and the open method, which may

Fig. 27-6. – Operative approaches to the prostate. **A,** transurethral; **B,** transperineal urethral; **C,** perineal; **D,** retropubic; **E,** suprapubic.

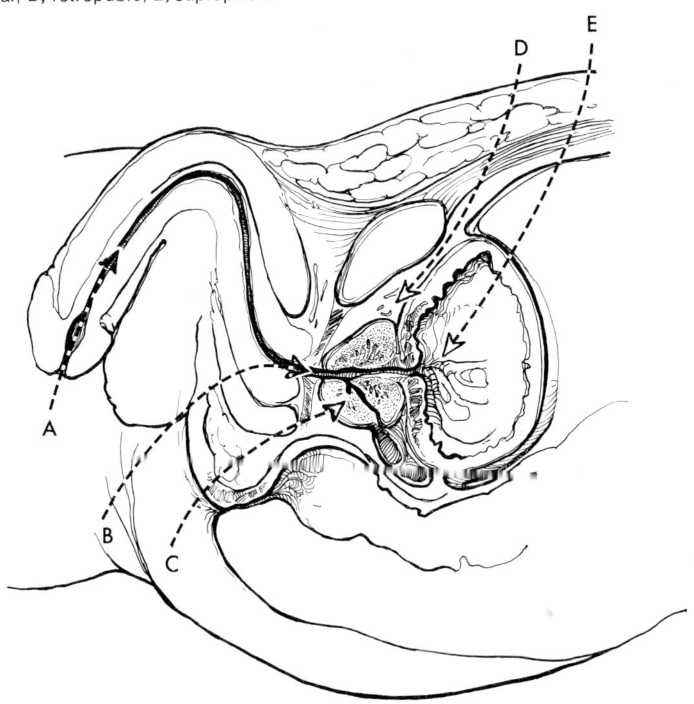

be by way of the suprapubic (Fig. 27-6, *E*), retropubic (Fig. 27-6, *D*) or perineal (Fig. 27-6, *C*) route. A variation of the transurethral route is the transperineal urethral method (Fig. 27-6, *B*), differing only by the route of entrance of the resectoscope, which traverses the perineal urethra rather than the urethral meatus.

HEMORRHAGE.—Hemorrhage, both operative and postoperative, is the single most common problem encountered in surgery of the prostate, particularly when the open route is employed. Several factors contribute to bleeding. The prostate gland develops a generous arterial and venous blood supply as hypertrophy develops. Present methods of prostatic enucleation leave large, raw surfaces in the prostatic capsule and bladder neck with multiple bleeding points which are difficult to identify. Many of these areas of bleeding may occur if the prostatic capsule fails to contract due to atony or chronic infection. Large arterial bleeders at 5 and 7 o'clock at the bladder neck, when identifiable, may be ligated, thus reducing hemorrhage. The prostate gland is normally rich in the enzymes euglobulinlysin and fibrinolysin and on occasion large amounts may be liberated during prostate surgery, with subsequent lysis of clots and severe hemorrhage.

Management of hemorrhage is initially, of course, dependent on precise hemostasis at surgery. Additional operative adjuncts include the temporary use of packing material such as gauze or Gelfoam and use of large displacement balloon catheters which tamponade the vesical neck area and prostatic fossa. Balloon catheter effectiveness will be enhanced by external traction. Traction devices should be employed only for short periods of 2–8 hours. Longer periods of use may produce severe external urinary sphincter ischemia and permanent urinary incontinence.

Significant blood loss should be corrected with whole blood. Pain and bladder spasms should be controlled and possibly eliminated, using adequate amounts of analgesics. Demerol used in large amounts is often not effective. Morphine, 10–15 mg., is usually more effective when given as often as every 3–4 hours. Belladonna and opium rectal suppositories every 3–4 hours are often quite helpful. Adequate drainage of urine and blood clots must be maintained by the use of continuous or intermittent irrigation with saline solution.

If increased fibrinolysin activity can be demonstrated, epsilon aminocaproic acid is the treatment of choice. Occasionally the use of nonspecific agents such as Premarin may be helpful.

Suprapubic pain and rigidity following transurethral resection, unaccompanied by obvious signs of severe bladder hemorrhage, may indicate perforation of the prostatic capsule with subsequent extravasation of irrigating fluid, urine and blood. If such a diagnosis is considered, it should be confirmed by retrograde cystography and if confirmed, immediate open drainage of the perivesical spaces and suprapubic cystostomy should be carried out. Failure to recognize and treat such a complication may be disastrous to the patient since untreated extensive extravasation will usually lead to sepsis, peritonitis and renal failure.

THE CREEVY SYNDROME.—Occasionally during or after a transurethral resection a patient who is otherwise doing well may experience a sudden rise in blood pressure, disorientation and confusion. This clinical picture may then be followed by pulmonary edema, shock and collapse. This condition, designated as the Creevy syndrome, has been attributed to absorption of excess quantities of irrigating fluid through the large venous sinuses in the prostatic cortex into the general circulation with subsequent hyponatremia. A blood sample drawn at this time will show hemolysis and hyponatremia. Recognition of the cause of this syndrome and prompt correction are mandatory. Management of the syndrome is fortunately in large part preventive. If the urologist encounters large venous sinuses during the operation, the use of isotonic irrigating fluids may preclude the development of this syndrome. Furthermore, since a certain amount of absorption occurs with all resections, the experienced urologist will reserve resection of the deep cortex, where most absorption occurs, until near the very end of the operation.

Once recognized, management of the syndrome usually does not require volume and salt replacement, since the lowered hematocrit and hyponatremia represent a relative rather than an absolute deficit. In general, these patients are in the older age group and have impaired cardiovascular reserve. Careful observation and judicious treatment, including small amounts of mannitol, are indicated to decrease the effect of hemolysis on the kidney and prevent renal failure. The use of Thorazine will aid in peripheral vasodilation and accommodation of excess fluid. If these measures are observed, spontaneous diuresis can be expected and correction of the process will occur.

The duration of catheter drainage following prostatectomy will vary depending on the amount of prostatic tissue removed and the method of prostatectomy employed. In general, no less than 7 days of catheter drainage is advisable after open prostatectomy; in instances of very large prostates, several more days of drainage may be desirable. When a TUR is performed, the catheter may be removed as early as the third day, but usually remains for 5 days. If a catheter should inadvertently be removed prior to the scheduled date, it should be reinserted, bearing in mind that the area of the prostate and vesical neck may be temporarily irregular and friable from surgery. It is better to employ a coudé catheter in these instances, and if resistance is encountered, the operating surgeon should negotiate this area himself.

SUPRAVESICAL URINARY DIVERSION

URETEROSIGMOIDOSTOMY.—Anastomosis of both ureters to the intact rectosigmoid (ureterosigmoidostomy, Fig. 27-7, *A*) is the only form of urinary diversion in which the patient may be expected to maintain

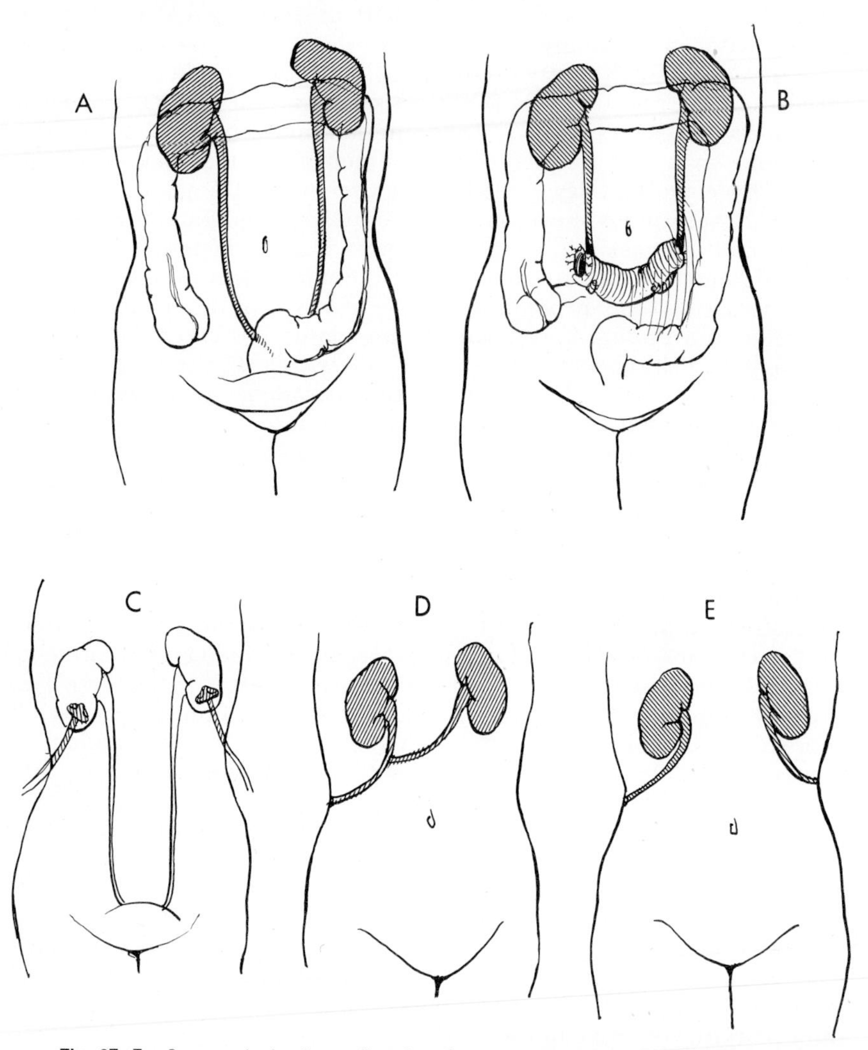

Fig. 27–7.—Supravesical urinary diversion. **A,** ureterosigmoidostomy; **B,** ureteroileostomy (ileal conduit); **C,** bilateral nephrostomy; **D,** ureteroureterostomy; **E,** bilateral cutaneous uretero-stomy. In **B, D** and **E** it is desirable to fit an external appliance to the stoma as soon as convenient following surgery.

urinary control without resorting to the use of external tubes and appliances. Unfortunately, the fecal stream is in direct continuity with the urinary tract; thus retrograde infection of the kidneys and renal failure are likely complications. Except in instances of exstrophy of the bladder, and short-term palliation, ureterosigmoidostomy has not been routinely practical.

A special hazard of this operation is electrolyte absorption from the colon with consequent elevation of serum chloride and acidosis. In more severe instances, pronounced dehydration, weight loss and vomiting may occur. The syndrome of hyperchloremic acidosis can occur in the immediate postoperative period or even months to years later. Correction may be difficult. Initially the use of a rectal tube serves to reduce further absorption from the colon. Antibiotics and fluids must be utilized to treat the infection and dehydration. The use of sodium or potassium citrate may help greatly in correction of the problem.

Ileal conduit (ureteroileostomy).—Implantation of the ureters into a segment of small intestine (ileum) is one of the most satisfactory methods of long-term upper urinary tract diversion (Fig. 27-7, *B*). The intestinal reservoir empties into an external appliance and is not associated with residual urine. In this way the problem of recurrent urinary infection and renal failure, common with other forms of diversion, is largely obviated. The ileal conduit would be employed in all instances in which supravesical diversion is indicated except for three reasons. (1) The operation is time-consuming and, especially when carried out in conjunction with other forms of extirpative pelvic surgery, is more hazardous in the elderly poor-risk patient. (2) The required use of an external appliance is inconvenient. (3) Stenosis of the ileal stoma, especially in children, is common.

The diagnosis of ileal loop complications requires meticulous postoperative observation and care. A progressively discolored purplish to black mucosa will indicate infarction of the ileal stoma and/or loop. The continued silent, distended abdomen may indicate extravasation of urine or intestinal anastomotic malfunction. Immediate or delayed occurrence of oliguria or anuria or the appearance of a cutaneous urinary fistula demands immediate exploration. An ileal loopogram should be performed promptly in any of the above instances. Using dilute radiopaque contrast instilled by a catheter into the stomal lumen under gravity, the entire reconstituted urinary tract can be readily outlined. Urinary extravasation, obstruction or non-filling of the ureters and the ureteroileal anastomosis may be seen. Delayed drainage films will demonstrate obstructed stomas, atonic, malfunctioning ileal conduits and impaired ureteral drainage.

Once demonstrated, small urinary leaks may be conservatively managed with such measures as catheter or suction drainage of the conduit. However, large amounts of extravasated urine must be drained surgically, possibly by diverting nephrostomy, ureterostomy and/or direct repair of the malfunctioning segment. Uncontrolled pyelonephritis without extravasation may require nephrostomy. Stomal slough, ischemia or extravasation may be managed by indwelling catheter drainage temporarily and later revised, but total ischemia of the conduit is an emergency which must be corrected by excision and replacement of the loop.

BILATERAL NEPHROSTOMY.—Bilateral nephrostomy (Fig. 27-7, *C*) provides immediate and direct urinary drainage by use of Foley or mushroom type catheters inserted directly into the renal pelvis. This form of urinary drainage is usually employed only as a temporary measure. It is important to remember that the accurate placement of catheters is mandatory for adequate drainage. Long-term nephrostomy drainage is unsatisfactory because of infection, stone formation and the necessity for changing drainage tubes. Proper drainage from nephrostomy tubes may be difficult to restore once a tube has been removed. With the passage of time the sinus tract becomes tortuous and accurate replacement of tubes becomes quite difficult.

URETEROSTOMY.—Cutaneous ureterostomy (Fig. 27-7, *D* and *E*) is employed as a permanent form of upper urinary tract diversion in instances of chronic ureteral dilatation. There are many variations of this procedure, but all involve the direct anastomosis of the ureter to the skin.

In the immediate postoperative period it is important that the stoma be kept as clean and dry as possible by means of a temporary diverting catheter. Careful observation to detect ischemia of the ureteral stoma is required. In general, as soon as adequate healing takes place, the catheter should be removed, since catheters are in themselves a source of chronic irritation and stricture formation. If a splinting ureteral catheter is dislodged, it should be immediately reinserted to maintain adequate drainage of urine from the kidney and to keep the area of surgery as dry as possible. The major disadvantage of cutaneous ureterostomy is the frequency of stricture formation at the skin level.

28

Treatment of Burns

RANDALL E. McNALLY, M.D.

Assistant Attending Surgeon, Rush-Presbyterian-St. Luke's Medical Center; Associate Professor of Surgery, Rush Medical College

A PLAN FOR care of the burn patient should be outlined directly after initial resuscitation. In general, burns of more than 15% of the body surface usually require intensive care. Selected smaller burns, however, may also necessitate such care, depending upon the anatomic location and presence of associated disease or injury. Burn victims in these categories should have the advantage of modern transportation to an intensive care facility in the early hours following injury. Resuscitation should be instituted in transit.

The emergency care of burns is most clearly stated in "Guide to initial therapy of burns," prepared by the Subcommittee on Burns, Committee on Trauma of the American College of Surgeons (Fig. 28-1). This guide should be displayed in all emergency rooms and all those who treat burns should be familiar with its recommendations.

Initial Evaluation

The history and physical examination are of prime importance. The collaboration of several physicians is usually necessary to evaluate the patient and simultaneously initiate resuscitation. The burn injury may be so obvious that care must be taken not to overlook associated life-threatening injuries.

Specific factors which affect treatment, survival and complications are age, pre-existing disease, causative agent, extent and depth of the burn and the anatomic location of the burn.

The extremes of age are associated with an increased morbidity and mortality. Maintenance of fluid and electrolyte balance requires extremely close supervision in those under 2 and over 60 years of age. Any complications which occur are potentially more lethal in this group.

BROOKE FORMULA

Fluids During First 24 Hours

A. Colloid (blood, plasma or dextran)—Wt. in kg. X % burned X 0.5 ml.

B. Electrolytes (lactated Ringer's solution)—Wt. in kg. X % burned X 1.5 ml.

C. Water (5 % dextrose in water)

Adults—2,000 ml.

Children—1 yr.—80 ml. per kg.
5 yr.—60 ml. per kg.
8 yr.—40 ml. per kg.

More than 50 per cent burn is calculated as 50 per cent. Little or no colloid is required in second-degree burns. Urine flow should be such that urine is cleared of gross hemoglobinuria.

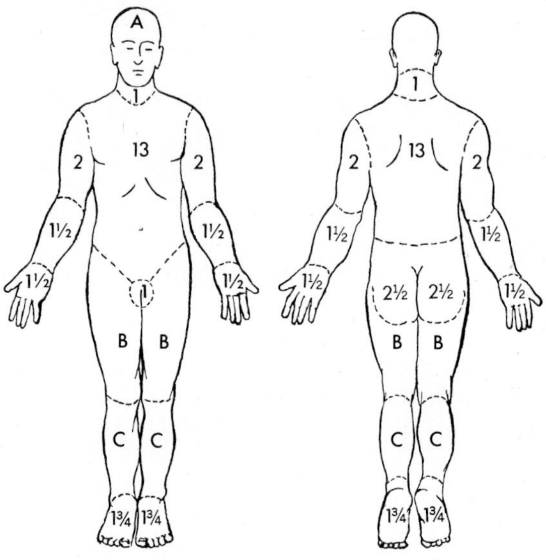

Relative percentage of areas affected by growth

	AGE IN YEARS					
	0	*1*	*5*	*10*	*15*	*adult*
A—½ of head	9½	8½	6½	5½	4½	3½
B—½ of one thigh	2¾	3¼	4	4¼	4½	4¾
C—½ of one leg	2½	2½	2¾	3	3¼	3½

Total per cent burned ______ 2°+ ______ 3°= ______

Fig. 28-1.—How to estimate per cent of burn (From Guide to initial therapy of burns, Bull. Am. Coll. Surgeons 52:196–197, 1967).

MINOR BURNS

A. Put on cap and mask
B. Consider cold packs for relief of pain
C. Give narcotic intravenously if necessary
D. Cleanse wound with bland soap and warm water
E. Dress with sterile, nonadherent fine-mesh gauze, and secure bulky dressing firmly in place
F. Have patient return in two days

SEVERE BURNS

A. Assure an adequate airway. This may require tracheostomy. Need most often occurs with:
   1. Respiratory tract injury from inhalation of noxious gases
   2. Deep burns of face and neck
B. Perform venipuncture with large-bore needle
   1. Obtain blood for crossmatch, hemoglobin, hematocrit, electrolyte, and blood urea nitrogen tests
   2. Start plasma, dextran, or lactated Ringer's solution
   3. Give morphine intravenously if needed
C. Do cut-down for burns over 20 per cent of body.
   1. Choose cephalic vein at shoulder or wrist, or long saphenous vein at medial malleolus
   2. Use long plastic catheter which accepts 16- or 18-gauge needle
   3. Infuse lactated Ringer's or colloid solution
D. Communicate with responsible attending physician

Pre-existing disease markedly alters the prognosis of burn victims. Cardiopulmonary, renal and hepatic disease are the major compromising illnesses. All too frequent is the association of alcoholism or epilepsy as the causative agent in the production of the injury. Diabetes mellitus is the most common metabolic disorder associated with burns. Ordinarily, the diabetes is not especially difficult to control, but wound healing is delayed and infections are more difficult to manage. Particular caution in fluid management is necessary in those patients with cardiopulmonary and renal disease. Regulation by central venous pressure monitoring is essential in this group.

Information regarding the agent causing the burn is of prognostic importance. Scalds of water are generally partial-thickness burns. In some cases clothing may retain the heat and inflict a full-thickness injury on the thin skin of the child or elderly person. Flame burns characteristically have a central area of full-thickness injury and a peripheral partial-thickness injury. Electrical and chemical burns are invariably the most deceptive in the estimation of extent and depth. In both there may be an inexorable progression which necessitates extensive debridement and, in the extremities, may require amputation.

The extent and depth of injury are the basis for current resuscitation formulas. Burns are classified by depth as: (1) first degree – erythema only; (2) second degree – blistering, mottled red and white weeping surface with viable dermal elements and (3) third degree – charred black or pearly white with destruction of all layers. A thrombosed venous pattern is invariably indicative of a third degree burn. A more recent classification describes partial-thickness burns as those which

---

E. Obtain adequate assistance, put on cap and mask
F. Remove patient's clothing, completely exposing all burned areas for evaluation
G. Obtain history, i.e., age; when, where, and how injury occurred; allergies; tetanus immunization status; previous health
H. Insert Foley catheter and send specimen to laboratory
I. Cleanse wound
   1. Use bland soap and warm water
   2. Gently remove dirt and loose devitalized shreds
   3. Irrigate chemical burns with copious amounts of water
J. Estimate per cent and depth of burn, making chart for estimation of per cent of burn as illustrated
K. Remember early photographs are desirable
L. Weigh patient or estimate weight
M. Expose, dress, or excise wound, as indicated – **Remember decompression incisions on circumferential extremity burns**
N. Immunize against tetanus
O. Write orders
   1. Nothing per mouth initially
   2. Record intake and output on chart
   3. Record blood pressure, pulse, and urine output hourly
   4. Cradle on bed if exposure method is used
   5. Mouth care
   6. Procaine penicillin, 600,000 units b.i.d. for five days
   7. Vitamin B complex
   8. Vitamin C (1,000 – 1,500 mg. daily)
   9. No narcotics after 24 hours except on special order
   10. Barbiturate or tranquilizer p.r.n.
   11. Nasogastric tube if patient vomits
   12. Humidified oxygen
   13. Culture of burn wound
   14. Watch for gastric dilatation
   15. Critical list? Special nurses?
   16. Calculate fluids, number all bottles

   Use any suitable formula, such as the Brooke, during first 24 hours

   17. If blood pressure decreases and urine output falls below 30 ml. per hour, increase colloid
   18. If blood pressure is stable but urine output falls below 30 ml. per hour, increase electrolyte solution
   19. If hourly urine output exceeds 50 ml. per hour, decrease fluid therapy unless a large volume is required to maintain urine free of hemoglobin
P. Laboratory work: hemoglobin and hematocrit daily; blood urea nitrogen, carbon dioxide combining power, potassium, sodium, and chloride every two days after second day

progress to healing from retained dermal elements and full-thickness burns as those which require grafting. Pinprick sensation is not completely accurate in the evaluation of depth when the examination is done early. Radioisotope and special dye studies are not necessary to determine extent or depth in the usual clinical situation, since the exact level is academic. For resuscitation the only burn injury calculated is second degree and third degree.

The extent of the injury is based on the "rule of nines," which, simply stated, is: 9% for the head and neck, 9% for each upper extremity, 18% for each lower extremity, 18% for the anterior torso, 18% for the posterior torso and 1% for the perineum. The rule of nines is valid only for adults. For infants and children more area is given to the head and less to the lower extremities.

Burns of certain areas require special attention. These areas include the extremities, the face, perineum and major joints. Appropriate local management of each area is a major factor in obtaining satisfactory functional results.

Burns of the face may compromise respiration and alimentation. Tracheostomy may be indicated for mechanical obstruction secondary to injury of the upper respiratory tract. Hand and foot burns usually require dressings, immobilization and elevation. Major joints are maintained in extension to prevent disabling flexion deformities. Due to repeated contamination, burns of the perineum are prone to sepsis, especially of the gram-negative variety. Circumferential burns of the trunk and extremities require careful evaluation to anticipate and treat respiratory or circulatory embarrassment. Escharotomy to the level of the fascia must be performed at the earliest indication of compromise to either of these essential functions.

Intensive Care of Burn Patient

Respiratory Tract Injury

Aside from incineration, respiratory tract injury is the major early cause of mortality in burn victims. The history of flame or explosion in a closed space increases the likelihood of this type of injury. Burns of the face, palate, pharynx and larynx result in edema and airway obstruction. Inhalation of noxious and hot gases may also cause pulmonary injury. Tachypnea, dyspnea, stridor, voice change and carbon particles in the sputum indicate a significant burn.

Tracheostomy.—On occasion acute respiratory distress requires immediate tracheostomy. The majority of respiratory burns can be managed by elevation of the head, oxygen and humidity. An additional group will benefit from temporary intubation. During this period the need for tracheostomy is re-evaluated and if tracheostomy is necessary, a soft, cuffed tube is used. The soft tube minimizes tracheal trauma and inflation of the cuff facilitates ventilatory assistance.

There is a high incidence of sepsis associated with tracheostomy in burn patients. Cultures are taken initially and every other day thereafter. Treatment includes frequent but gentle tracheobronchial toilet, systemic antiobiotics, mucolytics, bronchodilators and occasionally bronchoscopy. Large dose, short-term corticosteroids are frequently of benefit in the management of severe respiratory injuries.

A chest x-ray should be done as soon as practical. The majority of x-rays will be normal despite significant inhalation injury. Parenchymal involvement is indicative of severe injury.

Fluid Therapy

An intravenous route is established in a carefully selected vein. Because multiple intravenous sites are usually needed during the hospitalization, a proper sequence is necessary. A large polyethylene catheter is introduced centrally via the neck or upper extremities so that central venous pressure may be monitored, particularly during the early phase of resuscitation. The burn formulas are empirically derived estimations of fluid and electrolytes sequestered in and about the burn wound. The calculations are related to the extent and depth of the wound and the body weight.

The sequestered fluid is similar to plasma; consequently, this fluid would be the ideal replacement. The risk of hepatitis and the unavailability of pooled plasma dictate that balanced electrolyte solutions are best for replacement of losses. The Brooke formula is the most popular in use. For adults, according to the Brooke formula, the requirement during the first 24 hour period includes colloid, 0.5 ml./kg. of body weight for each per cent of body surface burned; electrolyte solution, 1.5 ml./kg. for each per cent of body surface burned, and 2,000 ml. of dextrose in water. During the first 24 hours 50% of the calculated losses is administered in the first 8 hours and 25% during each of the following 8 hour periods. The second 24 hour period requirements for colloids and electrolytes are about one-half those of the first 24 hours. In all formulas no number higher than 50 is used in the calculation of the extent of the injury. Approximately 10 L. is the maximum volume given in any 24 hours.

Dextran is the colloid of choice because of the risk of homologous serum hepatitis associated with the use of pooled plasma. Lactated Ringer's is the preferred electrolyte solution since it most closely resembles plasma. Saline may be used but often causes hyperchloremia.

The formulas are used only as a guide. The clinician must examine the patient hourly to re-evaluate progress and revise calculations according to clinical and laboratory information. The hourly urine output and specific gravity are the most reliable signs of the adequacy of resuscitation. Initially fluid therapy is vigorous, since frequently there is a lag of several hours from the time of injury to the initiation of fluid therapy. Once urine flow is established, it is maintained at 50 ml. per hour by regulation of the fluid intake.

A Foley catheter is essential to monitor the urine output. Most burns of the external genitalia also require catheter drainage. Urinary sepsis should be controlled with irrigation and systemic urinary antiseptics as indicated. Acute renal failure may supervene in burns of moderate severity if complicated by pre-existing renal disease, incompatible transfusion, drug reaction or crush trauma. In more severe burns, renal failure can occur if shock is untreated or undetected for variable periods. Hemolysis often accompanies severe thermal and electrical burns. It is vital to prevent hemoglobin precipitation in the tubules. Mannitol promotes diuresis, while sodium bicarbonate is used to alkalinize the urine and further decrease the tendency for pigment precipitation.

Anuria or oliguria associated with a rising central venous pressure indicates renal failure. If a rapid infusion of dextrose and water does not improve urine flow, a trial of diuretics is indicated for treatment or confirmation of the diagnosis. The indications for dialysis are discussed in Chapter 9.

In the otherwise uncomplicated case, spontaneous diuresis usually occurs between the third and fifth day following injury. This must be anticipated because injudicious intravenous therapy coupled with mobilization of fluid and electrolytes can result in pulmonary edema. Clinical and laboratory examinations are helpful in predicting this occurrence. The hematocrit on the day of injury may rise to 50–55%, but should be treated when more than 60%. Serum electrolyte and BUN values are determined daily for the first week. An early rise in the BUN may be anticipated with return to normal by the end of this period.

Initially most burn patients have a clouding of the sensorium. A clearing of the sensorium usually indicates correction of fluid and electrolyte imbalance.

Acute gastric dilatation, abdominal distention, nausea or vomiting may result from adynamic ileus in the early postburn phase. Gastric aspiration frequently is necessary and is almost routine in severe burns. This relatively common complication precludes alimentation for 3–5 days. Several days should elapse to allow the return of peristalsis prior to the resumption of feedings. Approximately 10% of hospitalized burn patients demonstrate gastrointestinal bleeding from a Curling ulcer. The peak incidence is 72 hours postburn. Stool examination for occult blood and nasogastric aspiration may allow earlier recognition and treatment of this entity. Surgery, even through burned tissue, is mandatory for uncontrollable hemorrhage or perforation.

A catabolic state exists from the time of injury until almost complete healing. Neither oral nor parenteral feedings can reverse this state. At least 4,000 calories daily by an oral diet with frequent supplementary feedings is considered optimal, and efforts to provide this amount of calories must be made. Intravenous hyperalimentation is a useful adjunct in the early catabolic phase. Most of the caloric loss is secondary to evaporative water loss through burned tissue and maintenance of body temperature.

Medication

Most medications, particularly analgesics, are administered intravenously for the first several days following injury. Since third degree burns are anesthetic, analgesics are not necessary for every patient. For those who require pain relief, morphine (2–6 mg.) or meperidine (25–50 mg.) is given by titration. Since the pain and length of hospitalization are prolonged, the possibility of addiction must be recognized. Barbiturates are the agents of choice for sedation. Hypoxia as the cause of restlessness and anxiety must be ruled out prior to administration of any sedative.

Procaine penicillin, 600,000 units, is given twice daily for the first 5 days to prevent streptococcal and clostridial infections. Additional antibiotics are administered during the postburn phase for specific bacterial infections as they become manifest. Fluid tetanus toxoid, 0.5 ml., is administered to all burn patients. If a history of prior tetanus immunization is questionable or absent, 250 units of hyperimmune human globulin is recommended every 3 weeks. This is also given to high-risk patients with buttock and perineal burns.

Despite the lack of confirmatory data, many clinicians favor digitalization in the high-risk groups and those with severe burns. Therapeutic doses of vitamin B complex and large doses of vitamin C are indicated to promote healing.

Wound Care

The objective of wound care is to promote early healing of partial-thickness burns, to prevent conversion of partial to full-thickness losses, to facilitate closure of full-thickness burns by split-thickness skin grafts and to maintain or restore function. In accomplishing these goals, complications are frequent obstacles.

Control of invasive infection requires constant attention until full healing occurs. For burn survivors contractures are the most common complication. The prevention of contracture is a primary goal of wound care.

There is universal agreement in the initial care of the burn wound. Caps, masks, sterile gloves and gowns all decrease contamination. Gentle cleansing with bland soap (Ivory, Dial, pHisohex) and copious amounts of water is performed with the patient on clean sheets. A wide area surrounding the burn is shaved. All devitalized epithelium is debrided. Anesthesia is usually not indicated for this initial phase of treatment.

At the completion of the cleansing phase, universal agreement in regard to wound care ceases. The goals remain as above but individualization of patient need becomes paramount. The surgeon may elect one or more of the following modalities of treatment to achieve early wound healing in a given patient. The facilities of an institution often dictate the mode of treatment.

Excision of a burn is restricted to the small full-thickness injury in an otherwise healthy individual. The advantage is obviously a shortened rehabilitation. The limiting feature of this procedure is the difficulty in early assessment of full-thickness losses. A prime example of this type of management is that of molten metal burns of the dorsum of the hand. In such cases the wound is excised 4–5 days postburn and covered with a split-thickness skin graft 1–2 days later. Excision of burn wounds of more than 15% of the body surface increases morbidity and mortality.

Another surgical maneuver in burn care is the use of escharotomy. This is occasionally indicated in constricting circumferential burns of the trunk and extremities. As the eschar contracts (especially with the exposure technique), circulatory and neurologic deficits may become manifest. Relaxing incisions to the level of the fascia relieve the compression. A constricting eschar of the thorax can limit respiratory excursion and require multiple vertical and horizontal incisions. Moist dressing techniques often obviate the need for escharotomy.

Skeletal suspension improves the efficiency of burn wound care. This method immobilizes the extremity, allows ready accessibility and prevents contact of the burned surface with bedclothes.

DRESSINGS.—The advantages of dressings are comfort, splinting and prevention of external contamination. Dressings allow accurate positioning and facilitate care. With the exception of the small joints of the hands, the commonest contractures are of the flexion (comfort) type. Accordingly, most injuries are initially dressed and later in the burn course splinted in extension.

The most common method utilizes fine mesh petrolatum or Furacin gauze as the first layer. The fine mesh gauze prevents adherence to the wound surface but permits egress of fluid. The next layer is fluffed gauze in generous amounts. ABD pads are placed over the fluffed gauze. An outer roll of bias-cut stockinette is then applied. Elastic bandages produce complications similar to those produced by a circumferential constricting eschar and are not recommended.

Hands and feet are often best treated with the dressing technique. Hands are dressed as usual in the position of function, except that metacarpophalangeal joints are flexed to 90 degrees. This marked flexion at the M-P joints prevents shortening of the collateral ligments. Cleanliness is essential in all surgical wounds. Burn dressings are changed as often as necessary. For the method described above, dressing changes would be necessary every 2–5 days, depending on the amount of drainage and the patient's general course.

EXPOSURE.—Exposure is the treatment of choice for burns of the face and perineum. Also well managed by this technique are burns of one surface of an extremity or one surface of the trunk.

The aim of the exposure method is the development of a dry surface which retards bacterial proliferation. A partial-thickness injury exudes a variable amount of serum, less as the injury deepens from the superficial level.

The exposure technique challenges the ingenuity of the medical and nursing personnel. Circumferential burns require circle beds or special frames. These often entail considerable discomfort. New plastic nonadherent dressings are being developed which will, hopefully, eliminate painful exposure. Air currents which cause pain with the open technique can be minimized by draping sheets over a cradle. These patients also complain of being cold and measures are necessary to combat this. The most useful is local control of the environment.

Infection usually supervenes at the interface of the eschar and viable tissue, requiring removal of this nonviable dried tissue, usually with scissors. The crust over a partial-thickness loss begins to separate at 8–10 days and is usually healed by 18–20 days after the burn. Full-thickness losses should have split skin grafts in the fourth week postburn. A significant deviation from this schedule requires re-evaluation of the patient's progress.

TOPICAL THERAPY.—A major advance in the treatment of burns is the use of topical agents such as Sulfamylon and silver nitrate. The use of these agents has decreased the need for elaborate isolation techniques. Neither silver nitrate nor Sulfamylon negate basic wound care of frequent cleansing and debridement; however, both agents significantly reduce the evaporative water loss through the burned tissue.

The reduction in invasive wound infection and in conversion of partial-thickness to full-thickness losses by infection has been impressive. In the average major thermal burn treated with these agents, approximately one-third less skin grafting is necessary. Pseudomonas aeruginosa, the most common pathogen isolated from burn wounds, has been minimized with the application of these agents.

Sulfamylon.—Sulfamylon is used as a 10% acetate water-soluble cream. It is applied with a gloved hand or applicator stick in a 5 mm. thickness to the burned area. Some pain is associated with its application. It is applied once or twice daily after cleansing and debridement in the Hubbard tank or shower. It is used more frequently when the exudate is excessive or when contact with clothes or linens removes the coating. Sulfamylon is subsequently not applied to areas of regenerating epithelium since it irritates and retards proliferation of new tissue.

In addition to its bacteriostatic action, Sulfamylon is also a carbonic anhydrase inhibitor. Because of this effect on the buffering system, the lungs assume a major role in acid-base balance. For this reason,

Sulfamylon must be used cautiously in patients with respiratory embarrassment.

Hyperchloremic acidosis is a not uncommon complication of Sulfamylon therapy. Absorption of the acid salt as well as inhibition of the carbonic anhydrase buffering system contribute to the metabolic acidosis. Compensatory respiratory alkalosis follows, and tachypnea and hyperpnea are a normal effect of this mechanism in patients undergoing Sulfamylon therapy. Inability to compensate is suggested by labored respiration and verified by serial blood gas, pH and electrolyte determinations. Significant aberrations require temporary interruption of therapy and correction of the base deficit with sodium bicarbonate. Following a satisfactory response, Sulfamylon application is resumed, usually on a once-daily basis.

Silver nitrate.—Silver nitrate is used in a 0.5% solution as a moist dressing. Saturated multiple-ply gauze without batting is used to cover the wounds. Plastic irrigation tubes are incorporated into the dressings and an impervious covering is then secured about the gauze layer with bias-cut stockinette. The gauze is kept moist by irrigation every 3–4 hours. The dressing is changed and mechanical debridement accomplished once or twice daily.

The electrolyte abnormalities which occur with silver nitrate therapy are essentially opposite to those associated with Sulfamylon. Covering the burned surface with hypotonic silver nitrate solution results in metabolic alkalosis with large plasma losses of sodium, chloride and potassium. This hypo-osmolar dilution can occur within hours following application of silver nitrate dressings, particularly in children and adults with major burns.

Serum electrolytes are determined once daily during the initial phase, then several times weekly after relative stabilization is obtained. Intravenous supplements of sodium and potassium may reach 2–3 times the ordinary daily requirements in patients with large weeping burns. Calcium and magnesium are added as indicated. As the epithelium regenerates, water and salt losses gradually decrease, lessening the need for salt supplements.

Although a minute quantity of silver is absorbed in patients treated for prolonged periods, the toxicity of this element is minimal. A major disadvantage of silver nitrate is the fact that it stains everything that it contacts and thereby complicates nursing and housekeeping. Since it does not penetrate the eschar, one must always remain alert for subeschar abscess formation. Klebsiella organisms are not affected by silver nitrate and occasionally become predominant. Despite the fact that a burn wound prepared with silver nitrate accepts and maintains a skin graft in the absence of obvious bacterial overgrowth, these wounds are not sterile. Many pathologic bacteria remain but are apparently maintained under control.

All burn wounds should be cultured at regular intervals to provide constant awareness of the bacterial flora. Clean granulating wounds are resurfaced with split-thickness skin grafts, usually starting in the third and fourth postburn weeks. Dermatomes and skin graft expanders facilitate this phase.

Summary

Guidelines for burn resuscitation and surgical principles of wound management have been described. Frequent re-evaluation of progress and flexibility in planning of therapy are essential to provide optimal care and restoration of function.

References

1. Artz, C. P., and Moncrief, J. A.: *The Treatment of Burns* (2d ed.; Philadelphia: W. B. Saunders Company, 1969).
2. Committee on Trauma, Subcommittee on Burns: Guide to initial therapy of burns, Bull. Am. Coll. Surgeons 52:196-197, 1967.
3. Monafo, W. W.: The Management of Burns: II. The Silver Nitrate Method, in *Current Problems in Surgery* (Chicago: Year Book Medical Publishers, Inc., February, 1969).
4. Shuck, J. M., and Moncrief, J. A.: The Management of Burns: I. General Considerations and the Sulfamylon Method, in *Current Problems in Surgery* (Chicago: Year Book Medical Publishers, Inc., February, 1969).
5. Stone, N. H., and Boswick, J. A.: *Profiles of Burn Management* (Miami, Fla.: Industrial Medicine Publishing Company, Inc., 1969).

Index

B

C

E

F

I

J

K

M

S

T